CLINICAL
ENDOCRINOLOGY

SECOND EDITION

The **Slide Atlas of Clinical Endocrinology** (Second Edition), based on the contents of this book, is available. In the slide atlas format, the material is divided into volumes, each of which is presented in a binder together with numbered 35mm slides of each illustration. Further information is available from:

Times Mirror International Publishers Limited
Lynton House
7-12 Tavistock Square
LONDON WC1H 9LB
UK

CLINICAL
ENDOCRINOLOGY

SECOND EDITION

G Michael Besser MD, DSc, FRCP
Professor of Medicine
Physician in Charge
Department of Endocrinology
St. Bartholomew's Hospital
London, UK

Michael O. Thorner MB BS, DSc, FRCP
Kenneth R. Crispell Professor of Medicine
Chief, Division of Endocrinology and Metabolism
University of Virginia
Charlotteseville
Virginia, USA

Foreword by
David N. Orth MD
Visiting Scientist
The Vollum Institute
Portland
Oregon, USA

Ⲙ Wolfe

Project Manager:	Claire Hooper
	Richard French
Designer:	Louise Bond
	Lee Riches
Illustration:	Lynda Payne
	Chris Read
	James Evoy
Production:	Jane Tozer
Index:	Laurence Errington

Copyright © 1984 Gower Medical Publishing.
Copyright © 1994 Times Mirror International Publishers Limited.
Published in 1994 by Mosby-Wolfe, an imprint of Times Mirror International Publishers Limited.

ISBN 1 56375 552 1

Cataloging in Publication data:
CIP catalogue records for this title are available from the British Library and US Library of Congress.

Text set in Galliard.
Captions set in GillSans.
Originated in Singapore by Chroma Graphics (Overseas) Pte. Ltd.
Produced by Grafos S.A. Arte sobre papel, Barcelona, Spain
Printed and bound in Spain, 1994.
10 9 8 7 6 5 4 3 2 1

For full details of all Times Mirror International Publishers Limited titles please write to: Times Mirror International Publishers Limited, Lynton House, 7–12 Tavistock Square, London WC1H 9LB, England.

CONTRIBUTORS

Eli Y Adashi MD
Professor of Obsterics/Gynecology & Physiology
University of Maryland School of Medicine
Baltimore, Maryland, USA

Peter H Baylis BSc, MD, FRCP
Consultant Physician and Professor of Experimental Medicine
Endocrine Unit, Royal Victoria Infirmary and
The University of Newcastle upon Tyne, UK

Stephen Bloom MA, MD, FRCP
Department of Medicine
Hammersmith Hospital
London, UK

Jamshed B Bomanji MD, MSc, PhD
Consultant Physician
Department of Nuclear Medicine
St. Bartholomew's Hospital
London, UK

Keith E Britton MD, MSc, FRCR, FRCP
Professor and Consultant in Charge
Department of Nuclear Medicine
St. Bartholomew's Hospital and Medical College
London, UK

Charles G D Brook MD, FRCP
Professor of Paediatric Endocrinology
University College London
Consultant Paediatrician
The Middlesex Hospital
London, UK

John D Brunzell MD
Professor of Medicine
Division of Metabolism, Endocrinology and Nutrition
Department of Medicine
University of Washington
Seattle, Washington, USA

Alan Chait MD
Professor of Medicine
Division of Metabolism, Endocrinology and Nutrition
Department of Medicine
University of Washington
Seattle, Washington, USA

Janet E Dacie FRCP, DMRD, FRCR
Consultant Radiologist
Department of Diagnostic Radiology
St. Bartholomew's Hospital
London, UK

Leslie J DeGroot MD
Professor of Medicine
Thyroid Study Unit, Department of Medicine
University of Chicago Medical Center
Chicago, Illinois, USA

Israel Doniach MD, FRCPath, FRCP
Emeritus Professor of Morbid Anatomy
University of London
Honorary Lecturer in Histopathology
St. Bartholomew's Hospital
London, UK

Christopher R W Edwards MA, MD, FRCP, FRCP(Ed), FRSE
Dean of Faculty of Medicine
University of Edinburgh Medical School
Edinburgh, UK

James E Griffin MD
Professor of Internal Medicine
The University of Texas Southwestern Medical Center
Department of Internal Medicine
Dallas, Texas, USA

Reginald Hall CBE, MD, FRCP
Professor of Medicine Emeritus
University of Wales College of Medicine
Cardiff, UK

Peter Hammond MD, MA, MRCP
Division of Endocrinology & Metabolism
Department of Medicine
Hammersmith Hospital
London, UK

Victor M Haughton MD
Professor of Radiology
Director of Neuroradiology Research
Medical College of Wisconsin
Froedtert Memorial Lutheran Hospital
Milwaukee, Wisconsin, USA

Vivian H T James PhD, DSc, FRCPath
Unit of Metabolic Medicine, Department of Chemical Pathology
St. Mary's Hospital Medical School
London, UK

Leighton P Mark MD
Consultant Radiologist
Medical College of Wisconsin
Froedtert Memorial Lutheran Hospital
Milwaukee, Wisconsin, USA

Vincent Marks MA, DM, FRCP, FRCPath, FIFST, MBAE
Professor of Clinical Biochemistry
School of Biological Sciences
University of Surrey
Guildford, Surrey, UK

Gregory R Mundy MD
Professor & Head
Division of Endocrinology & Metabolism
Department of Medicine, The University of Texas
Health Sciences Center at San Antonio
San Antonio, Texas, USA

Seymour Reichlin MD, PhD
Professor of Medicine
Tufts University School of Medicine
Division of Endocrinology, Diabetes, Metabolism and Molecular Medicine
New England Medical Center Hospitals
Boston, Massachusetts, USA

Peter H Sönksen MD, FRCP
Professor of Endocrinology
Chairman, Division of Endocrinology and Chemical Pathology
United Medical and Dental Schools of Guy's and St. Thomas' Hospitals
St. Thomas' Hospital
London, UK

Dennis M Styne MD
Professor and Chair, Department of Pediatrics
University of California, Davis Medical Center
Sacramento, California, USA

Tony E Torresani PhD
Biochemist, Chief of Protein Hormone Laboratory
Children's Hospital
Department of Endocrinology, University of Zürich
Zürich, Switzerland

Peter J Trainer BSc, MRCP
Lecturer, Department of Endocrinology
St. Bartholomew's Hospital
London, UK

John A H Wass MD, FRCP
Professor of Clinical Endocrinology
St. Bartholomew's Hospital
London, UK

F Elizabeth White MRCP, DMRD, FRCR
Consultant Radiologist
Royal Liverpool University Hospital
Liverpool, UK

Jean D Wilson MD
Professor of Internal Medicine
The University of Texas Southwestern Medical Center
Department of Internal Medicine
Dallas, Texas, USA

Robert J Witte MD
Consultant Radiologist
Medical College of Wisconsin
Froedtert Memorial Lutheran Hospital
Milwaukee, Wisconsin, USA

Ken Yamaguchi MD, PhD
Chief, Growth Factor Division
National Cancer Center Research Institute
Tokyo, Japan

FOREWORD

The Second Edition of this textbook maintains the lavish use of color illustration that characterized the First Edition, summarizes many of the advances that have been made since the publication of the First Edition, and improves upon the content of the First Edition by replacing some chapters and adding others. To cite three notable examples: Chapter 6, Lipids and Lipoproteins, sets forth our current knowledge about normal and abnormal lipid metabolism and the diseases that are associated with disordered lipid metabolism as lucidly as any treatise of which I am aware; Chapter 11, The Testis, is the finest summary of the development and the normal and abnormal function of the male reproductive system one is likely to find anywhere; and Chapter 21, Ectopic Humoral Syndromes, provides both a clear conceptual framework for understanding humoral manifestations of malignancy and a concise summary of the incidence, pathogenesis, diagnosis, and treatment of individual syndromes. Each of these chapters makes especially effective use of colored diagrams and patient photographs.

This textbook is an excellent and sometimes elegant summary of current thought concerning clinical endocrinology. It does not pretend to be a comprehensive treatise on the subject. Not all chapters, for example, reflect the recent explosion of detailed knowledge about molecular mechanisms of hormonal intercellular signal transduction and gene regulation, and the nature and results of genetic mutations of hormonal agonists, receptors and effectors. The bibliography, limited by intention, necessarily provides only a very cursory introduction to the relevant literature.

What clearly sets this textbook apart from all others is its uniquely generous use of color, color that is effectively used to highlight and clarify beautifully conceived and executed diagrams of anatomical and functional relationships. It thereby sets a standard that other texts are unlikely soon to emulate. However, color can often most effectively be

used to illustrate the clinical manifestations of disease. It is usually the patient's objective physical signs and subjective symptoms that suggest a specific syndrome of endocrine dysfunction and lead the clinician to perform appropriate diagnostic procedures. It does not require an endocrinologist to recognize a large goiter, severe exophthalmos, florid Cushing's syndrome, or chronic acromegaly. The skilled specialist must strive to detect these manifestations of disease in their earliest, most subtle forms, when effective treatment can often prevent the serious and sometimes irreversible sequelae of the disorders. Therefore, one wishes that the authors had responded more generously to Dr Jean D. Wilson's request, in his Foreword to the First Edition, that there be more photographs of patients "to illustrate the spectrum of changes between the normal and abnormal", rather than only florid, fullblown examples of the disorders. On the other hand, the illustrations of radiographs and scans with accompanying explanatory line drawings are outstanding.

This textbook's clear, concise, and highly visual presentation of the underlying concepts of endocrinology and their clinical consequences should make it especially useful for teaching medical students, house staff, and postdoctoral fellows. In a time when the lay public is increasingly concerned and informed about medical matters and physicians may first learn of the latest development by a patient who heard it on the morning news, a copy of this textbook should be in the office to be used as an aid educating and informing patients about their endocrine disorders.

David N. Orth, MD

PREFACE

The dramatic advances of recent years in the understanding of the normal physiology of human endocrinology and, as a consequence, of its pathological processes and their management, have continued unabated. This has largely been as a result of improvements in analytical techniques and in the specificity and sensitivity of hormone assays, and of the dramatic new knowledge acquired from application of the powerful molecular biological weapons. These innovations have allowed separation and accurate measurement of the relevant endocrine factors in blood, CSF and tissues, new imunocytochemical procedures for cellular localisation of hormones and identification of the structure and functions of genes, gene products, receptors and their ligands and their disturbances in disease. Neuroendocrinology has become a clinical science with elaboration of profound new concepts of the relationships between mind and body, and the mechanisms governing the body's homeostasis and its alterations in disease. These developments were behind the design of the first edition of this textbook originally planned with the late Andrew Cudworth, who tragically died so young. The principles have been continued and developed in this new second edition. As before the text is highly illustrated using the new techniques developed by the publishers. The work was initially conceived as a slide atlas and the principal messages of the book which have developed from it, are conveyed in

the diagrams and pictures, explained and expanded by the text. Normal physiology is the starting point of each section so that the pathological and clinical features of the disorders, their investigation and management can be based on this fundamental knowledge. Special attention has been given to the radiology and neuroradiology of endocrine diseases, and the inter-relationships between the behavioural and emotional features of the disorders and the chemical changes which have induced them. Wherever possible the molecular basis of the events considered are described. Diabetes mellitus and its closely related topics are not dealt with here as there is a sister book devoted to this subject. Disorder of lipids have now been included.

Many colleagues have contributed to this work and our thanks go to them for making it possible, and for their tolerance. The staff of Mosby–Year Book Europe Ltd. have been long-suffering during the production of the slide atlas and this textbook, and we wish to extend our gratitude to the for their expert attention and help, especially to Richard French, Pete Wilder, Louise Bond and Fiona Foley.

G.M.B.
M.O.T.

CONTENTS

1

Neuroendocrine Control of Pituitary Function

Seymour Reichlin, MD, PhD

Secretion of each of the known anterior pituitary hormones is controlled by one or more hypothalamic releasing or inhibitory factors, interacting with feedback effects of target gland hormones. All of the hormones are peptides, with the exception of dopamine which is a catecholamine and the principal prolactin-inhibiting factor (PIF). Thyrotrophin-releasing hormone (TRH) was the first of the hypophysiotrophic hormones to be chemically characterised (1969) and, between 1969 and 1982, all of the principal hypothalamic regulatory factors had been isolated and their structures elucidated. Furthermore, all have now been synthesised and introduced into clinical medicine. These discoveries validated the hypothesis proposed by Harris over four decades ago, that chemical substances carried from the hypothalamus to the anterior pituitary by way of the hypophysial–portal vessels are the means by which the brain controls pituitary function. These substances, and their analogues, can be used to stimulate or inhibit pituitary hormone secretion selectively for diagnostic and therapeutic purposes.

Pituitary regulatory substances of the hypothalamus are synthesised within specialised neurones by a process known as neurosecretion. The general concept of neurosecretion underlies our understanding of the way in which neural information is converted into chemical messages. The notion was first proposed by Scharrer and colleagues in the 1930s; they recognised that certain nerve cells in the brain of insects and fish, and in the neurohypophysial system of mammals, resembled gland cells. Scharrer suggested that some nerve cells were capable of acting like glands of internal secretion and so introduced the term neurosecretion to describe this phenomenon.

Two different types of neurosecretory neurones are found in the brain-neurohypophysial and hypophysiotrophic (Figs. 1.1(a)&(b)). Neurohypophysial neurones secrete the posterior pituitary hormones antidiuretic hormone (ADH, also known as vasopressin) and oxytocin into the general circulation, while hypophysiotrophic neurones secrete releasing factors into the blood that supplies the anterior pituitary. In general, all neurones are neurosecretory in that they release a synthesised product from their terminals, the difference being that in the central nervous system the neuronal product is released into the confines of the synaptic cleft instead of into the bloodstream (Fig. 1.1(c)). Conventional neurotransmitter and neuro-modulatory neurones synapse with the neurohypophysial and hypophysiotrophic neurones and regulate them by secretion of neurotransmitters and neuropeptides.

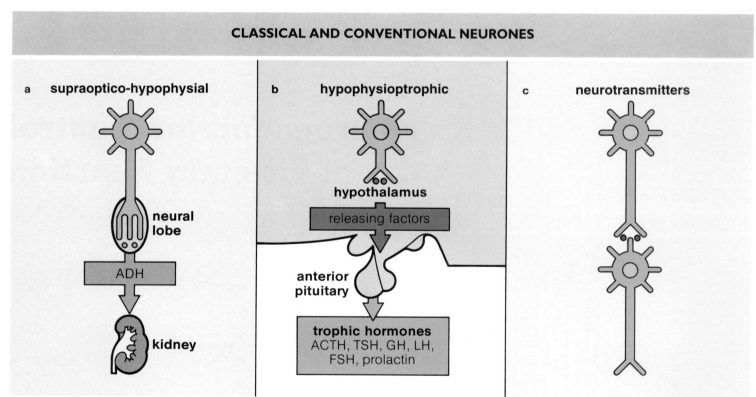

CLASSICAL AND CONVENTIONAL NEURONES

a supraoptico-hypophysial
b hypophysioptrophic
c neurotransmitters

hypothalamus

releasing factors

neural lobe

ADH

anterior pituitary

kidney

trophic hormones
ACTH, TSH, GH, LH, FSH, prolactin

Fig. 1.1 Neurosecretory peptidergic neurones involved in pituitary regulation and conventional neurotransmitter synapses. (a) The classical neurohypophysial system. Nerves project from cells of origin in the supraopticohypophysial and paraventriculohypophysial nuclei and end in the neural lobe. Oxytocin and ADH (vasopressin) are synthesised on the endoplasmic reticulum as part of a larger prohormone (which includes the specific oxytocin- and ADH-related neurophysins) and are then packaged into granules where they are stored in nerve endings and subsequently released into the peripheral blood. Since they affect tissues at a remote site, they are classified as neurohormones. (b) The hypophysiotrophic neurones that arise in the hypothalamus and terminate in the median eminence in contiguity to the specialised capillary blood vessels of the hypophysial–portal circulation. Their secretions are also considered to be neurohormones since they are secreted into blood and act remotely. (c) Conventional neurones may secrete the same substances as those that are released into the blood by the classical neurosecretory neurones. The main difference, however, is that their products are secreted into a synaptic cleft. At receptors on neurones, neuropeptides can act as classical neurotransmitters or as neuromodulators. A neuromodulator is a substance that modifies neuronal responses to neurotransmitters. Modified from Reichlin (1977); by courtesy of Raven Press.

ANATOMY OF THE HYPOTHALAMO–PITUITARY UNIT

The neural lobe of the pituitary gland (also known as the posterior pituitary or neurohypophysis) consists mainly of endings of nerve cells whose origins are in the hypothalamus (Fig. 1.2). The principal secretions of the neurohypophysis are oxytocin (uterus-contracting hormone/milk let–down hormone) and ADH; both are synthesised as part of prohormones that include distinctive neurophysins. The neurophysin–oxytocin and neurophysin–vasopressin prohormones are transported from the cell body peripherally in the form of packaged granules, to be stored in the nerve endings of the posterior pituitary. From their storage site, they are released in response to appropriate physiological signals: ADH release is determined by blood osmolality, effective blood volume, and stress; oxytocin is released during labour and in response to suckling. Secretion of both hormones is mediated by neural reflexes that are also modulated by the hormonal milieu.

ADH secretion is suppressed by glucocorticoids, while oxytocin secretion is stimulated by oestrogens.

The anterior pituitary (also known as the adenohypophysis) is also controlled by the brain but, unlike the neural lobe, does not have a direct nerve supply. Rather, neural information from the brain is translated into chemical messages by specialised hypothalamic cells and then released into the blood supply of the pituitary. Transfer of neuroregulators from hypothalamic neurones to the pituitary blood supply takes place in an anatomically specialised region of the ventral hypothalamus known as the median eminence or tuberoinfundibular region (Fig. 1.2). Neurones that project to this region are called tuberoinfundibular neurones. These terminate in proximity to capillary walls within the median eminence, which drain into a venous system that in turn, supplies the sinusoids of the pituitary. By analogy with the venous supply of the liver, this vascular system is referred to as the hypophysial–portal system.

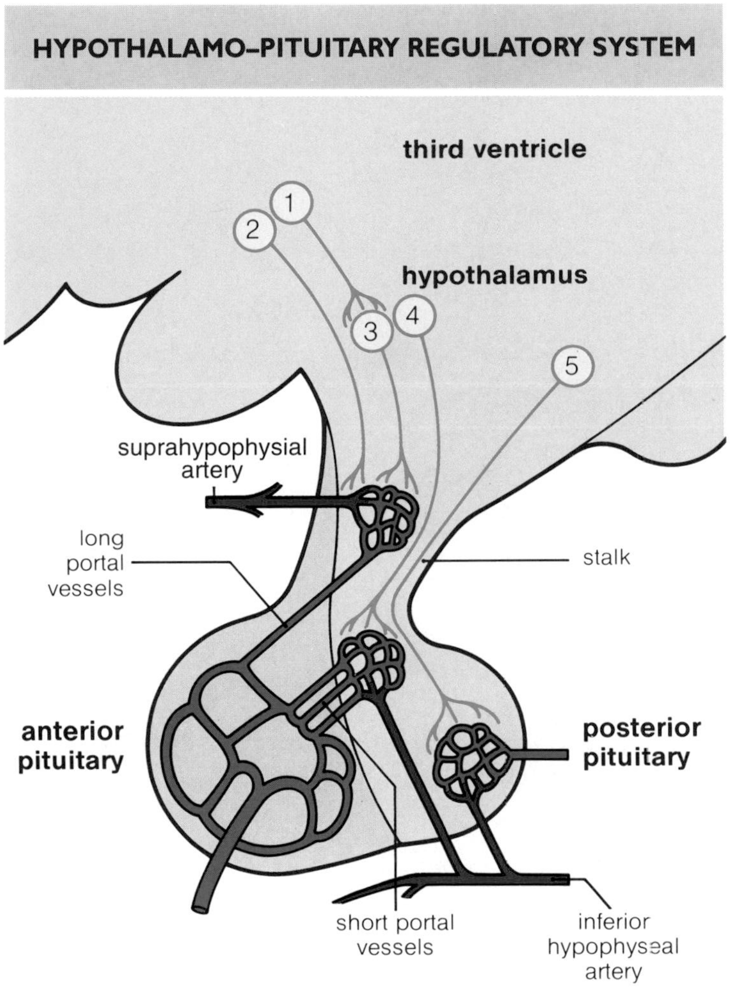

HYPOTHALAMO–PITUITARY REGULATORY SYSTEM

Fig. 1.2 Diagrammatic representation of the hypothalamo–pituitary regulatory system. The products of the posterior pituitary are synthesised in the supraoptic and paraventricular nuclei (5). After packaging, they are transported as granules, by axoplasmic flow, to the nerve terminals in the posterior pituitary where they are released directly into the circulation to act as classical neurohormones on distant target sites. The mechanism of anterior pituitary hormone secretion is entirely different. The pituitary hormone-releasing or releasing-inhibiting hormones of the hypothalamus are synthesised within the nuclei of the hypothalamus (1–4) and transported to the median eminence from where they travel to the anterior pituitary via the dense capillary network and the long portal veins. These hypothalamic factors occupy specific receptors on pituitary cells and lead either to the release or inhibition of the pituitary hormones. Modified from Gay (1972); by courtesy of the American Fertility Society.

The anatomical distribution of the tuberoinfundibular neurone system has been elucidated by retrograde tracing of markers injected in the median eminence (Fig. 1.3) and by immunohistochemical staining of neurones containing hypophysiotrophic peptides (Fig. 1.4). By using mRNA probes that code for the hypothalamic factors, *in situ* hybridisation methods can demonstrate the anatomical distribution of the hypothalamic hormones and determine the factors that regulate specific mRNA synthesis (Figs. 1.5 & 1.6).

Tuberoinfundibular neurones are influenced by nerve fibres from many parts of the brain; for example, those that integrate homeostasis, stress responses, mating, and reproduction. In addition, the tuberoinfundibular neurones are regulated by feedback effects of target gland hormones (thyroid, adrenal cortex, gonads).

The gross anatomical relations of the hypothalamus and pituitary, and abnormalities in disease, can be visualised by CT (computerised tomography) scanning and by nuclear magnetic resonance imaging (MRI) (Fig. 1.7).

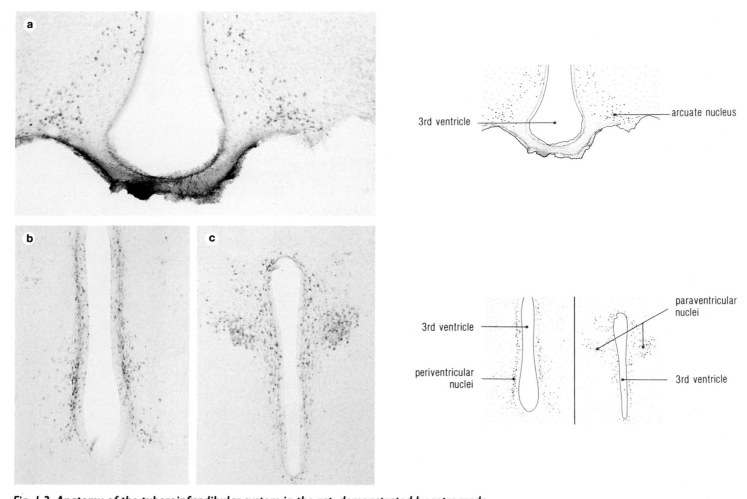

Fig. 1.3 Anatomy of the tuberoinfundibular system in the rat, demonstrated by retrograde transport of a tracer compound. A tracer compound, wheat germ agglutinin (which is taken up by nerve endings), was injected into the median eminence of a rat. Several hours later, the animal was killed and the brain sectioned and stained immunohistochemically with an antibody to wheat germ agglutinin. The tracer was found in cell bodies located in three main areas: (a) the arcuate nucleus; (b) the periventricular nucleus, which comprises a rich plexus that is several cells deep immediately under the ependymal layer of the third ventricle; and (c) the paraventricular nuclei. Many of the arcuate cells are dopaminergic, and most periventricular cells are somatostatinergic. The paraventricular nucleus is complex and includes cells that secrete ADH, oxytocin, TRH, somatostatin, neurotensin, CRH, VIP, and many other hormones. In addition to projecting to the median eminence (for control of anterior pituitary secretion), the paraventricular nucleus projects to other regions of the neuroaxis where other visceral regulating functions are carried out. By courtesy of Dr R Lechan.

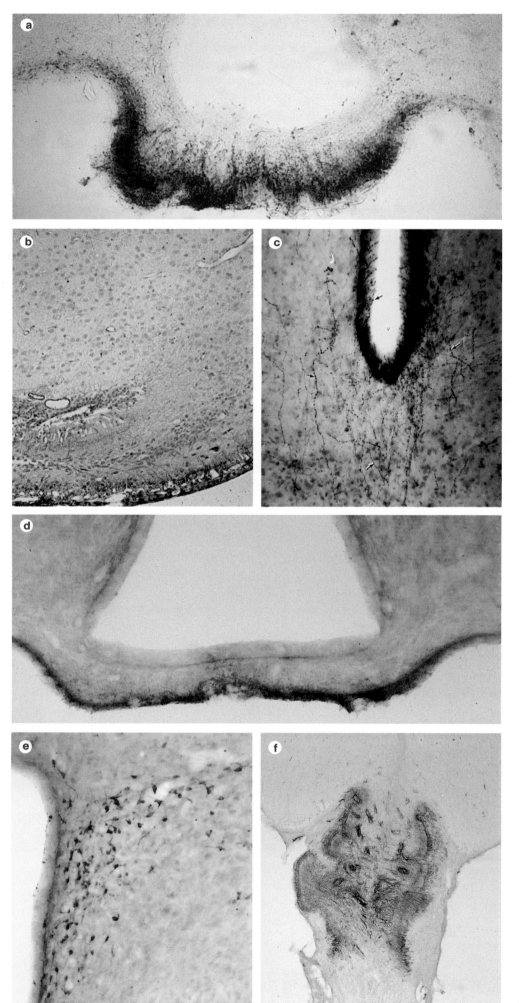

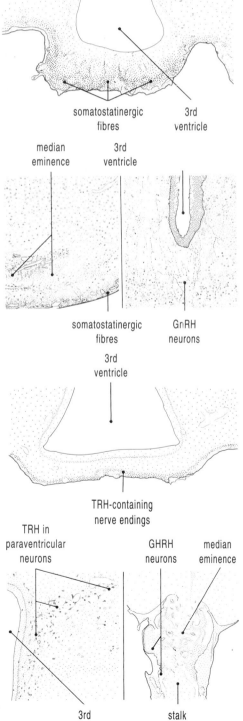

Fig. 1.4 Hypophysiotrophic neurones in the hypothalamus, demonstrated by immunohistochemical techniques using the Sternberger PAP method. (a) The immunohistochemical appearance of somatostatinergic fibres in a frontal section of the hypothalamus of the rat at the level of the median eminence. (b) The sagittal section of the hypothalamus of the rat showing somatostatinergic fibres. (c) GnRH peptidergic pathways in a horizontal section of the rat hypothalamus. (d) TRH-containing nerve endings in the median eminence of the rat (frontal section). (e) TRH containing neurones in the paraventricular nucleus of the rat (frontal section). (f) Anatomical localisation of GHRH in the stalk and median eminence of the rhesus monkey. By courtesy of Drs R Lechan, L Alpert, and J King.

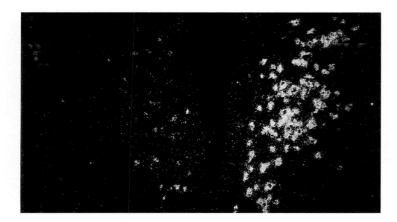

Fig. 1.5 In situ *hybridisation of TRH mRNA in the paraventricular nucleus of a hypothyroid rat.* The paraventricular nucleus on the left has been injected with a minute pellet of T_3, whereas an inert substance was injected into the right nucleus. The striking suppression of the hybridisation signal indicates that T_3 acted locally to suppress synthesis of mRNA and is thus indicative of a hypothalamic locus for the suppress on of the hypothalamic–pituitary–thyroid axis. By courtesy of *Endocrinology* and Dr R Lechan.

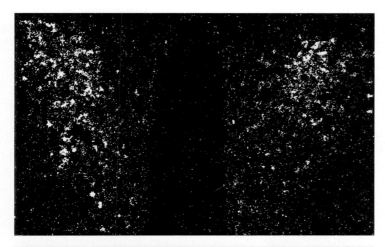

Fig. 1.6 **In situ *hybridisation of CRH mRNA in the paraventricular nucleus of a rat.*** (a) *In situ* hybridisation of CRH mRNA in the paraventricular nucleus of a normal rat. (b) Hybridisation of CRH mRNA in a rat following the intracerebroventricular administration of recombinant human IL-Ib (100ng, followed by an infusion of 20ng/h for 12 hours). When compared with (a), there is readily detectable activation of CRH neuronal activity. By courtesy of Drs I Kakuschka and R Lechan.

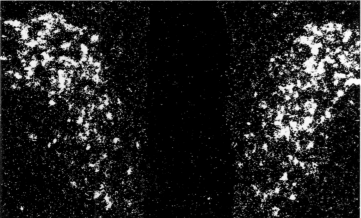

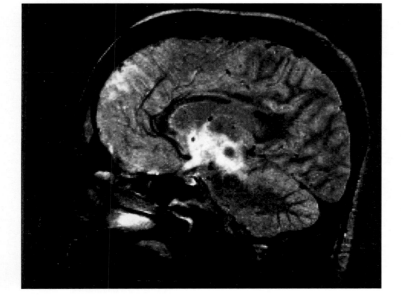

Fig. 1.7 **MRI scan of the brain and pituitary of a patient with eosinophilic granulomas that have densely infiltrated the hypothalamus and thalamus.** The patient was deficient in all anterior pituitary functions and had diabetes insipidus, but the lesion did not directly involve the pituitary region.

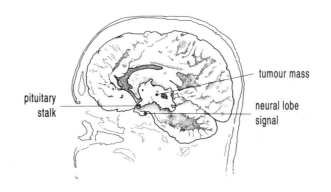

Each of the known anterior pituitary hormones is regulated by one or more hypothalamic hormones, and in some instances, a single hypothalamic hormone (sometimes referred to as 'releasing factor' or hypophysiotrophic hormone) can influence more than one pituitary hormone. The main pituitary hormones and their regulating hypothalamic hormones are listed in Fig. 1.8.

STRUCTURE OF THE HYPOPHYSIOTROPHIC HORMONES OF THE HYPOTHALAMUS

Isolation and chemical identification of hypothalamic factors with anterior pituitary-regulating properties has focused on extracts of

hypothalamic tissues. Initially, the factors were known as 'releasing factors' after the first description in 1955 of corticotrophin-releasing factor (CRF), now known as corticotrophin-releasing hormone (CRH). The term 'releasing factor' was introduced by Saffran and Schally to describe a substance extracted from the neural lobe, which stimulated the release of adrenocorticotrophic hormone (ACTH) from pituitary fragments maintained in organ culture. Twenty-six years later, the chemical nature of this substance was elucidated by Vale and colleagues (1981).

The chemical structure of the five principal peptide hypophysial-regulating hormones identified so far are shown in Fig. 1.9. They can also be referred to as hypophysiotrophic hormones, since they regulate differentiation and growth, as well as release of the pituitary hormones.

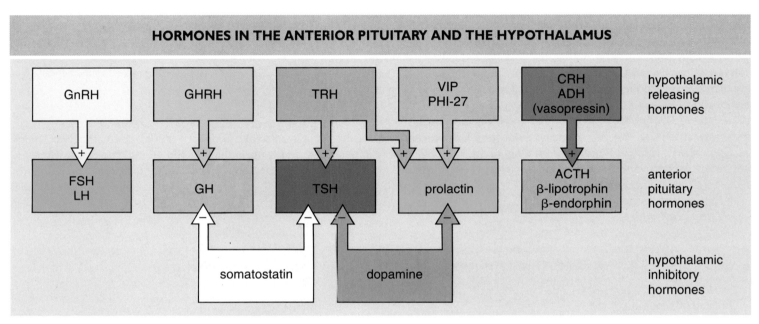

HORMONES IN THE ANTERIOR PITUITARY AND THE HYPOTHALAMUS

Fig. 1.8 *Summary of the hormones produced in the anterior pituitary and the hypothalamic hormones that regulate their secretion.*

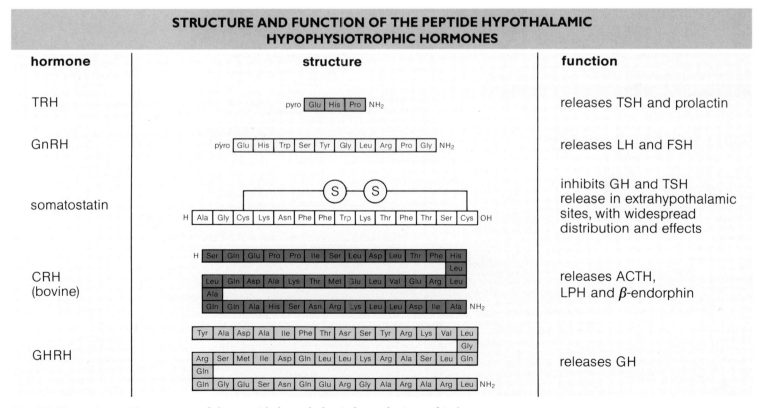

STRUCTURE AND FUNCTION OF THE PEPTIDE HYPOTHALAMIC HYPOPHYSIOTROPHIC HORMONES

hormone	structure	function
TRH	pyro Glu His Pro NH₂	releases TSH and prolactin
GnRH	pyro Glu His Trp Ser Tyr Gly Leu Arg Pro Gly NH₂	releases LH and FSH
somatostatin	H Ala Gly Cys Lys Asn Phe Phe Trp Lys Thr Phe Thr Ser Cys OH	inhibits GH and TSH release in extrahypothalamic sites, with widespread distribution and effects
CRH (bovine)		releases ACTH, LPH and β-endorphin
GHRH		releases GH

Fig. 1.9 *The amino-acid sequences of the peptide hypothalamic hypophysiotrophic hormones.*

Dopamine can also be classified as a hypophysiotrophic pituitary hormone since it is present in hypophysial–portal vessel blood in sufficient concentrations to duplicate all of its known inhibitory effects on the secretion of prolactin (Fig. 1.10). Several hormones thought to act as prolactin-releasing factors (PRFs) include TRH and vasoactive intestinal polypeptide (VIP), the latter also being found in the gut.

Many other active peptides and neurotransmitters can be isolated from the hypothalamus (Fig. 1.11) and, in some instances, are cosecreted with the known hypophysiotrophic hormones or are found in neurones that project into the hypothalamus from other parts of the brain. Indeed, the hypothalamus contains a wide variety, and a higher concentration, of neuropeptides and neurotransmitters than any other part of the brain.

Most of the peptides first isolated from the hypothalamus have now also been shown to be formed within pituitary cells where they form intrinsic paracrine (cell–to–cell) and autocrine (cell–to–itself) regulatory systems. They are also found outside the hypothalamus where they may act as mediators of affective state and biological rhythms; or as regulators of visceral function, activity, body temperature, and eating and drinking behaviour.

Some of the hypothalamic factors exert physiologically significant inhibitory actions on anterior pituitary function. These inhibitory factors interact with the respective releasing factor to exert dual control of secretion of prolactin, growth hormone (GH), and thyroid-stimulating hormone/thyrotrophin (TSH). The action of each

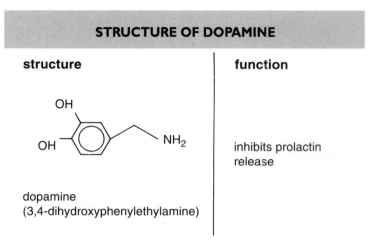

STRUCTURE OF DOPAMINE

structure	function
dopamine (3,4-dihydroxyphenylethylamine)	inhibits prolactin release

Fig. 1.10 The structure of dopamine, the principal PIF. Dopamine is a biogenic catecholamine secreted by a distinct group of cells in the ventral hypothalamus. It serves as an important neurotransmitter in other regulatory pathways of the brain which are not related to the pituitary.

of the hypophysiotrophic hormones is not limited strictly to a single pituitary hormone: for example, TRH (the physiological releaser of TSH) is a potent releaser of prolactin, and in some circumstances, releases ACTH and GH; gonadotrophin-releasing hormone (GnRH)

STRUCTURE OF SEVERAL HYPOTHALAMIC REGULATORY PEPTIDES

hypothalamic peptide	structure
substance P	Arg Pro Lys Pro Gln Gln Phe Phe Gly Leu Met NH₂
neurotensin	pyro Glu Leu Tyr Glu Asn Lys Pro Arg Arg Pro Tyr Ile Leu OH
angiotensin II	Asp Arg Val Tyr Ile His Pro Phe
leu-enkephalin	Tyr Gly Gly Phe Leu OH
met-enkephalin	Tyr Gly Gly Phe Met OH
α-endorphin	Tyr Gly Gly Phe Met Thr Ser Glu Lys Ser Gln Thr Pro Leu Val Thr OH
β-endorphin	Tyr Gly Gly Phe Met Thr Ser Glu Lys Ser Gln Thr Pro Leu Val/Thr — OH Glu Gly Lys Lys Tyr Ala Asn Lys Ile Ile Ala Asn Lys Phe Leu
γ-endorphin	Tyr Gly Gly Phe Met Thr Ser Glu Lys Ser Gln Thr Pro Leu Val Thr Leu OH
VIP	His Ser Asp Ala Val Phe Thr Asp Asn Tyr Thr Arg Leu Arg/Lys NH₂ Asn Leu Ile Ser Asn Leu Tyr Lys Lys Val Ala Met Gln

Fig. 1.11 The aminoacid sequence of several hypothalamic peptides. Many physiologically potent peptides have been isolated from the hypothalamus and are found to be localised in neurosecretory vesicles in hypothalamic neurones. They are also found in the brain outside the hypothalamus in many different projection systems where they perform functions unrelated to pituitary regulation. Changes in visceral function, appetite, and emotional state can be induced by these substances. Most of the peptides shown here are also secreted by pituitary cells themselves, where they form an intrinsic 'paracrine' (cell-to-cell) communicating system. The endogenous opioid peptides are a large group of substances that act like morphine by binding to various classes of opioid receptors. Included in this category are the enkephalins and the endorphins. All of the peptides listed (and many others not shown) influence pituitary activity, but their function in normal regulation is not fully understood. Acting on the hypothalamus, substance P stimulates the release of GH and LH; neurotensin stimulates the release of GH; angiotensin II stimulates the release of ACTH and ADH; and the endogenous opioids stimulate the secretion of ACTH, prolactin and GH, and inhibit LH. VIP is an important PRF responsible (at least in the rat) for response to stress and in part to suckling.

releases both luteinising hormone (LH) and follicle-stimulating hormone (FSH); and somatostatin inhibits secretion of GH, TSH, and a wide variety of other nonpituitary hormones. The principal inhibitor of prolactin secretion is dopamine, but this potent bioamine, acting directly on the pituitary, also inhibits TSH and gonadotrophin secretion. Additionally, under some circumstances, it inhibits GH secretion.

CHEMISTRY AND FUNCTION OF THE INDIVIDUAL HYPOTHALAMIC HORMONES

THYROTROPHIN-RELEASING HORMONE

The chemical structure of TRH was elucidated by groups of investigators led by Andrew Schally and by Roger Guillemin. Their work, which was the culmination of more than a decade of effort to identify the nature of the thyrotrophin-releasing activity of crude hypothalamic extracts, made neuroendocrinology credible to the general scientific and clinical community and was ultimately recognised by the award of a Nobel Prize. The discovery made the introduction of TRH into clinical medicine possible, vastly widened the scope of understanding of nonhypothalamic functions of hypothalamic peptides, and provided powerful incentive to efforts to identify other biological activities in hypothalamic extracts.

TRH, a tripeptide amide – (pyro)Glu-His–Pro–NH2 – is a relatively simple substance. Although some substituted forms are potent, an intact amide and the cyclised glutamic acid terminal are essential for activity. TRH is chemically stable, but it is rapidly degraded in plasma by circulating enzymes. Following injection of TRH in humans or rats, blood TSH levels rise rapidly and dramatically, a change being detected within three minutes; peak values are normally attained between ten and twenty minutes after injection in normal subjects (Fig. 1.12) and sometimes later in subjects with hypothalamic or pituitary disease. The hormone is very potent: as little as 15μg yields a detectable response, and maximal effects are achieved with a dose of 400μg. The standard clinical dose administered as an intravenous bolus injection is 200–500μg. Transient mild nausea, a sense of urinary urgency, and moderate (rarely marked) increases in blood pressure occur as side effects of injection. The surge of TSH release induced by TRH injection leads to a detectable rise in plasma triiodothyronine (T_3) and also an increase in thyroxine (T_4) release, although the latter is usually not large enough to be reflected in a significant increase in circulating levels of T_4.

A striking feature of the TRH-induced TSH response is that its effects are blocked by prior treatment with thyroid hormone. Indeed, the interaction of the negative feedback effects of thyroid hormone on the pituitary with the stimulating effects of TRH is a major element in the feedback control of TSH secretion (Fig. 1.13).

In addition to stimulating TSH release, TRH is also a potent PRF (Fig. 1.14). The time course of response of blood prolactin levels to TRH, and the dose–response characteristics and suppressibility (by thyroid hormone pretreatment) of TRH, all parallel changes in TSH secretion. Nevertheless, there is reason to believe that TRH is not an important regulator of prolactin secretion under normal circumstances; for example, the prolactin secretory response to breastfeeding (in women and experimental animals) is unaccompanied by changes in plasma TSH levels, thus suggesting that this neurogenic reflex does not involve TRH. The prolactin release-stimulating effects of TRH, however, may be responsible for the occasional occurrence of hyperprolactinaemia (with or without galactorrhoea) in patients with hypothyroidism. This finding can be attributed to increased sensitivity of prolactin-secreting cells to TRH in the hypothyroid state, and to an increase in TRH secretion.

In normal individuals, TRH has no influence on pituitary hormone secretion other than on TSH and on prolactin secretion. It can, however, stimulate release of ACTH in patients with Cushing's syndrome; and GH in acromegalics (Fig. 1.14).

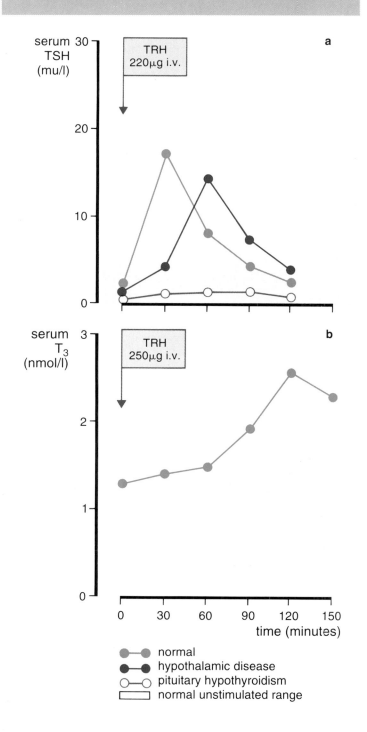

NORMAL AND ABNORMAL RESPONSE TO TRH

normal
hypothalamic disease
pituitary hypothyroidism
normal unstimulated range

Fig. 1.12 Normal and abnormal responses to TRH. (a) The delayed TSH response to TRH in a patient with hypothalamic disease. Peak plasma TSH values are reached at approximately 60 minutes following exogenous TRH, compared to the normal where the peak occurs at 20–30 minutes. In pituitary hypothyroidism, TSH reserve may be severely reduced and there may be only a slight, or no response, to exogenous TRH. (b) The normal rise in circulating plasma T_3 following an injection of TRH. The T_3 response lags behind the TSH response, reflecting the fact that T_3 rises secondary to stimulation of the thyroid gland by the released TSH.

The 'paradoxical' GH response is a useful indicator of acromegaly (occuring in 70% of patients) and of the state of remission after therapy. TRH also releases GH in some patients with depression.

The greatest diagnostic value of TRH is in the differential diagnosis of thyrotoxicosis in borderline cases of mild thyroid overactivity. Since thyroid hormones inhibit TSH response to TRH, TRH effects are blunted or blocked in the presence of even mild degrees of hyperthyroidism. In current practice, the TRH test, which had been widely used in the evaluation of difficult diagnostic problems, has been largely supplanted by the ultrasensitive TSH immunoassays that allow measurement of basal or unstimulated TSH values in the full range of normal and below.

It might have been anticipated that TRH would be useful as a diagnostic agent to differentiate between pituitary and hypothalamic causes of TSH deficiency. Indeed, many patients with disease of the hypothalamus which has caused TRH deficiency show responses to injected TRH, while others with pituitary disease fail to respond to TRH (see Fig. 1.12). There are, however, a sufficient number of cases not showing the classical or predicted response to prevent clear-cut differential diagnosis. In such cases, accurate radiological studies and other endocrine evaluations are required for diagnosis.

When TRH was chemically sequenced and synthesised, it became possible to use specific and sensitive methods to study its tissue distribution. One of the most surprising findings to arise from this work was that TRH was distributed widely outside of the classical thyrotrophic area of the hypothalamus. TRH has been found in virtually all parts of the brain, including the cerebral cortex; the spinal cord; nerve endings abutting upon the ventral motor horn cells and upon the intermediolateral column of the spinal cord; the neurohypophysis; and the pineal gland. TRH has also been found in pancreatic islet cells and in various parts of the gastrointestinal tract. Although present in low concentrations in these areas, the aggregate in extrahypothalamic tissue far exceeds the total amount in the hypothalamus.

The extensive extrahypothalamic distribution of TRH, its localisation in nerve endings, and the presence of TRH receptors in brain tissue suggest that this peptide acts as a neurotransmitter or neuromodulator outside the hypothalamus. In particular, its distribution in the spinal cord at nerve endings of the intermediolateral column, which contain the cells of origin of the sympathetic nervous system, may explain the elevation of blood pressure which follows injections

THE HYPOTHALAMIC–PITUITARY–THYROID AXIS

Fig. 1.13 The hypothalamic–pituitary–thyroid axis and its feedback control. The thyroid gland is stimulated by TSH secreted by the anterior pituitary. Secretion of TSH is stimulated in turn by hypothalamic TRH and is inhibited by the hypothalamic factor somatostatin. TSH secretion is also inhibited by the principal secretions of the thyroid $-T_4$ and T_3, thus forming a negative feedback loop. In addition to exerting direct inhibitory actions at the pituitary level, the thyroid hormones inhibit the secretion of TRH and stimulate the secretion of somatostatin, thus adding a hypothalamic level of negative feedback control of TSH secretion. The regulatory system is made even more complex by the intrahypothalamic and intrapituitary conversion of T_4 to the more-potent T_3, a process that is regulated by thyroid hormones and by the hypothalamic factors. Modified from Reichlin (1985); by courtesy of WB Saunders Company.

EFFECT OF TRH ON PROLACTIN AND GH RELEASE

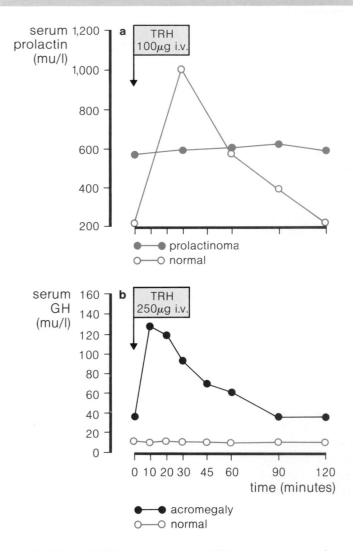

Fig. 1.14 Effect of TRH on prolactin and GH release in normal subjects and in patients with pituitary tumours. (a) TRH stimulates the release of prolactin in a normal subject, while having no effect in a patient with prolactinoma (the usual response in such patients). (b) TRH has no effect on plasma GH levels in a normal individual, while it stimulates GH release in a patient with acromegaly.

of TRH and may be relevant to clinical benefits claimed in treatment of shock and depression.

GONADOTROPHIN-RELEASING HORMONE

It had been known from the work of McCann (1960) and of Campbell and co-workers (1964) that extracts of hypothalamic tissue contain a biologically active substance capable of stimulating the release of gonadotrophic hormones from the pituitary. This material was isolated from the hypothalami of stockyard animals, and the structure was finally elucidated by Schally's group in 1971. Like TRH, the amino terminal of GnRH is a substituted amide. A terminal amide group is characteristic of a number of other small peptide hormones, including ADH, oxytocin, calcitonin, gastrin, and glucagon; in all of these hormones (including TRH and GnRH), the amide group is needed for full hormonal activity.

Following intravenous injection, GnRH triggers a prompt, dose-related increase of LH and FSH in humans (Fig. 1.15) and in all vertebrate species in which it has been tested. After a single bolus

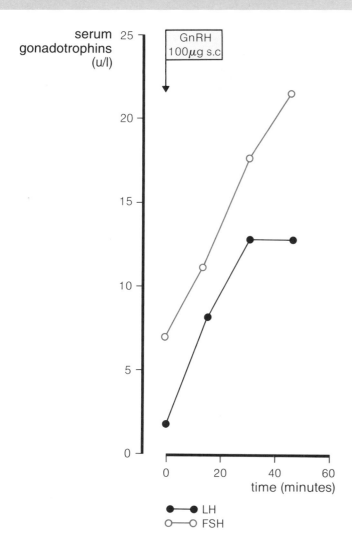

GONADOTROPHIN RESPONSE TO GnRH

GnRH 100μg s.c

serum gonadotrophins (u/l)

time (minutes)

●—● LH
○—○ FSH

Fig. 1.15 Gonadotrophin response to GnRH in a woman with galactorrhoea–amenorrhoea due to prolactinoma. This patient responded to an injection of GnRH with a brisk release of FSH and LH.

injection, FSH release is usually delayed compared with LH secretion, the values peaking ten to thirty minutes after injection. The response of LH and FSH to GnRH is markedly influenced by the prior GnRH secretory state, by the gonadal steroid milieu, by the state of gonadal activity, by the time course of GnRH injection (i.e. single dose, multiple pulse, or constant infusion), and by the patient's genetic sex. Through secondary effects of pituitary activation, and under appropriately defined conditions, GnRH can induce spermatogenesis and testosterone production in men with hypothalamic hypo-gonadotrophic hypogonadism, and ovulation in women with hypothalamic amenorrhoea.

Most reproductive neuroendocrinologists now believe that the GnRH decapeptide is the only hypothalamic gonadotrophin regulator and that observed dissociations of secretion of LH and FSH are due to the interacting effects of prior hormone status, steroid pretreatment, and patterns of GnRH administration.

GnRH has been extensively tested as a diagnostic agent in differentiating between the causes of hypogonadism. In patients with complete pituitary destruction, GnRH does not stimulate gonadotrophic hormone release, but in patients with lesser degrees of pituitary dysfunction associated with hypogonadism, GnRH may induce a gonadotrophin response within the normal range. Long-standing hypothalamic dysfunction can lead to poor or absent pituitary responsiveness. For these reasons therefore, a single bolus injection of GnRH is a poor differential diagnostic agent.

Intermittent injections of GnRH, which mimic the intermittent release of GnRH by the normal hypothalamus, will stimulate gonadotrophin secretion and lead to normal pituitary–testicular and pituitary–ovarian function in individuals with hypothalamic failure (Fig. 1.16). This application is clinically the most important of the hypothalamic hormones thus far and is widely used.

In contrast, administration of GnRH at a constant rate leads to reduced gonadotrophin secretion (Fig. 1.17). This phenomenon, attributed to downregulation of GnRH receptors, has been exploited for the treatment of idiopathic precocious puberty. In patients with this disorder, the use of a 'super agonist' of GnRH inhibits gonadal function to prepubertal levels. This approach has also been used to suppress ovarian function in patients with metastatic carcinoma of the breast and pituitary–testicular function in men with carcinoma of the prostate.

The stimulating actions of GnRH interact with the effects of the gonadal steroids and with peptide secretions of the gonads–termed inhibins (see Chapter 11). Under particular circumstances, oestrogens sensitise the pituitary to the stimulating effects of GnRH (the mechanism underlying the midcycle ovulatory surge), but can also inhibit GnRH responsiveness. Important negative feedback effects on the gonadotroph cells are exerted by the inhibins which selectively inhibit FSH secretion but not LH secretion.

Unlike TRH and somatostatin, almost all of the GnRH in the brain of mammals is restricted to the hypothalamus and related neural structures. Small amounts are found in the circumventricular organs of the brain, including the pineal gland. GnRH has also been found in milk, suggesting that the breast, a dermally derived structure, may have embryological origins analogous to the primitive neuroectoderm, the source of neuroendocrine cells. The most important central nervous system effect of GnRH may be that involved in the regulation of mating behaviour. Direct injection of GnRH into the hypothalamus has been reported to enhance female sexual responsivity, even in animals without a pituitary (which are therefore incapable of responding with gonadotrophin–ovarian hormone activation). Studies of the effect of GnRH on sex drive in humans have been unconvincing.

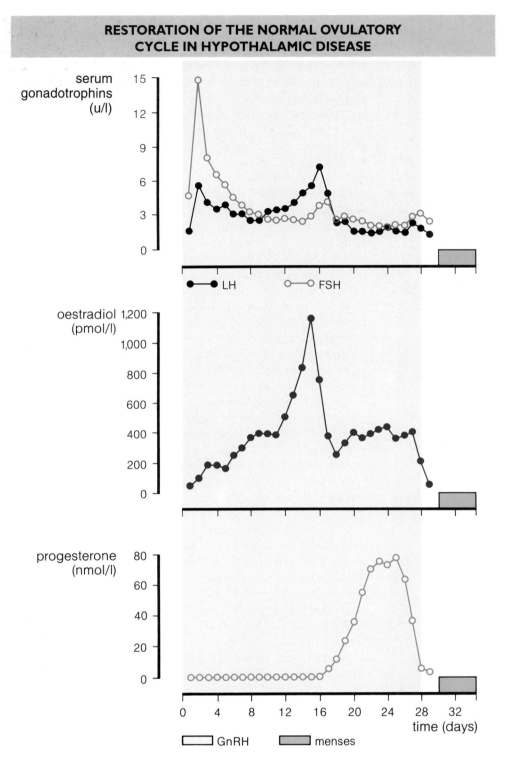

RESTORATION OF THE NORMAL OVULATORY CYCLE IN HYPOTHALAMIC DISEASE

Fig. 1.16 Restoration of a normal ovulatory cycle in a woman with hypothalamic disease, using intermittent GnRH injections. Intermittent doses of GnRH were administered at 90-minute intervals by a pump. These findings indicate that mimicking of the normal pulsating release of GnRH can restore normal cyclical function. Modified from Crowley and McArthur (1980); by courtesy of Williams and Wilkins Company.

GROWTH HORMONE-RELEASING HORMONE

Efforts to identify the chemical nature of GH-releasing hormone (GHRH) from hypothalamic extracts were unsuccessful for a long time. Nevertheless, a series of clinical insights, coupled with brilliant experiments, led, in 1982, to the elucidation of the structure of GHRH isolated from the pancreatic islet tumours of two patients with the rare disease of acromegaly due to ectopic secretion of GHRH. Two different molecules have been identified, one consisting of forty-four amino acids, and the other of forty amino acids. Identical hormones have been isolated from the hypothalamus.

Administration of GHRH stimulates a brisk release of GH after intravenous injection (Fig. 1.18). GHRH has been used to treat GH deficiency in hypopituitary patients with short stature. It can stimulate GH secretion in many patients with GH deficiency due to proven

hypothalamic disease, or in the syndrome of idiopathic GH deficiency. The most common form of acquired GH deficiency is due to hypothalamic disease or rupture of the pituitary stalk. Most cases of 'idiopathic' GH deficiency are of hypothalamic origin. In theory, such cases could be treated with GHRH as well as with GH.

SOMATOSTATIN

During the course of efforts to isolate GHRH from hypothalamic extracts, Krulich and McCann discovered a fraction that inhibited GH release from pituitary incubates, *in vitro*. They named the factor 'growth hormone release inhibitory factor' and postulated that GH secretion was regulated by a dual control system, one stimulatory, and the other inhibitory. Relatively little attention was paid to this concept when first described since it was thought by most workers to be a nonspecific effect. Several years later, however, Brazeau and collaborators, while working in Guillemin's laboratory on the attempted isolation of GH-releasing factor, again observed the inhibitory factor. With the background in methodology gained from earlier studies of TRH and GnRH, they were able, in a relatively short time, to isolate and identify a potent peptide from hypothalamic extracts, which inhibited GH release. The material, to which the name 'somatostatin' was applied, is a peptide containing fourteen amino acids, which lacks the amide and pyroglutamic acid termini that are characteristic of GnRH and TRH, but contains a disulphide bridge similar to that of ADH and oxytocin. Other molecular forms of somatostatin have been isolated, including a peptide of twenty-eight amino acids (the last fourteen amino acids are identical to those in somatostatin-14) and a still larger form, the prohormone, with a molecular weight of approximately 15,000.

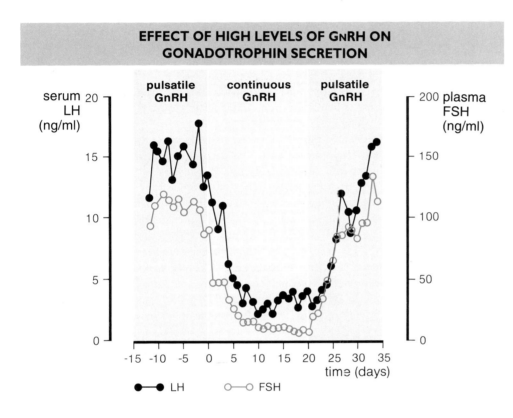

EFFECT OF HIGH LEVELS OF GₙRH ON GONADOTROPHIN SECRETION

Fig. 1.17 The effect of constant high levels of GnRH on gonadotrophin secretion. Data from a monkey with hypothalamic lesions (causing GnRH deficit) show that continuous infusions of GnRH suppress LH and FSH release, while pulsatile injections restore it. Similar suppressive actions can be exerted by long-acting 'super agonist' doses of GnRH. Modified from Belchez et al (1978); by courtesy of the AAAS.

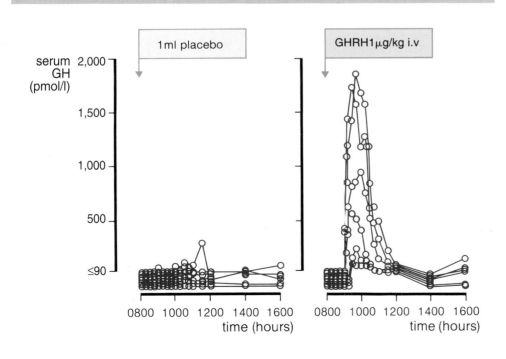

SECRETORY RESPONSE OF GH TO GHRH

Fig. 1.18 The secretory response of GH to GHRH administration. Human pancreatic GHRH was injected into six normal men and was shown to stimulate the release of GH. Modified from Thorner et al (1983); by courtesy of The Lancet.

REGULATION OF GH SECRETION

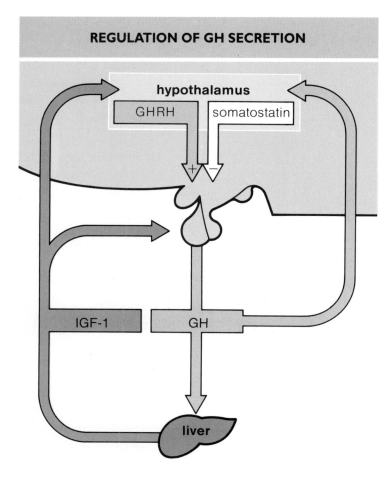

Fig. 1.19 Diagrammatic representation of the regulation of GH secretion. The secretion of GH is stimulated by GHRH from the hypothalamus and inhibited by somatostatin. The two hypothalamic hormones are secreted by distinct populations of tuberoinfundibular neurones. At the level of the pituitary, the stimulating effect of GHRH is modulated by insulin-like growth factor-1 (IGF-1), a peptide formed in the liver and in many other tissues that are under the influence of GH; thus, IGF-1 becomes part of the negative feedback loop control of GH secretion. The release of somatostatin by the hypothalamus is stimulated by both GH and IGI-1, thus comprising the hypothalamic component of the negative feedback loop for GH regulation. Modified from Reichlin (1985); by courtesy of WB Saunders Company.

Somatostatin has been shown to be an important physiological regulator of GH release (Fig. 1.19). It also inhibits the secretion of TSH and that of virtually all of the glands of the pancreas and gastrointestinal tract, including glucagon, insulin, gastric acid, and intestinal enzymes (Fig. 1.20). Furthermore, it inhibits salt/water transport across the intestine. Somatostatin is present in almost every tissue, in nerve terminals and/or in specialised glandular cells on which it acts. It is widely distributed in tissues where it acts in some situations as a paracrine secretion (i.e. control of one cell by secretion of an adjacent cell), and in others as a neuroendocrine secretion (e.g. as in the tuberohypophysial neurones of the hypothalamus).

Of the hypophysiotrophic hormones isolated so far, somatostatin has the most extensive extrahypothalamic distribution in other parts of the central nervous system and in extraneural structures, especially in the gastrointestinal tract. Since there is a relatively large amount of somatostatin in the brain, much effort has been made to determine its role in neural function, although no clear-cut generalisations have as yet emerged.

A highly potent somatostatin analogue, octreotide, which contains only eight amino acids, has been designed to be highly resistant to proteolytic digestion and now has an established use in the suppression of hormone secretion in acromegaly, carcinoid tumours, and hypersecretory tumours of the gastrointestinal tract (such as VIPomas and glucagonomas). Radiolabelled preparations of somatostatin analogues are selectively bound to tissues and organs that possess somatostatin receptors and have been used to image metastases from neuroendocrine tumours (Fig. 1.21). Somatostatin receptors are also expressed in several types of immunocompetent cells where they modulate immune function; radiolabelled octreotide has been used to outline and stage several forms of lymphoma.

CORTICOTROPHIN-RELEASING HORMONE
Although CRH (initially referred to as CRF) was the first of the hypophysiotrophic factors to be recognised and to be given the generic name 'releasing factor' (by Saffran and Schally, 1955), its chemical nature was not determined until 1981 by Vale and collaborators.

Patients injected with CRH respond with increased ACTH and plasma corticosteroid levels (Fig. 1.22). In addition, the peptides β-lipotrophin and endorphin are stimulated; these are synthesised in the corticotrophs, together with ACTH, as part of the precursor molecule POMC (pro-opiomelanocortin).

Fig. 1.20 Some of the biological actions of somatostatin outside the central nervous system.

SOME OF THE BIOLOGICAL ACTIONS OF SOMATOSTATIN OUTSIDE THE CNS

acts on	inhibits secretion of	other actions
pituitary	GH TSH	
gastrointestinal tract	gastrin secretin GIP motilin enteroglucagon VIP gastric acid pancreatic bicarbonate pancreatic enzymes	inhibition of gall bladder emptying, gastric emptying, intestinal absorption and gastrointestinal blood flow
pancreas	insulin glucagon	

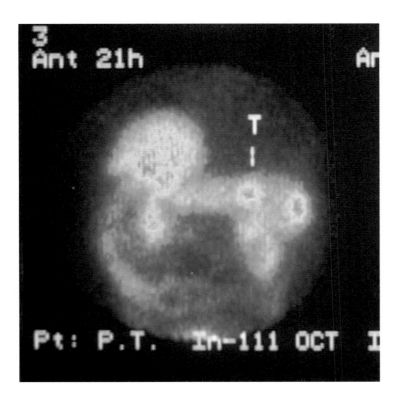

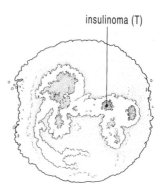

Fig. 1.21 Visualisation of a metastatic neuroendocrine tumour of the pancreas. An insulinoma (T) is shown utilising an ¹¹¹In radiolabelled octreotide preparation which binds selectively to the somatostatin receptor

insulinoma (T)

ACTH RELEASE IN RESPONSE TO CRH

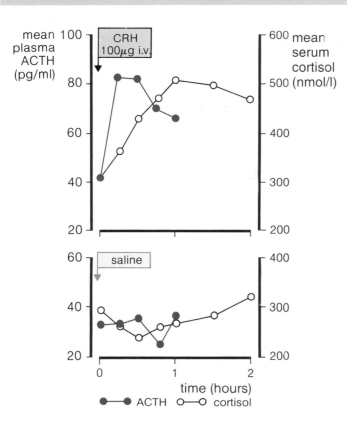

Fig. 1.22 ACTH release in response to synthetic CRH. Six normal men were injected with 100μg of CRH. The initial rise in mean plasma ACTH was followed by an increase in mean serum cortisol. Control values after saline injections are also shown. Modified from Grossman *et al* (1982); by courtesy of *The Lancet*.

The availability of synthetic CRH has made it possible to answer several classical questions about hypothalamic–pituitary–adrenal control. The effects of CRH on the pituitary are inhibited by cortisol, thus confirming a direct pituitary feedback effect (Fig. 1.23). ADH, which previously had been shown to have CRH-like activity, has now been shown to potentiate CRH action, and in some settings, may be even more important than CRF as a stimulator of ACTH release. An important element in the negative feedback control of ACTH secretion by cortisol is the striking inhibitory effect of this steroid on the synthesis and secretion of CRH and ADH.

Extrahypothalamic distribution of CRH, long suspected from results of bioassay studies, has now been confirmed by more specific methods. Its distribution indicates that CRH can be regarded (as is the case of TRH and somatostatin) as a gut–brain peptide. Unlike other hypophysiotrophic factors, CRH is bound in neurones and in blood (during pregnancy) to a specific binding protein.

PROLACTIN-REGULATING FACTORS

In keeping with the observation that the hypothalamus exerts tonic inhibitory effects on prolactin secretion, is the finding that crude hypothalamic extracts inhibit prolactin release. This bioactivity has been termed PIF by Meites (1966). PIF has been identified in portal vessel blood (1971), thus satisfying one of the critical requirements for proof of physiological significance of a hypophysiotrophic hormone. Although a number of substances that can inhibit prolactin release have been isolated from the hypothalamus, most workers believe that dopamine is the principal factor.

Evidence that acute prolactin release, as occurs in stress or in response to suckling, is due to a PRF is convincing. Several potent PRFs have been isolated, including VIP and TRH. In addition, evidence of a distinct PRF being present in posterior pituitary extracts has also been adduced. It is likely that chronic 'tone' of prolactin secretion is determined by dopamine and that in acute release situations, hypothalamic dopamine is suppressed and one or more of the PRFs is released.

NEUROTRANSMITTER REGULATION OF HYPOTHALAMIC HORMONES

The hypophysiotrophic neurones themselves are regulated by hormonal, neuropeptide, and neurotransmitter influences, the latter arising from well-defined bioaminergic pathways that originate in the hypothalamus and elsewhere in the brain (Fig. 1.24). The neurotransmitter dopamine is also a hypophysiotrophic hormone and arises in the hypothalamus from a group of tuberohypophysial neurones. It is secreted into the portal vessel blood and inhibits prolactin secretion. Biogenic amines (including dopamine) influence other pituitary secretions by their effects on hypophysiotrophic neurones.

The hypothalamic neurones that control the anterior pituitary gland are in turn influenced by neuropeptides, neurotransmitters, and the feedback effects of various hormones. These various influences are integrated with other mechanisms for control of visceral and homeostatic function.

Central adrenergic pathways are important, not only for regulation of pituitary function, but also for a number of important visceral and homeostatic functions. Ascending noradrenergic fibres stimulate gonadotrophin, ACTH, and GH secretion, regulate the level of alertness in the reticular activating system, and have important effects on eating and drinking behaviour. The ascending serotoninergic system stimulates GH, prolactin, and ACTH secretion. Central dopaminergic, noradrenergic, and serotoninergic systems are involved in determination of affective state and may also be involved in the pathogenesis of the major psychoses. Drugs that are used in clinical psychiatry and which modulate central bioaminergic function may also influence endocrine function: for example, dopamine agonists inhibit prolactin release, and dopamine antagonists stimulate prolactin release.

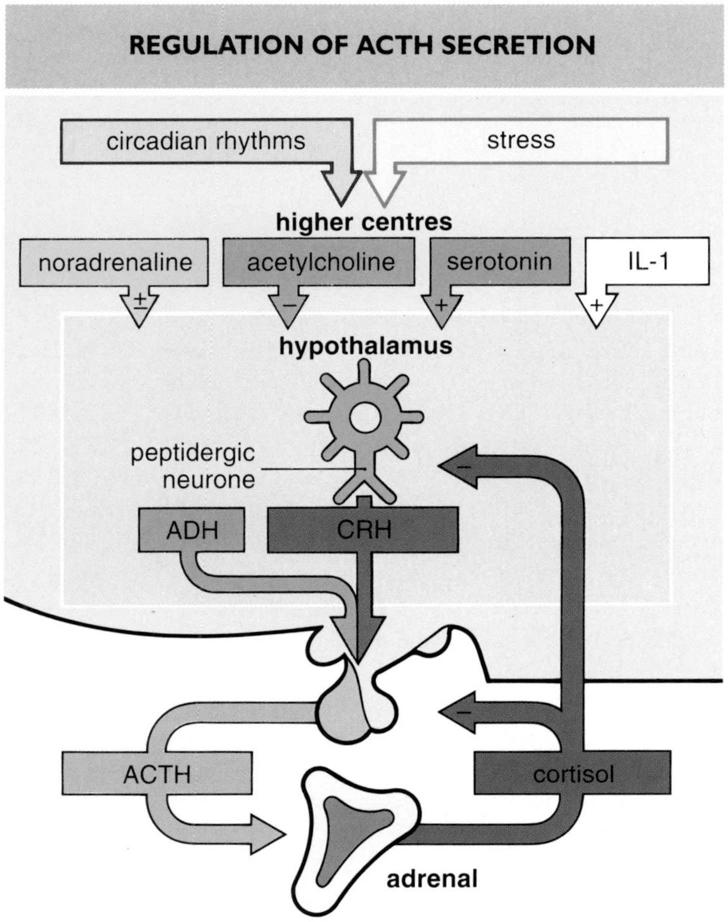

REGULATION OF ACTH SECRETION

Fig. 1.23 The regulation of ACTH secretion. The secretion of ACTH is stimulated by CRH and ADH acting synergistically and is inhibited by the feedback effects of cortisol exerted directly at the level of the pituitary. In addition, cortisol inhibits both CRH and ADH secretion, thus acting on the hypothalamus as well.

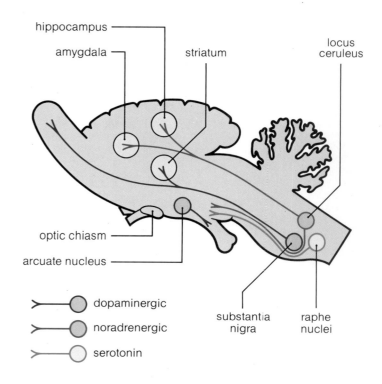

ASCENDING BIOAMINERGIC TRACTS INVOLVED IN HYPOTHALAMO–PITUITARY FUNCTION

Fig. 1.24 An outline of the ascending bioaminergic tracts involved in hypothalamopituitary function in the rat. Dopaminergic fibres comprise one group whose origin is in the *substantia nigra* in the midbrain, and project to the basal ganglia (forming part of the extrapyramidal motor system). An intrinsic tuberoinfundibular system is responsible for dopamine secretion into the hypophysial–portal vascular system, which tonically inhibits prolactin secretion. The mesolimbic dopamine system that innervates brain structures involved in affective states is not shown. Ascending fibres from the *locus ceruleus* bring noradrenergic influences into the hypothalamus, and fibres from the raphe nuclei carry serotoninergic signals into the hypothalamus and elsewhere. All of these pathways are involved in the regulation of the anterior and posterior pituitary and, in addition, have important effects on visceral function and behaviour. Modified from Martin *et al* (1977); by courtesy of FA Davis Company.

2

Hypopituitarism and Growth Hormone Deficiency

John AH Wass, MD,FRCP

Peter H Sönksen, MD,FRCP

HYPOPITUITARISM

Hypopituitarism means the partial or complete deficiency of anterior and posterior pituitary hormone secretion. It occurs frequently in clinical endocrine practice and causes a wide variety of symptoms and signs which are influenced by the aetiology and rate of onset of the disorder. When hypopituitarism is slow in onset, the diagnosis may be delayed, often for many years. Hypopituitarism may be associated either with pathological processes that destroy the pituitary itself or with those that destroy the hypothalamus and thus interfere with the hypothalamic hormone control of the pituitary gland (see Chapter 1).

CAUSES OF HYPOPITUITARISM

Hypopituitarism is most commonly caused by the presence of a pituitary tumour (Figs 2.1 & 2.2). The tumour is usually benign and most frequently arises from the anterior lobe. Pituitary carcinoma is very rare indeed, but in such cases metastases occur inside or outside the nervous system. Pituitary microadenomas, tumours less than 10mm in diameter, have a surprisingly high incidence and are present in approximately twenty-five per cent of all patients examined at autopsy. It is now known that, in life, only the minority (less than ten per cent) progress to form macroadenomas. Since microadenomas are small in size, such tumours are only very occasionally associated with hypopituitarism. Pituitary tumours range widely in size and may extend outside the pituitary fossa to compress surrounding structures (see below).

Pituitary Tumours

Pituitary tumours account for ten per cent of clinically significant intracranial tumours. Currently, they are most frequently classified as 'functioning' or 'nonfunctioning', depending on whether a known hormone (for example, prolactin, growth hormone (GH), or adreno-

corticotrophic hormone (ACTH)) is produced by the tumour. They are also classified according to their immunological and histochemical staining characteristics (Fig. 2.3). Since interpretation of tumour sections may be extremely subjective using the haematoxylin and eosin (H and E) stain, current practice is to use the periodic acid Schiff–orange G (PAS–OG) stain. Evaluation of the size of the intracellular granules by electron microscopy is also useful since prolactin- and GH-secreting adenomas have the largest intracellular granules (the prolactin granule has a mean diameter of 550nm).

Prolactinomas or Lactotroph Cell Tumours

Prolactinomas or lactotroph cell tumours (Fig. 2.4) are the most common pituitary tumours, accounting for approximately fifty per cent of all such tumours. For many years, these tumours were considered to be nonfunctioning; however, with the discovery of human prolactin, and with the development of radioimmunoassays, it has become clear that most of these so-called nonfunctioning pituitary tumours are prolactinomas. Pseudoprolactinomas are tumours that are usually functionless. They are associated with hyperprolactinaemia, since stalk compression interferes with the passage of dopamine from the hypothalamus to the pituitary. The incidence of truly nonfunctioning adenomas varies, but is usually approximately twenty per cent.

Somatotroph Cell Adenomas

Approximately fifteen per cent of pituitary tumours are usually associated with gigantism before epiphysial fusion or acromegaly after epiphysial fusion. Acromegaly is the more common manifestation since pituitary tumours occur most frequently in middle age and only rarely in childhood. Large tumours or macroadenomas, particularly those secreting prolactin and GH, are often locally invasive, rendering complete surgical removal difficult or impossible. Many pituitary tumours have mixed cell populations; for example, somatotroph and

CAUSES OF HYPOPITUITARISM

pituitary and
parapituitary tumours

trauma

radiotherapy

infarction (pituitary apoplexy)

infiltrations
e.g. sarcoidosis, Langerhans' cell histiocytosis (histiocytosis-X) and haemochromatosis

infections
e.g. tuberculosis
abscess, syphilis

Sheehan's syndrome
(post-partum pituitary necrosis)

Fig. 2.1 The causes of hypopituitarism.
Hypopituitarism is most commonly caused by the presence of a pituitary tumour.

PITUITARY AND PARAPITUITARY TUMOURS

anterior pituitary		parapituitary
functioning (adenoma or carcinoma)	non-functioning	germinoma/teratoma
prolactin-secreting	adenoma	primary choriocarcinoma
		ependymoma
GH-secreting		dermoid/epidermoid cyst
		A–V malformation
		chondrosarcoma
ACTH-secreting	carcinoma	craniopharyngioma
		chordoma
gonadotrophin or TSH-secreting	sarcoma	optic nerve glioma
		reticulosis
posterior pituitary		sphenoidal ridge meningioma
ganglioneuroma	astrocytoma (very rare)	secondary deposits, e.g. from breast and lung

Fig. 2.2 Pituitary and parapituitary tumours. The anterior pituitary tumours that produce hormones (i.e. prolactin-, GH-, ACTH-, TSH- and gonadotrophin-secreting tumours) are known as 'functioning' tumours.

lactotroph cells are associated with increased secretion of both GH and prolactin. With mixed-cell tumours, however, the same cell is only rarely found to contain both hormones.

Corticotroph Cell Adenomas

Around ten per cent of pituitary tumours are the cause of Cushing's disease. Such tumours (corticotroph cell adenomas), may be as small as 2mm in diameter and may be located in the centre of the gland. It is therefore unusual for these adenomas to be associated with a radiological abnormality of the pituitary fossa or with hypopituitarism.

Gonadotrophinomas

Gonadotrophinomas are more common than thyrotrophinomas (thyroid-stimulating hormone (TSH) producing adenomas), and are increasingly being recognised. Gonadotroph and thyrotroph cell adenomas, however, are rare and have a combined incidence of five per cent. Clinically, gonadotrophinomas are most often seen in middle-aged men who have a history of normal puberty and normal fertility (Fig. 2.5). Such patients come to medical attention because

they experience visual impairment, often caused by an enormous pituitary tumour. Examination shows normal virilisation, but the testes may be larger than normal. *In vivo*, they most commonly secrete follicle-stimulating hormone (FSH), often accompanied by excessive production of FSH β- and α-subunits. Intact luteinising hormone (LH) is much less commonly secreted (Fig. 2.6).

Hypopituitarism can occur as a result of compression of secretory cells in the normal gland by a pituitary tumour. Large nonsecreting tumours may also cause hypopituitarism by compressing the pituitary stalk and interfering with the delivery of hypothalamic hormones to the anterior pituitary. If dopamine secretion is interfered with in this way, hyperprolactinaemia may ensue.

Molecular Biology of Pituitary Tumours

Genetic factors play a role in some pituitary tumours and, in familial multiple endocrine neoplasia type I (MEN I), prolactin-, GH-, and ACTH-secreting tumours contribute one of the neoplastic components.

Recently, oncogenic mutations have been found in a subset of GH-producing adenomas, which are involved in their development.

CHARACTERISTICS OF THE FUNCTIONING ANTERIOR PITUITARY TUMOURS

tumour	staining characteristics		mean granule diameter (nm)
	H and E	**PAS–OG**	
GH-secreting	acidophil	yellow	550
prolactin-secreting	acidophil	yellow	450
ACTH-secreting β-LPH-secreting	basophil	magenta	360
LH-secreting FSH-secreting	basophil	magenta	200
TSH-secreting	basophil	magenta	135

Fig. 2.3 The staining characteristics and granule size of the functioning tumours of the anterior pituitary. The PAS–OG staining technique is less subjective than H and E staining. Evaluation of the size of intracellular granules by electron microscopy may also be useful.

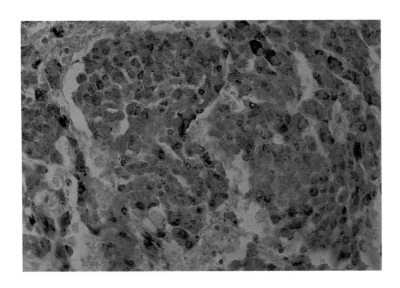

Fig. 2.4 Immunostaining of a histological section of a prolactinoma. The majority of the tumour cells contain fine, brown cytoplasmic granules, thus indicating a positive immunoperoxidase reaction with antiprolactin antibody. Immunoperoxidase and haematoxylin stain, magnification × 100. By courtesy of Prof I Doniach.

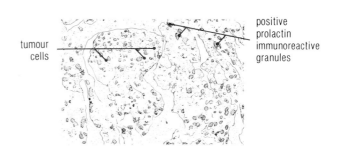

GH-releasing hormone (GHRH) regulates pituitary somatotroph function by interacting with specific membrane receptors that activate adenylyl cyclase via the stimulating G protein, Gs. The consequent increase in intracellular cAMP levels stimulates GH secretion and somatotroph proliferation. In some GH-secreting adenomas, intracellular cAMP concentration and secretory activity are elevated, even under nonstimulated conditions. In these tumours, oncogenic mutation in the chain genes of the Gs has been shown. The resulting activation of adenylyl cyclase bypasses the normal requirement of the cell to be activated by GHRH and is thus autonomous. Such exciting studies suggest that we are beginning to understand the pathogenesis of pituitary tumours.

Other Causes of Hypopituitarism

Parapituitary tumours are rare and of these, craniopharyngiomas, evolved embryologically from Rathke's pouch, are the most common (Fig. 2.7). They occur above or, more rarely, in the sella turcica and may be solid or cystic. The majority show calcification above the sella turcica (Fig. 2.8). These tumours may contain an oily fluid containing human chorionic gonadotrophin and cholesterol crystals, and are characteristically lined by squamous epithelial cells. Fifty per cent of cases occur in patients under the age of fifteen years, and patients commonly present with GH deficiency and diabetes insipidus, with or without visual field defects.

Other tumours may compress the pituitary stalk and cause hypopituitarism; these include meningiomas arising from the sphenoidal ridge and, very rarely, germinomas and chordomas. Metastases from lung and breast carcinomas to the hypothalamus and pituitary are well documented, but rare.

Operative surgery and irradiation for the treatment of pituitary tumours can also lead to hypopituitarism. Cranial irradiation for other reasons (for example, leukaemia) is an increasingly common cause of GH deficiency in children because of hypothalamic damage. Very rarely, severe head trauma causes pituitary insufficiency by severing the pituitary stalk. Previously, major postpartum haemorrhage with ensuing circulatory failure was a more common cause of hypopituitarism. The associated hypopituitarism resulted from pituitary infarction and is referred to as Sheehan's syndrome. This is now mainly confined to developing countries in which obstetric services are less well developed.

Several granulomatous or infiltrative processes, including sarcoidosis or Langerhans' cell histiocytosis (previously known as histiocytosis X or eosinophilic granuloma), may involve the hypothalamus and cause hypopituitarism, particularly diabetes insipidus. Infections such as tuberculosis are now seen only rarely but may cause hypopituitarism associated with basal meningitis.

Isolated disorders of pituitary hormone secretion can occur in the absence of structural lesions of either the hypothalamus or pituitary. Thus, GH, or LH and FSH deficiency, can occur as isolated phenomena. These disorders result from isolated defects in hypothalamic hormone secretion: GH deficiency is due to a congenital deficiency of GHRH; and LH and FSH deficiency results from deficient gonadotrophin-releasing hormone (GnRH) secretion (Kallmann's syndrome). Isolated TSH and ACTH deficiencies occur less commonly and are presumably associated with deficient thyrotrophin-releasing hormone (TRH) or corticotrophin-releasing hormone (CRH) secretion, respectively.

CLINICAL CHARACTERISTICS OF GONADOTROPHINOMAS

male >> female

> 40 years

previously normal gonadal function

large testes

large pituitary tumour (usually)

Fig. 2.5 The clinical characteristics of patients with gonadotrophinomas.

HORMONAL CHARACTERISTICS OF GONADOTROPHINOMAS

excessive secretion of :
FSH (usual)

FSH-β and α (often)

LH-β (occasional)

LH (rare)

Fig. 2.6 The hormonal characteristics of gondatrophinomas.

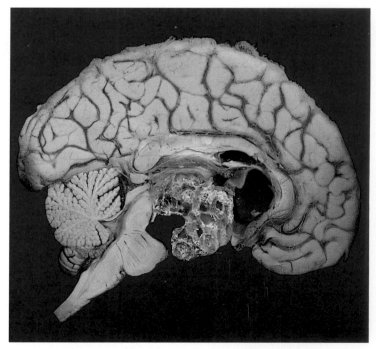

Fig. 2.7 Macropathology of a craniopharyngioma. This photograph shows a large, cystic, calcified craniopharyngioma in a hemisected brain. The lesion extends into the substance of the brain.

SYMPTOMS ASSOCIATED WITH HYPOPITUITARISM

Although symptoms may be caused by local pressure effects in patients with a pituitary or parapituitary tumour, the clinical picture of hypopituitarism results chiefly from pituitary hormone deficiency. Symptoms and signs vary widely, but early symptoms of hypopituitarism relate mostly to hypogonadism in both sexes.

In progressive hypopituitarism, for example due to an anterior pituitary tumour, there is a characteristic order in the development of hormone deficiency (Fig. 2.9). Usually, secretion of GH and LH fails first; this is followed later by failure of FSH and TSH secretion, and finally by that of ACTH secretion. Prolactin deficiency is rare except in Sheehan's syndrome, where it is associated with a failure of lactation. Antidiuretic hormone (ADH or vasopressin) deficiency is virtually unknown in patients with anterior pituitary tumours, although it may occasionally be seen in patients following head injury. The result is diabetes insipidus. The effects of severe hypopituitarism are illustrated in Fig. 2.10.

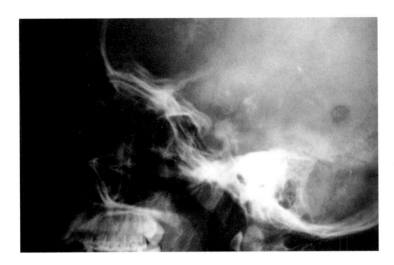

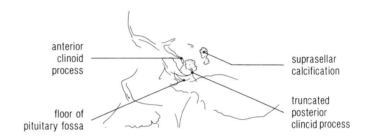

Fig. 2.8 A radiograph of a pituitary fossa in hypopituitarism.
A mass of amorphous calcification extends upwards from the tip of the dorsum sellae, which is typical of a craniopharyngioma.

anterior clinoid process

suprasellar calcification

floor of pituitary fossa

truncated posterior clincid process

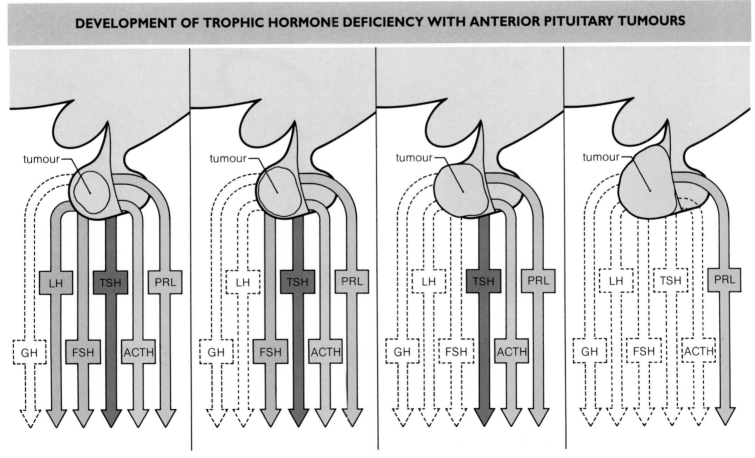

DEVELOPMENT OF TROPHIC HORMONE DEFICIENCY WITH ANTERIOR PITUITARY TUMOURS

Fig. 2.9 The development of trophic hormone deficiency with anterior pituitary tumours.
As the disease progresses, there is a characteristic order in the development of hormone deficiency. Usually, GH secretion fails first, with ACTH secretion failing much later on. Prolactin deficiency is rare, except when associated with an early failure of lactation in Sheehan's syndrome. ADH deficiency is virtually unknown in patients with anterior pituitary tumours, but may be seen with other causes of hypopituitarism (e.g. head trauma).

SYMPTOMS OF DEFICIENT ANTERIOR PITUITARY HORMONE SECRETION

GH deficiency causes short stature in children and sometimes retards bone development. It occurs most often as an isolated congenital defect (for example, isolated GHRH deficiency), in association with a craniopharyngioma or pituitary tumour, or after brain irradiation for malignancy. Effective treatment with parenteral biosynthetic GH or GHRH is now available, although the potential for catch-up growth decreases as the child becomes older. Early diagnosis is therefore essential. At birth, these children look normal. Growth failure can, however, usually be recognised between one and three years of age, but may only be detected much later. If the condition is untreated, growth continues at between fifty and sixty per cent of the normal

rate. Body and facial features remain immature, and the patient is usually fat due to the absent lipolytic action of GH (Fig. 2.11). Body proportions and mental development are normal and consistent with chronological age. Investigation of these children shows retarded bone age in parallel with their height. GH secretion is deficient on provocative challenge (such as insulin-induced hypoglycaemia or arginine stimulation). In adults, both abnormal fat distribution and reduced exercise capacity can be reversed with GH therapy (see below).

Gonadotrophin deficiency also occurs early in progressive hypopituitarism. Thus, patients with gonadal dysfunction should be investigated to avoid delayed diagnosis of a pituitary or parapituitary lesion. In women, gonadotrophin deficiency leads to inadequate oestrogen

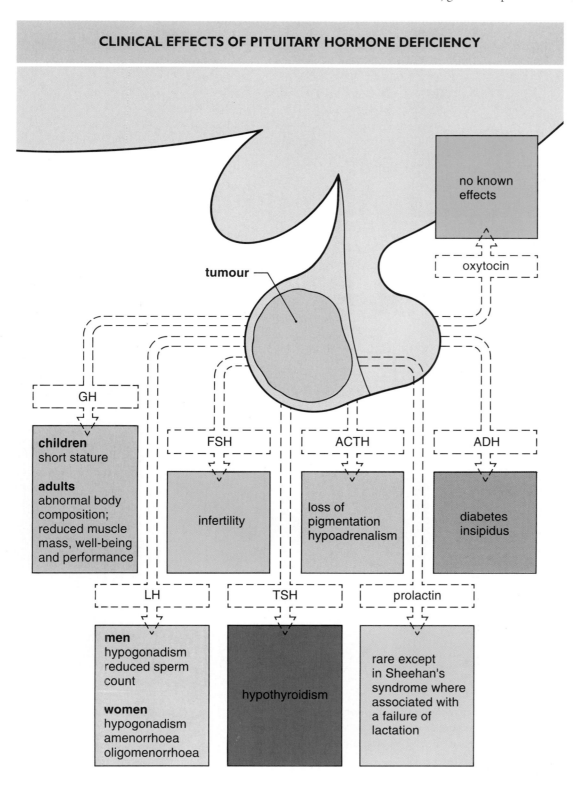

Fig. 2.10 The clinical effects of pituitary hormone deficiency in hypopituitarism.

secretion, which may result in amenorrhoea and infertility (Fig. 2.12). Oestrogen deficiency also causes dyspareunia and atrophy of the breasts. Loss of secondary sexual hair occurs in both sexes after several years (Fig. 2.13). In men, the principal symptoms of gonadotrophin deficiency are poor libido and impotence, with infertility resulting from a decrease in sperm production. The testicles become smaller and soft. Beard growth may take many years to regress and may be normal for some time after libido and sexual

function have been impaired. In both sexes, there is fine wrinkling of the skin, particularly around the mouth and eyes. If gonadotrophin secretion fails in childhood, while GH remains normal, there will be excessive linear growth due to failure of closure of the epiphyses. Thus, a eunuchoid proportion develops, with span exceeding height.

TSH- and ACTH-secreting cells are usually the last to fail in progressive hypopituitarism. TSH deficiency (Fig. 2.14) is associated with growth retardation in children. In adults, the most marked

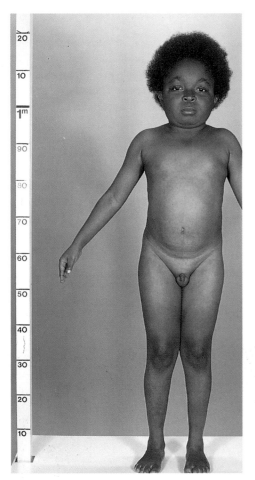

Fig. 2.11 A seventeen-year-old boy with GH deficiency associated with hypopituitarism. The patient has short stature for his age and underdeveloped genitalia.

SYMPTOMS OF GONADOTROPHIN DEFICIENCY

women

amenorrhoea/oligomenorrhoea

infertility

dyspareunia

breast atrophy

loss of secondary sexual hair

men

poor libido/impotence

infertility

small, soft testicles

loss of secondary sexual hair

Fig. 2.12 The symptoms of gonadotrophin deficiency in hypopituitarism.

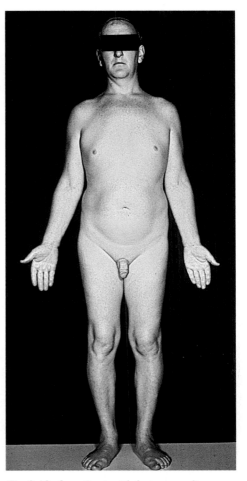

Fig. 2.13 A patient with hypogonadism resulting from a tumour. This hypopituitary patient has regression of secondary sexual characteristics and an absence of pubic hair as a result of the gonadotrophin deficiency caused by a pituitary tumour.

Fig. 2.14 The symptoms of TSH and ACTH deficiency. As well as the symptoms listed, in advanced hypopituitarism, TSH and ACTH deficiency may lead to collapse, coma, and death.

SYMPTOMS OF TSH AND DEFICIENCY

TSH deficiency	ACTH deficiency
in children growth retardation	weakness
	tiredness
in adults decrease in energy constipation sensitivity to cold dry skin weight gain	dizziness on standing pallor hypoglycaemia

features are constipation, a decrease in energy, an increased sensitivity to cold dry skin, and weight gain; however, the features are not as marked as in primary hypothyroidism since the deficiency is usually less severe. Lack of ACTH secretion produces the symptoms of hypoadrenalism, particularly weakness and tiredness, nausea and vomiting, and progression to dizziness on standing due to postural hypotension. ACTH deficiency results in reduced adrenal androgen secretion and contributes to the decreased libido and loss of secondary sexual hair seen in hypopituitarism. In pituitary ACTH deficiency, there is also pallor of the skin (Fig. 2.15). Hypoglycaemia can occur in hypoadrenalism for two reasons: first, because of increased insulin sensitivity due to a lack of cortisol (cortisol is an insulin antagonist), and, second, because adrenal insufficiency decreases hepatic glycogen reserves. In advanced hypopituitarism, collapse, coma and even death are possible due to a combination of hypoglycaemia, hypothyroidism, hypothermia and hypotension. Most patients with hypopituitarism, even in the advanced stage, are well nourished; however, severe prolonged hypopituitarism can produce extreme weight loss and an appearance of malnutrition ('pituitary cachexia') which may be clinically indistinguishable from anorexia nervosa.

The clinical appearance of hypopituitarism may be complicated. Patients with large tumours that secrete prolactin, GH or ACTH may have hypopituitarism despite oversecretion of one particular hormone. Thus, in the acromegalic patient shown in Fig. 2.16, the pallor and texture of the skin are consistent with coexistent hypopituitarism.

Symptoms Associated with Local Hypothalamic or Pituitary Lesions

Headaches are caused by local pressure from a tumour and probably result from stretching of the dura mater above the pituitary fossa in a patient with a pituitary tumour (Fig. 2.17). Rarely, they can be caused by a suprasellar tumour (for example, a craniopharyngioma), which compresses the aqueduct of Sylvius and thus prevents the passage of cerebrospinal fluid (CSF) between the third and fourth ventricles. This results in hydrocephalus and enlargement of the third and lateral ventricles. In general, headaches caused by pressure effects are variable in location and are intermittent.

If a large pituitary or parapituitary tumour compresses the optic chiasm, it may cause visual field defects. The nasal visual fields are transmitted by temporal retinal fibres. The temporal visual fields are transmitted by the nasal retinal fibres and these fibres cross at the optic chiasm. Therefore, if, as frequently is the case, a pituitary tumour grows upwards centrally towards the chiasm, the nasal central fibres become compressed, thus initially causing an upper outer quadrant field defect. If the pressure on the chiasm continues, a complete bitemporal hemianopia may occur. With long-standing compression, this will progress to irreversible optic atrophy and blindness. The growth of the tumour and the resultant visual field defects may, however, be asymmetrical. Further upward extension may cause a hypothalamic disturbance and produce disturbed consciousness, abnormal thirst, hyperphagia, or abnormal temperature regulation.

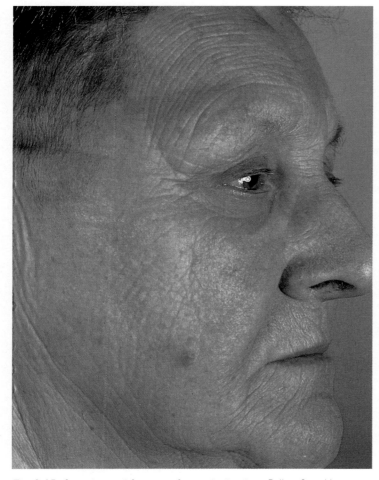

Fig. 2.15 A patient with severe hypopituitarism. Pallor, fine skin wrinkling, and absence of facial hair can be clearly seen.

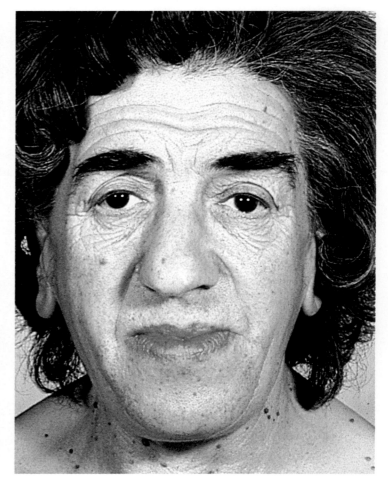

Fig. 2.16 A patient with concomitant acromegaly and hypopituitarism. The presence of a GH-secreting pituitary tumour was the cause of the symptoms in this patient.

LOCAL SYMPTOMS OF A PITUITARY TUMOUR AND OF HYPOPITUITARISM

upward

headaches

(a) stretching of dura
by tumour

(b) hydrocephalus (rare)

visual field defects
nasal retinal fibres
compressed by tumour

sideways

**cranial nerve
palsies and temporal
lobe epilepsy**
lateral extension
of tumour

downward

**cerebrospinal fluid
rhinorrhoea**
downward extension
of tumour

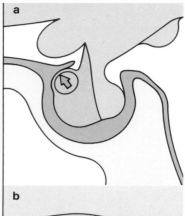
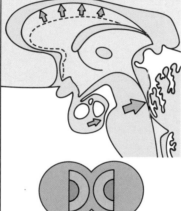
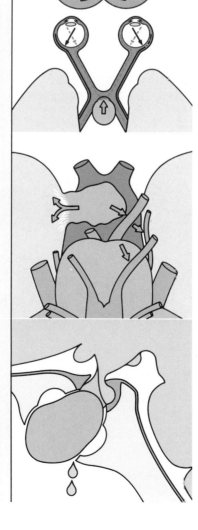

**Fig. 2.17 *The local symptoms of a pituitary tumour, in addition to
hypopituitarism.*** Headaches are caused only rarely by hydrocephalus.
Visual field defects caused by extension of the tumour are readily plotted
using the Goldmann perimeter.

Lateral extension of parapituitary or pituitary tumours is less common. In approximately five per cent of patients with a pituitary tumour, there is extension into the cavernous sinus; this may cause cranial nerve palsies due to compression of the third, fourth, or sixth cranial nerves. Very rarely, pituitary tumours extend into the temporal lobe of the brain to cause epilepsy. If a tumour extends downwards, it may erode the sphenoid bone through to the sphenoid sinus and postnasal space, and so the patient may present with CSF rhinorrhoea. In contrast to the fluid discharged with the 'runny nose' of the cold, in this instance the fluid contains glucose.

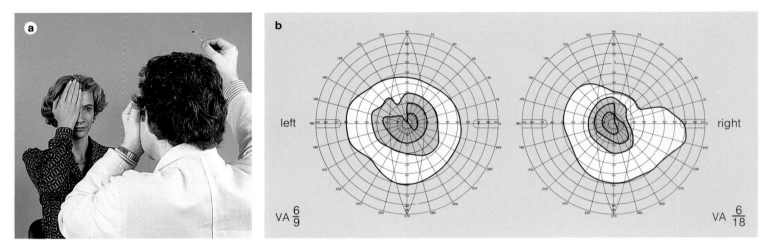

Fig. 2.18 *The clinical assessment of visual field defects.* Visual fields are tested accurately using a red pin (a), and the results are recorded on a Goldmann field plot as in (b), which also shows visual acuity (VA). In this patient, bitemporal field defects were found. Classically, this results from chiasmal compression by a suprasellar extension.

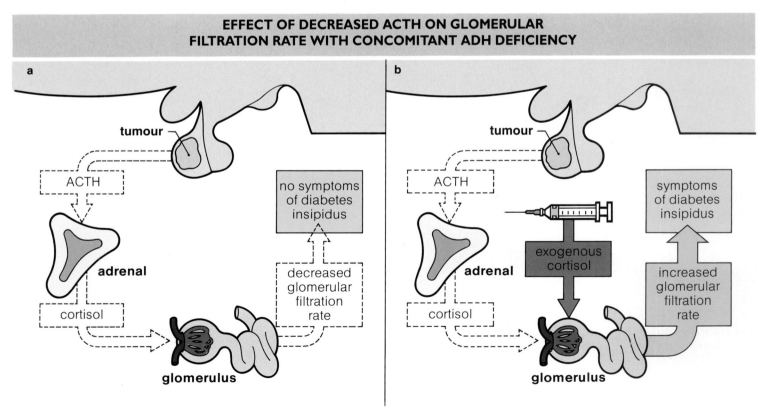

EFFECT OF DECREASED ACTH ON GLOMERULAR FILTRATION RATE WITH CONCOMITANT ADH DEFICIENCY

Fig. 2.19 *The effect of decreased ACTH on glomerular filtration rate, with concomitant ADH deficiency.* (a) The symptoms of diabetes insipidus are obscured by ACTH deficiency. These symptoms may appear for the first time with administration of cortisol (hydrocortisone), either orally or intramuscularly as shown in (b).

DIAGNOSIS OF HYPOPITUITARISM
Investigation of Patients with Space-occupying Lesions that cause Hypopituitarism

Both the anatomical and physiological aspects of the pituitary should be considered when investigating a patient with suspected hypopituitarism. From the anatomical point of view, the most important tests are those used for visual fields, since they may indicate chiasmal compression (for example, resulting from a pituitary tumour). For early diagnosis of such lesions, peripheral vision is assessed using a red pin, where patients inform the doctor when the colour red appears in their outer field of view (Fig. 2.18). Red-colour perception is lost before perception of other colours or white light. Additionally, visual fields should be plotted objectively: for example, by using the Goldmann perimeter. Typical Goldmann plots showing bitemporal field defects are illustrated in Fig. 2.18.

Plain radiography of the pituitary region is essential, and lateral and anteroposterior (AP) views of the pituitary fossa should be taken. Frequently, pituitary tumours increase the overall size of the fossa and cause blistering or ballooning of the floor of the pituitary fossa (see Chapters 23 & 24). Suprasellar calcification may be seen if a craniopharyngioma is present. The AP view is also helpful when looking at the pituitary region. Normally, the floor of the pituitary fossa is flat; an obvious dip in the floor of the sella turcica may indicate the presence of a tumour. The position of this indentation may also show the location of the tumour within the pituitary gland. The presence of a normal pituitary fossa does not preclude the presence of a pituitary tumour, since ninety per cent of patients with Cushing's disease, and twenty per cent of prolactinoma patients, also have normal fossae. With parasellar lesions causing hypopituitarism, the plain skull radiographs may be normal, and an abnormality may be revealed only using computerised tomography (CT) scanning or magnetic resonance imaging (MRI) (see Chapter 24).

CT scanning with facilities for reconstruction has revolutionised the assessment of patients with hypopituitarism. More recently, MRI has been introduced and may be more useful in the diagnosis of microadenomas (for example, Cushing's disease). With CT scanning, radiographic attenuation values that are obtained from a scan are processed by computer to determine the density of each tissue that appears on the scan, and results are shown in the form of a cross-sectioned picture on the viewing screen. This technique is useful for delineating pituitary tumours with suprasellar and lateral extensions,

as well as with parasellar lesions. In the 'empty sella' syndrome, an enlarged pituitary sella is usually filled with CSF. This classically occurs in obese women who have headaches, but may also occur in symptom-free patients where the radiographic appearance is often found incidentally. The aetiology is unclear but it may result from herniation of arachnoid through the diaphragma sellae. Pituitary function is usually normal. In some patients, an enlarged empty sella may represent a partially or completely infarcted tumour, in which case the empty sella syndrome may be associated with hyperprolactinaemia, acromegaly, Cushing's disease, or a nonfunctioning tumour with or without hypopituitarism.

Endocrine Assessment of Patients with Hypopituitarism

When assessing pituitary function in the hypopituitary patient, anterior pituitary function should be tested and corrected before function of the posterior pituitary. The reason for this is that decreased ACTH secretion and consequent reduction in cortisol from the adrenal gland decrease the glomerular filtration rate, which can thus obscure the symptoms of polyuria in diabetes insipidus (Fig. 2.19). Basal hormone levels yield much information; it is therefore important to measure directly, by radioimmunoassay, serum concentrations of prolactin, TSH, thyroxine (T_4), cortisol, LH, FSH, testosterone in men, and oestradiol in women (Fig. 2.20). The correlation between levels of the pituitary hormone and the target organ hormone will help to establish the cause of underactivity in a target gland (Fig. 2.21); for example, in a patient with hypothyroidism, low or normal TSH levels combined with low T_4 levels imply pituitary gland malfunction or pituitary hypothyroidism. High TSH concentrations combined with a low T_4 level indicate disease in the thyroid gland itself (that is, primary hypothyroidism).

After the assessment of basal hormone levels, dynamic tests are used to assess hormonal reserves. GH and ACTH secretion in most cases can be tested using the insulin hypoglycaemia test (Fig. 2.22), where insulin is given intravenously. Hypoglycaemia causes symptoms of neuroglycopenia, such as sweating and tachycardia, with concomitant ACTH and GH release. Provided that adequate hypoglycaemia is induced (blood glucose $\leq$2.2mmol/l), cortisol levels should rise to 580nmol/l (21µg/100ml) or above, and GH levels to above 20mu/l (10ng/ml). If these levels are not achieved, the patient is deficient in either ACTH or GH.

BASAL HORMONE LEVELS TO BE MEASURED IN SUSPECTED HYPOPITUITARISM
testosterone or oestradiol
LH & FSH
GH
prolactin
thyroxine
cortisol (0900)
TSH
osmolalities of plasma and urine (early morning)

Fig. 2.20 Basal hormone levels to be measured in a patient with suspected hypopituitarism.

Patients unable to undergo insulin hypoglycaemia tests (for example, those with a history of epilepsy or ischaemic heart disease) can instead be given 1mg glucagon, subcutaneously. This causes a transient rise in blood glucose and, during the subsequent fall, ACTH and GH are released. Glucagon is a less-reliable stimulus than insulin, and in approximately ten per cent of patients, there is no rise in ACTH or GH levels, even in the presence of normal reserves of these hormones. Arginine infusion stimulates GH secretion and may be used to assess GH reserves in some cases.

Assessment of Posterior Pituitary Hormone Secretion

The rise in plasma osmolality resulting from lack of fluid for a period of several hours stimulates ADH secretion; this forms the basis of the standard eight-hour water deprivation test that is used in the diagnosis of diabetes insipidus (Fig. 2.23). The test should be performed during the day when careful observation is possible, since severe fluid and electrolyte depletion can occur. Urine and plasma osmolality are measured for eight hours, after which time a synthetic analogue of ADH, desmopressin, is given intramuscularly. The urine osmolality is then remeasured. As ADH is secreted, water is normally absorbed, with

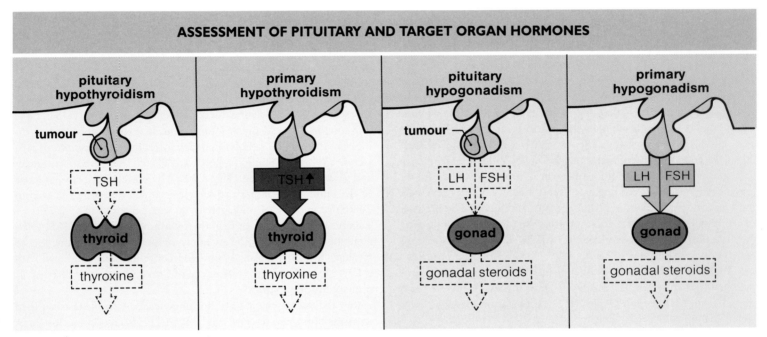

ASSESSMENT OF PITUITARY AND TARGET ORGAN HORMONES

Fig. 2.21 The assessment of pituitary and target organ hormones in the diagnosis of hypopituitarism. The importance of simultaneous measurements of pituitary and target organ hormone levels should be emphasised. In hypothyroidism, low TSH in conjunction with low thyroxine implies pituitary failure, in contrast to low thyroxine with elevated TSH which implies thyroid failure. Similarly, hypogonadal patients with low testosterone or oestradiol in the presence of (inappropriately) low gonadotrophins, have hypopituitarism.

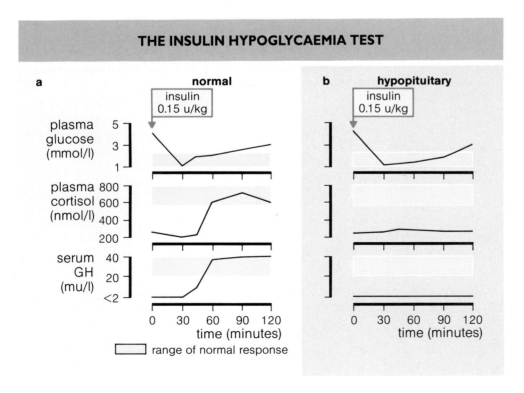

THE INSULIN HYPOGLYCAEMIA TEST

Fig. 2.22 The insulin hypoglycaemia test in the diagnosis of hypopituitarism. Plasma glucose, plasma cortisol, and serum GH levels are shown in a normal (a) and a hypopituitary (b) subject. GH levels should rise to a minimum of 20mu/l and cortisol to 580nmol/l, provided that adequate hypoglycaemia is reached with blood glucose concentrations ≤2.2mmol/l.

the subsequent elevation of urine osmolality. Following desmopressin administration, only a small additional rise in osmolality is observed. In diabetes insipidus, the urine fails to concentrate to twice the plasma osmolality due to lack of ADH, hence plasma osmolality rises. The urine concentrates adequately only after administration of desmopressin. Desmopressin therefore has no effect on patients with nephrogenic diabetes insipidus where the renal tubules are unresponsive to ADH. Diabetes insipidus may be masked in untreated hypopituitarism, sometimes being revealed only after hormone replacement, particularly with cortisol.

Occasionally, in patients with mild cranial diabetes insipidus, urine concentrations do rise to twice that of plasma. More prolonged dehydration may be required to demonstrate the defect (Fig. 2.24b).

TREATMENT OF HYPOPITUITARISM

The many causes of hypopituitarism have to be dealt with individually; thus, a pituitary tumour may be treated by surgery, radiotherapy, or medical treatment. Surgical decompression is usually required to relieve pressure effects on parapituitary structures (such as the optic chiasm or contents of the cavernous sinus) when the lesion cannot be shrunk medically (for example, a prolactinoma). This is the case with functionless tumours when after surgery, radiotherapy may be used to prevent regrowth of the tumour.

Regimens of hormone replacement therapy for gonadotrophin deficiency are shown in Fig. 2.25. In women, a typical regimen involves the administration of ethinyloestradiol (30µg daily) or oestradiol valerate (2mg daily) for three weeks out of four and, for ten days in each calendar month, medroxyprogesterone (5mg daily), after which time a withdrawal bleed occurs. In men, depot mixtures of

testosterone esters can be given intramuscularly in doses of 250–750mg every two to four weeks. The dose varies widely from 125mg every two weeks to 500mg every four weeks. Occasionally polycythaemia can develop on testosterone replacement therapy and the haemaglobin concentration should be monitored during treatment. A safe oral testosterone preparation (testosterone undecanoate 40–80mg three times daily) is also available. In women, libido, vaginal dryness and breast atrophy are remedied. If hypopituitarism develops at a young age, osteoporosis will be prevented by adequate sex steroid treatment. In men, strength, vigour, libido and potency are all improved.

If ovulation or spermatogenesis is required, treatment may be given either with human menopausal gonadotrophin (such as menotrophin) or with GnRH delivered intermittently with a pump (see Chapter 10). If carefully monitored, these treatments usually result in ovulation in women and spermatogenesis in men, the latter after a minimum of three months' treatment.

GH deficiency in childhood is treated with biosynthetic human GH, which is now widely available. Two to four units should be given subcutaneously, daily, and linear growth plotted on a growth chart. With plentiful supplies of GH, therapy in adults with GH deficiency is now possible, and its effects are being studied in detail. Early results suggest that muscle volume and strength may increase, and adipose tissue may decrease, with GH treatment. Furthermore, there may be an improvement in wellbeing (see below).

Replacement hydrocortisone can be administered twice daily in doses of 20mg on waking and 10mg in the early evening in patients who need replacement for ACTH deficiency. The levels of cortisol obtained should be monitored by assessing a profile of serum cortisol

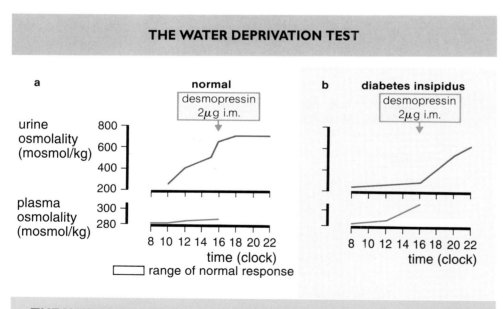

THE WATER DEPRIVATION TEST

a

normal

desmopressin 2µg i.m.

b

diabetes insipidus

desmopressin 2µg i.m.

urine osmolality (mosmol/kg)

plasma osmolality (mosmol/kg)

range of normal response

Fig. 2.23 The water deprivation test used in the diagnosis of hypopituitarism. (a) The sequence of events during normal testing. (b) The hypopituitary response to this test. The patient with ADH deficiency fails to concentrate urine in the presence of a rising plasma osmolality until desmopressin is given. Normally, the peak urine osmolality exceeds twice that of urine before desmopressin administration.

THE WATER DEPRIVATION TEST

1 free access to water overnight, then:
2 no water for eight hours
3 urine and plasma osmolality measured over eight hours
4 desmopressin given intramusculary after eight hours
5 urine osmolality measured after desmopressin

in multiple samples that are obtained via an indwelling needle throughout the day, since the needs of individual patients vary from 15 to 60mg daily. Oral therapy should be increased during a febrile illness and, with vomiting or surgery, hydrocortisone should be given parenterally. In such situations it is prudent to issue a steroid card and instruct patients to wear a MedicAlert (or equivalent) bracelet. Mineralocorticoid replacement is unnecessary since aldosterone secretion is not ACTH dependent.

T$_4$ should be given to patients who are TSH-deficient. The usual dose varies from 0.1 to 0.2mg daily and it is rarely necessary to exceed this. Adequate replacement therapy is indicated by serum triiodothyronine (T$_3$) in the upper part of the normal range.

Posterior pituitary replacement is best achieved using an enzyme-resistant analogue of ADH, which itself has a short duration of action and may cause intense vasoconstriction. For this reason, the drug desmopressin is given (10–20μg once or twice daily, intranasally),

since it is devoid of vasoconstrictor actions at therapeutic doses. Recently, it has become clear that this drug is also effective orally (100μg three times daily). In partial ADH deficiency, a reduction in urine volume can be achieved by using chlorpropramide, which increases the sensitivity of the renal tubules to endogenous ADH. This can, however, cause hypoglycaemia, particularly in the elderly, who should be warned to eat before retiring to bed.

With the correct hormone replacement therapy, symptoms such as lack of libido, hair growth and general wellbeing are alleviated in most hypopituitary patients. Hypopituitarism requires early diagnosis, which can be difficult unless care is taken when documenting patients' history. Women tend to present earlier than men because of menstrual abnormalities. Once the diagnosis has been made, deficient hormones can be adequately replaced to achieve complete symptomatic relief. Additionally, if a pituitary tumour is present, treatment must be directed at arresting and reversing tumour growth.

PROTOCOL FOR MODIFIED WATER DEPRIVATION TEST

PROTOCOL

1   patients suspected of mild diabetes insipidus (DI) should be nil by mouth from 1800h on the evening before the test

2   at 0800h the patient is weighed and blood and urine samples taken for osmolality measurements

3   urine is collected hourly for osmolality measurements

4   blood is collected 2-hourly for osmolality measurements and the patient is weighed 2-hourly

5   when the urine osmolality becomes constant, with less than 30mosmol/kg increase between consecutive samples, blood is taken for plasma osmolality measurement; the patient is given 2μg DDAVP (desmopressin) im and allowed to drink

6   plasma and urine samples are collected 60 minutes after DDAVP

if at any stage the patient's body weight falls by more than 3% of the initial value, results should be reviewed and consideration given to terminating the test

INTERPRETATION

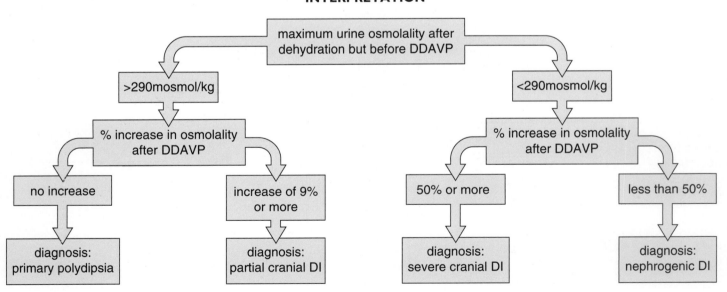

Fig. 2.24 The modified water deprivation test and test to detect mild diabetes insipidus.
The instructions are set out in the upper half and the interpretation in the lower half. Assessment of the maximum osmolality achieved after dehydration allows the differentiation of primary polydipsia, partial cranial diabetes insipidus and nephrogenic diabetes insipidus.

GROWTH HORMONE DEFICIENCY IN ADULTS

The specific effects of GH deficiency in adults, and the importance of GH secretion in adult life, have only recently been elucidated and documented with the help of carefully controlled clinical trials involving patients on GH replacement therapy. Previously, adults with panhypopituitarism on 'full' hormone replacement therapy were considered to be restored to 'normal', but recently it has been shown that, as a group, they have a marked increase in premature 'total' and 'cardiovascular' mortality, and also often have major abnormalities in body composition, physical performance, and quality of life. Replacement therapy with GH in deficient adults is still experimental, however, and its role has not yet been accepted by all authorities.

THE DEFINITION OF THE GROWTH HORMONE DEFICIENCY SYNDROME IN ADULTS

The features of the GH deficiency syndrome have been deduced from placebo-controlled trials of GH replacement therapy given to adults with GH deficiency who are receiving full and adequate replacement of all other hormones. A summary of the clinical and biochemical features that have to date been identified as being attributable to GH deficiency is given in Fig. 2.26.

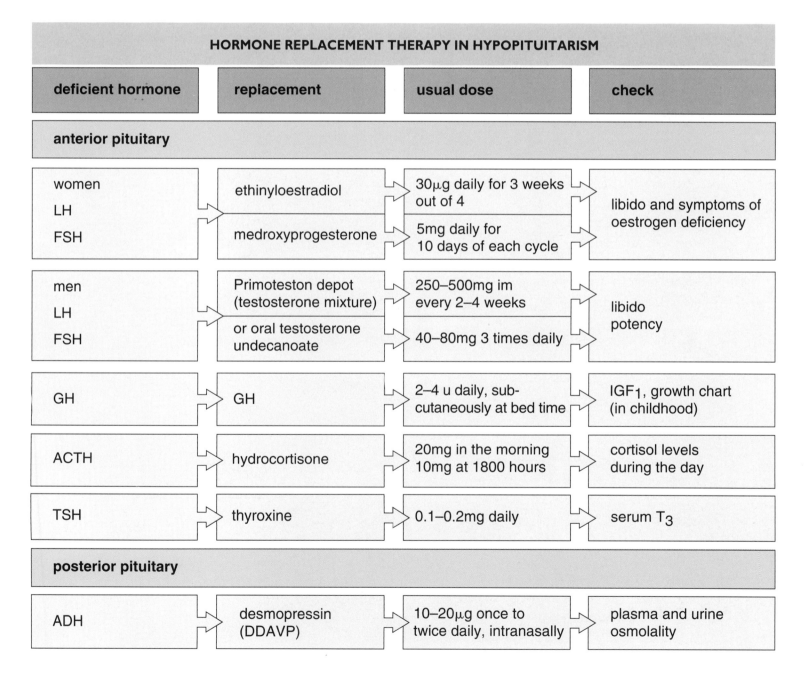

HORMONE REPLACEMENT THERAPY IN HYPOPITUITARISM

deficient hormone	replacement	usual dose	check
anterior pituitary			
women LH FSH	ethinyloestradiol	30µg daily for 3 weeks out of 4	libido and symptoms of oestrogen deficiency
	medroxyprogesterone	5mg daily for 10 days of each cycle	
men LH FSH	Primoteston depot (testosterone mixture)	250–500mg im every 2–4 weeks	libido potency
	or oral testosterone undecanoate	40–80mg 3 times daily	
GH	GH	2–4 u daily, sub-cutaneously at bed time	IGF$_1$, growth chart (in childhood)
ACTH	hydrocortisone	20mg in the morning 10mg at 1800 hours	cortisol levels during the day
TSH	thyroxine	0.1–0.2mg daily	serum T$_3$
posterior pituitary			
ADH	desmopressin (DDAVP)	10–20µg once to twice daily, intranasally	plasma and urine osmolality

Fig. 2.25 Regimens of hormone replacement therapy in the treatment of hypopituitarism.
The normal replacement doses for men and women are indicated.

CHANGES IN BODY COMPOSITION

Some of the most dramatic effects of GH deficiency and GH treatment are on body composition. Lean body mass of adults with GH deficiency that was acquired in adult life is reduced by approximately eight per cent (corresponding to some 4kg of lean tissue) but is completely restored following six months' replacement therapy with GH (Fig. 2.27), with the majority of this increase occurring in the first month of therapy. Skeletal muscle mass increases with GH replacement by between five and eight per cent (Fig. 2.28), and left ventricular wall mass also increase by a similar amount (Fig. 2.29). Additionally, extracellular fluid volume, glomerular filtration rate and renal plasma flow all increase substantially with GH replacement.

In adults with GH deficiency, body fat is excessive and is distributed in a more central (abdominal) than peripheral pattern. With GH replacement, body fat decreases in parallel with the increase in lean body mass (see Fig. 2.27); a mean 5kg loss of body fat in the first month of GH replacement therapy has been reported, and this loss is particularly marked from 'central' sites (Fig. 2.30).

FEATURES OF GH DEFICIENCY

symptoms

known pituitary pathology

impaired psychological wellbeing

   poor health

   impaired emotional reaction

   depressed mood

   impaired self-control

   anxiety

   reduced vitality and energy

   increased social isolation

increased abdominal adiposity

reduced strength and exercise capacity

intolerance to the cold

signs

mixed truncal/generalised obesity

increased waist:hip ratio

thin, dry skin; cool peripheries; poor venous access

minor reductions in muscle strength

moderate reductions in exercise performance

psychological state characterised by low labile mood

tests

stimulated GH level below 5mu/l

low or low/normal IGF-I level

hypercholesterolaemia, high LDL-cholesterol level

low glomerular filtration rate and renal plasma flow

reduced lean body mass/increased fat mass/increased waist:hip ratio

reduced basal metabolic rate/kilogram body weight

reduced bone density

Fig. 2.26 Features that indicate the presence of GH deficiency in adults. All of the symptoms and signs that are listed have been shown to disappear in trials involving patients on GH replacement therapy under placebo-controlled conditions. Modified from Cuneo et al. (1992) with permission.

CHARACTERISTICS OF PHYSICAL PERFORMANCE

Isometric quadriceps force has been shown to be significantly impaired in GH-deficient adults when compared with carefully matched controls; however, although data from other muscle groups have shown a reduction in force, this was not statistically different. Following GH replacement therapy, none of the double-blind studies has so far been able to demonstrate a statistically significant increase in force, despite significant increases in thigh cross-sectional area (probably because of a 'type II' error). Longer-term but uncontrolled follow-up has, however, been able to demonstrate an increase in quadriceps force when therapy has been continued for over twelve months.

Exercise performance has also been shown to be impaired in patients with GH deficiency and, in one study, maximal oxygen uptake (VO$_2$max) was found to be significantly reduced (mean seventy-two to eighty-two per cent of that predicted from age, sex, and height); power output was also reduced. Following GH replacement, maximal and submaximal exercise performance improved markedly. Moreover, VO$_2$max increased to a mean of ninety-seven per cent of the predicted value, and maximal power output increased proportionally (Fig. 2.31). Submaximal exercise performance, measured as anaerobic threshold, also increased significantly, in keeping with the patients' observations that activities that were performed during daily life could be accomplished with less stress and would leave them less exhausted.

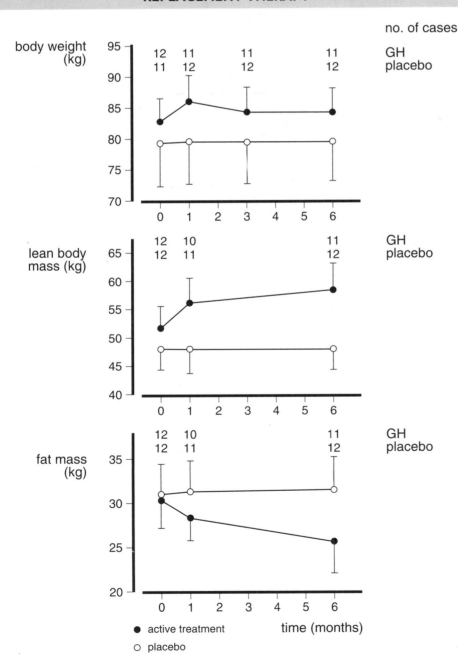

CHANGES IN BODY COMPOSITION DURING GH REPLACEMENT THERAPY

Fig. 2.27 Changes in body composition in adults with GH deficiency during six months of GH replacement therapy. Lean body mass increased by 4.1kg at one month and by 6.2kg at six months. Fat mass fell by 2.2kg at one month and by 5kg at six months. Redrawn from Salomon et al. (1989) with permission.

Histological appearances in muscle biopsies from adults with GH deficiency have been essentially normal, with no signs of myopathy. Treatment with GH results in no detectable changes, in line with the suggestion that improvements in muscle function are primarily related to increased muscle mass and possibly metabolic performance.

CARDIOVASCULAR AND RENAL EFFECTS

The antinatriuretic action of GH has been known for a long time but is seldom a problem in the treatment of children. Clinical evidence of the effects of GH on sodium and water retention has been evident in nearly all of the studies that have been performed in adults with GH deficiency. Weight gain, dependent oedema, and symptoms of carpal tunnel syndrome have been found to occur early (often within days or weeks) in patients on GH replacement, and usually resolve promptly (within days or weeks) on dose reduction, or more slowly (after several months) with no dose reduction. Despite these obvious and quite marked effects on sodium retention, changes in blood pressure are much less obvious, with hypertension being an uncommon side effect which responds quickly to a dose reduction.

Small but statistically significant increases in resting left ventricular end-diastolic and stroke volumes, probably related to the increase in extracellular volume, have been found on echocardiography: a direct association has been shown to exist between the increase in end-diastolic volume at rest and VO_2max. Two case reports have been published demonstrating dramatic improvements in cardiac function in hypopituitary patients with severe cardiomyopathy and highlight the importance of GH in cardiac function in adult life. The renal effects of GH replacement include a marked increase in glomerular

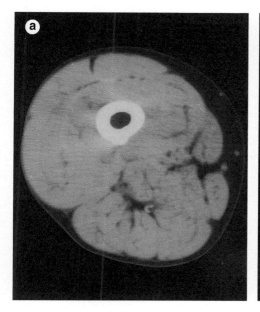
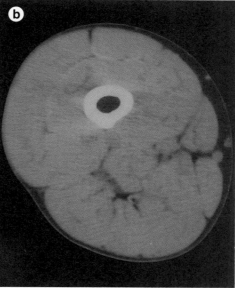

Fig. 2.28 Changes in thigh muscle mass after six months of GH replacement therapy. The midthigh CT scan before (a) and after (b) replacement therapy demonstrates the increase in muscle size, as well as a (less marked) decrease in fat (both intramuscular and subcutaneous).

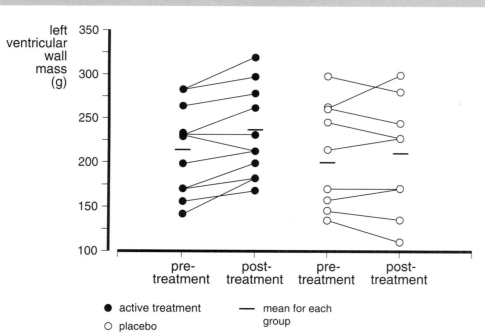

GH REPLACEMENT THERAPY ON LEFT VENTRICULAR WALL

- ● active treatment
- ○ placebo
- — mean for each group

Fig. 2.29 Changes in left ventricular wall mass after six months of GH replacement therapy. Echocardiography showed a small but significant increase in left ventricular wall mass ($P < 0.05$) despite no change in mean arterial pressure. Modified from Cuneo et al. (1991c) with permission.

filtration rate and renal plasma flow. Filtration fraction and albumin excretion have been shown to be unaffected.

The mechanism behind the antinatriuretic and other renal effects of GH is not clear, but the parallel time course of renal effects, and the increase in levels of plasma insulin-like growth factor (IGF-I), suggest that it may be IGF-I mediated. In addition, significant activation of the renin–angiotensin–aldosterone system following GH treatment has been found to occur (Fig. 2.32).

METABOLIC EFFECTS
Energy Expenditure
The anabolic effect of GH is associated with a marked rise in energy expenditure. In one study, basal metabolic rate (BMR) increased twenty-two per cent after one month of GH replacement therapy and was still sixteen per cent higher than baseline after six months of treatment. The action of GH to increase the peripheral conversion of T_4 to T_3 may also contribute to the early increase in BMR, while part of the increase in BMR is accounted for by the increase in lean body mass.

Carbohydrate Metabolism
Levels of fasting plasma glucose are normal in adults with GH deficiency, but those of fasting insulin and C-peptide are increased, particularly in patients who are overweight, suggesting a state of insulin resistance. Plasma glucose, insulin and C-peptide levels rise following GH replacement therapy and remain elevated after six months. The insulin:C-peptide ratio increases progressively, thus suggesting an alteration in postsecretory insulin metabolism, possibly related to the reduction in abdominal fat. No changes in HbA1 have been noted.

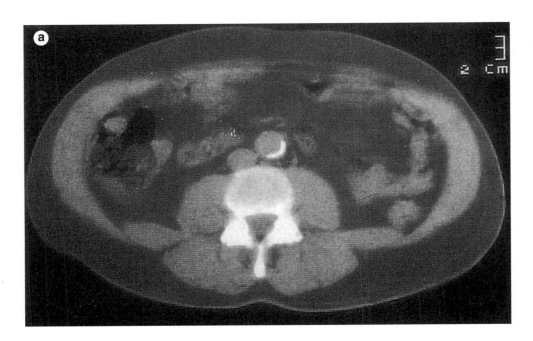

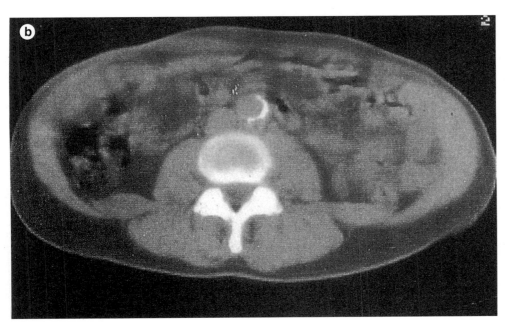

Fig. 2.30 Changes in subcutaneous and intra-abdominal fat after six months of GH replacement therapy. CT scan of the abdomen before (a) and after (b) treatment with GH demonstrates the predominant loss of 'central' as opposed to 'peripheral' fat (see Fig. 2.27). This is also reflected in a fall in waist:hip ratio and skin-fold thickness. By courtesy of Dr B-Å Bengtsson.

Lipid Metabolism

Slight increases in levels of low-density lipoprotein (LDL) and total cholesterol have been reported in adults with GH deficiency. Replacement with GH results in a significant reduction in levels of total cholesterol, LDL-cholesterol, and apolipoprotein B, with a rise in the level of high-density lipoprotein-cholesterol. Furthermore, replacement of GH causes substantial loss of body fat, predominantly from abdominal sites, probably through direct stimulation of lipolysis. This is accompanied by a significant fall in waist:hip ratio (see Fig. 2.30).

Protein Metabolism

GH has an important physiological role in the regulation of whole-body protein metabolism in adults. Recent placebo-controlled dynamic tracer studies using ^{13}C leucine have shown that GH stimulates protein synthesis directly (Fig. 2.33), in contrast to insulin which contributes to the regulation of protein metabolism by inhibiting proteolysis. The increase in protein synthesis is accompanied by a reduction in leucine oxidation.

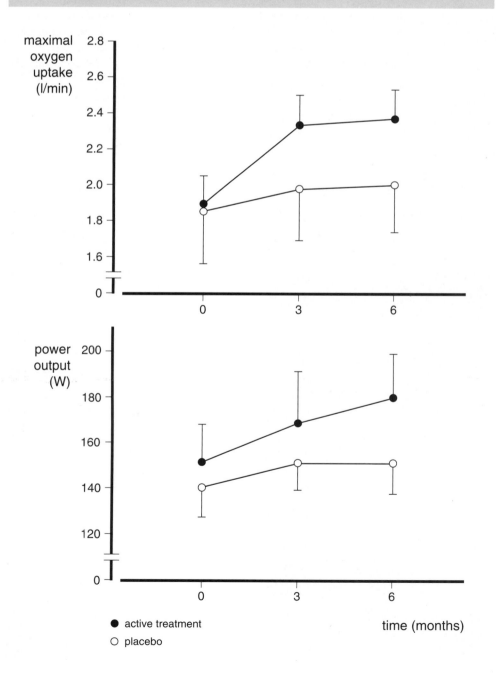

GH REPLACEMENT THERAPY AND EXERCISE PERFORMANCE

Fig. 2.31 *Effect of six months of GH replacement therapy on exercise performance.* Maximal oxygen uptake and maximal power output were significantly impaired in adults with GH deficiency but normalised following six months' replacement therapy with GH. Modified from Cuneo *et al.* (1992) with permission.

● active treatment
○ placebo

time (months)

PSYCHOLOGICAL EFFECTS

Detailed assessment of quality of life using several well-validated questionnaires that compare GH-deficient adults with matched controls has shown that GH-deficient patients perceive themselves as having much greater physical and psychological health problems: over one-third scored in the range that was consistent with psychiatric disturbance requiring therapy. Particular areas of concern were poor energy, emotional lability, low mood and social isolation. Following GH therapy in strictly placebo-controlled conditions, psychological wellbeing improved and returned to normal over a period of six months.

SIDE EFFECTS OF GROWTH HORMONE THERAPY

Arthralgias and muscle aches, likened to 'growing pains', are encountered by several patients after commencing GH therapy. Some patients develop symptoms of carpal tunnel syndrome, and ankle oedema and hypertension can also occur in the first weeks of therapy, but all disappear within a week or two after reduction in dose. Most, if not all, of these side effects can be avoided by initiating replacement therapy at a low dose and thereafter increasing the dose gradually.

GH REPLACEMENT THERAPY AND THE RENIN–ANGIOTENSIN SYSTEM

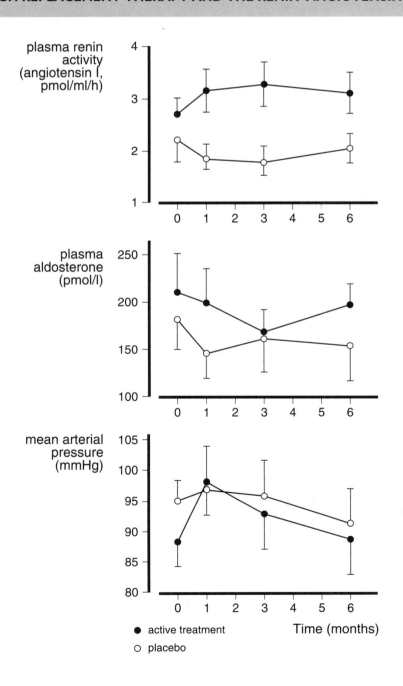

Fig. 2.32 Effects of six months of GH replacement therapy on some components of the renin–angiotensin system. There was a significant rise in plasma renin activity but no significant change in either mean arterial pressure or plasma aldosterone concentration. Modified from Cuneo et al. (1991c) with permission.

● active treatment
○ placebo

EFFECTS OF GH REPLACEMENT THERAPY ON PROTEIN METABOLISM

	placebo group (n=9)		treament group (n=9)	
	baseline	2 months post-treatment	baseline	2 months post-treatment
age (years)	44.4 ± 2.9		48.8 ± 1.4	
lean body mass (kg)	46.3 ± 1.9	47.8 ± 2.3	54.9 ± 5.1	58.6 ± 5.4*
fasting insulin (mu/l)	10.2 ± 1.4	12.4 ± 1.1	11.8 ± 3.7	20.3 ± 6.0*
IGF-I (nmol/l)	15.5 ± 1.4	13.7 ± 1.3	16.9 ± 2.3	45.9 ± 4.5**
steady-state plasma leucine concentration (μmol/l)	133 ± 4	132 ± 4	129 ± 4	135 ± 6
leucine Ra (μmol/min/kg body weight)	1.44 ± 0.09	1.41 ± 0.08	1.40 ± 0.08	1.65 ± 0.08**
leucine oxidation rate (μmol/min/kg body weight)	0.18 ± 0.01	0.18 ± 0.01	0.24 ± 0.02	0.18 ± 0.01*
nonoxidative leucine Rd (μmol/min/kg body weight)	1.25 ± 0.08	1.22 ± 0.07	1.16 ± 0.07	1.46 ± 0.08**

data are mean ± SEM. Significant difference baseline *$P<0.02$; **$P<0.01$

Fig. 2.33 Effects of two months of GH replacement therapy on indices of protein metabolism in adults with GH deficiency. No change in protein breakdown occurred, but there was a significant increase in protein synthesis and reduction in amino-acid oxidation, resulting in the increase in lean body mass. Modified from Russell-Jones et al. (1993) with permission.

3

Acromegaly

John A H Wass, MD, FRCP

Acromegaly is the clinical condition which results from prolonged, excessive circulating levels of growth hormone (GH) in adults (Fig. 3.1). The rare clinical counterpart of acromegaly, which occurs in younger patients before epiphyseal fusion, is called pituitary gigantism (Fig. 3.2).

Acromegaly was first described in 1886 by Pierre Marie, who noted 'a striking noncongenital hypertrophy of the extremities' including the face, hands and feet. In 1891 Minkowski noted that this hypertrophy was always accompanied by an enlarged pituitary, which Tamburine in 1894 recognised as a pituitary adenoma. However, Harvey Cushing, in 1909, was the first to use the word 'hypopituitarism' to describe the condition. This was confirmed in 1922 by Evans, who demonstrated that the parenteral injection of extracts of the anterior lobe of the pituitary gland causes true gigantism in rats, whose epiphyses never fuse, and acromegalic-like features in dogs, whose epiphyses do.

AETIOLOGY

Benign pituitary tumours are by far the most common cause of acromegaly; however, very rarely, pituitary carcinomas may be responsible. Pituitary tumours may be associated with other endocrine adenomas (e.g. multiple endocrine neoplasia Type I) which most commonly involve the parathyroid glands, resulting in hypercalcaemia.

Carcinoid tumours, usually of the pancreas or lung, may rarely be the cause of acromegaly due to ectopic secretion of hypothalamic growth hormone releasing hormone (GHRH). However, instead of a pituitary tumour, these patients have somatotroph hyperplasia in the pituitary, which nevertheless may enlarge the fossa.

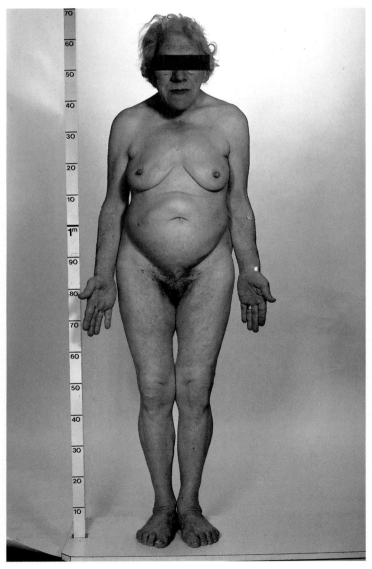

Fig. 3.1 A female patient with acromegaly. The facial features have become coarse with progression of the disease.

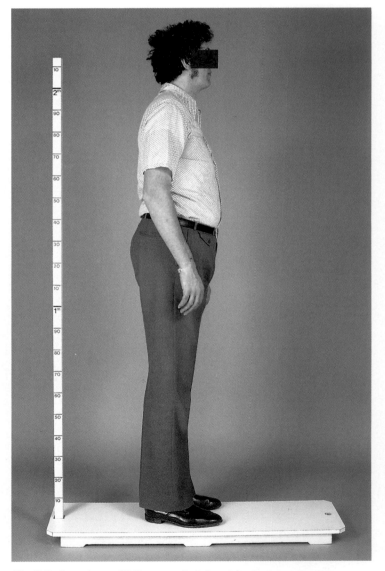

Fig. 3.2 A patient of 2.3 metres height with pituitary gigantism. Gigantism is the rare, clinical counterpart of acromegaly and occurs in the young before epiphyseal fusion has taken place.

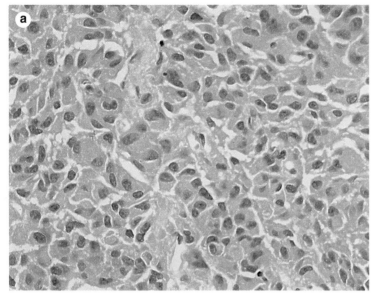

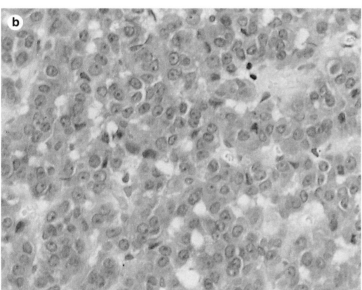

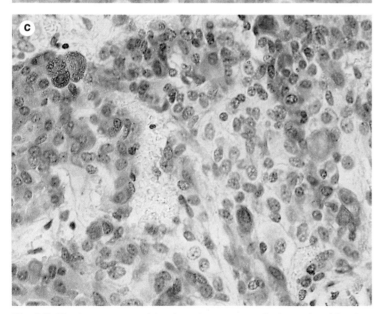

Fig. 3.3 Pituitary tumour histology in acromegaly. In section (a), using haematoxylin and eosin (H and E) stain, the eosinophils contain cytoplasmic red granules. The illustration shows a tumour consisting entirely of such cells. In section (b), using periodic acid–Schiff and orange G (PAS–OG) stain, the acidophils stain yellow or orange and the nuclei stain black. This stain is less subjective than H and E. Section (c), an immunostain for GH in a GH secreting tumour, shows somatotrophs stained brown.

HISTOPATHOLOGY OF ACROMEGALY-ASSOCIATED PITUITARY TUMOURS

Microadenomas are rare and the tumours associated with acromegaly are more commonly intrasellar or extrasellar macroadenomas. While these tumours are usually acidophilic on conventional haematoxylin and eosin histological staining (Fig. 3.3), acromegaly can also result from chromophobe adenomas. The secretion from pituitary adenomas usually consists of GH alone, but the tumour may also be of mixed cell types and thirty per cent of acromegalic patients are also hyperprolactinaemic. Very occasionally GH and prolactin may originate from the same cell.

Growth hormone cell adenomas occur in both sparsely and densely granulated forms. The latter look very similar to normal somatotrophs and the cells stain with acid dyes, representing the eosinophil adenoma in the conventional classification. By contrast, the sparsely granulated somatotroph adenoma represents the chromophobe adenoma. Clinically, the sparsely granulated somatotroph adenomas tend to be more aggressive, the cells show less differentiation and the tumour is more invasive.

AETIOLOGY OF PITUITARY TUMOURS

In some patients with acromegaly, as described previously, somatotroph hyperplasia may occur because of excessive secretion of GHRH from a hypothalamic hamartoma (a tumour-like lesion, usually present at birth, which ceases to grow when general body growth ceases), hypothalamic gangliocytoma (a tumour of mature gangliocytes), or carcinoid tumour of the lung or pancreas. However, over ninety-nine per cent of patients have a primary pituitary tumour. Genetic factors may play a role in some tumours, such as in multiple endocrine neoplasia (MEN) syndrome type 1, where GH-secreting adenomas may constitute one of the neoplastic components.

Many receptors alter the level of intracellular cyclic nucleotides. Such receptors do not interact directly with the cyclase enzymes but work through an intermediate protein which binds guanosine 5'-triphosphate (GTP), called a GTP-binding protein, or more simply, a G-protein. Recently, a subset of GH-secreting human pituitary tumours have been discovered, which carry somatic mutations of G-protein α-chains that inhibit GTPase activity in somatotroph cells. The resulting activation of adenylate cyclase within GH-secreting adenoma cells bypasses the normal requirement of the cell to be activated by GHRH and thus, it is autonomous. Such an oncogenic mutation may promote tumour growth by producing an autonomous action of proteins that normally transmit the proliferative signals initiated by extracellular factors.

DIAGNOSIS

Acromegaly is a disease of the whole organism in which everything but the central nervous system enlarges. Although the diagnosis is often made coincidentally, the patient usually presents complaining of a change in appearance of the face, hands or whole body, headaches, sweating, goitre or symptoms related to renal stones. Early diagnosis is important but this depends on a high index of suspicion. It often helps to look at old photographs, but a delay in diagnosis of many years may occur (Fig. 3.4). The condition is most frequently diagnosed in the third decade but may be found from the teenage years up until the eighth decade.

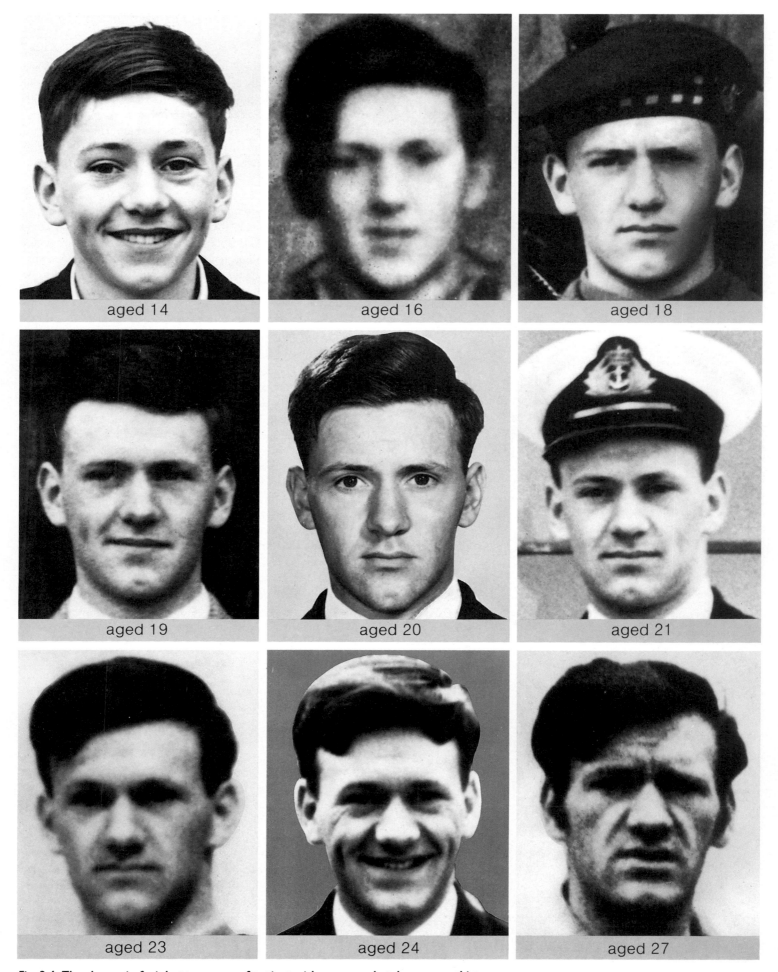

aged 14   aged 16   aged 18

aged 19   aged 20   aged 21

aged 23   aged 24   aged 27

Fig. 3.4 The change in facial appearance of patient with acromegaly taken over a thirteen year period. The development of an acromegalic appearance is seen, with enlargement of the supraorbital ridges and nose, thickening of the lips and generalised coarsening of the features. From Belchetz (1984), by courtesy of Chapman and Hall Ltd.

CLINICAL FEATURES

The clinical features of acromegaly (Fig. 3.5) result from (i) over-secretion of GH, which has both clinical and metabolic sequelae, and (ii) effects of the pituitary tumour which are both local and endocrine. Several groups have noted that young patients with acromegaly tend to present with larger tumours, which appear to behave more aggressively, than those that present in patients over the age of fifty years. Pituitary giants often have features of acromegaly as well as tall stature, especially when they present after the age of sixteen or seventeen years (see Fig. 3.2).

CLINICAL EFFECTS OF GROWTH HORMONE OVERSECRETION

The typical facial appearance of an acromegalic patient shows coarsening of the features with enlargement of the supraorbital ridges, a broad nose and also thickening of the soft tissues (Fig. 3.6). Sweating is excessive, sebaceous activity increases, papillomas and seborrhoeic warts occur; acne and hirsutism may also be present in women. Lips thicken and prognathism occurs, together with increased dental separation and macroglossia (Fig. 3.7). Using skull radiography, prognathism (where there is loss of angle of the mandible) can be seen, as well as a thickened skull vault, enlargement of the sinuses and,

CLINICAL FEATURES OF ACROMEGALY	
coarse facial features	headaches
enlargement of supraorbital ridges	'spade-like' hands
soft tissue thickening e.g. lips	excessive sweating
separation of teeth	kyphosis
prognathism	hypertension
macroglossia	goitre
	impaired glucose tolerance

Fig. 3.5 The clinical features of acromegaly.

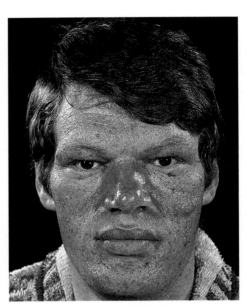

Fig. 3.6 The characteristic facial features of a male acromegalic patient.

Fig. 3.7 Prognathism (a) and macroglossia (b) in acromegaly. These are shown with a tongue of normal size (c) for comparison.

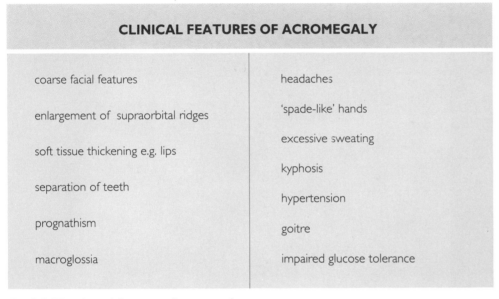

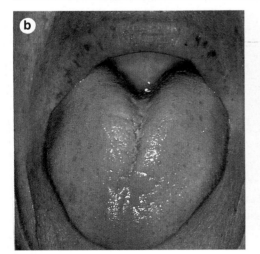

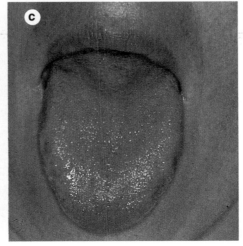

in more than ninety-five per cent of patients, an abnormal and enlarged pituitary fossa (Fig. 3.8).

The hands also become enlarged in acromegaly and the fingers look short and fat (Fig. 3.9). Heel pad and skin thickness are increased, and the latter is clearly visible on the dorsum of the hand (Fig. 3.10). Carpal tunnel syndrome often occurs due to the compression of the median nerve by soft tissue and bony overgrowth around the median

nerve (see Fig 3.9). Kyphosis may be present in long-standing acromegaly or pituitary gigantism and lumbar spondylosis is common. Myopathy is frequent and, paradoxically, these patients are weak despite their muscular appearance.

Radiographs of the hands show characteristic 'tufting' of the terminal phalanges. This may occur normally in heavy manual labourers, but the increase in the joint spaces due to the cartilaginous

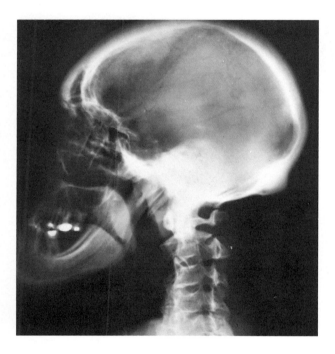

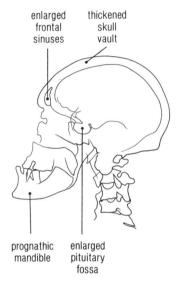

Fig. 3.8 Skull radiograph of an acromegalic patient. The enlarged pituitary fossa and sinuses, thickened skull vault and prognathism with loss of angle of the mandible can be seen.

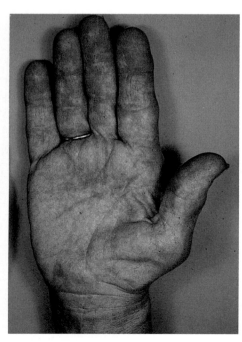

Fig. 3.9 The enlarged hand of an acromegalic patient. The hand is big and the fingers appear short because they are broad. There is thenar wasting because of long-standing compression of the median nerve in the carpal tunnel.

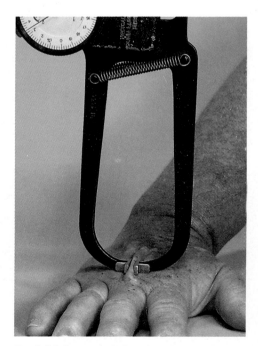

Fig. 3.10 Increased skin thickness can be measured on the dorsum of the hand in acromegaly with skin fold calipers.

overgrowth, typical of acromegaly, does not (Fig. 3.11). Degenerative arthropathy occurs prematurely, particularly in the spine and other weight-bearing joints such as the hips and knees. The joints enlarge due to synovial overgrowth and cartilaginous thickening. The lumbar spine may also show characteristic changes with scalloping of the posterior vertebral margins and anterior new bone formation (Fig. 3.12).

Acromegalic patients may also have cardiomegaly related either to coronary artery disease, the incidence of which is increased in acromegaly, or to hypertension which occurs in thirty-five per cent of acromegalic patients. In the absence of these, cardiomegaly may be related to a primary cardiomyopathy. Hypertension is usually 'essential' but may be caused by a coexistent phaeochromocytoma or Conn's tumour.

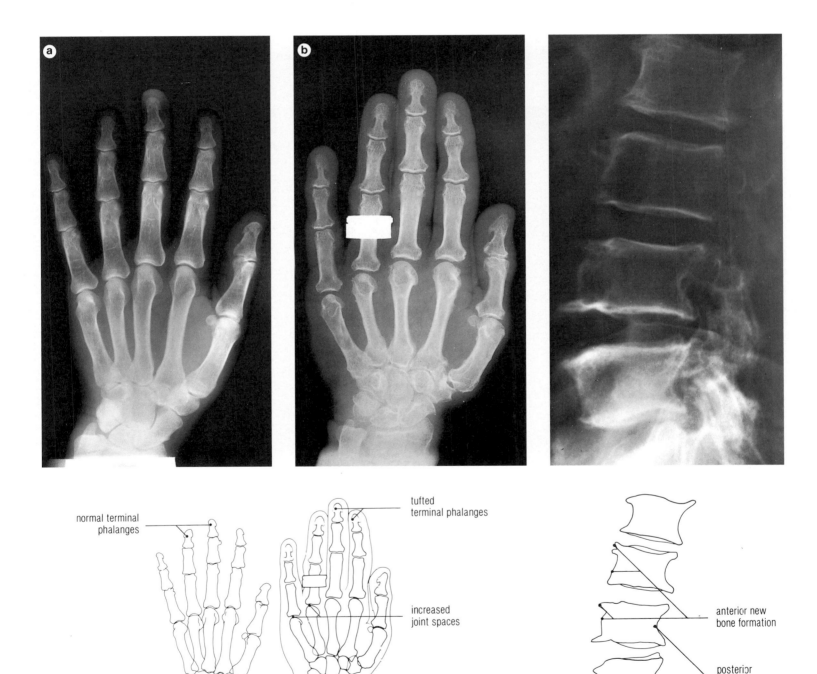

Fig. 3.11 Comparison of radiographs of (a) a normal and (b) an acromegalic hand. The characteristic tufting of the terminal phalanges in the acromegalic patient is shown together with an increase in joint space due to cartilaginous overgrowth.

Fig. 3.12 Radiographic appearance of the lumbar spine in acromegaly. Scalloping of the posterior margin of the vertebrae and anterior new bone formation are present.

Diabetes mellitus occurs in approximately twenty per cent of patients and is secondary to insulin resistance as a consequence of raised GH levels. Hypercalcaemia occurs in five to ten per cent of patients usually resulting from parathyroid adenomas or hyperplasia (MEN type 1). There is also a five per cent increased incidence of urinary calculi resulting from hypercalciuria, even in the absence of hypercalcaemia. Hypercalciuria occurs in eighty per cent of acromegalic patients because GH is facultative in the synthesis of vitamin D and levels of 1,25-dihydroxycholecalciferol are raised.

CLINICAL EFFECTS OF PITUITARY TUMOURS

Patients may present with headaches due to dural stretching. The pituitary fossa is enlarged in over ninety-five per cent of cases (Fig. 3.13).

Upward extension of the pituitary tumour, when present, may cause a characteristic bitemporal field defect best found with the Goldmann perimeter. The enlarged supraorbital ridges may produce technical problems with visual field plotting; this is therefore best performed by tilting the head backwards by twenty degrees. Lateral extension of the tumour may cause third, fourth and sixth cranial nerve palsies and, more rarely, temporal lobe epilepsy. Erosion into the sphenoid sinus may be associated with cerebrospinal fluid (CSF) rhinorrhoea.

Hyperprolactinaemia is common; females may present with amenorrhoea and galactorrhoea or infertility and males with low libido and impotence. Hyperprolactinaemia is more commonly due to the coexistent production of prolactin by the tumour than to pituitary stalk compression by it. Stalk compression can lead to functional disconnection of the normal pituitary prolactin-secreting cells from the dopaminergic prolactin-inhibiting influence of the hypothalamus, this is then called a 'pseudoprolactinoma'. Hypopituitarism also occurs and this most frequently affects gonadotrophin production. Later in the development of the disease, hypothyroidism and adrenocortical insuffiency may occur due to decreased thyroid stimulating hormone (TSH) and adrenocorticotrophic hormone (ACTH) reserves.

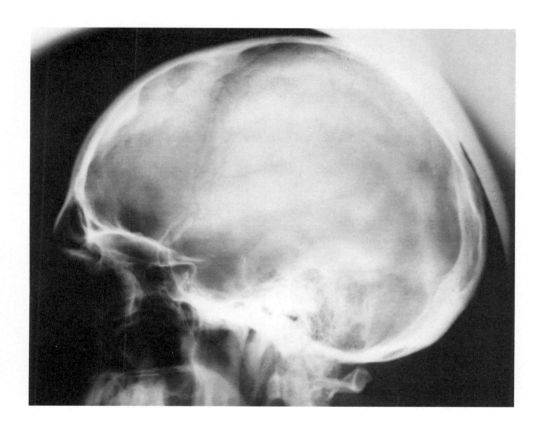

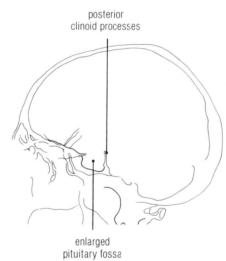

Fig. 3.13 The skull radiograph of an acromegalic patient with an enlarged pituitary fossa and thinning of the posterior clinoid processes. The expansion of the pituitary fossa occurs in over 95 per cent of patients with this disease and is best seen on the lateral view.

posterior clinoid processes

enlarged pituitary fossa

Fig. 3.14 The relationship between serum IGF-1 and serum GH levels in acromegaly. The natural logarithm of serum GH concentration (mu/l) is plotted against the concentration of serum IGF-1 (u/ml).

IGF-I AND GH LEVELS IN ACROMEGALY

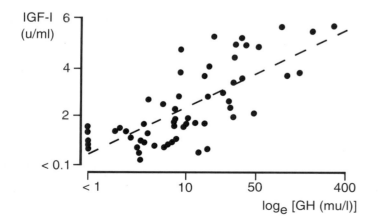

Hypopituitarism may be due to pressure on the stalk by the tumour but is more often due to pressure of the tumour on normal pituitary tissue in the fossa. Diabetes insipidus, resulting from upward extension of the tumour into the hypothalamus is exceedingly rare.

GROWTH HORMONE SECRETION IN ACROMEGALY

Basal GH levels are elevated and fluctuate widely but do not correlate well with any clinical manifestation of the disease. GH stimulates the production of insulin-like growth factor I (IGF-I) and levels of IGF-I are often, though not invariably, elevated in acromegaly (Fig. 3.14). In normal subjects, GH levels are mostly undetectable in the serum, apart from intermittent pulses of secretion, lasting approximately ninety minutes, which occur five or six times during the day and more frequently at night. This pulsatile nature of GH secretion in normal subjects means that it may not be possible to distinguish between normal and some acromegalic patients using basal GH concentrations; dynamic tests are therefore necessary.

A rise in circulating glucose normally causes a suppression of GH to below 1mu/l (0.5ng/ml) but this is not the case in acromegaly (Fig. 3.15). Usually, only a slight or no fall in serum GH occurs in acromegaly and there may even be a paradoxical rise. This phenomenon is not specific to acromegaly and may also occur in severe hepatic or renal disease, in anorexia nervosa, in Laron's syndrome and in patients on heroin or L-dopa. Dopamine and related drugs cause a rise in serum GH levels in normal subjects. In 1972 L-dopa was first found to cause a paradoxical suppression of GH in many patients with acromegaly; bromocriptine, a long-acting dopamine agonist, also has this property. These effects are antagonised by haloperidol, pimozide and metoclopramide which are specific dopamine antagonists. The hypothalamic hormone, somatostatin, also decreases GH secretion in acromegaly. Unfortunately, its short half-life means that its effects wear off after a few minutes. Recently, long-acting analogues of somatostatin (e.g. octreotide) have become available for use in the treatment of acromegaly.

Thyrotrophin releasing hormone (TRH) and gonadotrophin releasing hormone (GnRH) may also cause GH secretion in many acromegalic patients, twenty and thirty per cent respectively, but not in normal subjects.

PROGNOSIS AND TREATMENT

Mortality is approximately doubled in acromegaly compared with the normal population (Fig. 3.16). The main reason for this is the presence of cardiovascular and cerebrovascular disease secondary to hypertension and diabetes mellitus. Respiratory disease also occurs

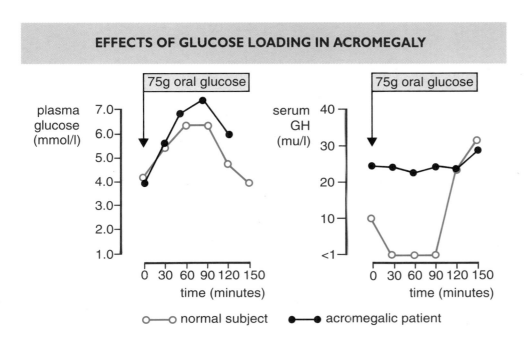

Fig. 3.15 The effects of a 75g glucose load on blood glucose and GH levels in a normal subject and an acromegalic patient. GH levels are acutely suppressed in normal subjects following a glucose load, whereas in acromegaly there is either no suppression or occasionally there is even a paradoxical rise. Carbohydrate tolerance is normal in both of the subjects shown.

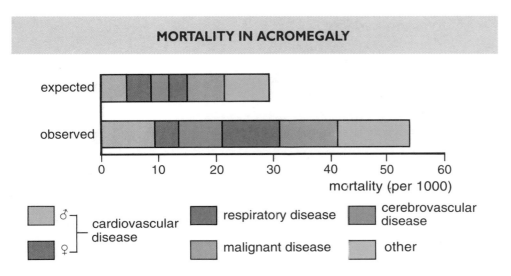

Fig. 3.16 Mortality in acromegaly. It can be seen that the observed mortality compared to that expected for normal patients is approximately double. Significant differences were seen in cardiovascular disease in men, and in cerebrovascular and respiratory disease (after Wright et al., 1970).

with increased frequency. Early treatment is therefore recommended.

Aims of treatment should be the relief of symptoms, the reversal of the somatic changes occurring with acromegaly, together with reversal of the associated metabolic abnormalities. The ideal treatment should cause the minimum disturbance to the patient with no side effects, particularly that of hypopituitarism. Early treatment avoids the subsequent complications of diabetes mellitus, enlargement of the tumour, hypopituitarism, osteoarthritis and cardiomyopathy.

Regrettably, there is no agreed definition of 'cured' acromegaly. Serum GH is less than 1mu/l (0.5ng/ml) in the circulation of normal subjects, except during stress or spontaneous brief pulses which occur during the day. In assessing activity, some authors use basal serum GH levels at 0900h, whilst others measure the mean GH concentration during a glucose tolerance test. It seems most logical to take several measurements during a normal day to assess the average serum GH level to which the patient's tissues are exposed as an indicator of the response to treatment. The treatments available fall into three groups (Fig. 3.17): (i) surgery, via the transsphenoidal or transfrontal route; (ii) radiotherapy using a linear accelerator, a cobalt source or a proton beam, and (iii) medical therapy using a long-acting somatostatin analogue (e.g. octreotide) or a dopamine agonist (e.g. bromocriptine).

SURGERY

Surgery is the primary treatment of acromegaly. It most rapidly accomplishes a reduction in GH levels. The transsphenoidal route is mostly used and was the route first used by Harvey Cushing (Fig. 3.18). Small, medium-sized and some large tumours, with suprasellar extensions of up to 1cm, can be removed by this route. Removal of the latter can improve field defects, if present for a short period, once

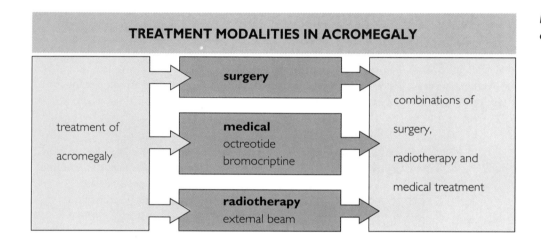

Fig. 3.17 *Possible treatment modalities in acromegaly.*

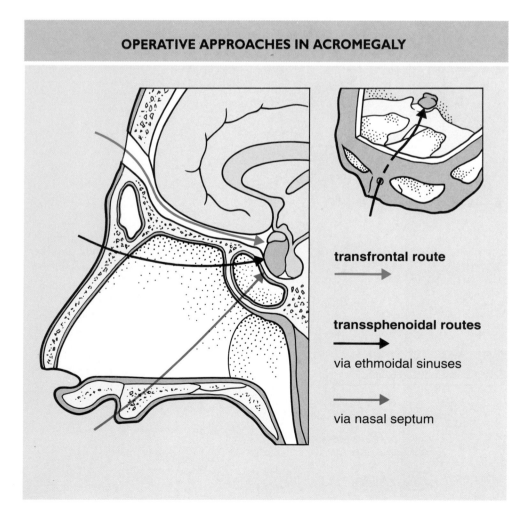

Fig. 3.18 *Operative approaches in acromegaly:* transfrontal, transethmoidal and transsphenoidal.

pressure on the optic chiasm is released. Cure by the transsphenoidal route is most often achieved with small tumours of under 1cm in diameter. Cure is less frequent, and postoperative hypopituitarism more frequent, with larger tumours, in part because the tumours have a tendency to infiltrate, locally, the bone and the dura (Fig. 3.19). A significant proportion of tumours recur after surgery so in any patient with GH levels that are detectable postoperatively, radiotherapy should be considered. Side effects of transsphenoidal surgery include operative bleeding, meningitis, pulmonary embolism, postoperative diabetes insipidus, hypopituitarism and local nasal complications.

The transethmoidal approach to the sphenoid sinus is rarely used nowadays. Transfrontal surgery is necessary for very large extrasellar extensions, and this is most often seen in young acromegalics presenting with rapidly growing tumours. Cure of acromegaly using this operative approach is virtually unknown due to the difficulty in clearing the pituitary fossa of tumourous tissue, and postoperative radiotherapy is necessary. Field defects may be relieved, but the morbidity of this operative approach is higher as it involves craniotomy, frontal lobe retraction and section of an olfactory nerve.

RADIOTHERAPY

Radiotherapy is an effective treatment for acromegaly but its effects are slow in onset. Although the greatest fall occurs in the first year after treatment, GH levels, if still raised, continue to fall for at least fifteen years. A great deal of skill and careful planning is necessary to ensure success without complications. Best results occur using a linear accelerator and a three field technique, which allows the largest dose of radiation to be delivered safely to the tumour; this is not the case using the simpler two field, parallel opposed field technique. Pretreatment high resolution computed tomography (CT) (Fig. 3.20) is necessary to completely delineate the upper, lower and lateral margins of the tumour. A dose of 4,500cGy should be delivered over

TRANSSPHENOIDAL SURGERY IN ACROMEGALY

	number of patients	success rate (GH < 20mu/l)	incidence of hypopituitarism
microadenomas	17	82%	0%
diffuse adenomas	38	68%	23%
invasive adenomas	25	54%	24%
total	80	66%	19%

Fig. 3.19 The improvement of GH levels and the incidence of hypopituitarism following transsphenoidal surgery for acromegaly. For all types of pituitary tumours, transsphenoidal surgery leads to an improvement in GH levels in 66 per cent of patients. The incidence of hypopituitarism following transsphenoidal surgery is lowest in microadenomas. Redrawn from Laws *et al.* (1979), by courtesy of the American Association of Neurological Surgeons.

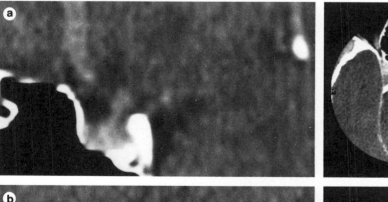

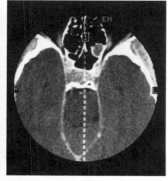

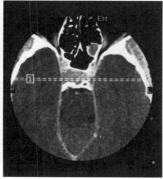

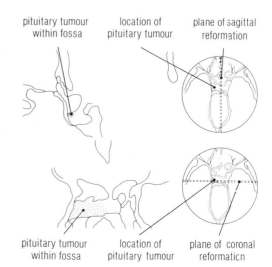

Fig. 3.20 Pituitary tumour in acromegaly. High resolution post-contrast CT scans: (a) lateral and (b) frontal projections. This technique is used to show the precise location of a pituitary tumour.

pituitary tumour within fossa   location of pituitary tumour   plane of sagittal reformation

pituitary tumour within fossa   location of pituitary tumour   plane of coronal reformation

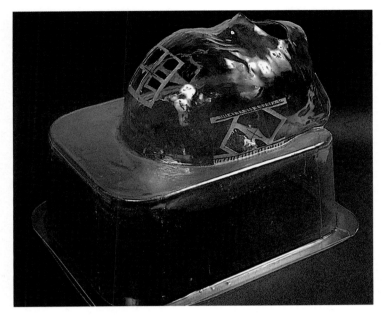

Fig. 3.21 *An individual head mask used to position the patient accurately during radiotherapy.* Three fields are used and the daily dose of radiation should not exceed 180cGy.

twenty-six treatment days using five fractions per week, each fraction consisting of no more than 180cGy. Using this technique no radiation-induced neurological damage has been recorded by the author. During treatment, an individual head mask is used to encompass and immobilise the whole of the patient's head; this improves accuracy and safety (Fig. 3.21).

With external pituitary irradiation using a linear accelerator, a mean fall in GH levels of seventy-seven per cent after five years has been obtained (Fig 3.22), and, at the end of ten years, eighty-one per cent of patients have serum GH concentrations of less than 20mu/l (10ng/ml). The effect is more rapid if the initiating serum GH level prior to radiotherapy is lower. Thus, if GH levels are greater than 50mu/l (25ng/ml) the time taken for there to be a fall of the average serum GH to less than 5mu/l (2.5ng/ml) is longer: six years versus four years if pretreatment serum GH is below 50mu/l. Recurrence of tumour growth is very rare after radiotherapy – less than one per cent. Hypopituitarism occurs after external pituitary irradiation in approximately ten per cent of patients, and may develop gradually, becoming apparent some years after treatment. Thus, it is imperative to measure pituitary function regularly after the administration of pituitary irradiation.

RADIOTHERAPY IN ACROMEGALY

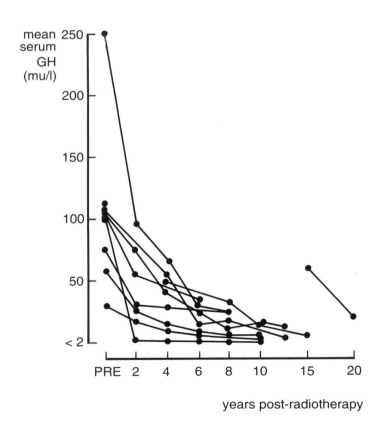

SOMATOSTATIN AND OCTREOTIDE

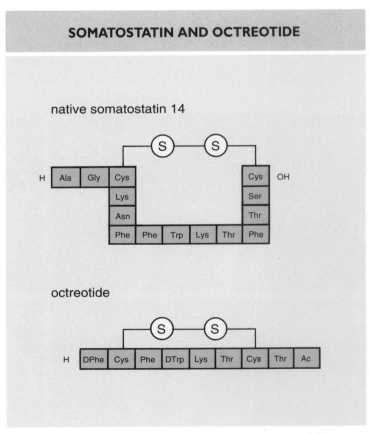

Fig. 3.22 *Growth hormone levels after radiotherapy in patients with acromegaly.*

Fig. 3.23 *Comparison of the structures of native somatostatin and the long-acting somatostatin analogue octreotide.*

SOMATOSTATIN, OCTREOTIDE AND GH SECRETION

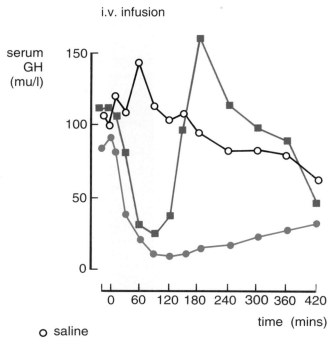

Fig. 3.24 Comparison of the effects of an intravenous infusion of octreotide, native somatostatin and saline on serum GH secretion in an acromegalic patient.

MEDICAL THERAPY

Medical treatment of acromegaly is given either using octreotide, a synthetic long-acting analogue of somatostatin (Fig. 3.23), or the dopamine agonist bromocriptine.

Natural somatostatin, present in the hypothalamus, gastrointestinal tract and pancreas, suppresses GH and insulin release for equal, brief periods. Octreotide has a longer duration of action on GH secretion than native somatostatin (Fig. 3.24) but insulin and glucagon suppression is of shorter duration than that of GH. In the majority of acromegalics, if octreotide is administered subcutaneously in doses of 300–600µg per day (100–200µg eight hourly), GH levels are suppressed (Fig. 3.25) such that fifty-five per cent of patients have average levels below 10mu/l, compared to fourteen per cent with bromocriptine. In the same patients octreotide proves more effective than bromocriptine (Fig. 3.26) and, unlike bromocriptine, causes no suppression of prolactin secretion except in some rare, mixed secretory mammosomatotroph tumours. Usually, carbohydrate tolerance does not worsen with octreotide administration, despite transient insulin suppression. Symptomatic relief is good and headaches may be dramatically reduced. Fifty per cent of tumours shrink in size (Fig. 3.27) but this is not as great in volume, nor as rapid, as the effect of

SERUM GH LEVELS AND OCTREOTIDE THERAPY

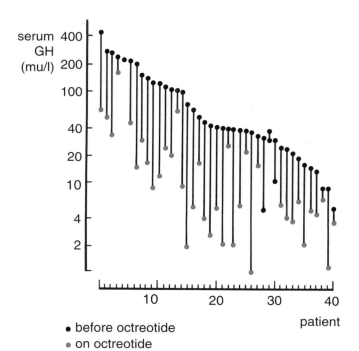

Fig. 3.25 Reduction in mean serum GH levels in acromegalic patients receiving long-term octreotide therapy in doses of 150–600µg per day.

BROMOCRIPTINE VERSUS OCTREOTIDE

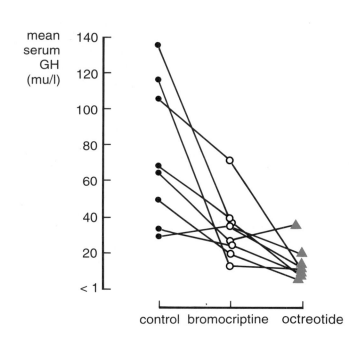

Fig. 3.26 Comparison of the effects of octreotide and bromocriptine on serum GH levels in the same acromegalics.

bromocriptine in prolactinoma. Side effects do occur with octreotide (Fig. 3.28). Initial diarrhoea and abdominal pain usually settle with time. Gallstones have been found with increased frequency in patients on octreotide, due to a combination of factors including gallbladder stasis, induced by octreotide, as well as biliary saturation with cholesterol. The gallstones are usually without clinical effects. Some patients have been found to have gastritis, histologically, but without symptoms.

In normal subjects, dopamine agonists raise GH levels but, paradoxically, lower them in acromegalics (Fig. 3.29). Bromocriptine, a dopamine agonist, suppresses GH levels in about seventy per cent of acramegalics, but only rarely are GH levels reduced to normal. Doses of 10–60mg per day, in four divided doses, are used.

In all patients treated with bromocriptine, prolactin levels fall to normal. Pituitary tumour size decreases in about fifty per cent of cases, particularly those with mixed GH and prolactin-secreting tumours in whom, because of this effect, bromocriptine should probably be used first. Although, in most patients, the response of the GH level to octreotide is better than to bromocriptine, there are occasional acromegalic patients who respond better to bromocriptine. Bromocriptine may be administered orally, but side effects include postural hypotension, nausea and vomiting. These may be avoided by starting with a low dose (e.g. 1.25mg per day), increasing the dosage slowly (i.e. every three days) and advising patients to take the drug during meals.

Choice of Different Treatments in Acromegaly
Acromegalics have either mixed GH and prolactin secreting tumours (thirty-five per cent) or pituitary tumours that secrete GH alone. Clinical experience suggests that there is a spectrum of disease ranging from young patients, who often have very large, aggressively behaving tumours associated with very high levels of GH, to older patients who have much smaller tumours with slower progression and lower levels of GH. Often all the available modalities of treatment are needed in a single patient (Fig. 3.30), particularly with aggressive tumours.

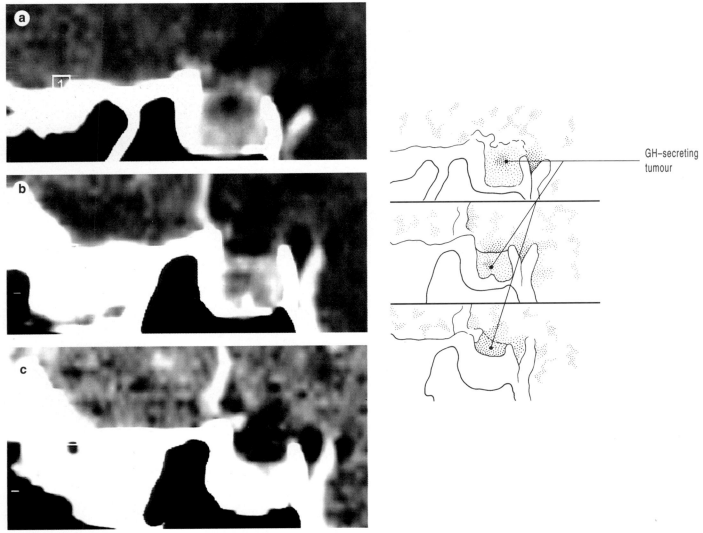

GH–secreting tumour

Fig. 3.27 Effect of octreotide on tumour size in an acromegalic patient with a pure GH-secreting tumour. CT scan (a) was taken at the commencement of treatment, (b) and (c) at 24 and 43 weeks respectively. No other treatment was given.

It is clear that surgery results in a rapid fall in GH levels but, equally, it is not always successful or permanent, particularly in patients with large tumours in whom there is a significant incidence of surgically-induced hypopituitarism and occasional recurrence. In most cases, surgery may be performed via the transsphenoidal route.

Pretreatment of pituitary tumours may cause tumour shrinkage such that the tumour is more readily excised surgically; certainly, surgical results are better with smaller tumours, both in terms of cure rate and the incidence of hypopituitarism.

If surgery is not curative, then external radiotherapy is advised and will eventually be effective in the majority of cases, though it may take several years to be fully effective. In the meantime, either octreotide or bromocriptine can be given to keep GH levels as near normal as possible. These should be regularly withdrawn, each year, to assess the effects of pituitary irradiation on GH secretion. At these times the residual pituitary function should also be assessed (see Chapter 2).

CONCLUSIONS

Acromegaly is an insidious disease which requires a high degree of suspicion on the part of the clinician for early diagnosis to be made. This is important because of the greater mortality associated with this condition which is twice that of normal.

No treatment currently available satisfies all the requirements of an ideal therapy. Surgery, if successful, rapidly reduces GH levels to normal, but may not eradicate circulating GH and may cause hypo-pituitarism, particularly with large tumours. Radiotherapy is successful but takes time to act and causes hypopituitarism in a proportion of cases. Medical treatment with octreotide or bromocriptine is only rarely used alone and, although it improves symptoms, it does not always reduce GH levels to normal. Its main use is as an adjunct to ablative treatment of the pituitary tumour. Often, after careful judge-ment, all three types of treatment may be needed to reduce GH levels to normal.

SIDE EFFECTS OF OCTREOTIDE

local	stinging
biochemical	antibody formation
gastroenterological	
short term:	diarrhoea
	abdominal pain
long term:	gallstones
	gastritis
endocrinological	rarely, worsening of carbohydrate tolerance
	hypoglycaemia
	pituitary tumour enlargement

Fig. 3.28 Side effects of octreotide. Stinging occuring at the site of the injection is transient and may be obviated by warming the solution prior to injection. Gallstones and gastritis are usually without clinical effects.

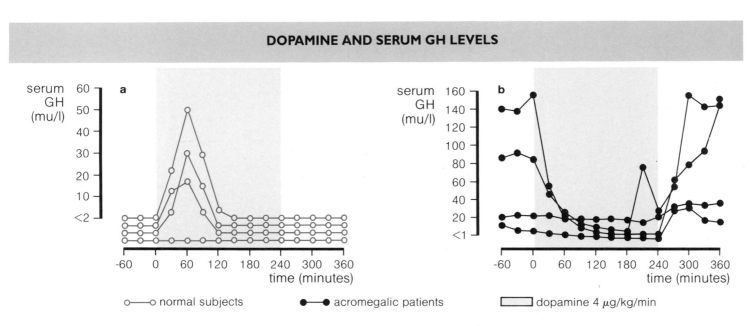

DOPAMINE AND SERUM GH LEVELS

o——o normal subjects   ●——● acromegalic patients   ▭ dopamine 4 μg/kg/min

Fig. 3.29 The effects of intravenous dopamine on serum GH levels. The contrasting responses of (a) normal subjects and (b) acromegalic patients are shown.

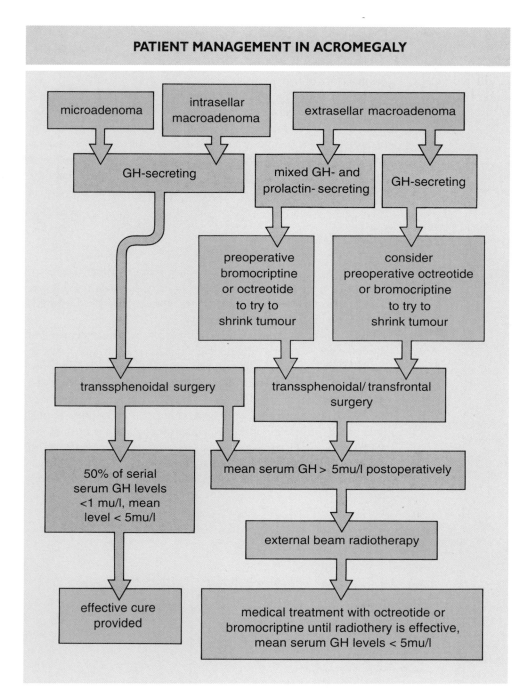

PATIENT MANAGEMENT IN ACROMEGALY

microadenoma

intrasellar macroadenoma

extrasellar macroadenoma

GH-secreting

mixed GH- and prolactin- secreting

GH-secreting

preoperative bromocriptine or octreotide to try to shrink tumour

consider preoperative octreotide or bromocriptine to try to shrink tumour

transsphenoidal surgery

transsphenoidal/ transfrontal surgery

50% of serial serum GH levels <1 mu/l, mean level < 5mu/l

mean serum GH > 5mu/l postoperatively

external beam radiotherapy

effective cure provided

medical treatment with octreotide or bromocriptine until radiothery is effective, mean serum GH levels < 5mu/l

Fig. 3.30 *The place of various treatment modalities in the management of an individual acromegalic patient.*

4

Hyperprolactinaemia

Michael O Thorner, MB BS, DSc, FRCP

PROLACTIN SECRETION

Prolactin is secreted by the lactotroph cells of the anterior pituitary. The control of its secretion, like that of other anterior pituitary hormones, is regulated by the hypothalamus. Unlike the other anterior pituitary hormones, however, the hypothalamic influence is of tonic inhibition (Fig. 4.1).

The hypothalamus secretes two hypothalamic factors to control prolactin secretion: a prolactin-releasing factor (PRF) and a prolactin release-inhibiting factor (PIF). The latter is almost certainly the catecholamine dopamine, although the possibility of the existence of noncatecholamine PIFs cannot be excluded. Additionally, γ-aminobutyric acid (GABA) may play a role as an inhibitor, and there may well also be one or more PIF peptides. The nature of PRF

is unclear, although it is known that thyrotrophin-releasing hormone (TRH) can act as a PRF. Other candidates that may be involved in the release of prolactin include vasoactive intestinal peptide (VIP) and PHM-27, the latter being a peptide with structural homology to VIP (see Chapter 1).

CAUSES OF HYPERPROLACTINAEMIA

The causes of hyperprolactinaemia may be considered, in a simplified fashion, as resulting from four basic abnormalities of prolactin secretion (Fig. 4.2). In some patients, however, it is not possible to elucidate the cause of hyperprolactinaemia.

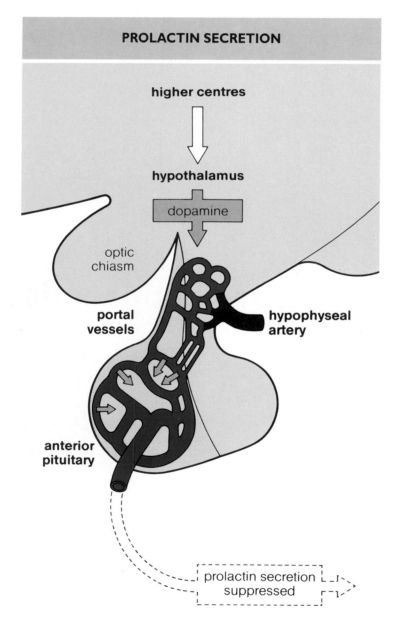

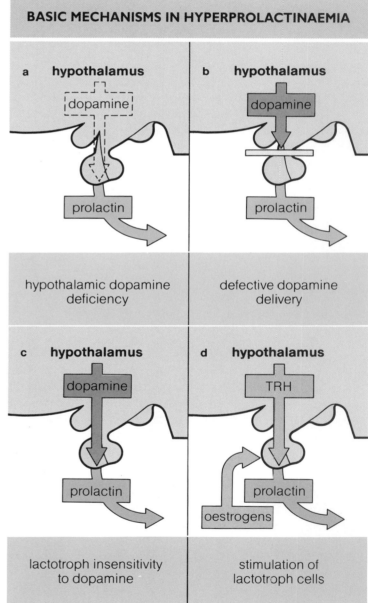

Fig. 4.1 Prolactin secretion. Dopamine is formed in the hypothalamus and stored in the median eminence. It is secreted into the hypothalamo-hypophysial portal vessels to inhibit prolactin release tonically from pituitary lactotrophs. Any disruption of this pathway may therefore result in hyperprolactinaemia.

Fig. 4.2 Four basic mechanisms in hyperprolactinaemia.
(a) Inadequate synthesis and/or secretion of dopamine from the hypothalamus. (b) Interpretation of the hypothalamo-hypophysial portal circulation. (c) Decreased sensitivity of the dopamine receptors. (In such cases, lactotrophs will be released from dopaminergic inhibition, thereby permitting the release of prolactin.) (d) Stimulation of prolactin secretion by oestrogens or by excess TRH in hypothyroidism.

HYPOTHALAMIC DOPAMINE DEFICIENCY

Diseases of the hypothalamus, such as tumours, arteriovenous malformations, and inflammatory processes, might be expected to result in either diminished synthesis or release of dopamine. Furthermore, certain drugs (e.g. α-methyldopa and reserpine) are capable of depleting the central dopamine stores.

DEFECTIVE TRANSPORT MECHANISMS

Section of the pituitary stalk results in deranged transport of dopamine from the hypothalamus to the lactotrophs; it is also possible to speculate that pituitary or stalk tumours with abnormal blood supplies, or their pressure effects, may interfere with the circulatory pathways to the normal lactotrophs or to those within the tumour.

LACTOTROPH INSENSITIVITY TO DOPAMINE

Although dopamine receptors have been found on human pituitary adenoma cells, it is not certain if they are functionally intact. Receptor sensitivity to dopamine may be diminished, which would explain the lack of response to increased endogenous dopamine stimulation; however, the obvious response of the receptors to pharmacologic dopamine agonists makes this possibility less likely. Certain drugs act as dopamine receptor-blocking agents, including phenothiazines (e.g. chlorpromazine), butyrophenones (haloperidol), and benzamides (metoclopramide, sulpiride, and domperidone). These drugs block the effects of endogenous dopamine and thus release lactotrophs from their hypothalamic inhibition. This sequence of events results in hyperprolactinaemia.

STIMULATION OF LACTOTROPHS

Hypothyroidism may be associated with hyperprolactinaemia. If hypothyroidism results in increased TRH production, then TRH (which can act as a PRF), could lead to hyperprolactinaemia.

Oestrogens act directly at the pituitary level causing stimulation of lactotrophs and thus enhance prolactin secretion. Furthermore, oestrogens increase the mitotic activity of lactotrophs.

Injury to the chest wall can also lead to hyperprolactinaemia. The mechanism is unclear but probably results from abnormal stimulation of the reflex associated with the rise in prolactin that is seen normally in lactating women during suckling.

CLINICAL MANIFESTATIONS OF HYPERPROLACTINAEMIA

The symptoms associated with hyperprolactinaemia may be due to several factors: either to the direct effects of excess prolactin, such as the induction of galactorrhoea or hypogonadism or to the effects of the structural lesion causing the disorder (i.e. the pituitary tumour) leading to, for example, headaches, visual field defects, or external ophthalmoplegia; or to associated dysfunction of secretion of other anterior pituitary hormones (Fig. 4.3).

The incidence of galactorrhoea in hyperprolactinaemic patients is between thirty and eighty per cent, depending on the care with which the physician looks for this sign. Approximately fifty per cent of women with galactorrhoea, however, have normal prolactin and, as mentioned below, it is particularly those patients with very high prolactin levels, that is, greater than 100ng/ml (2,000mu/l), who often have no galactorrhoea – thus, it is a poor marker of hyperprolactinaemia. Normal prolactin levels are below 18ng/ml (360mu/l).

Women with hyperprolactinaemia usually present with menstrual abnormalities: amenorrhoea or oligomenorrhoea; or regular cycles with infertility. Occasionally, patients may present with menorrhagia.

In contrast, men often present late in the course of the disease with symptoms of expansion of their pituitary tumour (i.e. headaches, visual defects, and external ophthalmoplegia) or symptoms from secondary adrenal or thyroid failure. These men, however, have usually been impotent for many years before their presentation.

Occasionally, the syndrome may occur in prepubertal or peripubertal children, when it may present with delayed or arrested puberty.

DIFFERENTIAL DIAGNOSIS

The theoretical causes of hyperprolactinaemia have already been discussed. In practice, however, it is important to exclude two causes of hyperprolactinaemia: hypothyroidism, and the ingestion of drugs that either deplete central dopamine or block dopamine receptors. Having excluded these two important causes, three diagnostic possibilities remain (Fig. 4.4): the patient may have a microadenoma, a macroadenoma, or no tumour at all. If patients do not harbour an

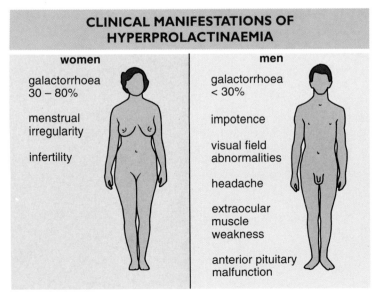

Fig. 4.3 Symptoms associated with hyperprolactinaemia. A variable incidence of galactorrhoea is reported in different studies.

DIAGNOSIS IN HYPERPROLACTINAEMIA

no tumour	microadenoma	macroadenoma
	presence of a microadenoma cannot be excluded by current biochemical or radiological tests	

Fig. 4.4 Differential diagnosis in hyperprolactinaemia.

identifiable tumour, they are described as having idiopathic hyper-prolactinaemia.

A microadenoma is described as having a maximum diameter of up to 10mm, and a macroadenoma as having a diameter in excess of this. The normal pituitary diameter does not exceed 10mm (Fig. 4.5). A microadenoma is often visualised using modern computed tomographic (CT) scanning or magnetic resonance imaging (MRI). Usually, the serum prolactin level is below 200ng/ml (4,000mu/l). A macroadenoma that secretes prolactin is usually associated with a serum prolactin level of more than 200ng/ml (4,000mu/l). The macroadenoma is visualised with CT or MRI. If the patient has a macroadenoma and a serum prolactin level of less than 200ng/ml (4,000mu/l), consideration should be given to the possibility that a nonfunctioning pituitary adenoma is present; here, the hyperprolactinaemia results from deprivation of some lactotrophs of dopaminergic inhibition. Enlargement of the pituitary fossa on a skull X-ray may represent the expansion of the fossa by the macroadenoma, but care should be exercised to exclude the possibility of cisternal herniation (a partially empty fossa) as a cause for the enlargement. CT and MRI scans are proving useful here (see Fig. 4.7) (see Chapter 24).

CHANGES IN THE BREAST DUE TO PROLACTIN

A woman with amenorrhoea due to hyperprolactinaemia does not develop the breast atrophy seen in postmenopausal women or in amenorrhoeic women who are gonadotrophin deficient or have primary ovarian failure. On examination, the breast is well developed and the Montgomery tubercles are hyperplastic (Fig. 4.6). If the breast is correctly examined, first by expressing it from the periphery towards the areola to empty the milk ducts, followed by squeezing and lifting the areola (rather than the nipple itself) to empty the milk sinuses, galactorrhoea can usually be found.

In patients with extremely high prolactin levels, galactorrhoea may not be found. In male patients with hyperprolactinaemia, there is usually no gynaecomastia, but milk may be expressed from an entirely normal-sized male breast. The incidence of galactorrhoea in men with hyperprolactinaemia is low, however, being less than thirty per cent (i.e. it is much less common than in women).

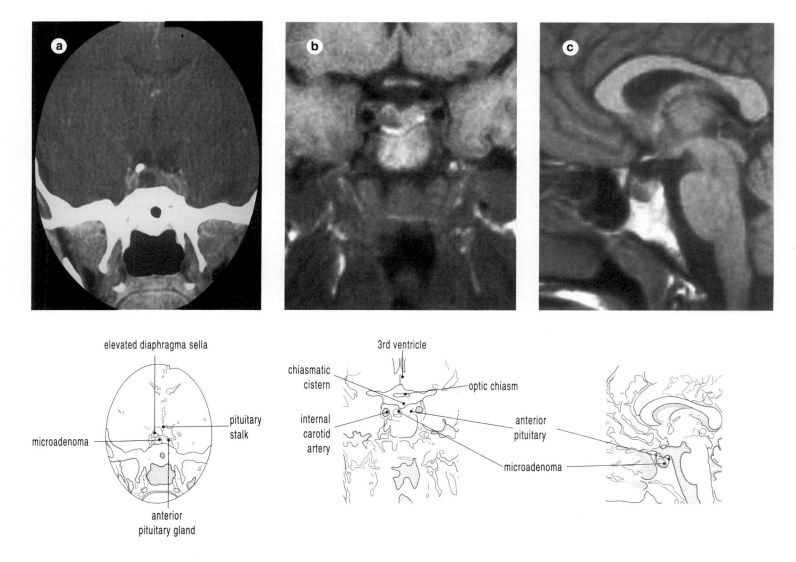

Fig. 4.5 CT and MRI scans of a microadenoma. (a) This post-contrast coronal CT scan demonstrates a 1cm mass of low density; note the elevation of the diaphragma sella on the right side. (b) Coronal and (c) sagittal MRI scans.

RADIOLOGY OF THE PITUITARY FOSSA

The radiologic evaluation of the pituitary fossa should include a skull radiograph to demonstrate the floor of the pituitary fossa. The routine use of tomography is no longer necessary since many of the minor abnormalities that were detected probably represent normal variants rather then being the pathognomonic changes of small tumours. Tomography of the sella, however, may be necessary if there are difficulties in visualising the floor of the fossa, for instance due to overlying shadows or to the lack of pneumatisation of the sphenoid sinus, or if the patient is about to undergo transsphenoidal surgery. Patients who have macroadenomas usually have expanded pituitary fossae One caveat, however, is necessary–the patient may have cisternal herniation (a partially empty fossa). The aetiology of this condition is unknown but it may be due to a defect in the diaphragma sellae, allowing the transmitted pressure changes of the cerebrospinal fluid to extend into the fossa, thereby expanding it. Another explanation may be that the fossa once contained a pituitary tumour that subsequently infarcted and therefore become smaller. The presence of cisternal herniation may be diagnosed either by CT scanning or MRI (Fig. 4.7).

TREATMENT OF HYPERPROLACTINAEMIA

Patients with hyperprolactinaemia and small pituitary tumours may be treated either by surgery, using the transsphenoidal approach, or medically, with dopamine agonist drugs. For microadenomas, the results, in the hands of most experienced surgeons, are similar. (In this discussion, the relative advantages of medical therapy and surgery will not be dealt with; the emphasis, reflecting our expertise, will be on medical therapy.)

TRANSSPHENOIDAL SURGERY

The transsphenoidal technique for approaching the pituitary gives the most satisfactory surgical results and often allows selective removal of the adenomas (Fig. 4.8). The operating microscope, image intensification (allowing video radiographic monitoring), and the advent of antibiotics (minimising postoperative meningitis) are advances enabling this to be performed.

Transsphenoidal Surgery: Microadenoma

Stages in the identification and removal of a prolactin microadenoma from the right side of the gland are shown in Fig. 4.9. The figure shows the exposed but undisturbed gland (Fig. 4.9(a)), the microadenoma being manipulated from the gland (Fig. 4.9(b)), and the complete tumour just before excision from the lateral aspect of the gland (Fig. 4.9(c)). The patient in this example was a 28-year-old women with a two-year history of amenorrhoea and galactorrhoea. Preoperatively, serum prolactin was 159ng/ml (3,180mu/1).

Transsphenoidal Surgery: Macroadenoma

A macroadenoma during surgery is shown in Fig. 4.10. The patient in the example had a mass effect with bitemporal hemianopia. The figure shows the large tumour immediately upon opening the dura, before any of the tumour has been removed (Fig. 4.10(a)), as well as the tumour completely excised leaving the thin pituitary gland intact (Fig. 4.10(b)). The bluish structure, anterior to the gland, is the diaphragma sellae. In this case, the removal of a moderately large adenoma was achieved with preservation of the gland.

BROMOCRIPTINE THERAPY

The first dopamine agonist ergot compound to be used in clinical practice was bromocriptine, a peptide ergot.

The *In Vitro* Effects of Bromocriptine

Bromocriptine has the advantage of having a long duration of action, which can be demonstrated using an *in vitro* system. Anterior pituitary cells of a prolactinoma from a female patient were dispersed, placed in a perfusion apparatus, and perfused continuously. When the cells were exposed to dopamine, prolactin secretion was inhibited, but within ten minutes after the withdrawal of dopamine, prolactin secretion increased, becoming maximal after approximately fifteen minutes. Prolactin secretion was inhibited on exposure of the cells to bromocriptine. When the bromocriptine was withdrawn, however, prolactin secretion remained suppressed for over three hours. On re-exposure to dopamine, prolactin secretion was once more inhibited, recovering again on withdrawal of dopamine. These results are summarised graphically in Fig. 4.11.

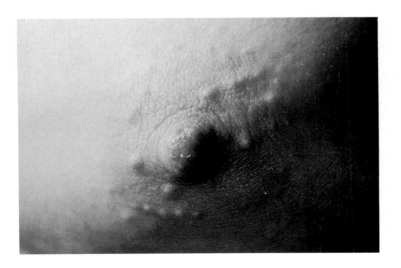

Fig. 4.6 Changes in the breast due to prolactin secretion. Prominent Montgomery tubercles are seen in the breast of a woman with hyperprolactinaemia.

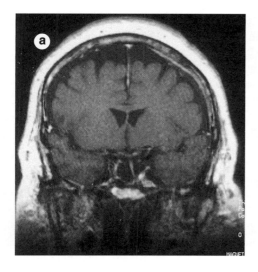

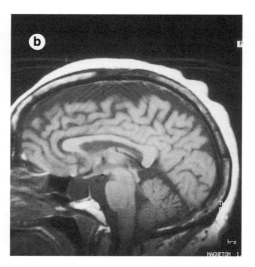

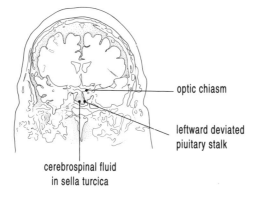

optic chiasm

leftward deviated piuitary stalk

cerebrospinal fluid in sella turcica

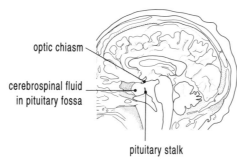

optic chiasm

cerebrospinal fluid in pituitary fossa

pituitary stalk

Fig. 4.7 Cisternal herniation shown by MRI. (a) Coronal MRI scan, which shows a deviated pituitary stalk reaching the floor of the pituitary fossa, and (b) a sagittal view in the same patient.

TRANSSPHENOIDAL SURGERY

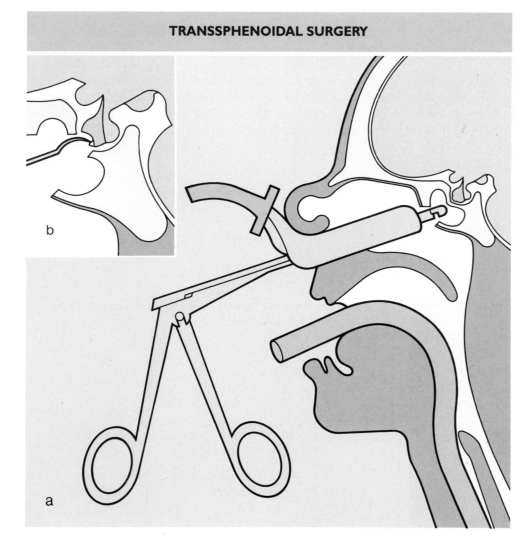

Fig. 4.8 Transsphenoidal surgery. (a) The sphenoidal sinus is reached by a transnasal route, and the floor of the sella and dura is opened, exposing the pituitary. This method allows the selective excision of adenomas (adenomectomy) (b).

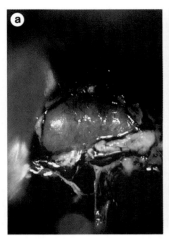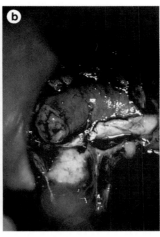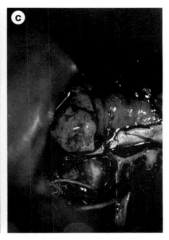

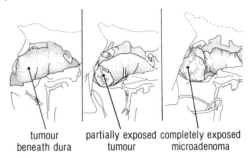

Fig. 4.9 Stages in the surgical removal of a microadenoma. (a) The exposed, undisturbed gland. (b) The tumour being manipulated from the gland. (c) The completely exposed tumour just before excision.

tumour beneath dura | partially exposed tumour | completely exposed microadenoma

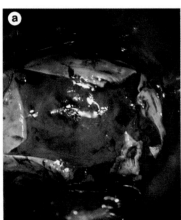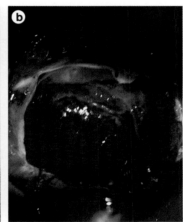

Fig. 4.10 Stages in the surgical removal of a macroadenoma. (a) The appearance of a macroadenoma after the dura has been opened. (b) The appearance of the pituitary gland after removal of the tumour. The bluish structure anterior to the gland is the diaphragma sellae.

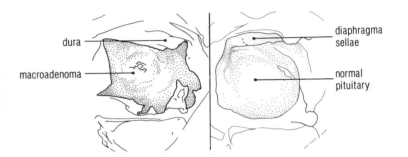

dura — macroadenoma — diaphragma sellae — normal pituitary

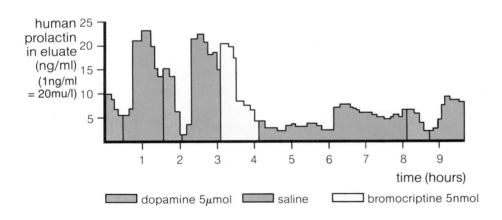

THE IN VITRO RESPONSE OF A PROLACTINOMA TO DOPAMINE AND BROMOCRIPTINE

human prolactin in eluate (ng/ml) (1ng/ml = 20mu/l)

time (hours)

dopamine 5μmol — saline — bromocriptine 5nmol

Fig. 4.11 The in vitro response of dispersed prolactinoma cells to dopamine and bromocriptine. Both drugs suppressed prolactin secretion but, whereas prolactin secretion became maximal within fifteen minutes after withdrawal of dopamine, the effect of bromocriptine was longer lasting, with prolactin levels remaining suppressed for three hours following withdrawal.

The In Vivo Effects of Bromocriptine

Bromocriptine has a similar mode of action to dopamine in stimulating dopamine receptors on the prolactin-secreting pituitary cells. Stimulation of these receptors leads to inhibition of both prolactin secretion and synthesis. After a single 2.5-mg dose of bromocriptine administered at 0900 to women with hyperprolactinaemia, prolactin secretion was inhibited within two hours and reached nadir at seven hours. When patients are treated chronically using 2.5mg three times per day, prolactin levels are maintained within the normal range, that is, less than 20ng/ml (400mu/l), throughout a twenty-four-hour period (Fig. 4.12).

Effects of Bromocriptine in Men

The first male patient commenced bromocriptine treatment at St Bartholomew's Hospital, London, in 1971, and his case illustrates a number of important points (Fig. 4.13). Initially, the prolactin levels of the patient were extremely elevated, but the administration of bromocriptine lowered them into the normal range (undetectable by bioassay); this was associated with cessation of galactorrhoea. Bromocriptine therapy normalised the patient's prolactin levels and gonadal function, restoring potency. Following withdrawal of bromocriptine, hyperprolactinaemia recurred, with associated galactorrhoea and impotence. After restoration of bromocriptine therapy, prolactin levels rapidly returned to normal, galactorrhoea ceased, and potency was restored.

Effects of Bromocriptine in Women

The second patient to be treated with bromocriptine was a woman with a large pituitary tumour and extremely high prolactin levels. Bromocriptine lowered her prolactin levels into the normal range, galactorrhoea ceased, and menstruation returned within one month of starting therapy, even though the patient had been amenorrhoeic for several years.

The third patient had post-oral contraceptive amenorrhoea and galactorrhoea associated with hyperprolactinaemia. Bromocriptine therapy lowered the prolactin levels to normal and led to cessation of the patient's galactorrhoea and to normal menstruation (Fig. 4.14).

Bromocriptine in Amenorrhoea

From experience of treating a large number of amenorrhoeic hyperprolactinaemia women, the results of treating the first fifty-eight appear to be representative of the success that can be achieved with bromocriptine therapy. (Fig. 4.15). Within one month of starting therapy, a regular menstrual cycle is restored in approximately twenty-five per cent of patients. Within two months, regular menstrual cycling can be restored in over sixty per cent, and within ten months, in some eighty per cent. Those patients who did not have restoration of regular menstrual cycles (with only one or two exceptions) had previously undergone surgery or radiotherapy for their pituitary tumour – this rendered them gonadotrophin deficient. Thus, if hyperprolactinaemia is the cause of amenorrhoea, the chances of restoring normal gonadal function by medical therapy alone are extremely good.

Long-term Effects of Bromocriptine

To study the long-term effects of bromocriptine on prolactin secretion, a group of patients was carefully evaluated (Fig. 4.16). Ten blood samples were taken from each patient before treatment; at three, six, and twelve months on therapy; and two months following drug withdrawal. All patients were treated with the same dose of bromocriptine (2.5mg three times per day). In all cases, bromocriptine lowered prolactin levels, and in nine of the twelve patients, prolactin secretion was suppressed throughout the year. After withdrawal of bromocriptine, prolactin levels rose in all patients to levels similar to those seen prior to therapy. The three patients in whom the prolactin levels were not lowered into the normal range, nevertheless, regained normal gonadal function.

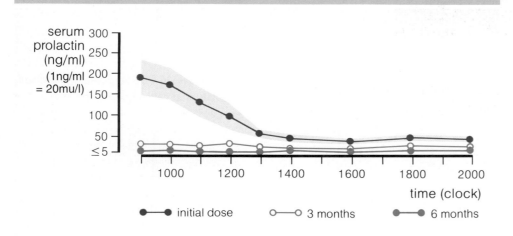

THE IN VIVO RESPONSE TO BROMOCRIPTINE

serum prolactin (ng/ml)
(1ng/ml = 20mu/l)

time (clock)

●—● initial dose   ○—○ 3 months   ●—● 6 months

Fig. 4.12 The effects of bromocriptine in vivo. After a single 2.5-mg dose of bromocriptine administered at 0900, prolactin secretion was inhibited within two hours, and reached nadir at seven hours. With chronic treatment (2.5mg three times per day) at three and six months, prolactin levels were maintained within the normal range throughout a 24-hour period.

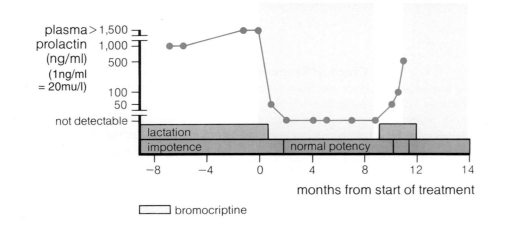

EFFECTS OF BROMOCRIPTINE IN A MALE PATIENT

plasma prolactin (ng/ml)
(1ng/ml = 20mu/l)

lactation
impotence   normal potency

months from start of treatment

▭ bromocriptine

Fig. 4.13 The effects of bromocriptine in a male patient with prolactinoma. Normalisation of serum prolactin by bromocriptine was associatec with cessation of galactorrhoea and with restoration of potency. On discontinuation of treatment, however, both galactorrhoea and impotence returned, only to disappear after reinstitution cf bromocriptine therapy.

EFFECTS OF BROMOCRIPTINE IN FEMALE PATIENTS

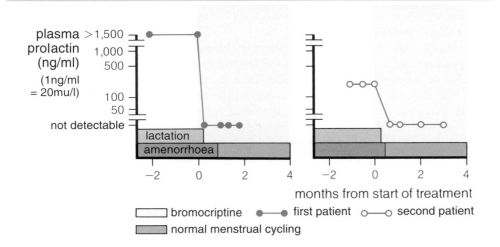

Fig. 4.14 The effects of bromocriptine in female patients. The first female patient treated with bromocriptine had hyperprolactinaemia associated with a large pituitary tumour, and the second had post-oral contraceptive amenorrhoea and galactorrhoea with hyperprolactinaemia. In both cases, bromocriptine therapy led to cessation of galactorrhoea and the return of normal menstrual cycling.

THE SUCCESS RATE OF BROMOCRIPTINE IN AMENORRHOEA

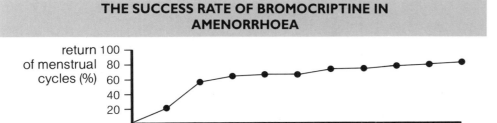

Fig. 4.15 The success rate of bromocriptine in amenorrhoea. If hyperprolactinaemia is the cause of amenorrhoea, the chances of restoring normal gonadal function with bromocriptine are very good. After one month of treatment, one woman in four will return to normal menstrual cycling; within two months, this number will increase to six out of ten, and after ten months, eight out of ten women will be menstruating normally. (Most of the remaining twenty per cent have had pituitary surgery and irradiation therapy and were gonadotrophin deficient).

LONG-TERM EFFECTS OF BROMOCRIPTINE THERAPY

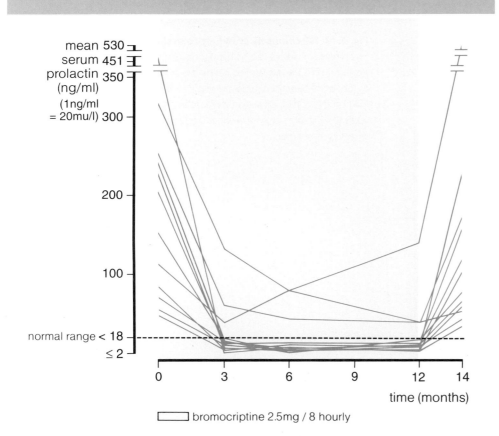

bromocriptine 2.5mg / 8 hourly

Fig. 4.16 The long-term effects of bromocriptine therapy. Prolactin levels in a group of patients on long-term bromocriptine therapy were tested before therapy; after three months, six months, and one year of treatment (during which time all patients received bromocriptine 2.5mg three times per day); and two months after cessation of treatment. In all cases, prolactin remained suppressed throughout the year, and in most cases, prolactin levels were held within the normal range. Gonadal function was restored, even in patients whose prolactin levels did not return to normal.

Hyperprolactinaemia and Ovulation

Ovulation is normally associated with a dip in basal body temperature, and normal luteal function with a temperature rise. Basal body temperature is therefore a useful means of documenting ovulation. When hyperprolactinaemic patients have had their prolactin levels and periods restored to normal by bromocriptine therapy, they usually demonstrate a biphasic temperature pattern. One patient had suffered from polymenorrhoea for many years and was found to be hyperprolactinaemic. Bromocriptine normalised her periods, and therapy was withdrawn after one year. During therapy, the basal body temperature chart (Fig. 4.17) showed a normal biphasic pattern, but following withdrawal of bromocriptine, prolactin levels rose to more than 100ng/ml (2,000mu/l), galactorrhoea returned, and the temperature pattern immediately became monophasic. Although the patient did not become amenorrhoeic, she developed irregular (presumably anovulatory) periods. Following reinstitution of therapy, two weeks, the patient ovulated, demonstrating a postovulatory temperature rise. She has subsequently had a regular cycle and three successful pregnancies, each with the help of bromocriptine.

Hyperprolactinaemic Hypogonadism

The pathogenesis of the hypogonadal state in hyperprolactinaemia is poorly understood. In men, testosterone levels may be normal or low, while in women, a hypo-oestrogenic state may occur, with loss of ovulation. The clinical features in hyperprolactinaemic women, however, differ from those in the postmenopausal state since breast atrophy is absent and gonadotrophin levels are not elevated.

Proposed explanations for the suppression of gonadal function in hyperprolactinaemia include suppression of gonadotrophin secretion; inhibition of positive oestrogen feedback on luteinising hormone

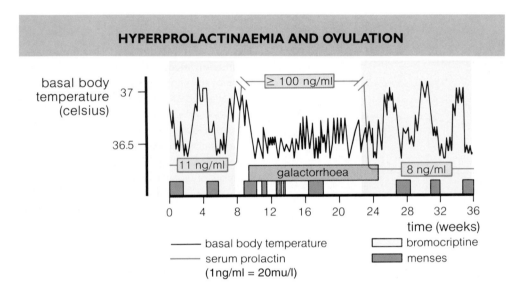

HYPERPROLACTINAEMIA AND OVULATION

basal body temperature (celsius)

≥ 100 ng/ml

11 ng/ml   galactorrhoea   8 ng/ml

time (weeks)

—— basal body temperature   ☐ bromocriptine
—— serum prolactin   ▨ menses
(1ng/ml = 20mu/l)

Fig. 4.17 Hyperprolactinaemia and ovulation. Normal ovulation and luteal function are associated with a biphasic basal body temperature. When patients have their prolactin levels and periods restored to normal with bromocriptine therapy, their temperature charts demonstrate the normal biphasic pattern. When therapy is withdrawn, the temperature chart shows a monophasic pattern, becoming biphasic again on reinstitution of bromocriptine.

MECHANISMS OF HYPERPROLACTINAEMIC HYPOGONADISM

hypothalamus

↓GnRH   ↑PIF (DA)   ↑PRF (TRH)

PRL   ↓LH   ↓FSH

breast
lactation

gonad   gonadal steroids

adrenal   ↑androgens

Fig. 4.18 Mechanisms of hyperprolactinaemic hypogonadism. Hyperprolactinaemia causes hypogonadism by several mechanisms: high prolactin (PRL) levels lead to partial suppression of GnRH release, as well as loss of its pulsatility; prolactin also interferes with the action of LH and FSH on the gonad, causes an increase in adrenal androgen secretion, and leads to inhibition of positive oestrogen feedback on GnRH and LH secretion in women.

(LH) secretion in women; an increase in adrenal androgen secretion; and blockade of the effects of gonadotrophins at the gonadal level (Fig. 4.18). It is probable that an important mechanism is prolactin feedback at the hypothalamus, which alters secretion of gonadotrophin-releasing hormone (GnRH), thus causing LH and follicle-stimulating hormone (FSH) secretion to become inappropriately low, relative to gonadal steroid levels. Abnormalities in LH pulsatility also occur. Prolactin may interfere with LH and FSH action at the gonad, blocking progesterone synthesis, and may stimulate adrenal androgen secretion.

Size Reduction of Prolactinomas

Since surgical therapy of large prolactin-secreting pituitary tumours normalises serum prolactin levels or gonadal function in less than twenty per cent of patients, particularly those with high prolactin levels, there is a need for another approach to the problem. Three major lines of evidence suggest that medical therapy may help in the treatment of these large tumours:

•Visual field defects due to prolactinomas pressing on the optic chiasm have improved with bromocriptine therapy alone.
•Dopamine agonist therapy has been shown, by neuroradiologic evaluations, to reduce the size of prolactinomas.
•Bromocriptine reduces DNA turnover and the mitotic index in the *in situ* pituitary of the rat.

Bromocriptine reduces pituitary tumour size in seventy-five to eighty per cent of patients with large prolactin-secreting tumours, even with gross extrasellar extension. The type of results that can be expected are illustrated by a patient with a large prolactin-secreting tumour, who was treated with bromocriptine alone. The patient had a suprasellar extension and visual field defects. Visual field plots from this patient before and during treatment, as well as after withdrawal and reinstitution of bromocriptine therapy, are illustrated in Fig. 4.19. Before therapy (baseline), the patient had a bitemporal hemi-

anopia, complete in the left eye and incomplete in the right eye. The visual fields were greatly improved after ten days, and only an equivocal superior bitemporal quadrantic defect to the low intensity object was present after nearly one year. Thirteen days after withdrawal of medical treatment, the tumour had enlarged again and the field defects recurred as an almost complete temporal hemianopia in the left eye and a partial temporal hemianopia in the right. Progressive improvement in visual fields was again observed over the subsequent six months after reintroduction of therapy.

Changes in Pituitary Volume During Bromocriptine Therapy

Coronal CT head scans (postenhancement) from the patient whose visual fields are shown in Fig. 4.19, are shown in Fig. 4.20. The left panel CT scan, performed on a Delta 25 scanner, illustrates the situation before therapy; the right panel shows a scan performed on a GE 8800 scanner two weeks after starting bromocriptine therapy, 2.5mg three times per day. Before therapy (Fig. 4.20(a)), the scan shows an enlargement of the pituitary fossa and an enhancing mass extending inferiorly into the sphenoid sinus, superiorly into the chiasmatic cistern, and abutting on the third ventricle. Two weeks post-treatment (Fig. 4.20(b)), the scan shows a marked reduction in tumour size, with regression of the suprasellar extension. The chiasmatic cistern is now largely free of tumour, apart from a finger-like process to the left of the midline. The intrasellar high density is present in the preenhancement scan and represents calcification within the tumour. Within the short space of two weeks, therefore, there was marked reduction in the size of the pituitary and a consequent decompression of the optic chiasm, which explains the rapid improvement in visual fields observed in this patient.

In sixteen patients with large prolactin-secreting tumours, thirteen showed similar changes. The three patients in whom these changes were not observed consisted of:

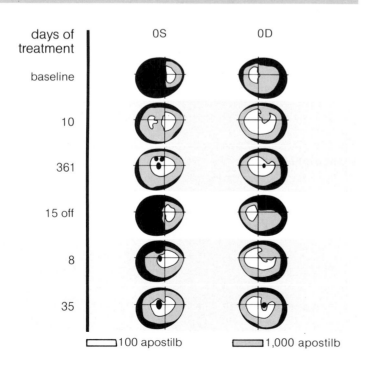

VISUAL FIELD PLOTS IN HYPERPROLACTINAEMIA

days of treatment | OS | OD

baseline, 10, 361, 15 off, 8, 35

100 apostilb   1,000 apostilb

Fig. 4.19 Visual field plots of a patient with hyperprolactinaemia. The visual fields shown here were plotted using a Goldmann perimeter, under identical conditions, with a 0.25mm² object at two different light intensities: 1,000 apostilb (I₄) and 100 apostilb (I₂). The black periphery indicates a normal visual field for comparison. An almost complete bitemporal hemianopia (pretherapy), which had almost disappeared after one year of treatment with bromocriptine, returned on cessation of therapy and began to subside after reinstitution of bromocriptine.

•A patient with a pituitary cyst that was associated with a small prolactin-oma, but in whom the majority of the pituitary mass was the cyst.

•A patient with an extremely large tumour that was reduced in size but still remained large. (The patient's serum prolactin level fell by ninety per cent but still remained elevated at 328ng/ml (6560mu/l) at the end of nine months of therapy).

•A patient who had only been treated for six weeks and in whom there was as yet only equivocal evidence of reduction in the size of the tumour.

Other groups have had similar results. It seems that some sixty-five per cent of macroadenomas with large extrasellar extensions may be treated with bromocriptine alone to shrink the tumours and to relieve the mass effects and the hormonal excess.

Changes in Serum Prolactin Levels

In patients with macroadenomas, the serum prolactin levels can be readily suppressed with bromocriptine therapy. Figure 4.21 shows serum prolactin levels throughout the day after an initial 2.5-mg oral dose of bromocriptine administered at 0900 to the patient whose visual field plots and CT scans are shown in Figs. 4.19 and 4.20, respectively, as well as those from a patient with a similar problem. After a single dose of bromocriptine, the prolactin levels fell by approximately ninety per cent. The mean and absolute range of prolactin levels in samples taken at the same time intervals before therapy (baseline) and during bromocriptine therapy, 7.5 mg/d, are also shown in Fig. 4.21. In the first patient, the prolactin levels were suppressed into the normal range (less than 18ng/ml (360mu/l)) and in the second patient, prolactin levels, although lowered, did not return to normal. With treatment over one year, however, the levels continued to fall to 78ng/ml (1560mu/l). In these patients, as with the patients with microadenomas, gonadal function is usually restored to normal. As previously noted, when therapy was withdrawn at one year, visual field defects recurred in the first patient and this was associated with prolactin levels rising again to 2,580ng/ml (51.6u/l) at thirteen days in comparison to the pretreatment level (3,940ng/ml (78.8u/l)). It should be noted, however, that in male patients on bromocriptine, prolactin levels usually fall rapidly and easily into the normal range. If this does not occur, gonadal function may not return to normal.

Side Effects

Side effects of bromocriptine therapy occur only at the start of treatment and disappear with continued therapy. There are no long-term problems associated with chronic treatment at the doses used for hyperprolactinaemia–usually 7.5mg/d, and rarely more than 15mg/d.

If treatment is started with full doses or increased too quickly, dizziness, nausea, and postural hypotension may occur. To avoid such effects, bromocriptine must always be taken during a meal. Administration should be started at night, with a sandwich and glass of milk, when the patient retires to bed. After taking half a tablet (1.25mg) for three nights, half a tablet is added with breakfast. After a further three days an additional half a tablet is added with lunch. At intervals of three days, additional half tablets (1.25mg increments) may be progressively added until achievement of the usual dose of one tablet (2.5mg) taken three times daily, in the middle of breakfast, lunch, and the evening meal. If side effects still occur, longer intervals and smaller increments should be used.

The only group of patients who do not suffer from such side effects if given the full dose immediately is puerperal women. They may be given bromocriptine 2.5mg two or three times daily to suppress puerperal lactation, without side effects, if treatment is started within twenty-four hours of delivery. The reasons for this difference are unknown.

There are several other dopamine agonists that lower serum prolactin levels and reduce tumour size to a similar extent to bromocriptine. These drugs include pergolide, lisuride, CV 205-502 (mesulergine), and cabergoline. These compounds are associated with a similar side effect profile to that observed with bromocriptine. Cabergoline has the advantage that it only needs to be taken once per week. With the exception of bromocriptine, safety during pregnancy has not been demonstrated. Bromocriptine may also be given now as a monthly depot intramuscular injection (50 or 100mg per dose), but this formulation is not available in all countries.

Pregnancy and Bromocriptine

Many hyperprolactinaemic women would like to fall pregnant and, since the administration of bromocriptine lowers the prolactin levels

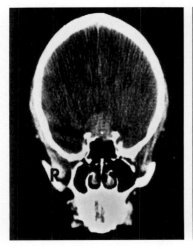
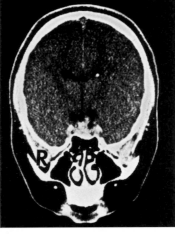

Fig. 4.20 Coronal CT head scans before and during treatment with bromocriptine. Scan (a), taken before therapy, shows enlargement of the pituitary fossa and an enhancing mass extending inferiorly into the sphenoid sinus, superiorly into the chiasmatic cistern, and abutting on the third ventricle. Scan (b), taken after two weeks of therapy, shows a marked reduction in tumour size, with regression of the suprasellar extension.

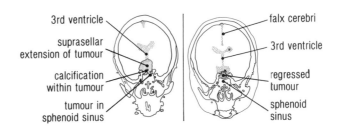

and restores gonadal function, conception presents little difficulty. There are, however, several important considerations that must be recognised by both physician and patient, including the possible teratogenic sequelae of fetal exposure to bromocriptine.

There is no evidence for teratogenicity in animal studies, and in one thousand four hundred women who were taking bromocriptine when they conceived, there is no evidence of increased incidence of abortion, multiple pregnancy, or fetal abnormalities. Until these babies have lived their own complete life cycles, however, the possibility of unexpected late effects cannot be excluded.

In order to minimise fetal exposure to bromocriptine, it is suggested that patients should use mechanical contraception. Once three regular menstrual cycles have occurred, contraceptive precautions are discontinued. In this way, pregnancy can be suspected as soon as a menstrual period is forty-eight hours overdue. At that time, a serum human chorionic gonadotrophin-β assay should be performed to confirm the pregnancy, and the patient should discontinue bromocriptine therapy. In this way, the fetus is exposed to bromocriptine for a theoretical maximum of sixteen days.

There is little doubt that patients with pituitary tumours run a small, but significant, risk of expansion of the tumour during pregnancy. It is very difficult, however, to assess the absolute risk. With microadenomas, the incidence seems to be less than one per cent and probably less than 0.5 per cent. In patients with macroadenomas, the incidence is probably higher, perhaps between five and twenty per cent. This risk is unrelated to bromocriptine therapy prior to pregnancy but may occur when fertility is induced with other drugs, including exogenous gonadotrophins and clomiphene, and even when no drug therapy has been employed in patients with pre-existing pituitary adenomas.

In practice, the problem of pregnancy is not great since the vast majority of women who present with hyperprolactinaemia only have microadenomas. To avoid major problems, it is extremely important that patients undergo careful endocrine, neuroradiological, and neuro-ophthalmological evaluation prior to treatment. If there is no suprasellar extension, and if the patient harbours only a microadenoma, then the risk of swelling of the pituitary is extremely small; it is therefore suggested that the patient is evaluated clinically at bimonthly intervals throughout the pregnancy. If the patient has a macroadenoma and suprasellar extension, a strong case can be made for trans-sphenoidal decompression of the tumour prior to pregnancy. It is, however, possible even for these patients to go through pregnancy without developing visual disturbances and, furthermore, even if visual disturbances occur in one pregnancy, the problem may not recur in subsequent pregnancies.

Thus, the approach to the patient with the prolactin-secreting macroadenoma who desires pregnancy can be either expectant or prophylactic. The author believes that as the risk of swelling of the adenoma is less than twenty per cent, it is reasonable to adopt an expectant policy. Others suggest that pituitary decompression should be performed surgically, and still others recommend that external pituitary irradiation is given. It is not clear whether external pituitary irradiation or decompression of the pituitary by surgery, or both, completely prevent symptom-generating pituitary enlargement. It should be stressed that so far, no patient has become permanently blind following expansion of the tumour during pregnancy.

If visual field defects or headaches from tumour expansion do occur during pregnancy, a number of therapeutic options are available. Following termination of the pregnancy, either by abortion or delivery

CHANGES IN SERUM PROLACTIN LEVELS AFTER BROMOCRIPTINE ADMINISTRATION

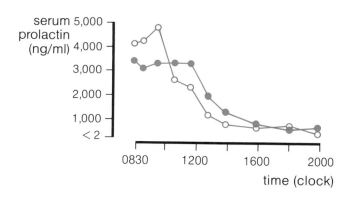

Fig. 4.21 *Changes in serum prolactin levels.* The effect on serum prolactin levels throughout the day, of a single 2.5-mg oral dose of bromocriptine at 0900 is shown. Case one is the patient whose visual field chart and CT scans are shown in Figs. 4.19 and 4.20, respectively. Case two is a patient with a similar problem. In patients such as these, even when prolactin levels do not come down to the normal range, gonadal function is usually restored.

serum prolactin (ng/ml)	mean	range
case 1		
baseline	3,940	1,730–5,700
3 months	2.2	1.7–3.0
6 weeks	2.3	1.4–3.2
case 2		
baseline	2,630	1,640–4,940
1 month	182	93–296
(1ng/ml = 20mu/l)		

of the baby, tumours have become smaller and such symptoms and headaches have resolved in all cases. Thus, if such symptoms occur early in pregnancy, abortion may be indicated. If they occur in the eighth month of pregnancy, premature delivery of the baby may be decided upon, although if field defects and symptoms are minor, careful observation may be all that is required. The most problematic situation arises when symptoms occur in the middle trimester. At that time, it is suggested that bromocriptine therapy is restarted in the hope of reducing the tumour size or at least preventing further swelling. If this is unsuccessful, high-dose dexamethasone can be used to achieve the same ends. Dexamethasone also reduces the chances of fetal respiratory distress occurring should premature delivery be needed. As a last resort, transsphenoidal surgery during pregnancy can, and has been, used to decompress the tumour. Since such complications are extremely rare, however, little data have to date been accumulated.

CONCLUSION

Dopamine agonist therapy for hyperprolactinaemia, such as with bromocriptine, leads to a reversal of the hyperprolactinaemic hypo-gonadal state without risk of the development of pituitary insufficiency. Dopamine agonist therapy is effective not only in patients with microadenomas, but also in the majority of patients with large prolactin-secreting tumours in reducing tumour size; however, the tumour size will increase (as will prolactin levels) after withdrawal of therapy. This may give rise to problems due to compression of vital structures by the tumour.

5

The Posterior Pituitary

Peter H Baylis, BSc, MD, FRCP

The pituitary is a composite gland, the anterior lobe being derived from an evagination of the stomodeal ectoderm known as Rathke's pouch, while the posterior lobe is an extension of the forebrain. The weight of the adult human gland is approximately 620mg; in women, twenty per cent, and in men, twenty-five per cent, of this gland is posterior pituitary. Nervous tissue is the principal component of the posterior pituitary.

The immediate anatomical relationship of the pituitary gland with surrounding structures is seen in Fig. 5.1. The gland lies in a bony fossa, and its stalk pierces the fibrous diaphragma sellae. The lateral wall of the fossa is made up of the cavernous sinus in which lie the carotid syphon and the cranial nerves III, IV and VI. The optic chiasm is situated immediately above the pituitary fossa, anterior to the pituitary stalk. The hypothalamus lies above the pituitary stalk and extends to the lateral walls of the third ventricle. Bounded anteriorly by the anterior commissure and posteriorly by the mammillary body,

it is composed of many sets of nuclei and neuronal tracts, a number of which terminate in the median eminence.

NEURONAL TRACTS FROM THE PARAVENTRICULAR AND SUPRAOPTIC NUCLEI

Two major nuclei in the hypothalamus – the supraoptic and paraventricular nuclei – synthesise the peptides vasopressin (antidiuretic hormone (ADH)) and oxytocin (Fig. 5.2). Smaller groups of neurones that synthesise these neurohypophysial hormones are clustered in the suprachiasmatic region in some, but not all, mammals. Each neurone in these nuclei synthesises either oxytocin or vasopressin as part of a larger precursor molecule. In the rostral (anterior) part of the supraoptic nucleus, oxytocin and vasopressin neurones are equally distributed, but in the caudal part, only oxytocin neurones are found. Additionally, both hormones are present in the rostral paraventricular nucleus. In the caudal region of the

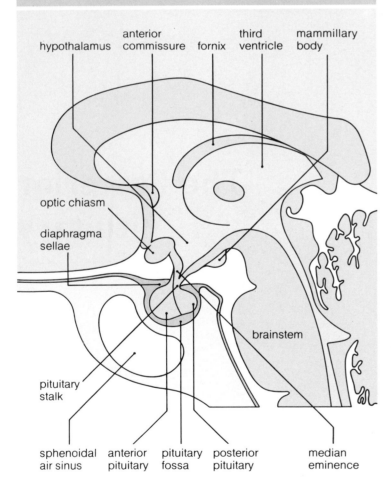

ANATOMICAL RELATIONSHIP OF THE POSTERIOR PITUITARY AND HYPOTHALAMUS WITH SURROUNDING STRUCTURES

Fig. 5.1 The anatomical relationship of the posterior pituitary and hypothalamus with surrounding structures. The diagram represents a sagittal section through the pituitary and hypothalamus.

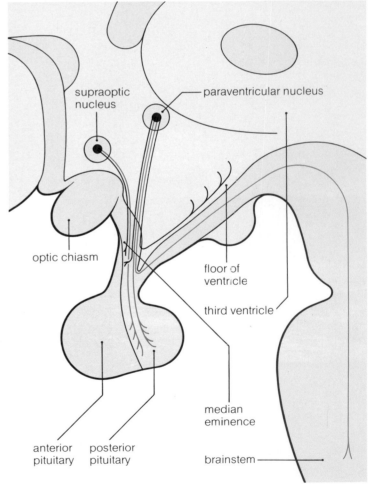

NEURONAL PATHWAYS FROM THE PARAVENTRICULAR AND SUPRAOPTIC NUCLEI

Fig. 5.2 Schematic representation of the neuronal pathways from the paraventricular and supraoptic nuclei. Neuronal tracts from the paraventricular and supraoptic nuclei connect with the posterior pituitary, the median eminence, the floor of the third ventricle, and the brainstem.

paraventricular nucleus, however, the neurones close to the third ventricle contain oxytocin, while those more laterally situated contain vasopressin.

At least four neuronal tracts arise from the supraoptic and paraventricular nuclei. The main pathway terminates in the posterior pituitary to release its peptides into the systemic circulation. Both vasopressin and oxytocin are found in the zona externa of the median eminence, and the majority of fibres to this region arise from the paraventricular nucleus. From the median eminence, the peptides are secreted into the hypothalamopituitary portal circulation. A third tract passes to the floor of the third ventricle. It is still unknown, however, if the peptide hormones are actively secreted via this tract into the cerebrospinal fluid. The final neuronal pathway terminates in the brainstem in close proximity to the vasomotor centre, and a few fibres pass down the spinal cord.

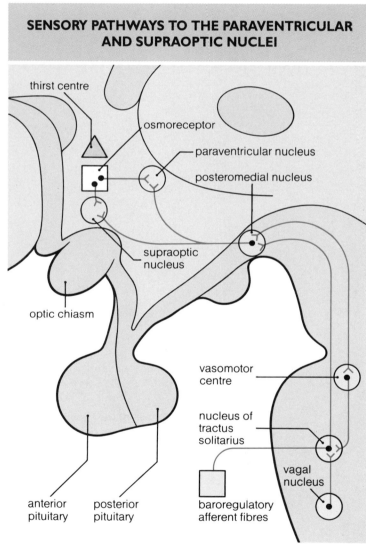

Fig. 5.3 The sensory pathways to the paraventricular and supraoptic nuclei. Changes in blood tonicity are recognised by osmoreceptors in the circumventricular organs of the anterior hypothalamus. Afferent fibres connect the osmoreceptor to the neurones that synthesise vasopressin. Baroregulatory information, from afferent fibres that terminate in the brainstem nuclei, is relayed to the paraventricular and supraoptic nuclei via the posteromedial nucleus of the hypothalamus.

SENSORY TRACTS TO THE PARAVENTRICULAR AND SUPRAOPTIC NUCLEI

Changes in blood tonicity are recognised by osmotically sensitive cells that are situated in the circumventricular organs of the anterior hypothalamus, probably the subfornical organ and/or the organum vasculosum of the lamina terminalis. There is evidence for the existence of two distinct osmoreceptors: one controls vasopressin secretion, principally from the supraoptic nucleus; the other that serves thirst appreciation (Fig. 5.3). Baroregulatory afferent fibres arise in low-pressure receptors that are sited in the atria of the heart and the great veins of the chest, and in high-pressure receptors that are present in the carotid body and arch of the aorta. These fibres terminate in a group of nuclei within the brainstem. They then relay in the posteromedial nucleus of the hypothalamus before ending in the paraventricular and supraoptic nuclei.

The potent stimulatory effect of vomiting on vasopressin release is probably mediated by the vagus nerve. It remains unclear whether the effects of hypoglycaemia are monitored by a hypothalamic glucostat and whether an angiotensin sensor exists to appreciate changes in blood angiotensin concentration. The release of oxytocin by suckling is a neurohormonal reflex, the afferent fibres being carried by the vagus nerve from the breast.

ARTERIAL SUPPLY TO THE HYPOTHALAMUS AND PITUITARY GLAND

The greater part of the arterial blood supply to the hypothalamus and pituitary gland arrives via the internal carotid artery or its branches (Fig. 5.4). The posterior lobe is supplied by the inferior hypophysial artery and the artery of the trabecula (a branch of the superior hypophysial artery). There is no direct arterial supply to the anterior pituitary and all of its blood arises from the long and short hypophysial portal vessels that drain the median eminence. Branches from the circle of Willis supply the hypothalamus, which is extremely well perfused. The paraventricular and supraoptic nuclei receive blood from branches of the suprahypophysial, anterior communicating, anterior cerebral, posterior communicating, and posterior cerebral arteries. Venous blood draining from the anterior and posterior lobes of the pituitary enters the dural, cavernous, and inferior petrosal sinuses.

CHEMISTRY OF VASOPRESSIN AND OXYTOCIN

The genes encoding vasopressin and oxytocin are tightly linked on chromosome 20. The structure of the neurohypophysial hormones vasopressin and oxytocin (Fig. 5.5) was elucidated, and their synthesis completed, by 1954. Arginine vasopressin (AVP) is the antidiuretic hormone of most mammals, although the pig family uses lysine vasopressin. The vasopressins are basic molecules with isoelectric points in the region of pH 9–10, while oxytocin is more neutral. The ring is essential for biological activity. Position 8 plays a key role in determining oxytocic or vasopressor characteristics. The more basic the amino acid in this position, the more vasopressor activity the molecule possesses.

Structure and activity data on a large number of analogues have facilitated the design of substances that possess desired biological properties. An example is the synthesis of a long-acting antidiuretic molecule, 1-deamino-8-D-arginine vasopressin (desmopressin or DDAVP), which has little pressor activity and is ideal for the treatment of cranial diabetes insipidus. Other modifications should lead to the formation of vasopressin antagonists that are suitable for the treatment of disorders associated with vasopressin excess.

After secretion by exocytosis from the neurohypophysis, the peptides circulate unbound to plasma proteins. Their plasma half-life is extremely short (Fig. 5.5) due to efficient clearance by the kidney and liver (for vasopressin), and by the uterus, kidney, and liver (for oxytocin). This clearance is so rapid that changes in plasma concentration are usually a reflection of changes in secretion rather than clearance rate. In pregnancy, the plasma enzyme oxytocinase rapidly degrades both oxytocin and vasopressin.

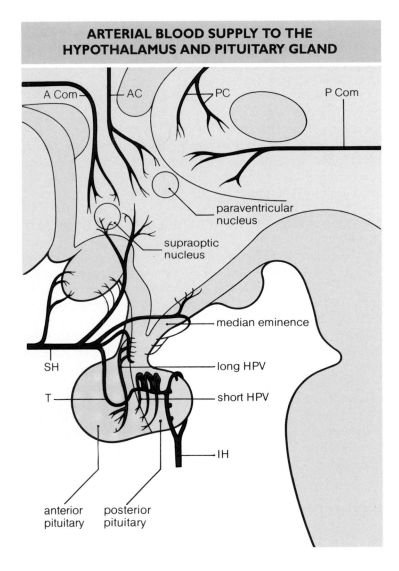

ARTERIAL BLOOD SUPPLY TO THE HYPOTHALAMUS AND PITUITARY GLAND

Fig. 5.4 The arterial blood supply to the hypothalamus and pituitary gland. Most of the blood supply to the hypothalamus and pituitary arises from the internal carotid artery or its branches. The posterior lobe of the pituitary is supplied by the inferior hypophysial artery (IH) and the artery of the trabecula (T), while the anterior lobe is supplied indirectly via the hypophysial portal vessels (HPV). Branches from the circle of Willis supply the hypothalamus, and the paraventricular and supraoptic nuclei in particular are served by branches from the suprahypophysial (SH), the anterior communicating (A Com), the anterior cerebral (AC), the posterior communicating (P Com), and posterior cerebral (PC) arteries.

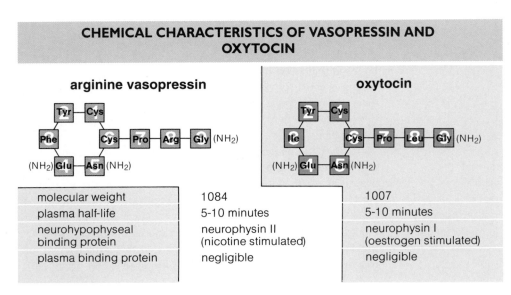

CHEMICAL CHARACTERISTICS OF VASOPRESSIN AND OXYTOCIN

	arginine vasopressin	oxytocin
molecular weight	1084	1007
plasma half-life	5-10 minutes	5-10 minutes
neurohypophyseal binding protein	neurophysin II (nicotine stimulated)	neurophysin I (oestrogen stimulated)
plasma binding protein	negligible	negligible

Fig. 5.5 Comparison of the chemical characteristics of vasopressin and oxytocin. Arginine vasopressin (AVP) is the antidiuretic hormone found in most mammals. The vasopressins are basic molecules (pH 9–10), while oxytocins are more neutral. The more basic the amino acid in position 8, the more vasopressor activity the molecule possesses.

NEUROSECRETION OF NEUROHYPOPHYSIAL HORMONES

The principal sites of biosynthesis of vasopressin and oxytocin are the magnocellular neurones of the supraoptic and paraventricular nuclei (Fig. 5.6). Each neurone synthesises either oxytocin or vasopressin as part of a larger precursor molecule (pro-oxyphysin and propressophysin, respectively). In contrast to the oxytocin precursor molecule, the vasopressin precursor has a glycoprotein portion attached to the C-terminal end. Neurophysin–nonapeptide complexes migrate, as neurosecretory granules, along the axons of the neurones from each nucleus at a rate of 1–3mm/h. The complex is then stored as granules at the end of the neuronal tracts to be released under the influ-ence of specific stimuli. The common final pathway of these stimuli is phasic electrochemical 'firing' of the neurones themselves. The neurosecretory granules then fuse with the plasmalemma of the axon, and the nonapeptide and its specific neurophysin are released separately by exocytosis. The membrane of the granule is subsequently recaptured by micropinocytosis. Once released into the circulation, the neurophysin no longer appears to have any physiological function. The distribution of vasopressin in neurosecretory granules within a rat neurohypophysis, demonstrated by immunocytochemical reactions that are specific for AVP, is shown in Fig. 5.7.

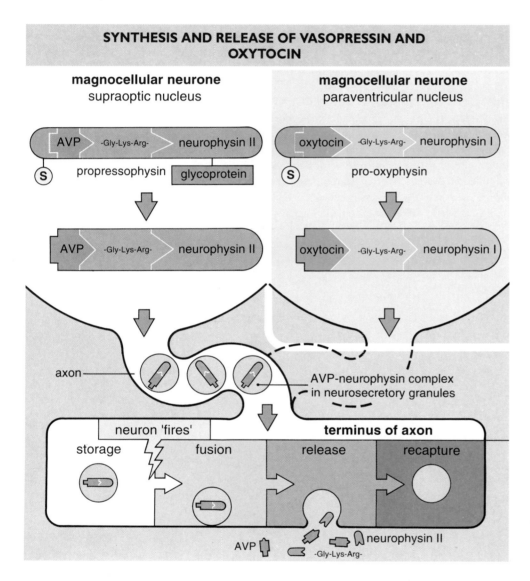

SYNTHESIS AND RELEASE OF VASOPRESSIN AND OXYTOCIN

Fig. 5.6 The synthesis and release of vasopressin and oxytocin. Vasopressin (AVP) and oxytocin are synthesised in the magnocellular neurones of the supraoptic and paraventricular nuclei. Each neurone synthesises either oxytocin or vasopressin. These peptides arise from the precursor molecules prooxyphysin and propressophysin, respectively. The neurophysin–nonapeptide groups migrate, in the form of neurosecretory granules, along the axons of the magnocellular neurones, to be stored at the ends of the neuronal tracts. When the neurones 'fire', the granules fuse with the axonal plasmalemma and each nonapeptide and its specific neurophysin are subsequently released separately. Once released, the neurophysin has no apparent physiological function.

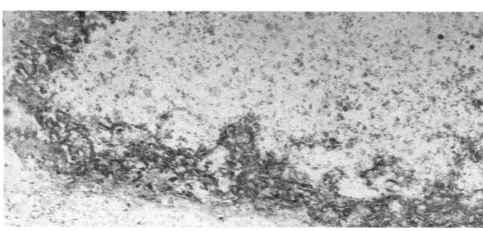

Fig. 5.7 A histological section of a rat neurohypophysis. The distribution of vasopressin in the form of neurosecretory granules is demonstrated by immunocytochemical reactions that are specific for AVP.

FUNCTIONS OF VASOPRESSIN AND OXYTOCIN

The functions of vasopressin and oxytocin are shown diagrammatically in Fig. 5.8. The main physiological role of vasopressin is the reduction of free-water clearance by the kidney to produce concentrated urine. Vasopressin acts on the distal nephron to increase water permeability of the tubular cell so that solute-free water may pass along the osmotic gradient from the lumen of the nephron to the renal interstitial medulla. At supraphysiological plasma concentrations, vasopressin contracts smooth muscle, resulting in pressor activity. Again at high concentrations, it activates liver glycogen phosphorylase to convert glycogen to glucose. Lipolysis is also increased. The secretion of vasopressin into the portal circulation of the hypothalamopituitary region, together with the secretion of corticotrophin-releasing factor from the median eminence, controls the release of adrenocorticotrophic hormone (ACTH) from the anterior pituitary gland. Recent studies suggest that intracerebral vasopressin may modify behaviour and improve memory in animals.

Oxytocin has no definite known role in men, although it may aid contraction of the seminal vesicles of the testis. In women, it contracts the pregnant uterus, although it is not the sole initiator of parturition. During lactation, oxytocin promotes milk ejection by contraction of smooth muscle in the breast ducts – an effect that is mediated by a neurohormonal reflex. Oxytocin also influences ovarian function. Like vasopressin, oxytocin is released from the median eminence and may affect the anterior pituitary. The response of gonadotrophins to the gonadotrophin-releasing hormone (GnRH) appears to be modified by oxytocin. There is tentative evidence to suggest that oxytocin increases lipolysis in the adipocyte and that it may affect cerebral function.

REGULATION OF VASOPRESSIN SECRETION

The factors that regulate vasopressin secretion have been clearly defined (Fig. 5.9), the major determinant being plasma osmolality. Different solutes, however, have varying abilities to stimulate vasopressin release. Sodium and mannitol appear to be the most potent solutes, while glucose has little or no effect on vasopressin secretion. Large quantities of vasopressin are released after marked hypotension, hypovolaemia, and vomiting. Angiotensin II and hypoglycaemia both appear to be specific stimuli of vasopressin secretion. Although many other factors have been reported to stimulate vasopressin release (e.g. pain, stress, profound emotion), it remains controversial whether vasopressin is a true stress hormone.

FACTORS REGULATING OXYTOCIN SECRETION

The factors that control oxytocin secretion in men and in nonpregnant, nonsuckling women are unclear (Fig. 5.10). Recent studies in animals show that osmotic stimulation releases oxytocin in similar quantities to vasopressin, but that the quantity of oxytocin released after haemorrhage is considerably smaller than the quantity of vasopressin released. Oxytocin secretion appears to increase with the duration of pregnancy, but the regulating factors that are involved

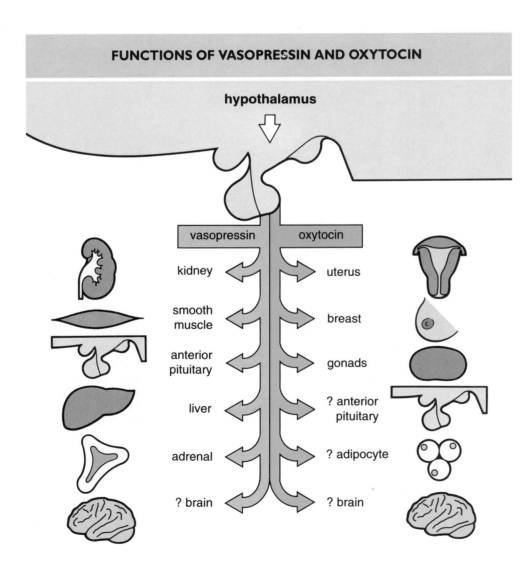

FUNCTIONS OF VASOPRESSIN AND OXYTOCIN

hypothalamus

vasopressin | oxytocin

kidney — uterus
smooth muscle — breast
anterior pituitary — gonads
liver — ? anterior pituitary
adrenal — ? adipocyte
? brain — ? brain

Fig. 5.8 The functions of vasopressin and oxytocin. The most important function of vasopressin is the reduction of free-water clearance by the kidney. At high concentrations, it contracts smooth muscle and initiates the conversion of glycogen to glucose in the liver. Secretion of vasopressin into the hypothalamopituitary circulation modulates the release of adrenocorticotrophic hormone (ACTH) from the anterior pituitary. Oxytocin aids contraction of the pregnant uterus and assists milk ejection during lactation. There is evidence that oxytocin may aid contraction of the seminal vesicles of the testis, may influence ovarian function, may have some effect in the anterior pituitary on the response of gonadotrophins to gonadotrophin-releasing hormone (GnRH), and may also increase lipolysis in the adipocyte.

are unknown. Suckling is a specific stimulus for oxytocin release. Plasma oxytocin concentrations rise to very high values at the end of parturition, release being stimulated by cervical dilatation (the Ferguson reflex).

Osmoregulation of Vasopressin Secretion and Thirst

Slow infusion of hypertonic saline into healthy individuals causes a linear increase in plasma osmolality, which in turn stimulates vasopressin release and thirst (Fig. 5.11). Conversely, a fall in plasma osmolality induced by an oral water load suppresses vasopressin secretion, with plasma concentrations becoming undetectable, and inhibits thirst. Under normal circumstances, healthy individuals maintain their plasma osmolality within the range 282–295mosmol/kg, with plasma vasopressin concentrations varying between 0.3 and 4pmol/l, thus allowing the formation of maximally dilute and concentrated urine, respectively.

The relationship between plasma vasopressin (pAVP) and plasma osmolality (pOS) is linear, the average regression line being defined by the function:

$$pAVP = 0.41 \, (pOS - 284), \quad r = 0.96, \quad P < 0.001.$$

The slope of the line is a measure of the sensitivity of the osmoreceptor and vasopressin-releasing unit. The abscissal intercept defines the mean theoretical threshold for vasopressin release. Using visual analogue scales to assess thirst, a similar linear relationship exists between plasma osmolality (pOS) and thirst (Th), defined by the function:

$$Th = 0.30 \, (pOS - 281), \quad r = 0.91, \quad P < 0.001.$$

The functional analysis of osmotically mediated vasopressin release is helpful in defining disorders of vasopressin secretion. Abnormalities in the sensitivity of the vasopressin-releasing unit and in the threshold of vasopressin secretion have been defined.

RELATIONSHIP BETWEEN PLASMA OSMOLALITY AND PLASMA VASOPRESSIN, AND BETWEEN PLASMA OSMOLALITY AND THIRST

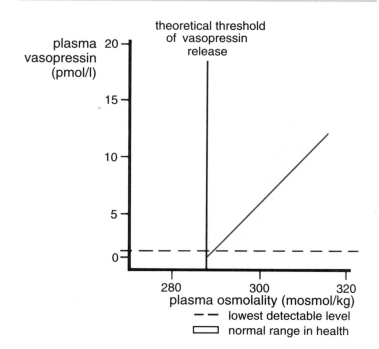

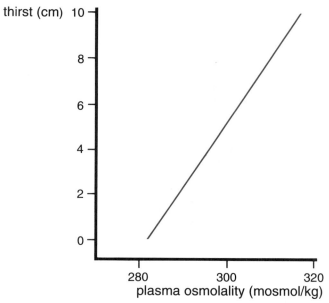

Fig. 5.11 The relationship between plasma osmolality and plasma vasopressin (upper), and between plasma osmolality and thirst (lower). Thirst is measured in arbitrary units along a linear scale. Plasma vasopressin rises in a linear fashion in response to increasing plasma osmolality. The abscissal intercept represents the theoretical threshold for vasopressin release, and the slope of the line represents the sensitivity of the osmoreceptor–vasopressin-synthesising unit. Healthy individuals maintain their plasma osmolality within the range 282–295mosmol/kg, with plasma vasopressin concentrations varying from 0.3–4pmol/l. There is a similar progressive increase in thirst sensation with rises in plasma osmolality.

FACTORS REGULATING VASOPRESSIN RELEASE

osmotic regulation	nonosmotic regulation
stimulatory solutes: sodium, mannitol, urea	haemodynamic: hypotension, hypovolaemia
nonstimulatory solutes: glucose	nausea and/or vomiting
	hypoglycaemia
	renin – angiotensin
	pain, stress, emotion?

Fig. 5.9 Factors regulating vasopressin release.

FACTORS REGULATING OXYTOCIN RELEASE

physiological regulation largely unknown

suckling

pregnancy and parturition

osmotic and haemodynamic factors?

Fig. 5.10 Factors regulating oxytocin release.

Baroregulation of vasopressin secretion

An acute fall in blood pressure or blood volume causes release of vasopressin. Whether hypertension or hypervolaemia affect vasopressin secretion is not known. The exponential rise in plasma vasopressin concentrations in response to progressive hypotension induced in healthy normal subjects by the infusion of the ganglion-blocking drug trimetaphan, over periods of fifteen to thirty minutes, is shown in Fig. 5.12. Similar large increases in the concentration of plasma vasopressin have been demonstrated in normal humans who have been rendered hypotensive after tilting, or hypovolaemic after phlebotomy.

Minor fluctuations in blood pressure appear to have very little effect on plasma vasopressin concentration. A fall in blood pressure of ten per cent or more must be attained before a significant rise in vasopressin is achieved. A forty per cent reduction in pressure, however, produces plasma vasopressin levels approximately one hundred times greater than the normal basal concentrations.

RENAL ACTION OF VASOPRESSIN

The major physiological function of vasopressin is the concentration of urine. The hormone binds to a specific receptor (V_2 receptor) on the contraluminal aspect of the tubular cells of the distal collecting duct of the nephron; its gene is on chromosome X, Xq28. Adenyl cyclase is activated to generate cAMP, which in turn stimulates a protein kinase, resulting in rearrangement of intracellular microtubules and microfilaments. Consequently, luminal tubular pores (water channels) open to allow hypotonic fluid in the nephron to flow across the cell into the hypertonic renal interstitium, thus concentrating the urine.

As the concentration of plasma vasopressin rises, a reduction in urine flow rate and an increase in urinary osmolality (Fig. 5.13) occur. Maximum antidiuresis occurs at plasma vasopressin concentrations of the order of 4pmol/l, while maximum diuresis in humans occurs with values of 0.5pmol/l or less.

CAUSES OF POLYURIA AND POLYDIPSIA

The only three basic disorders that can account for polyuria (arbitrarily defined as a persistent twenty-four-hour urine volume greater than 2.5l) and polydipsia (excessive thirst) are delineated in Fig. 5.14. These disorders are:
- Primary polydipsia.
- Cranial diabetes insipidus.
- Nephrogenic diabetes insipidus.

RELATIONSHIP BETWEEN MEAN ARTERIAL PRESSURE AND VASOPRESSIN RELEASE

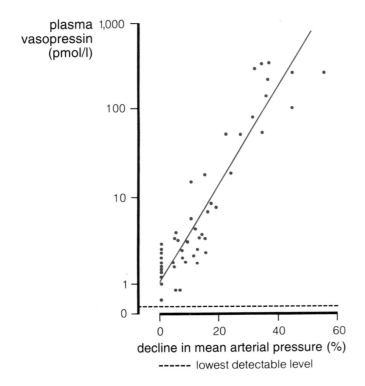

RELATIONSHIP BETWEEN PLASMA VASOPRESSIN CONCENTRATION AND URINE OSMOLALITY

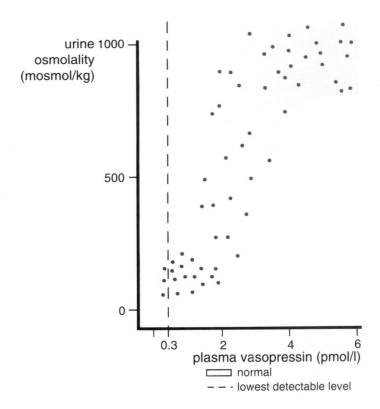

Fig. 5.12 The relationship between mean arterial pressure and vasopressin release. An acute fall in blood pressure or volume causes release of vasopressin. The graph shows the exponential rise in vasopressin in response to progressive hypotension induced (in normal subjects) by infusion of the ganglion-blocking drug trimetaphan over periods ranging from 15 to 30 minutes. Blood pressure must be reduced by at least ten per cent before any significant rise in vasopressin secretion occurs, although a forty per cent reduction in blood pressure leads to plasma vasopressin concentrations of some one hundred times the normal basal level.

Fig. 5.13 The relationship between plasma vasopressin concentration and urine osmolality. Maximum diuresis with minimal urine osmolality occurs in response to low or undetectable plasma vasopressin concentration. Maximum antidiuresis with maximal urine osmolality results from plasma vasopressin concentrations greater than 2–4pmol/l.

PRIMARY POLYDIPSIA

Primary polydipsia may occur for no apparent reason, but more often is related to some form of psychiatric illness. Mouth dryness caused by drugs (e.g. monoamine oxidase inhibitors) or mouth-breathing must be distinguished from true polydipsia. Vasopressin secretion is normally suppressed by the low plasma osmolality in primary polydipsia, but its renal action may also be impaired if excessive fluid intake is prolonged, since the solute concentration within the renal interstitial medulla is reduced by a 'washout' effect. This leads to a reduction in the osmotic gradient across the renal tubular cell. Thus, even when there is maximum tubular permeability under the action of vasopressin, free water is unable to flow normally from the lumen to the medulla and, consequently, urinary concentrating ability is impaired. Any cause of polyuria may result in this renal defect.

NEPHROGENIC DIABETES INSIPIDUS

Acquired nephrogenic diabetes insipidus is probably the most common cause of polyuria, particularly in association with the osmotic diuresis of diabetes mellitus. The hereditary, sex-linked form of nephrogenic diabetes insipidus is extremely rare. In all instances, there is resistance to the renal action of vasopressin and, consequently, plasma vasopressin is inappropriately high with respect to urine osmolality. Renal infection, postobstructive uropathy, vascular lesions, electrolyte disturbances (hypokalaemia and hypercalcaemia), amyloid, and sickle-cell anaemia are among the most common causes of nephrogenic diabetes insipidus.

CRANIAL DIABETES INSIPIDUS

Cranial diabetes insipidus is an uncommon condition characterised by an absolute, or (more often) a relative, lack of osmoregulated vasopressin. (The causes are listed in Fig. 5.15.) The majority of patients have measurable plasma vasopressin, but its concentration is inappropriately low for the concomitant plasma osmolality.

The familial forms of the disorder are very rare. It may be inherited as a dominant or recessive trait in patients with the isolated vasopressin deficiency. These patients become obviously polyuric in the

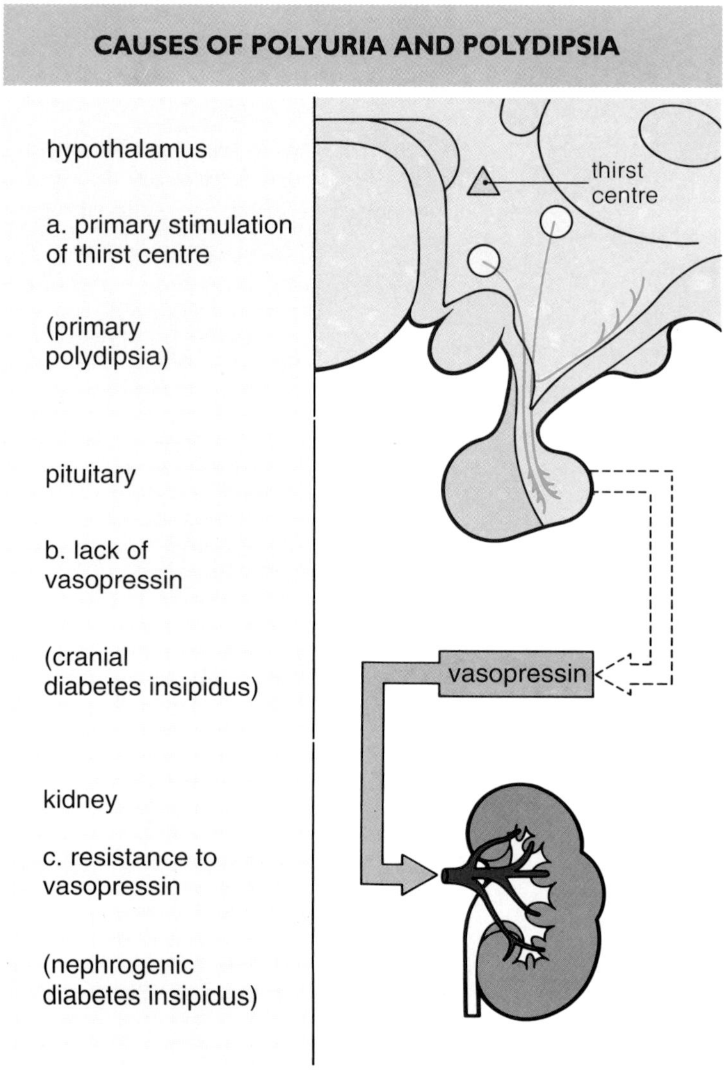

CAUSES OF POLYURIA AND POLYDIPSIA

hypothalamus

a. primary stimulation of thirst centre

(primary polydipsia)

thirst centre

pituitary

b. lack of vasopressin

(cranial diabetes insipidus)

vasopressin

kidney

c. resistance to vasopressin

(nephrogenic diabetes insipidus)

Fig. 5.14 The causes of polyuria and polydipsia. (a) Primary polydipsia is usually related to psychiatric illness. Vasopressin secretion is suppressed by low plasma osmolality induced by the excessive water intake which, if prolonged, may also affect the kidney. (b) Cranial diabetes insipidus is due to a shortage or absence of vasopressin. (c) In nephrogenic diabetes insipidus, there is resistance to the renal action of vasopressin, with a consequent rise in the plasma vasopressin concentration to a level that is inappropriately high relative to urine osmolality.

CAUSES OF CRANIAL DIABETES INSIPIDUS

familial

as isolated defect

or in association with diabetes mellitus, optic atrophy, nerve deafness, bladder and ureter atonia (DIDMOAD syndrome)

acquired

idiopathic (approx. 50% of patients)

trauma (head injury, surgery to hypothalamopituitary region)

rare

tumour (pituitary macroadenoma, craniopharyngioma, metastatic carcinoma)

granulomata (sarcoid, eosinophilic granuloma)

infection (pyogenic or tuberculous basal meningitis, encephalitis)

vascular (peripartum hypotension, aneurysm)

external irradiation

Fig. 5.15 The causes of cranial diabetes insipidus. All patients have polyuria and inappropriately low plasma vasopressin concentrations relative to their plasma osmolality. Idiopathic cranial diabetes insipidus may be due to autoimmune disease in some patients.

first year or two of life. Plasma vasopressin is undetectable under basal conditions, but it may be released following profound osmotic stimulation. The polyuria in patients with the DIDMOAD (diabetes insipidus, diabetes mellitus, optic atrophy, and [nerve] deafness) syndrome is less profound than in those with the isolated defect. No specific cause can be found for some fifty per cent of patients with acquired cranial diabetes insipidus, although approximately one-third of these patients may have circulating antibodies to the vasopressin-synthesising neurone, thus suggesting an autoimmune aetiology.

A pituitary tumour (or surgery to it) may cause cranial diabetes insipidus if there is injury to the hypothalamus or the upper part of the pituitary stalk; this accounts for a large proportion of cases. The other causes of cranial diabetes insipidus are rare.

All patients have a low or undetectable plasma vasopressin concentration in relation to their plasma osmolality.

THE WATER DEPRIVATION TEST

The water deprivation test has long been the 'cornerstone' for differentiating between the causes of polyuria. The protocol for a modified Dashe dehydration test, combined with an assessment of response to exogenous vasopressin, is shown in Figs 5.16 & 5.17. Patients with moderate or severe cranial diabetes insipidus are clearly distinguished from others by the observation of consistently hypotonic urine during fluid restriction, together with concentrated urine after the administration of exogenous vasopressin. Hypotonic urine following exogenous vasopressin strongly suggests nephrogenic diabetes insipidus. Interpretation of the water deprivation test is outlined in Fig. 5.18.

Difficulty is often experienced when differentiating between primary polydipsia, mild cranial diabetes insipidus and nephrogenic diabetes

WATER DEPRIVATION TEST

preparation of patient

fluid intake encouraged during night before test

light breakfast, no tea, coffee, alcohol or smoking for 12 hours before test

patient to be supervised throughout test

dehydration test

no fluids for 8 hours: allow only dry snacks

weigh patient hourly: consider stopping test if there is more than 3% loss of initial body weight

sample urine hourly to measure volume and osmolality

draw venous blood every 2 hours to measure plasma osmolality, and vasopressin if possible

patient to be supervised throughout test

Fig. 5.16 The procedure followed in preparation of the water deprivation test. In order to avoid excessive dehydration, patients must be encouraged to drink overnight before the test. They should also be closely supervised during the test, to prevent clandestine drinking.

WATER DEPRIVATION TEST

response to exogenous vasopressin

after period of dehydration (see Fig. 5.16) administer desmopressin 4μg intramuscularly

patient allowed to eat and drink, but avoid excessive fluid intake

sample urine at 3, 5 and 16 hours after desmopressin to measure volume and osmolality

draw venous blood at 5 and 16 hours after desmopressin to measure osmolality

patient to be supervised throughout test

Fig. 5.17 The test of response to exogenous vasopressin. This test should follow on immediately after fluid deprivation. Patients must avoid excessive fluid intake after injection of desmopressin to avoid sudden profound hyponatraemia.

insipidus. This is due to the fact that many polydipsic patients have a minor concentrating defect secondary to the solute loss from the renal interstitial medulla. Measurement of plasma vasopressin in response to osmotic stimulation, and the relationship of endogenous plasma vasopressin with urine osmolality after overnight dehydration, aids in the differentiation of these disorders.

The water deprivation test is difficult to perform correctly, unpleasant for the patient (who may drink surreptitiously during the test), and relies heavily on the patient's ability to empty the bladder completely. For these reasons, it is far from ideal. Furthermore, the stimulus to vasopressin secretion is a combination of hypertonicity and hypovolaemia, especially towards the end of the period of dehydration.

DIFFERENTIATION BETWEEN THE CAUSES OF POLYURIA

The most precise way to diagnose the three basic causes of polyuria rests on the measurement of plasma vasopressin, plasma osmolality, and urine osmolality after osmotic stimulation and/or dehydration. It can be seen in Fig. 5.19a that after infusion of five per cent hyper-

tonic saline, patients with cranial diabetes insipidus have values that fall to the right of the normal range, while those with primary polydipsia or nephrogenic diabetes insipidus remain in the normal range.

Nephrogenic diabetes insipidus (Fig. 5.19b) can be readily distinguished by the inappropriately high plasma vasopressin levels in relation to the low urine osmolality attained after dehydration.

Occasionally, polydipsic patients have features of nephrogenic diabetes insipidus. In such cases, one week's treatment with desmopressin restores the responsiveness of the renal tubule to endogenous vasopressin is restored. Indeed, these patients may even develop hyponatraemia because of persistent inappropriate drinking·in the presence of exogenous vasopressin. This observation has been recommended as the basis of a specific test for primary polydipsia.

TREATMENT OF CRANIAL DIABETES INSIPIDUS

Many patients with mild cranial diabetes insipidus (i.e. twenty-four-hour urine volume up to 4 litres) decide to have no therapy, and appear to remain well. These patients rely on their thirst mechanisms

INTERPRETATION OF RESULTS FROM WATER DEPRIVATION TEST

urine osmolality (mosmol/kg)		diagnosis
after dehydration	after desmopressin	
>750	>750	normal
<300	>750	CDI
<300	<300	NDI
300–750	<750	partial CDI, NDI or PP

Fig. 5.18 *The interpretation of results from the water deprivation test.* Results of many polyuric patients fall into the urine osmolality ranges of 300–750mosmol/kg after dehydration and to less than 750mosmol/kg after administration of desmopressin. The test, therefore, often fails to distinguish between partial forms of cranial diabetes insipidus (CDI) and nephrogenic diabetes insipidus (NDI), and primary polydipsia (PP).

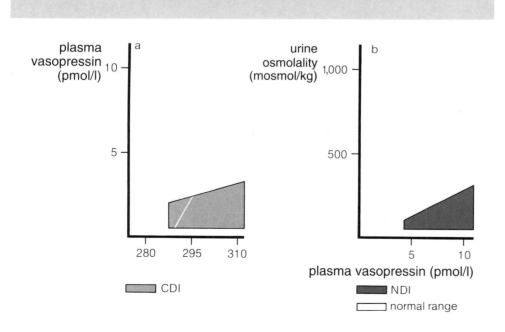

DIFFERENTIATING CAUSES OF POLYURIA

▢ CDI

▮ NDI
▢ normal range

Fig. 5.19 *Measurements used to differentiate between the causes of polyuria.* (a) After osmotic stimulation with five per cent hypertonic saline, patients with cranial diabetes insipidus (CDI) exhibit values to the right of the normal range, while those with nephrogenic diabetes insipidus (NDI) and primary polydipsia will show values within the normal limits. (b) After overnight dehydration, NDI is usually distinguishable from primary polydipsia by the inappropriately high levels of plasma vasopressin relative to urine osmolality.

to maintain water homeostasis. If an untreated patient is unable to obtain fluid or loses thirst awareness (e.g. is in a coma), the condition can be life-threatening. Furthermore, long-standing severe cranial diabetes insipidus can lead to hydroureter and hydronephrosis, and possibly to a degree of nephrogenic diabetes insipidus due to solute 'washout' from the kidney. There are therefore arguments for treating all patients whose urinary output exceeds 4 litres/24h.

Desmopressin, is a long-acting vasopressin analogue, is the treatment of choice (Fig. 5.20). In comparison with the native hormone, desmopressin has greater antidiuretic potency and little (if any) pressor activity. It can be administered intranasally, as a spray or by nasal tube, parenterally, or orally. Care must be taken to avoid overdosage since persistent antidiuresis with continual fluid intake will eventually lead to profound hyponatraemia. It is therefore wise to allow the patient to develop polyuria for a short period each week. Lysine vasopressin is a poor substitute for desmopressin because its therapeutic action lasts for only one to three hours and it retains pressor activity.

Although use of nonhormonal drugs (Fig. 5.20) has been recommended in the past, their high incidence of significant side effects and limited antidiuretic effect have restricted their use. Chlorpropamide

appears to act by increasing renal tubular sensitivity to circulating endogenous vasopressin, while carbamazepine probably increases vasopressin secretion. These drugs are suitable only for patients with partial cranial diabetes insipidus, who still secrete vasopressin but in insufficient quantities. The mechanism of action of thiazide diuretics is probably related to the reduction in extracellular sodium and decreased glomerular filtration. All oral preparations reduce the polyuria by twenty-five to fifty per cent.

THE SYNDROME OF INAPPROPRIATE ANTIDIURESIS

The syndrome of inappropriate antidiuresis (SIAD) is a common cause of hyponatraemia (Fig. 5.21); it falls into the category of normovolaemic (i.e. clinically normal extracellular volume) hyponatraemia. Although total water is increased in SIAD, it is not clinically demonstrable since water is distributed throughout intracellular and extracellular compartments. In contrast, hypervolaemic hyponatraemia is recognised by features of extracellular fluid overload, e.g.

TREATMENT OF CRANIAL DIABETES INSIPIDUS

vasopressin analogues		nonhormonal oral drugs	
desmopressin:		chlorpropamide	250–500mg daily
intranasal	5–60μg daily		
intramuscular	1–4μg daily	carbamazepine	200–400mg daily
oral	100–600μg daily	thiazide diuretic	
lysine vasopressin: intranasal	5–20 units daily	e.g. bendrofluazide	5mg daily

Fig. 5.20 *Drugs used in the treatment of cranial diabetes insipidus.* Desmopressin is the treatment of choice.

CLASSIFICATION OF HYPONATRAEMIA

type	hypervolaemic	normovolaemic	hypovolaemic
mechanism	extracellular sodium content increased body water greatly increased	extracellular sodium content normal body water increased	extracellular sodium content decreased body water slightly decreased
examples of causes	heart failure	SIAD	gastrointestinal losses
	cirrhosis	glucocorticoid deficiency	excessive sweating
	nephrotic syndrome	hypothyroidism	Addison's disease
	renal failure		renal salt wasting

Fig. 5.21 *Clinical classification of hyponatraemia.* The three groups are distinguished by differences in extracellular volume status. The syndrome of inappropriate diuresis (SIAD) is the most common cause of normovolaemic hyponatraemia.

dependent oedema and hypovolaemic hyponatraemia by signs of dehydration and hypotension. In all types of hyponatraemia there is an excess of water relative to extracellular sodium, and the three categories of hyponatraemia are distinguished by the extracellular sodium content. Examples of causes of the different types of hyponatraemia are given in Fig. 5.21.

The cardinal features of SIAD were described by Bartter and Schwartz (Fig. 5.22). These criteria must be fulfilled before a diagnosis of SIAD can be made. The measurement of plasma vasopressin does not aid the diagnosis of SIAD because over ninety per cent of all patients with hyponatraemia, irrespective of their extracellular volume status or underlying cause, have detectable or elevated vasopressin concentrations.

CAUSES OF SIAD

Many conditions have been described in association with the cardinal manifestations of SIAD (Fig. 5.23). Four main groups of disorders emerge: neoplastic, central nervous, respiratory, and drug related.

TYPES OF SIAD

Following extensive osmoregulatory studies of vasopressin secretion in hyponatraemic patients who all fulfilled the criteria for SIAD, four patterns of vasopressin secretion emerged (Fig. 5.24).

The first and most common pattern (type I), accounting for approximately forty per cent of patients with SIAD, is characterised by excessive and erratic vasopressin secretion that is totally unaffected by changes in plasma osmolality. Although neoplastic conditions

FEATURE OF THE SYNDROME OF INAPPROPRIATE ANTIDIURETIC HORMONE

hyponatraemia and hypotonicity of plasma

urine osmolality greater than plasma osmolality

excessive renal excretion of sodium

absence of volume depletion or oedema-forming states

normal renal and adrenal function

Fig. 5.22 Criteria for the diagnosis of SIAD. All criteria should be fulfilled before a diagnosis of SIAD can be made.

Fig. 5.23 Some causes of SIAD. The lists give a selection of the more common causes, and are not comprehensive.

CAUSES OF SIAD

tumours	drugs
carcinoma – especially of the lung	vasopressin
thymoma	oxytocin
lymphoma	vincristine
leukaemia	vinblastine
sarcoma	cyclophosphamide
mesothelioma	chlorpropamide
	carbamazepine
respiratory disorders	clofibrate
	thiazide diuretics
pneumonia	monoamine oxidase inhibitors
tuberculosis	phenothiazines
empyema	nicotine
pneumothorax	
asthma	
positive-pressure ventilation	
central nervous system disorders	**miscellaneous**
meningitis	psychosis
encephalitis	hypothyroidism
head injury	glucocorticoid deficiency
brain abscess	postoperative
brain tumour	idiopathic
subarachnoid haemorrhage	
cerebral thrombosis	
Guillain–Barré syndrome	
acute intermittent porphyria	

often demonstrate this pattern, many other causes of SIAD show the same abnormality. The pathogenesis of this type of defect is unknown, but several different mechanisms are possible. Ectopic production of vasopressin by neoplasms might be expected to cause random release. Rapidly fluctuating nonosmotic stimuli (e.g. hypotension) might also be responsible. Electrical instability of the neurogenic pathways that control vasopressin, or the neurohypophysis itself, is a further possible mechanism.

The type II pattern is the second most common osmoregulatory defect and has been termed the 'reset osmostat'. Patients with the type II defect continue to regulate water excretion about a lowered plasma osmolality. This pattern of vasopressin secretion is observed in patients with neoplasms, chest disease, and nervous disorders. The pathogenesis of the pattern remains unknown, but interruption of the afferent limb of the baroregulatory reflex arc that normally inhibits vasopressin secretion is one possible mechanism.

The type III defect is characterised by normal and appropriate osmoregulation of the hormone except under conditions of plasma hypotonicity when there is constant nonsuppressible vasopressin secretion. It is rarely seen in malignant disease. The abnormality may be due to a persistent 'leak' of vasopressin resulting from neurohypophysial damage, loss of inhibitory osmoregulatory neurones, or persistent nonosmotic stimulation.

Type IV is uncommon, accounting for less than ten per cent of all cases. Osmoregulated vasopressin secretion is entirely normal, yet patients still fulfil the criteria of SIAD. Antidiuretic hormones other than vasopressin (e.g. vasotocin) may be responsible. Alternatively, the defect may lie within the kidney.

TREATMENT OF SIAD

Asymptomatic or mild degrees of hyponatraemia due to SIAD may not require specific treatment. If therapy is deemed necessary, treatment of the underlying cause of SIAD may be sufficient to correct the hyponatraemia. Fluid restriction to 500ml/24h remains the mainstay of SIAD-induced hyponatraemia (Fig. 5.25). In the long-term management of SIAD, fluid restriction may be inconvenient or unpleasant for the patient, so administration of drugs that inhibit the renal action of vasopressin has been advocated. Demeclocycline is preferable to lithium since it is less toxic, but its maximum effect may take three weeks to achieve. Phenytoin may occasionally suppress abnormal vasopressin secretion from the pituitary. To date, there are no specific antidiuretic receptor (V_2) antagonists available for clinical use to block the renal action of vasopressin.

Isotonic or hypertonic saline infusion must be used with extreme caution to treat hyponatraemia and should be reserved for emergency situations such as associated fits, stupor, or marked confusion. Great care should be taken to avoid rapid correction of hyponatraemia, irrespective of the manner of treatment, or central pontine myelinolysis (osmotic demyelination syndrome) may ensue. The rate of increase in plasma sodium should not exceed 0.5mmol/l/h (12mmol/l/24h).

VASOPRESSIN LEVELS IN THE FOUR TYPES OF SIAD

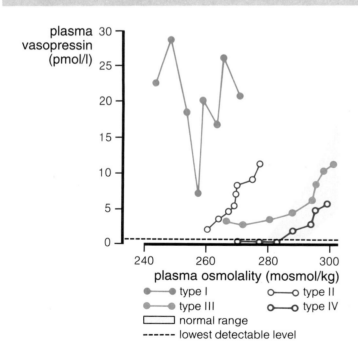

plasma vasopressin (pmol/l)

plasma osmolality (mosmol/kg)

●—● type I   ○—○ type II
●—● type III   ○—○ type IV
▭ normal range
----- lowest detectable level

Fig. 5.24 Vasopressin measurements found in the four types of SIAD. Type I SIAD accounts for some forty per cent of cases and is characterised by excessive and erratic vasopressin secretion unrelated to changes in plasma osmolality. Type II SIAD ('reset osmostat') is the second most common variant. Patients continue to regulate water excretion about a lowered plasma osmolality. Type III SIAD is characterised by normal osmoregulation of vasopressin except when the plasma is hypotonic, when there is constant and nonsuppressible vasopressin secretion. Type IV SIAD accounts for less than ten per cent of cases. Osmoregulation of vasopressin secretion is entirely normal and yet patients fulfil the criteria for SIAD.

TREATMENT OF THE SYNDROME OF INAPPROPRIATE ANTIDIURESIS

fluid restriction

500ml/24h or less (as long as plasma remains dilute)

drugs

induction of partial nephrogenic diabetes insipidus with demeclocycline or lithium

inhibition of vasopressin release by phenytoin or oxilorphan

induction of osmotic diuresis with oral urea

saline infusion

isotonic or hypertonic to be used in emergency situation only

infuse slowly; plasma sodium concentration should not increase more quickly than 0.5mmol/l/h

Fig. 5.25 Forms of management of SIAD. Long-term fluid restriction may be inconvenient and unpleasant for the patient; drug therapy may be a more useful solution. Hypertonic saline infusion should be used only in emergencies.

6

Lipids and Lipoproteins

Alan Chait, MD

John D Brunzell, MD

CLINICAL SIGNIFICANCE OF LIPIDS AND LIPOPROTEINS

Hyperlipidaemia, defined as an increase in levels of plasma cholesterol or triglyceride, or of both, is one of the most common metabolic disorders that occurs in industrialised societies. It results from genetic and acquired derangements in the metabolism of plasma lipoproteins. The major significance of hyperlipidaemia, particularly hypercholesterolaemia, is that it is one of the main risk factors for the development of premature atherosclerotic complications (Fig. 6.1), with the principal lipoprotein-related cardiovascular risk factors being increased levels of low-density lipoproteins (LDL) and low levels of high-density lipoproteins (HDL). The role of hypertriglyceridaemia as a risk factor is more complex and may be related more to the cause, rather than to the extent, of the condition (see below).

Recognition and treatment of the atherogenic disorders of lipoprotein metabolism can be of value in the prevention of atherosclerosis, and in some cases, can even result in regression of established lesions. The diagnosis and management of disorders of lipoproteins require an understanding of lipoprotein structure, function, and metabolism.

LIPOPROTEIN PHYSIOLOGY

LIPOPROTEIN STRUCTURE

Lipoproteins are composed of a central core in which the more lipophilic components, cholesterol esters and triglycerides, are sequestered from the aqueous environment of plasma by a surface comprised of unesterified (free) cholesterol, phospholipids, and

apolipoproteins (Fig. 6.2). These components exist in distinct proportions in the different lipoprotein classes, thereby permitting their separation by operational means such as ultracentrifugation and electrophoresis. There is, however, considerable heterogeneity within each lipoprotein class (Fig. 6.3). Several apolipoproteins are found in the different lipoprotein classes (see Figs 6.2 & 6.3), each having three major functions: structural; as ligands for receptors; and as enzyme cofactors.

LIPOPROTEIN FUNCTION

As can be deduced from their structure, lipoproteins sequester lipids during their transport through plasma. Triglycerides are transported from sites of synthesis and absorption, to sites of utilisation and storage. Cholesterol is transported to cells of the body where it forms part of critical structural components of cell membranes (all cells), or is used for bile acid synthesis (liver), for steroidogenesis (adrenals, gonads), and as a precursor for vitamin D (skin). These functions are achieved by the exogenous (Fig. 6.4) and endogenous (Fig. 6.5) metabolic pathways of lipoprotein metabolism and by the metabolism of HDL.

LIPOPROTEIN METABOLISM
Exogenous Pathway

Apo CII is a cofactor for lipoprotein lipase (LPL), an enzyme that hydrolyses the triglycerides in the triglyceride-rich lipoproteins, leading to the formation of partially triglyceride-depleted chylomicron remnants. Free fatty acids that are liberated by the action of LPL are taken up and re-esterified for storage as triglycerides in adipose tissue

MAJOR CARDIOVASCULAR RISK FACTORS	
Modifiable	**Fixed**
hypercholesterolaemia	age
hypertriglyceridaemia*	male gender
low HDL*	family history*
hypertension*	
cigarette smoking	
diabetes*	

* often associated with central obesity and insulin resistance

Fig. 6.1 Major cardiovascular risk factors.

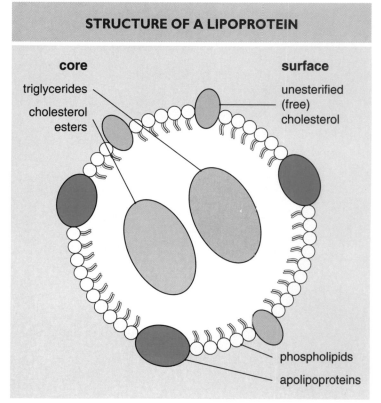

STRUCTURE OF A LIPOPROTEIN

core — triglycerides, cholesterol esters

surface — unesterified (free) cholesterol, phospholipids, apolipoproteins

Fig. 6.2 The structure of a lipoprotein particle. The central core contains the more lipophilic components – triglycerides and cholesterol esters – which are sequestered from the aqueous environment of plasma by a surface layer of free cholesterol, phospholipids, and apolipoproteins.

COMPOSITION OF THE MAJOR CLASSES OF LIPOPROTEINS

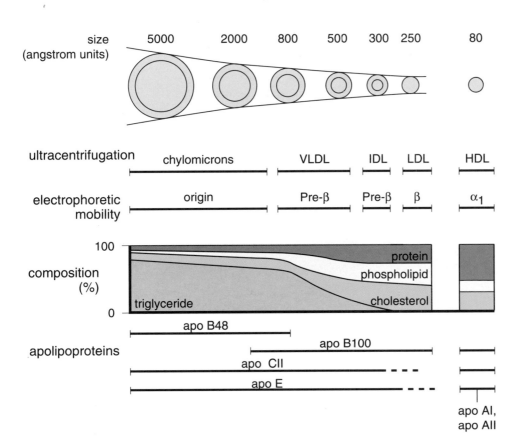

Fig. 6.3 The composition of the major classes of plasma lipoproteins. Although each of the lipoproteins is distinct with respect to its relative proportions of cholesterol, triglycerides, phospholipids and apolipoproteins, considerable heterogeneity exists within each lipoprotein class. Lipoproteins are graded according to their density: very low (VLDL), low (LDL), intermediate (IDL) or high (HDL).

EXOGENOUS PATHWAY OF LIPOPROTEIN METABOLISM

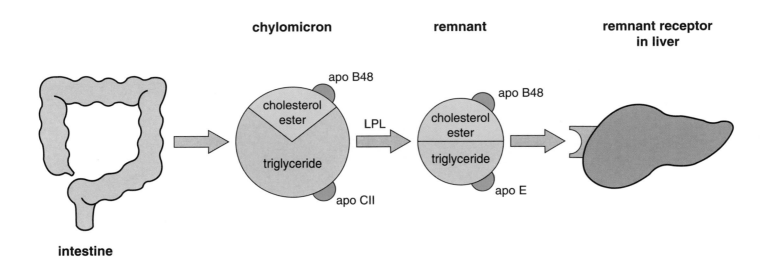

Fig. 6.4 The exogenous pathway of lipoprotein metabolism. Chylomicrons are formed in response to the consumption of dietary fat. They subsequently enter plasma where their triglyceride component is hydrolysed by LPL. The triglyceride-depleted chylomicron remnant is taken up by receptors on the liver, which recognise apo E.

(Fig. 6.6). The chylomicron remnants then lose apo CII and acquire apo E, which is shuttled to and from HDL (see below). Apo E mediates the binding of chylomicron remnants to chylomicron remnant receptors on the liver. The remnants then deliver cholesterol to the hepatocyte for synthesis of bile acid and very low-density lipoproteins (VLDLs).

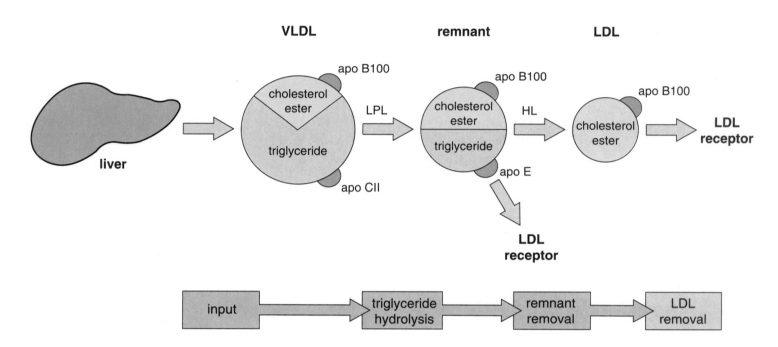

ENDOGENOUS PATHWAY OF LIPOPROTEIN METABOLISM

Fig. 6.5 The endogenous pathway of lipoprotein metabolism. VLDL particles enter plasma after being secreted by the liver, and VLDL triglycerides are hydrolysed by lipoprotein lipase (LPL). Some VLDL remnants are taken up and degraded by the liver, while others are converted into LDL.

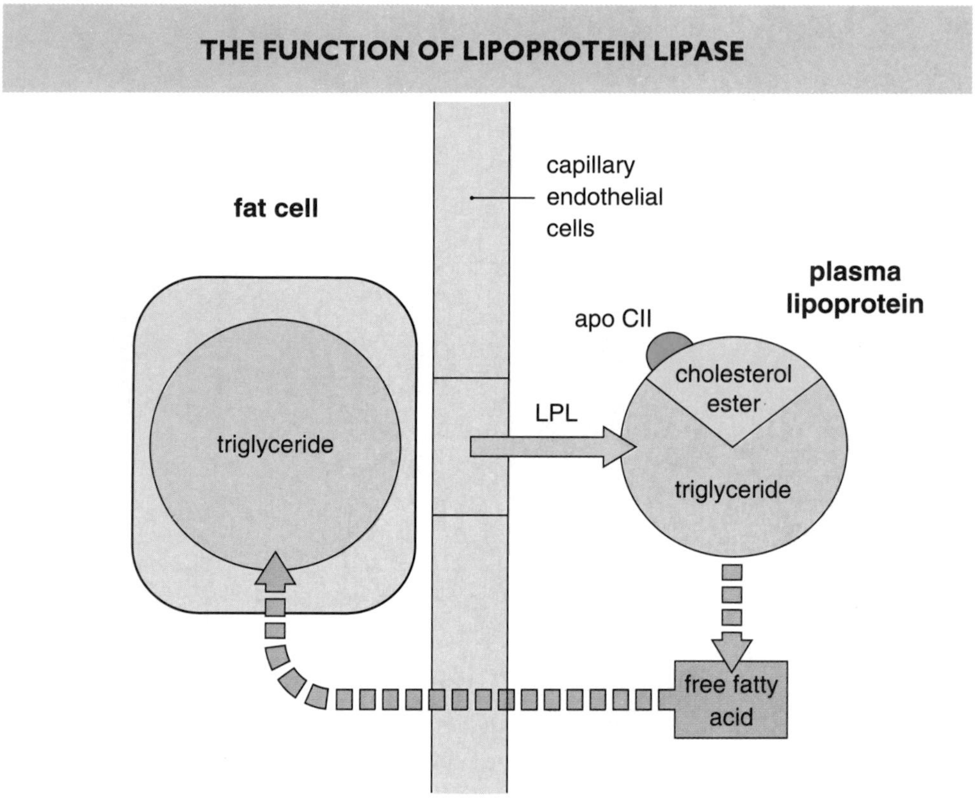

THE FUNCTION OF LIPOPROTEIN LIPASE

Fig. 6.6 The function of lipoprotein lipase LPL works on the luminal side of endothelial cells where it hydrolyses triglycerides in chylomicrons and VLDL particles. The free fatty acids that are liberated are translocated into adipocytes where they are re-esterified to form fat droplets.

Endogenous Pathway

In the liver, VLDL particles are formed using triglyceride that is synthesised from circulating free fatty acids or from those that are newly formed by lipogenesis. VLDL-cholesterol is derived largely from cholesterol that is delivered in chylomicron remnants. VLDL particles combine with apo B100, their major structural apolipoprotein, and are subsequently secreted into plasma (see Fig. 6.5). There they acquire apo CII, undergo triglyceride hydrolysis by LPL, and become remnant particles that acquire apo E in a similar manner to that described in the exogenous pathway. Some VLDL remnants are taken up and can be degraded by the liver after their apo E component binds to the LDL receptor (rather than to the chylomicron remnant receptor as occurs with chylomicron remnants). Other VLDL remnants are converted into LDL (see Fig. 6.5) by a process that is not well understood, but which probably involves another lipase, hepatic triglyceride lipase. A single molecule of apo B100 is present in each particle in this metabolic cascade. The apo B in LDL binds to LDL receptors on cells throughout the body, thereby supplying them with cholesterol when required. The major site of LDL metabolism is the liver, where the level of expression of LDL receptors largely determines the rate of catabolism of plasma LDL.

High-density Lipoprotein Metabolism

HDL is synthesised in the liver and intestines and secreted as bilayers of apo AI, apo AII and phospholipid. HDL acquires cholesterol from two major sources. During the catabolic pathways described earlier, lipoprotein surface components (particularly unesterified cholesterol) that become redundant as the particle size decreases are transferred to HDL. Additionally, excess cellular cholesterol is picked up by lipophilic particles. The cholesterol is subsequently esterified by the enzyme lecithin-cholesterol acyltransferase (LCAT). The hydrophobic cholesterol ester that results moves into the core of the HDL particle, leading to the formation of a spherical particle (Fig. 6.7). Cholesterol ester transfer protein (CETP) mediates transfer of cholesterol esters

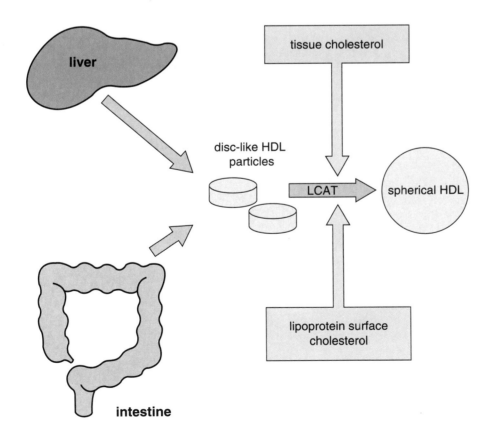

THE FORMATION OF HIGH-DENSITY LIPOPROTEIN

liver

tissue cholesterol

disc-like HDL particles

LCAT

spherical HDL

lipoprotein surface cholesterol

intestine

Fig. 6.7 The formation of high-density lipoprotein. Surface cholesterol that is made redundant during lipoprotein metabolism, and excess tissue cholesterol, is taken up by disc-like HDL particles that are secreted from the liver and intestine. Cholesterol esters that are formed as a result of LCAT activity enter the core of the HDL particle, which then becomes spherical.

to VLDL and LDL, which can then acquire apo E from HDL. Apo E is a ligand for hepatic lipoprotein receptors, which allows cholesterol to be delivered to the liver from where it can be secreted. This process is known as reverse cholesterol transport (Fig. 6.8).

In addition, apolipoproteins are shuttled between HDL and the triglyceride-rich lipoproteins in response to metabolic needs. Thus, the nascent triglyceride-rich lipoproteins acquire apo CII from HDL to form mature triglyceride-rich lipoproteins. Following LPL-mediated

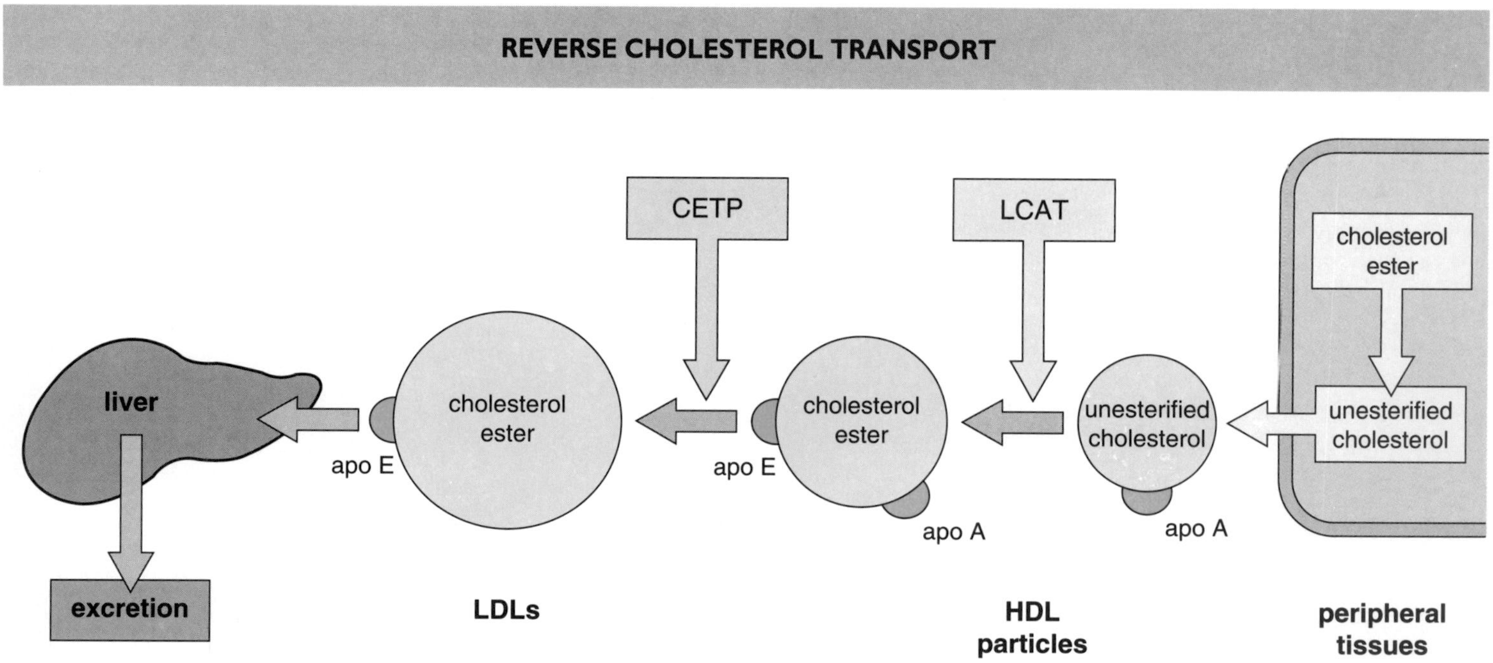

REVERSE CHOLESTEROL TRANSPORT

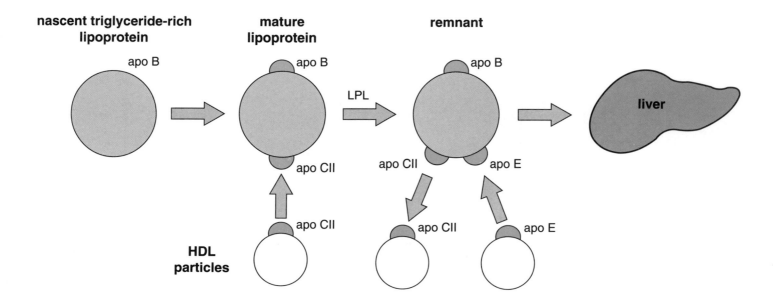

Fig. 6.8 Reverse cholesterol transport. Excess unesterified cellular cholesterol from cells is picked up by HDL particles and esterified by LCAT. The cholesterol esters in HDL are transferred to lower-density lipoproteins (VLDL and LDL) by CETP. These lipoproteins deliver cholesterol by apo-E-mediated mechanisms to the liver, from where they can be excreted.

SHUTTLING OF APOLIPOPROTEINS BY HIGH-DENSITY LIPOPROTEINS

Fig. 6.9 Shuttling of apolipoproteins by high-density lipoproteins. Nascent HDL particles mature after acquiring apo CII from HDL. Apo CII then activates LPL and is subsequently shuttled back to HDL. Apo E, which is then shuttled from HDL to remnant lipoproteins, is used for remnant uptake by hepatic receptors.

hydrolysis of triglycerides, apo CII, which is no longer required by the remnant lipoprotein, transfers back to HDL, which then donates the apo E required for hepatic remnant uptake (Fig. 6.9).

PATHOPHYSIOLOGY

Acquired and genetic forms of hyperlipidaemia can occur as a result of disturbances at four main sites in the endogenous pathway: increased input of VLDL and impaired LPL-mediated triglyceride

ACQUIRED FORMS OF HYPERLIPIDAEMIA		
VLDL	**Combined VLDL and/or LDL**	**LDL**
diabetes	hypothyroidism	anorexia
uraemia	nephrotic syndrome	fibrates
beta-blockers	diuretics	
alcohol	glucocorticoids	
oestrogens		
retinoids		
resins		

Fig. 6.10 Acquired forms of hyperlipidaemia.

removal can cause hypertriglyceridaemia; impaired remnant removal results in a combined elevation of cholesterol and triglyceride levels of approximately equal extent; and accumulation of LDL due to impaired LDL receptor-mediated clearance leads to hypercholesterolaemia.

ACQUIRED (SECONDARY) HYPERLIPIDAEMIA
Several underlying disorders or drugs can lead to disturbances at four major sites of regulation of lipoprotein metabolism. Acquired hyperlipidaemia tends to manifest either as hypertriglyceridaemia alone or as combined elevations of cholesterol and triglyceride levels (Fig. 6.10). It usually responds to treatment of the underlying condition, where possible, or to discontinuation of the responsible drug.

GENETIC FORMS OF HYPERLIPIDAEMIA
Very Low-density Lipoprotein Overproduction
Two major genetic forms of hyperlipidaemia result from increased VLDL – input familial hypertriglyceridaemia and familial combined hyperlipidaemia. In the former condition the VLDL particles that enter plasma are large and triglyceride-enriched, while in the latter they are smaller and less rich in triglycerides.

The primary defect in familial hypertriglyceridaemia is overproduction of cholic acid, which is related to increased hepatic triglyceride synthesis. In familial combined hyperlipidaemia this defect is unknown, although the disorder is characterised by overproduction of apo B (Fig. 6.11): apo B is overproduced in VLDL, leading primarily to hypertriglyceridaemia; occasionally in LDL, leading primarily to hypercholesterolaemia; and occasionally in both VLDL and LDL, leading to combined elevations of cholesterol and triglyceride

PATHOPHYSIOLOGICAL DEFECTS IN FAMILIAL HYPERTRIGLYCERIDAEMIA AND FAMILIAL COMBINED HYPERLIPIDAEMIA

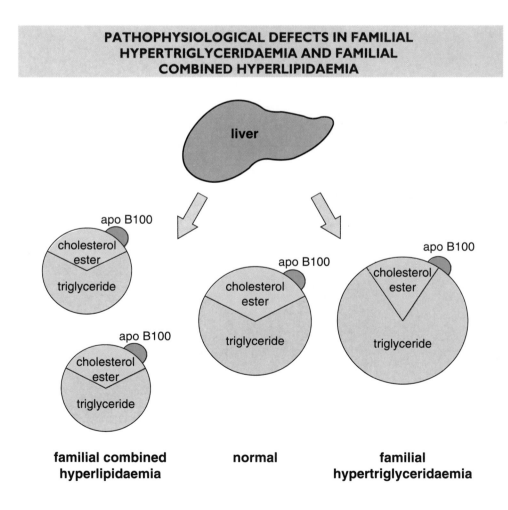

familial combined hyperlipidaemia   **normal**   **familial hypertriglyceridaemia**

Fig. 6.11 Pathophysiological defects in familial hypertriglyceridaemia and familial combined hyperlipidaemia.
Familial hypertriglyceridaemia is primarily due to overproduction of triglycerides, whereas familial combined hyperlipidaemia is primarily characterised by increased production of apo B. Both lead to an increased input of VLDL into plasma, although the composition of the VLDL particles differs in the two disorders.

levels. Thus, affected family members with familial hypertriglyceridaemia all have hypertriglyceridaemia, whereas affected individuals from families with familial combined hyperlipidaemia may have hypercholesterolaemia alone, hypertriglyceridaemia alone, or elevations of cholesterol and triglyceride levels (Fig. 6.12). The lipoprotein pattern in individuals with familial combined hyperlipidaemia frequently changes.

While some individuals with familial hypertriglyceridaemia may be at increased risk of atherosclerosis, most do not appear to be so. Conversely, familial combined hyperlipidaemia markedly increases cardiovascular risk. Both disorders are probably heterogeneous but further classification must await a better understanding of their pathogenetic mechanisms.

A common gene has been proposed to be associated with LDL particles that are small and dense (phenotype B), which is distinct from phenotype A where the particles are larger and more buoyant (Fig. 6.13). Small, dense LDL particles are found in association with high-to-normal plasma triglyceride levels, increased levels of remnant lipoproteins, and reduced levels of a subclass of HDL. The genotype may interact with other genes that raise levels of lipids and apo B, to cause familial combined hyperlipidaemia.

Lipoprotein Lipase Defects

Multiple mutations have now been described which impair the action of LPL. These include mutations in which there is no functional protein, defects that result in the production of nonfunctional enzyme, and mutations that result in the formation of an enzyme that does not bind normally to glycosaminoglycans on endothelial cells (the normal site of action of LPL). Rarely, defective LPL function results from a mutation in the gene for apo CII, which is a necessary cofactor for LPL (see Fig. 6.6). These defects usually result in marked hypertriglyceridaemia in early childhood due to the inability to hydrolyse triglycerides in ingested milk. Occasionally, affected individuals present for the first time in adult life.

Genetic defects in LPL or apo CII result in grossly impaired clearance of exogenous and endogenous triglycerides and the features of the chylomicronaemia syndrome (see later).

Remnant Removal Disease

Genetic defects in remnant catabolism are uncommon and result from mutations in the apo E gene. Multiple mutations have been described, although arginine–cysteine substitution at residue 158 of the gene is the most common. Most of the mutations described result in a charge change that can be detected by isoelectric focusing. More recently, polymerase chain reaction (PCR) techniques have been used to characterise defects in apo E.

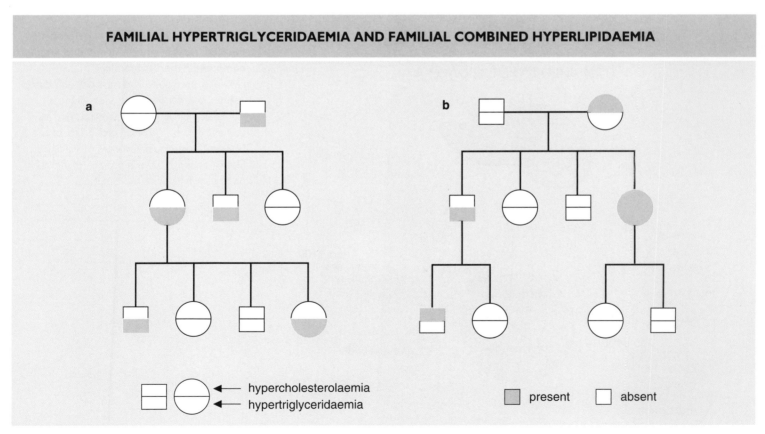

FAMILIAL HYPERTRIGLYCERIDAEMIA AND FAMILIAL COMBINED HYPERLIPIDAEMIA

hypercholesterolaemia
hypertriglyceridaemia

present   absent

Fig. 6.12 Pedigree of families with familial hypertriglyceridaemia and familial combined hyperlipidaemia. All affected individuals with familial hypertriglyceridaemia have hypertriglyceridaemia alone (a), while affected individuals from a family with familial combined hyperlipidaemia have hypercholesterolaemia alone, hypertriglyceridaemia alone, or elevations of both cholesterol and triglyceride level (b).

Although most cases of remnant removal disease result from inheritance of an abnormal gene from both parents, autosomal dominant forms of apo E defects have also been described. Remnant removal disease occurs as a result of a combination of a defect in the apo E gene, leading to a defect in apo E structure, and an abnormality leading to VLDL overproduction (for example, familial combined hyperlipidaemia or occasionally diabetes mellitus) (Fig. 6.14). The disorder is also known as broad-beta disease because of the electrophoretic appearance of the remnant accumulation, dysbetalipoproteinaemia, and type III hyperlipoproteinaemia. Very rarely, a total absence of apo E will result in remnant removal disease.

Low-density Lipoprotein-cholesterol Removal

Genetic defects of LDL-cholesterol removal are relatively common, occurring in approximately one in five hundred of the population. Many mutations have been described at the LDL-receptor gene locus, leading to the clinical manifestations of familial hypercholesterolaemia. These mutations, when inherited from one parent, result in approximately a fifty per cent reduction in LDL-receptor activity, known as heterozygous familial hypercholesterolaemia. Very occasionally (roughly one in a million cases), an individual inherits an abnormal gene for the LDL receptor from both parents, leading to homozygous familial hypercholesterolaemia in which there are essentially no functional LDL receptors. This situation is associated with very high levels of LDL and very accelerated atherosclerotic complications.

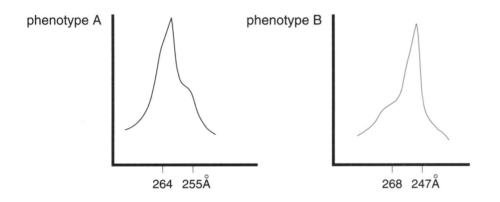

PARTICLE SIZE DISTRIBUTION OF LOW-DENSITY LIPOPROTEINS

phenotype A   phenotype B

264   255Å   268   247Å

Fig. 6.13 Particle size distribution of low-density lipoproteins. LDL particle size and density have been measured by nondenaturing gradient gel electrophoresis. Particle size distribution falls into two major patterns: large, buoyant LDL particles are characteristic of phenotype A, while smaller, more dense particles are characteristic of phenotype B.

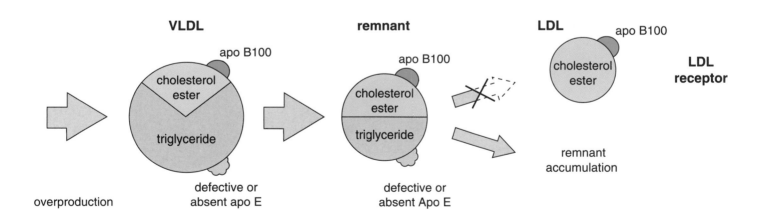

PATHOPHYSIOLOGY OF REMNANT REMOVAL DISEASE

VLDL   remnant   LDL

apo B100   apo B100   apo B100

cholesterol   cholesterol   cholesterol   LDL
ester   ester   ester   receptor

triglyceride triglyceride

overproduction   defective or   defective or   remnant
                 absent apo E   absent Apo E   accumulation

Fig. 6.14 Pathophysiology of remnant removal disease. For hyperlipidaemia to occur, there must be overproduction of VLDL, and the apo E structure must be absent or defective.

Recently, a genetic mutation of apo B, which also results in defective removal of LDL via the LDL-receptor pathway, has been described. The frequency of familial defective apo B is somewhat less than familial hypercholesterolaemia. The condition results in an identical clinical picture to that seen in heterozygous familial hypercholesterolaemia.

Hyper-apo B

Several genetic disorders can lead to increased levels of plasma apo B (apo B100), which can now be measured by immunochemical techniques. Such disorders include familial hypercholesterolaemia, familial defective apo B, and familial combined hyperlipidaemia.

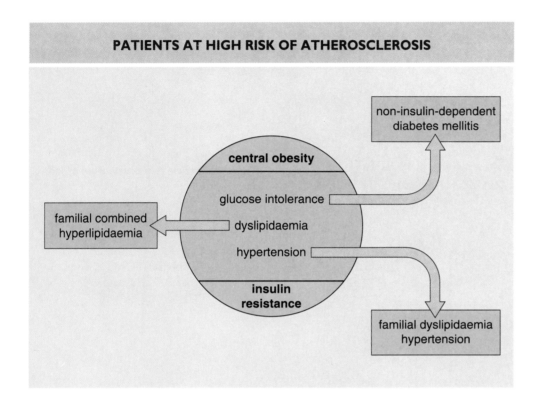

PATIENTS AT HIGH RISK OF ATHEROSCLEROSIS

Fig. 6.15 Glucose intolerance, dyslipidaemia, and hypertension relationships in individuals at high risk of atherosclerosis. A feature common to all of these conditions is the presence of central obesity and insulin resistance.

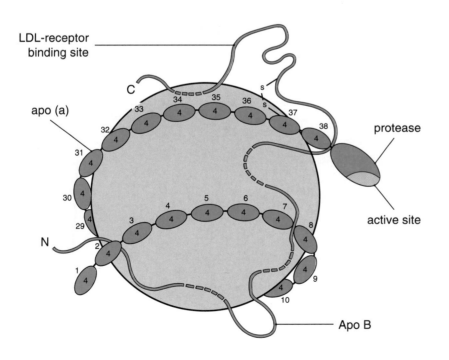

STRUCTURE OF Lp (a)

Fig. 6.16 The structure of Lp(a). Lp(a) consists of a particle that resembles LDL in structure and composition but which has an additional apolipoprotein, apo (a), attached to apo B by a disulphide bond.

Small, dense LDL particles are often found, together with high-to-normal triglyceride levels, modest increases in remnant lipoproteins, decreased levels of HDL, and elevated levels of apo B. This 'dyslipidaemic' pattern is quite common and occurs in association with central obesity and often with hypertension and insulin resistance (and occasionally non-insulin-dependent diabetes) to yield a very atherogenic group of disorders (Fig. 6.15). Apo B levels can also be increased as a result of excessive levels of Lp(a), a lipoprotein that consists of apo (a) in disulfide linkage with LDL (Fig. 6.16). The source, fate, and precise function of Lp(a) are not yet known, although the primary determinant of Lp(a) levels appears to be genetic. Apo (a) has considerable structural homology with plasminogen. Lp(a) may therefore play a physiological role in modulating fibrinolysis; high levels are associated with an increased risk of atherosclerosis.

GENETIC AND ACQUIRED FORMS OF HYPERLIPIDAEMIA
Occasionally, genetic and acquired forms of hyperlipidaemia coexist in the same patient, thereby resulting in hyperlipidaemia of a greater degree than would result from each alone. This is particularly important with respect to the several common genetic and acquired conditions that can affect triglyceride secretion and removal from plasma. The coexistence of genetic and acquired disorders at these sites can saturate LPL. The removal of further chylomicrons that enter plasma is thereby impaired, resulting in extremely elevated triglyceride levels with unique consequences (see later).

CLINICAL MANIFESTATIONS OF HYPERLIPIDAEMIA

There are three main clinical manifestations of hyperlipidaemia: increased clinical consequences of atherosclerosis; cutaneous manifestations of hyperlipidaemia; and the chylomicronaemia syndrome that can occur when chylomicrons accumulate chronically.

INCREASED ATHEROSCLEROSIS RISK
There is consensus that elevated plasma LDL levels and reduced HDL levels are associated with an increased atherosclerosis risk. The role of hypertriglyceridaemia as a cardiovascular risk factor is more complex. Hypertriglyceridaemia may be a marker for other lipoprotein abnormalities such as increased levels of LDL, the presence of an LDL subclass phenotype B, low levels of HDL, or remnant accumulation. When associated with familial combined hyperlipidaemia, with the small, dense LDL phenotype, and with diabetes mellitus, hypertriglycerdaemia appears also to be associated with increased cardiovascular risk. However, other forms may not be associated with increased cardiovascular risk.

The precise mechanisms whereby increased levels of LDL result in increased atherosclerosis risk is unclear. Recent studies, however, have suggested that LDL needs to be modified, especially oxidatively, before it can become atherogenic. Oxidised LDL has many biological properties that may cause it to become atherogenic (Fig. 6.17). The antiatherogenic properties of HDL are probably related to its postulated role in reverse cholesterol transport.

XANTHOMATA AND OTHER EXTERNAL MANIFESTATIONS
Several forms of xanthomata give important clinical clues to the nature of the underlying pathophysiological defect. Thus, tendon xanthomata typically occur in familial hypercholesterolaemia and in familial defective apo B. Their presence in the Achilles tendons (Fig. 6.18) or the extensor tendons of the hand (Fig. 6.19) is pathognomonic of genetic defects in interactions of LDL with its receptor.

OXIDISED LPL AND ATHEROGENESIS

cytotoxicity

stimulation of monocyte adhesion to endothelium

stimulation of monocyte chemotaxis

stimulation of colony-stimulating factor expression

foam cell formation

modulation of growth factor and cytokine expression

inhibition of endothelial-derived relaxation
  factor-mediated vasodilatation

stimulation of tissue-factor expression

Fig. 6.17 Biological effects of oxidised LPL which may affect atherogenesis.

Fig. 6.18 Achilles tendon xanthomata.

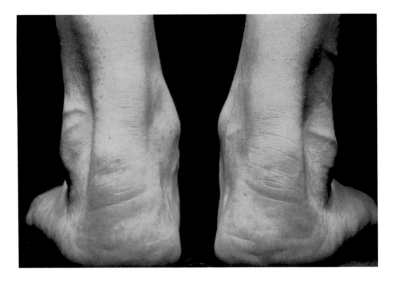

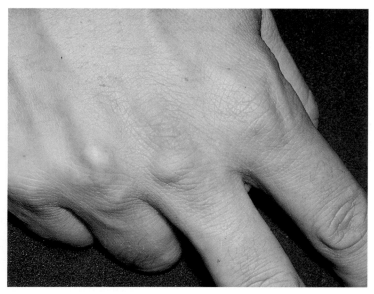

Fig. 6.19 Xanthomata on the extensor tendons of the hands.

Occasionally, xanthomata are seen on the patellar tendon. Since xanthomata are often subtle, careful examination of these sites is required for their detection. Eruptive xanthomata (Fig. 6.20) are indicative of chronic and long-standing chylomicronaemia. They occur most frequently on the buttocks and the extensor surfaces of the upper limb, only rarely being found on the face, soles, and palms. Palmar or planar xanthomata (Fig. 6.21) are pathognomonic for remnant removal disease, which can also can manifest with tuberoeruptive xanthomata (Fig. 6.22). Palmar xanthomata may be difficult to see and should be carefully sought using good lighting.

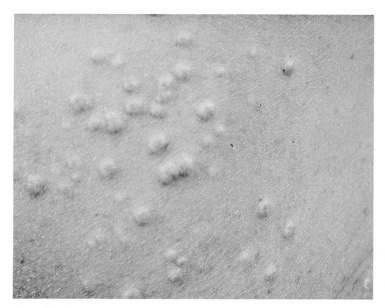

Fig. 6.20 Eruptive xanthomata on the buttocks. Note the erythematous base around the raised xanthomata.

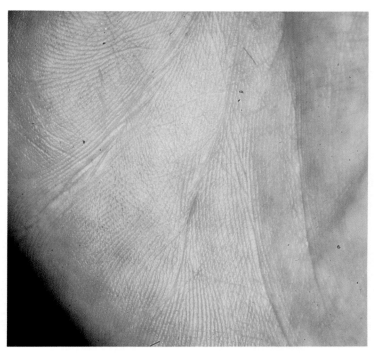

Fig. 6.21 Palmar or planar xanthomata.

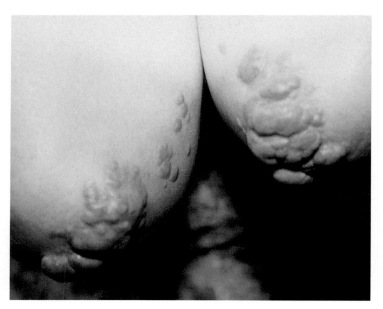

Fig. 6.22 Tuberoeruptive xanthomata of the elbow. The pink colour of these xanthomata is characteristically seen in remnant removal disease.

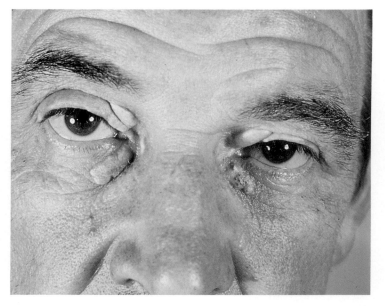

Fig. 6.23 Xanthelasma.

Several other external manifestations of hyperlipidaemia are more nonspecific but should, nonetheless, alert the clinician to the possibility that disorders of lipoprotein metabolism may have occurred. These include the presence of xanthelasma and corneal arcus. Xanthelasma (Fig. 6.23) can occur in familial hypercholesterolaemia, diabetes, and chronic obstructive liver disease, and may even signify more subtle abnormalities of plasma lipoproteins, such as those seen in apo E or hyper-apo B. Early corneal arcus is seen superiorly and inferiorly in the eyes and later becomes totally circumferential (Fig. 6.24). Arcus occurs fairly frequently in the elderly (arcus senilis). Its presence before the age of fifty warrants evaluation of plasma lipids and lipoproteins.

CHYLOMICRONAEMIA SYNDROME

A constellation of signs and symptoms, the chylomicronaemia syndrome, occurs in association with long-standing chylomicronaemia (Fig. 6.25). The most important consequence is acute pancreatitis, which is often recurrent. Pancreatitis is believed to be due to the release of free fatty acids and lysolecithin from chylomicrons in the capillaries of the pancreas by pancreatic lipase (Fig. 6.26). More chronic abdominal pain probably results from expansion of the liver capsule by fatty infiltration, which often accompanies chylomicronaemia. Eruptive xanthomata are frequently present, and the retinal vessels occasionally demonstrate lipaemia retinalis (Fig. 6.27). A reversible loss of memory, particularly for recent events, and peripheral

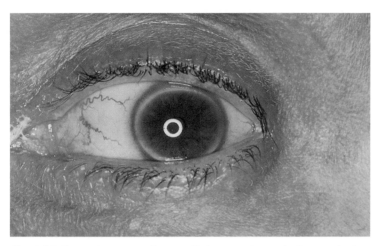

Fig. 6.24 Extensive corneal arcus. Early corneal arcus is characterised by deposition of cholesterol at the superior and inferior aspects of the cornea. With time the arcus may become totally circumferential, as illustrated.

THE CHYLOMICRONAEMIA SYNDROME

abdominal pain/acute pancreatitis

eruptive xanthomata

reversible memory loss/mental confusion

dysaesthesia

lipaemia retinalis

Fig. 6.25 Manifestations of the chylomicronaemia syndrome.

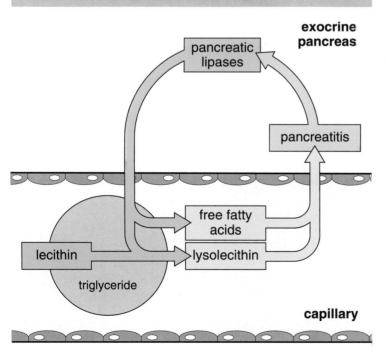

PROPOSED MECHANISM OF PANCREATITIS IN CHYLOMICRONAEMIA

exocrine pancreas

pancreatic lipases

pancreatitis

free fatty acids

lecithin

lysolecithin

triglyceride

capillary

Fig. 6.26 The proposed mechanism of pancreatitis due to prolonged chylomicronaemia. Pancreatic lipase hydrolyses chylomicron triglycerides and phospholipids (lecithin) to free fatty acids and lysolecithin, respectively. Both of the latter can cause chemical pancreatitis. Pancreatitis leads to the liberation of additional lipase, which leads to more free fatty acids and lysolecithin, and so the cycle continues.

neuropathy, which sometimes mimics the carpal tunnel syndrome, also occur. These clinical manifestations can be prevented or reversed by keeping the triglyceride level below approximately 10mmol/l. Eruptive xanthomata resolve in six to twelve weeks. The acute pancreatitis can be fatal and is often recurrent until low triglyceride levels are maintained permanently.

The chylomicronaemia syndrome occasionally occurs when LPL is inactive as a result of a genetic defect in the enzyme or its cofactor, apo CII. Much more commonly, it is due to saturation of the capacity of LPL to remove triglyceride, a result of the coexistence of a genetic form of hypertriglyceridaemia with a disorder of plasma triglyceride metabolism. The latter may be due to one or more diseases, or to drugs (Fig. 6.28).

ASSESSMENT OF HYPERLIPIDAEMIC PATIENTS

Hyperlipidaemia may present to the clinician in several ways. Unfortunately, the first manifestation is often a cardiovascular event. Lipids and lipoproteins should not be evaluated for three months following a major illness such as a myocardial infarction, since they can be markedly altered by the clinical event. As screening for hyperlipidaemia becomes more commonplace, asymptomatic cases are being detected more frequently. It is particularly important to screen young and middle-aged adult relatives of individuals who have presented with manifestations of premature cardiovascular disease. Occasionally, individuals present with cutaneous manifestations or with signs and symptoms of the chylomicronaemia syndrome.

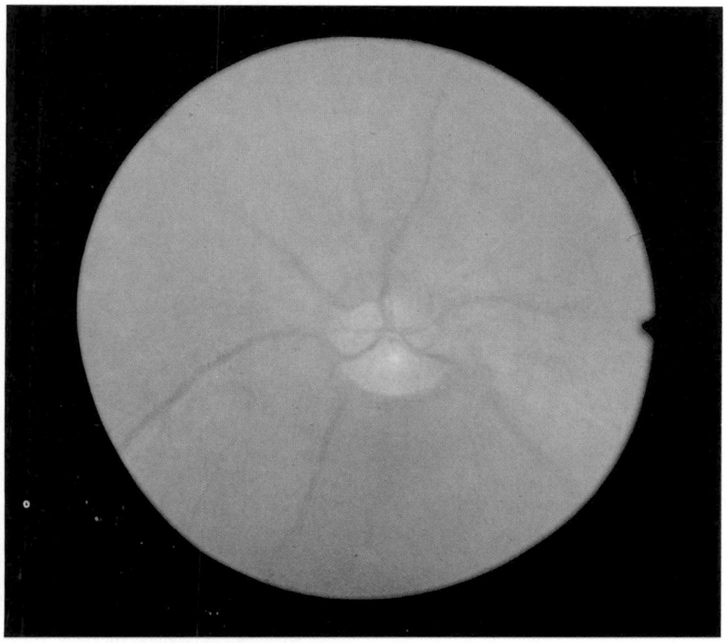

Fig. 6.27 *Lipaemia retinalis seen in association with marked hypertriglyceridaemia.* Note the pale colour of the retinal vessels (due to circulating chylomicrons) against the pink background of the retina.

GENETIC AND ACQUIRED FORMS OF HYPERTRIGLYCERIDAEMIA

genetic	acquired
familial hypertriglyceridaemia familial combined hyperlipidaema	**various disorders** diabetes mellitus hypothyroidism uraemia obesity **drugs** alcohol oestrogens glucocorticoids beta-blockers

Fig. 6.28 *Genetic and acquired forms of hypertriglyceridaemia that can lead to marked hypertriglyceridaemia when present in combination.*

ASSESSMENT OF HYPERLIPIDAEMIC PATIENTS

- confirm hyperlipidaemia

- exclude secondary causes

- evaluate for genetic causes

- decide whether to treat

- decide how to treat
  diet alone
  diet and drugs

Fig. 6.29 *Assessment of hyperlipidaemic patients.*

ESTIMATION OF LDL–CHOLESTEROL LEVELS

$$\text{LDL-cholesterol (mmol/l)} = \frac{\text{total cholesterol} - \text{triglycerides} - \text{HDL-cholesterol}}{2.2}$$

or

$$\text{LDL-cholesterol (mg/dl)} = \frac{\text{total cholesterol} - \text{triglycerides} - \text{HDL-cholesterol}}{5}$$

Fig. 6.30 *Formula used to estimate LDL-cholesterol levels.* The estimation requires the use of a plasma sample taken from a fasted patient. It is valid for triglyceride levels of <5mmol/l.

Once hyperlipidaemia has been discovered, it should be confirmed (Fig. 6.29), and lipoproteins should be evaluated by using appropriate methods (see below). Acquired forms of hyperlipidaemia need to be excluded, and genetic forms should be sought by careful family history. Special emphasis should be placed on the mother's side of the family, since atherosclerotic complications manifest later in females. Information concerning the mother's male siblings and father may therefore prove valuable in arriving at a genetic diagnosis.

The decision will then need to be made as to whether to treat the condition. The objective of treatment is prevention of atherosclerosis or of features of the chylomicronaemia syndrome. With respect to atherosclerosis, guidelines for the detection, evaluation and treatment of hyperlipidaemia have been provided by major organisations such as the Adult Treatment Panel of the National Cholesterol Education Program in the USA, and the European Atherosclerosis Society in Western Europe. Other risk factors (see Fig. 6.1) should be taken into account when considering whether, and how aggressively, to treat. Despite some differences in approach, the US and European guidelines essentially target the same patients for therapy. Diet is advocated initially; however, if compliance with a lipid-lowering diet fails to yield the desired results, drug therapy may also need to be initiated. Treatment of chylomicronaemia is geared towards prevention of the features of the chylomicronaemia syndrome and is discussed below.

LABORATORY TESTS

A detailed description of the various laboratory tests that are available is beyond the scope of this chapter. Generally, however, therapeutic decisions aimed at atherosclerosis prevention are based on determination of LDL and HDL levels. Estimation of LDL levels using a particular formula (Fig. 6.30) is adequate when triglyceride levels are below 5mmol/l. When they are higher, however, ultracentrifugation of plasma is necessary. There is no place in routine practice for lipoprotein electrophoresis, although electrophoresis of VLDL is useful in the diagnosis of remnant removal disease (Fig. 6.31); this also requires ultracentrifugation of plasma.

Diagnosis of the disorder requires assessment of the apo E phenotype. As measurements of apolipoproteins become better standardised, their use will no doubt become widespread. Methods to measure apo B will soon be widely available and may be useful diagnostic tools, particularly in detecting at-risk individuals with high apo B levels and LDL-cholesterol values approaching the top of the normal range. Measurement of apo B, however, will not enable distinction of the several causes of elevation of this apolipoprotein. Measurement of Lp(a) can be a useful addendum in assessing cardiovascular risk. At present, a high level of Lp(a) should best be considered in the same context as risk factors such as hypertension and smoking when considering therapy of the hyperlipidaemia.

A simple test that can be used to diagnose marked hypertriglyceridaemia is inspection of the plasma. A milky or creamy appearance is indicative of extreme elevations of triglyceride levels (Fig. 6.32). At present, assessment of the size of the LDL particle using gradient gel electrophoresis remains a research tool.

REMNANT REMOVAL DISEASE

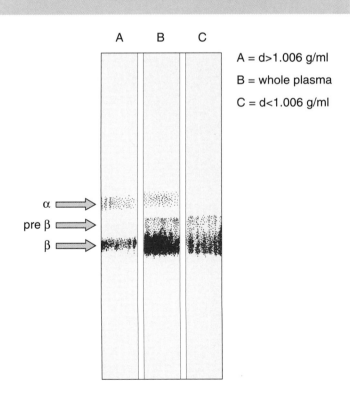

A = d>1.006 g/ml
B = whole plasma
C = d<1.006 g/ml

α
pre β
β

Fig. 6.31 Electrophoresis of plasma showing the d<1.006g/ml fraction of plasma from a patient with remnant removal disease. Lipoproteins are stained with Oil Red O, which stains neutral lipids such as cholesterol esters and triglycerides. Note the β-migrating band in the d<1.006g/ml fraction. This fraction normally contains only pre-migrating material.

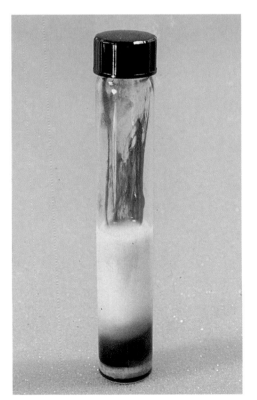

Fig. 6.32 Appearance of plasma from a patient with marked hypertriglyceridaemia.

TREATMENT

DIETARY TREATMENT

A diet low in saturated fat and cholesterol (both of which suppress LDL-receptor activity), will reduce elevated cholesterol levels substantially in most cases. Reductions of ten to twenty per cent can be achieved by long-standing compliance with this type of diet, although the response will, to some extent, be determined by patients' baseline diet and their degree of compliance. Compliance can be markedly enhanced if patients are offered counselling by a qualified dietitian or nutritionist who should try to make the diet as appetising as possible and tailor it to the taste of individual patients. Lack of adequate compliance is the most common cause of failure of diet therapy.

The American Heart Association has recommended two diets for the treatment of hypercholesterolaemia. Treatment should be commenced with a Step I diet, in which less than ten per cent of calories are derived from saturated fat, and cholesterol consumption is <300mg/d. If the desired response is not obtained after an adequate period of good compliance, the Step II diet should be applied whereby saturated fats should provide less than seven per cent of calories, and cholesterol consumption should be <200mg/d. Similar diets have been recommended by many other organisations. Overall, however, the diets should be nutritionally sound and appetising, and should contain abundant fruits, vegetables, grains, pasta and legumes. Attention should also be given to weight control since obesity, particularly central obesity, is associated with many cardiovascular risk factors.

MAJOR LIPID-LOWERING DRUGS

group	drug	usual daily dose	major effect	other effects on lipoproteins	side effects	comments
bile-acid binding resins	*cholestyramine	8–32g	↓ LDL	slightly ↑ HDL ↑ TG	constipation, interferes with absorption of drugs	hypertriglyceridaemia: relative contraindication, take other drugs 1 hour before or 4 hours after resin
	*colestipol	10–40g				
nicotinic acid	*nicotinic acid (niacin)	1.5–6g	↓ TG ↓ LDL ↑ HDL	↓apo B	flushing, itching, ↑ insulin resistance, ↑ liver function tests	need to increase dose slowly, take with food, avoid hot drinks
HMG CoA reductase inhibitors	*lovastatin	20–80mg	↓ LDL	slightly ↓ TG slightly ↑ HDL	occasionally liver function test abnormalities, occasionally myopathy especially when used in combination with cyclosporin, fibrates, or niacin	
	*pravastatin	10–40mg				
	*simvastatin	10–40mg				
fibric acid derivatives	gemfibrozil	600mg twice per day	↑TG ↑HDL	slightly ↓ LDL sometimes ↑ LDL	gallstones gastrointestinal symptoms myopathy especially in patients with chronic renal failure	
	bezafibrate	200mg three times per day				
	clofibrate	1g twice per day				
antioxidants	probucol	500mg twice per day	↓LDL ↓HDL	prevents lipoprotein oxidation	diarrhoea ↑ QT interval	

*response is dose-dependent
TG = triglycerides

Fig. 6.33 Major lipid-lowering drugs.

DRUG THERAPY

Drug therapy may need to be initiated when target lipid levels are not achieved with diet alone. Most patients with a genetic form of hyper-lipidaemia will need to take drugs in addition to following a diet. The effects of diet and drugs are independent and additive; consumption of an appropriate diet can reduce the dose of drug required. Drug therapy may also be of value in patients with established coronary artery disease; recent trials have demonstrated that the progression of atherosclerotic lesions can be halted or even regress with substantial lowering of plasma lipid levels. A complete review of the available lipid-lowering drugs and their indications, dosages, and side effects is beyond the scope of this chapter. An understanding of their mechanisms of action is, however, useful and provides important insights into their use.

MECHANISM OF ACTION OF LIPID-LOWERING DRUGS

Several groups of lipid-lowering drugs are available (Fig. 6.33), and their mechanism of action on lipoprotein metabolism is reviewed briefly. As discussed earlier, LDL-cholesterol levels are determined by the relative rates of input and removal of this class of lipoprotein from plasma. Removal of LDL occurs primarily via LDL receptors in the liver. Hepatocytes derive their cholesterol from exogenous sources via the LDL receptor, and by endogenous synthesis from HMG CoA. A major use of cholesterol by the liver is for the synthesis

of bile acids, which undergo enterohepatic circulation after secretion into the intestinal tract (Fig. 6.34a). Bile acid-binding resins can interrupt the enterohepatic circulation of bile acids, leading to a compensatory increase in LDL receptors and cholesterol synthesis (Fig. 6.34b). HMG CoA reductase inhibitors inhibit endogenous cholesterol synthesis, which is also associated with an increase in hepatic LDL-receptor activity (Fig. 6.34c). Combined use of bile acid resins and HMG CoA reductase inhibitors leads to a marked increase in LDL-receptor activity (Fig. 6.34d).

Niacin (nicotinic acid) has a different mechanism of action. Its major effects are to reduce the production of the apo B-containing lipoproteins and to inhibit the mobilisation of free fatty acids from adipose tissue (Fig. 6.35). Use of niacin leads to a reduction in VLDL and LDL levels and is also associated with an increase in HDL-cholesterol levels.

The fibric acid derivatives (fibrates) primarily affect VLDL metabolism, whereby VLDL input is reduced and removal is enhanced. Their major use therefore is for the treatment of hypertriglyceridaemia, in which they also increase HDL levels.

Probucol reduces LDL and HDL levels. It is also a powerful anti-oxidant and has been shown to inhibit lipoprotein oxidation and the extent of atherosclerosis in experimental animals. Its use as an anti-oxidant in man is, however, premature.

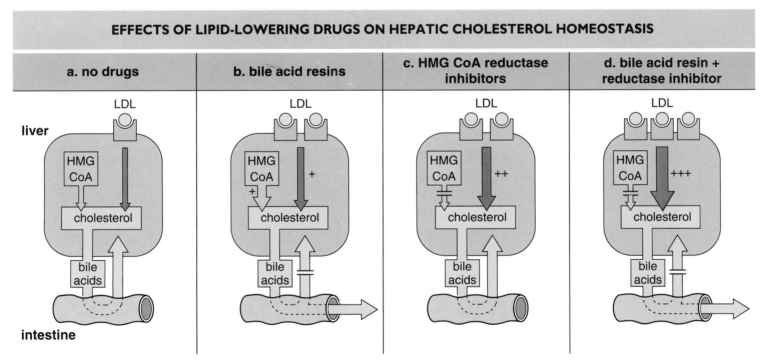

EFFECTS OF LIPID-LOWERING DRUGS ON HEPATIC CHOLESTEROL HOMEOSTASIS

a. no drugs	b. bile acid resins	c. HMG CoA reductase inhibitors	d. bile acid resin + reductase inhibitor

Fig. 6.34 The effect of lipid-lowering drugs on hepatic cholesterol homeostasis.
(a) The hepatocyte derives cholesterol for bile acid synthesis via the LDL receptor and by endogenous synthesis. Bile acids enter the intestinal tract from where they are reabsorbed for reutilisation. (b) Interruption of the enterohepatic circulation by bile acid-binding resins leads to an increase in LDL-receptor activity and cholesterol synthesis. (c) HMG CoA reductase inhibitors inhibit cholesterol synthesis and are associated with an increase in hepatic LDL receptors. (d) The combined use of a bile acid resin and HMG CoA reductase inhibitor leads to a marked increase in LDL-receptor levels by inhibiting the increase in cholesterol synthesis that occurs when resins are used alone.

OTHER CARDIOVASCULAR RISK FACTORS

Atherosclerosis is a multifactorial disease for which hyperlipidaemia is but one of several important risk factors. Other risk factors should therefore also be evaluated and treated in their own right. In particular, cigarette smoking should be discouraged in the strongest possible terms. Smoking cessation is also associated with an increase in HDL-cholesterol levels. Hypertension should be treated when indicated, although it should be noted that use of diuretics and beta-adrenergic blocking agents may aggravate hyperlipidaemia. Lipid neutral or beneficial antihypertensive agents therefore may be more appropriate.

CHYLOMICRONAEMIA SYNDROME

Management of the chylomicronaemia syndrome requires special consideration. Since marked hypertriglyceridaemia usually results from a combination of genetic and acquired causes of hypertriglyceridaemia, identification and treatment of treatable secondary causes are essential. Furthermore, administration of triglyceride-raising drugs should be discontinued where possible and a trial of alcohol restriction should be attempted. If triglyceride levels remain elevated, fibric acid derivatives should be used to lower them. Symptoms of the chylomicronaemia syndrome and risk of recurrence of pancreatitis can be prevented by maintaining triglyceride levels of below 20mmol/l and 10mmol/l, respectively.

POSTULATED MECHANISM OF ACTION OF NIACIN

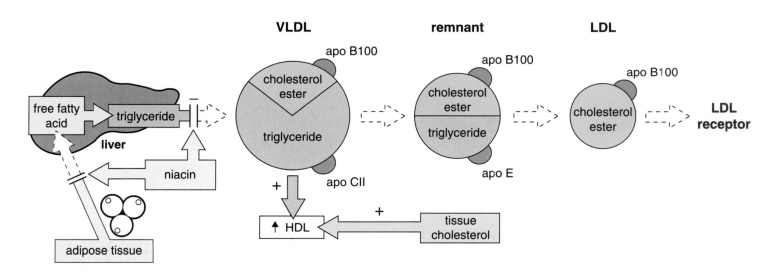

Fig. 6.35 The postulated mechanism of action of niacin. The primary effect of niacin is to reduce the production of the apo B-containing lipoproteins..

7

Adrenal Cortex Physiology

Vivian HT James, PhD, DSc, FRCPath

The human adrenal glands are paired structures, situated at the upper pole of each kidney. Each gland is shaped roughly like a cocked hat, is highly vascularised, and weighs approximately 4–5g in a normal healthy adult. The outer cortex, comprising ninety per cent of the gland, surrounds the central medulla. The cortex is a zonated structure (Fig. 7.1) and is covered by a thin capsule, below which isolated groups of glomerulosa cells are found. Most of the cortex is made up of the zona fasciculata and the zona reticularis, the latter adjoining the medulla. The blood supply is derived from the inferior phrenic artery, the aorta, and the renal arteries, and is largely subcapsular. The venous circulation within the gland is complex and is thought to play an important role in regulating steroid synthesis. The central vein from the right adrenal is short and enters the inferior vena cava directly, whereas that from the left adrenal drains into the left renal vein.

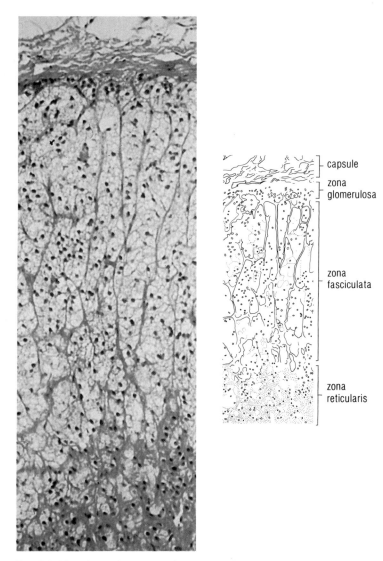

Fig. 7.1 Histological section of an adrenal gland. The medulla represents ten per cent of the gland, while the remaining ninety per cent is made up of cortical tissue – the zonae glomerulosa, fasciculata, and reticularis. The whole gland is surrounded by a fibrous capsule below which the zona glomerulosa cells appear only focally. Haematoxylin and eosin stain, magnification × 250.

HORMONE PRODUCTION IN THE GLOMERULOSA CELLS

The adrenal cortex produces three major types of steroid hormones: mineralocorticoids, glucocorticoids, and androgens. The source of the mineralocorticoids (aldosterone and, in part, deoxycorticosterone) is the zona glomerulosa. The major factor controlling aldosterone secretion is angiotensin, but increased plasma potassium concentration is also an efficient aldosterone-stimulating agent (Fig. 7.2). The role of corticotrophin (adrenocorticotrophic hormone: ACTH) is less clear; it is more effective in salt-depleted subjects than in those with normal salt balance, and is probably relatively unimportant in the normal situation. There is also evidence of the existence of other factors, as yet unknown.

Angiotensin I is formed from angiotensinogen substrate by the action of renin. Renin synthesis occurs in the juxtaglomerular cells of the kidney and is released in response to changes in tubular sodium concentration, renal arteriolar blood pressure, and stimulation via sympathetic nerves. The decapeptide angiotensin I is converted into the octapeptide angiotensin II by a converting enzyme (angiotensin-converting enzyme: ACE); this conversion takes place primarily, but not exclusively, in the lungs. The heptapeptide angiotensin III is also formed and can stimulate aldosterone secretion, although a physiological role for it has not yet been established.

HORMONE PRODUCTION IN THE FASCICULATA AND RETICULARIS CELLS

Cortisol and the adrenal androgens are derived from the fasciculata and reticularis cells. The only known important control mechanism is by means of ACTH (Fig. 7.3). This anterior pituitary hormone regulates adrenocortical growth; it also mediates the rate at which steroid biosynthesis occurs. Other fragments of the ACTH precursor, pro-opiomelanocortin (POMC), may also have a trophic effect on the adrenal, and antidiuretic hormone (ADH/vasopressin) may act synergistically with ACTH to stimulate steroid biosynthesis.

The effect of ACTH is rapid, occurring within a few minutes. The release of ACTH, leading to the secretion of cortisol and androgen, occurs episodically throughout the twenty-four-hour cycle in a circadian pattern. ACTH release occurs in response to low circulating levels of cortisol (as in Addison's disease) and is inhibited by high circulating levels of cortisol or synthetic glucocorticoids (as in corticosteroid therapy). This negative feedback probably occurs at hypothalamic and pituitary sites. ACTH is also released in response to stress (such as trauma, surgery, anxiety and emotional disturbance).

MECHANISM OF ACTION OF ADRENOCORTICOTROPHIC HORMONE

ACTH acts on the adrenal gland by binding to a specific receptor in the membrane of the cell (Fig. 7.4). This results in the stimulation of the membrane-bound adenylate cyclase enzyme, leading to rapid production of intracellular cyclic AMP (cAMP), a mechanism that may also involve calcium entry into the cell. Other cyclic nucleotides such as cGMP may also be important. cAMP, in turn, activates a protein kinase (by dissociating an active subunit), which then stimulates a number of protein-phosphorylation processes using ATP. The role of the phosphoproteins that are formed is not yet clearly defined, but they appear to mediate cholesterol ester hydrolysis and side-chain cleavage of cholesterol to form pregnenolone. The increased concentration of pregnenolone subsequently leads to increased biosynthesis of cortisol and the androgens.

Angiotensin II binds to specific high-affinity sites in the plasma membrane of the adrenal glomerulosa cell. Unlike ACTH, cAMP does not appear to be a 'second messenger' in aldosterone biosynthesis. Sensitivity to angiotensin is increased by sodium deficiency, with the formation of more angiotensin receptors and an increase in binding affinity. The major pathway involved in the biosynthesis of aldosterone is probably as shown in Fig. 7.5, although others almost certainly exist and may be important in particular conditions.

Cortisol and androgens are synthesised from cholesterol that is mainly derived from circulating cholesterol esters, although intracellular cholesterol biosynthesis also occurs (Fig. 7.6). Low-density lipoprotein (LDL) is an important source of cholesterol, particularly during ACTH stimulation.

Specific enzymes and cofactors are required for glucocorticoid and androgen biosynthesis. These enzymes are located either in the smooth endoplasmic reticulum or in the mitochondria within each cell. Movement of substrate between these organelles is therefore necessary, and this mechanism of intracellular transport may require

specific steroid-binding proteins. Thus, intracellular feedback effects of intermediates in the earlier biosynthetic steps may be of importance in regulating cholesterol biosynthesis.

Hydroxylation steps in the biosynthesis of adrenal steroids (Fig. 7.7) require NADPH, molecular oxygen, and an enzyme complex. The complex consists of a flavoprotein dehydrogenase, a nonhaem iron-containing protein (adrenodoxin), and cytochrome P_{450} (so called since a characteristic high absorption is observed when it complexes with carbon monoxide). This oxidase system is essentially similar for 11β-, 20,22-, 17α- and 18-hydroxylation, and it appears that specificity is achieved through differences in the respective P_{450} cytochromes. Hydroxylation is mediated by the introduction of one electron into the electron transport chain, with the introduction of one atom of oxygen into the steroid. The remaining oxygen atom combines with hydrogen to form water. This system is known as a 'mixed-function oxidase'.

Biosynthesis of the adrenocortical steroids is thus effected by the interaction of the various steroid hydroxylases: P_{450} scc, P_{450} C21,

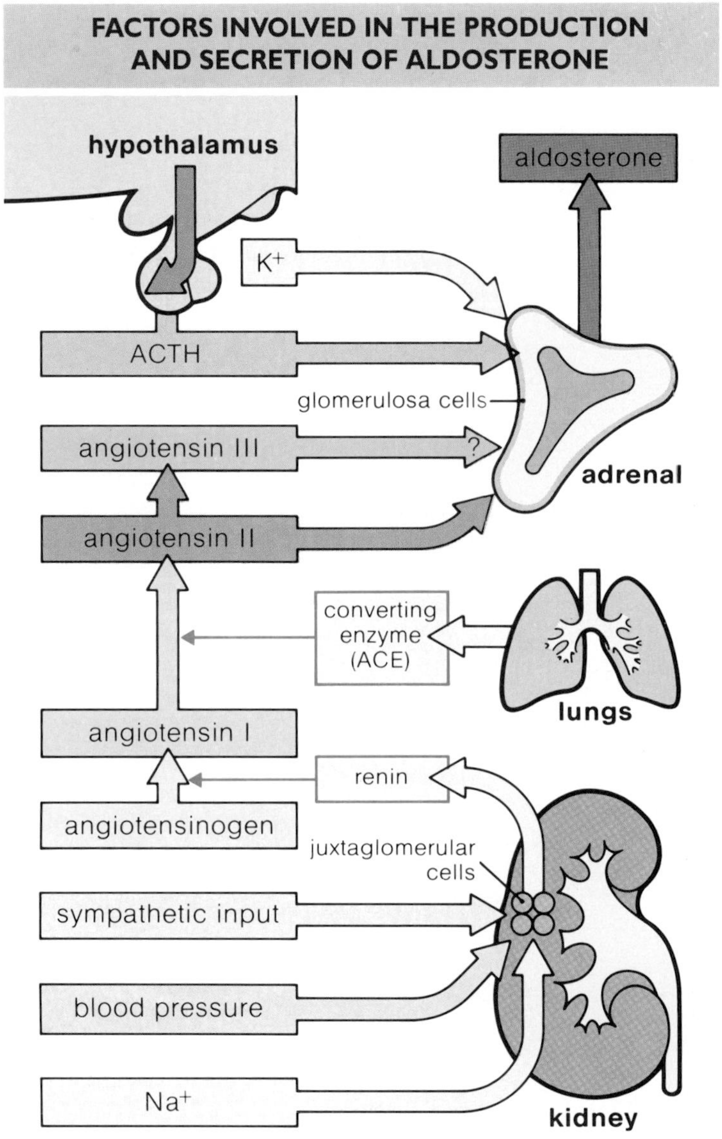

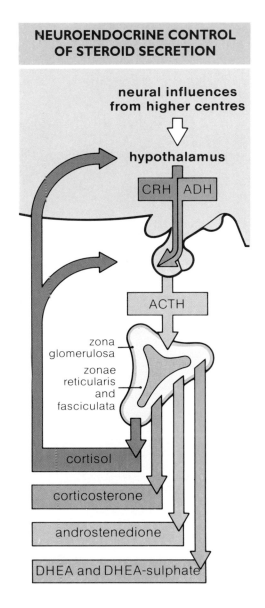

FACTORS INVOLVED IN THE PRODUCTION AND SECRETION OF ALDOSTERONE

NEUROENDOCRINE CONTROL OF STEROID SECRETION

Fig. 7.2 Physiological mechanisms governing the production and secretion of aldosterone. The major factor influencing aldosterone secretion is angiotensin, although an increased plasma potassium concentration also contributes. Renin output, in turn, is regulated by sympathetic tone, blood pressure, and tubular sodium concentration.

Fig. 7.3 The neuroendocrine control of steroid secretion from the adrenal cortex. Negative feedback in the hypothalamus and pituitary operates through cortisol and, to a minor extent, through corticosterone. Thus high cortisol levels suppress ACTH output, whereas low cortisol levels stimulate ACTH production by increasing the release of CRH and also by increasing the sensitivity of ACTH to CRH.

P_{450} C17α, and P_{450} C11β. In addition, 3β-hydroxysteroid dehydrogenase isomerase is required to change the structure in ring A to the important 4-ene-3-one configuration. P_{450} C21 appears to be capable only of effecting hydroxylation at C21 (for example, of 17-hydroxyprogesterone to 11-deoxycortisol), whereas other hydroxylases are multifunctional. Thus, P_{450} scc effects hydroxylation at C20 and C22, and also acts as a 20,22 lyase. P_{450} C17α mediates hydroxylation at C17α and also acts as a 17,20 lyase. This enzyme is absent from the zona glomerulosa cells, which limits the steroidogenic capacity of the cells to mineralocorticoid production. P_{450} C11β causes hydroxylation at C11, C18, and C19, and can also act in some species as an aromatase.

Molecular biological techniques have been employed with considerable effect to widen our knowledge of the structure of the steroid hydroxylase genes and of the mechanism of action of ACTH. Human P_{450} scc, P_{450} C17α, and P_{450} C21 are encoded by a single mRNA species, some 2kb in length. Bovine P_{450} C11β is encoded by three mRNAs, with the smallest being 4.3kb in length. Exposure of adrenocortical cells to ACTH (or cAMP) causes the accumulation of all four P_{450} steroidogenic enzymes, as well as of adrenodoxin and adrenodoxin reductase. Chronic exposure to ACTH involves transcription of the genes for steroid hydroxylases. The structure of the genes has now been elucidated: P_{450} C11β contains nine exons and is located on chromosome 15; and P_{450} C17α also contains nine exons,

and is located on chromosome 8. There are possibly two gene products of P_{450} C11β: one that uses 11-deoxycortisol as a substrate to produce cortisol, and the other being involved in the final synthesis of aldosterone. The P_{450} C17α gene is on chromosome 10 and contains eight exons; and the P_{450} C21 gene contains ten exons and is closely united to a pseudogene on chromosome 6 in the histocompatibility leucocyte antigen locus.

The steroid hydroxylases represent three gene families in the P_{450} superfamily. It seems likely that these genes have evolved from a common progenitor, several hundred million years ago, into distinct steroid hydroxylase gene families that now catalyse specific reactions.

CONTROL OF ANDROGEN SECRETION

The main adrenal androgens are androstenedione, dehydroepiandrosterone (DHEA), 11β-hydroxyandrostenedione, and DHEA-sulphate. The possible control mechanisms involved in the secretion of these androgens are shown in Fig. 7.8. Although ACTH is capable of stimulating adrenal androgen secretion, there are several well-documented situations in which secretion of cortisol and androgen appears to be dissociated. This has resulted in the concept of the existence of an additional factor, adrenal androgen-stimulating hormone (AASH – as yet undefined), which can specifically stimulate adrenal androgen secretion. Prolactin has been invoked as such a factor since hyperprolactinaemia is associated with increased production of DHEA-

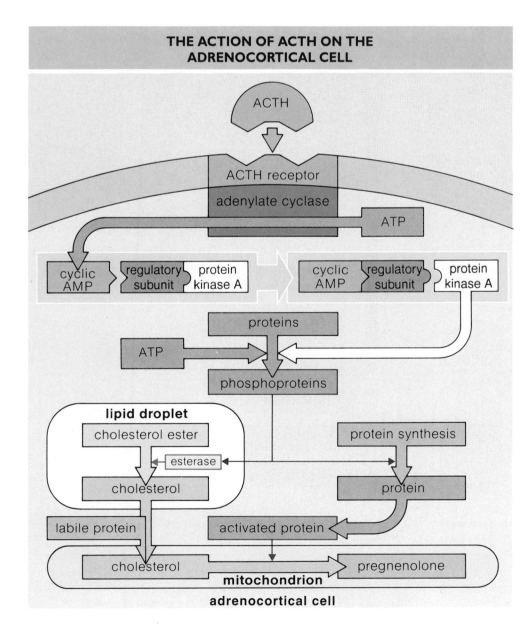

THE ACTION OF ACTH ON THE ADRENOCORTICAL CELL

ACTH

ACTH receptor

adenylate cyclase

ATP

cyclic AMP | regulatory subunit | protein kinase A

cyclic AMP | regulatory subunit | protein kinase A

proteins

ATP

phosphoproteins

lipid droplet

cholesterol ester

esterase

cholesterol

protein synthesis

protein

labile protein

activated protein

cholesterol

pregnenolone

mitochondrion

adrenocortical cell

Fig. 7.4 Simplified mechanism of action of ACTH on the adrenocortical cell. The ACTH receptor is linked to the adenylate cyclase membrane enzyme system which is responsible for cAMP production. This 'second messenger' triggers the intracellular events that are responsible for steroid production and secretion. Pregnenolone is subsequently converted to other corticosteroids (see Figs 7.6 and 7.12).

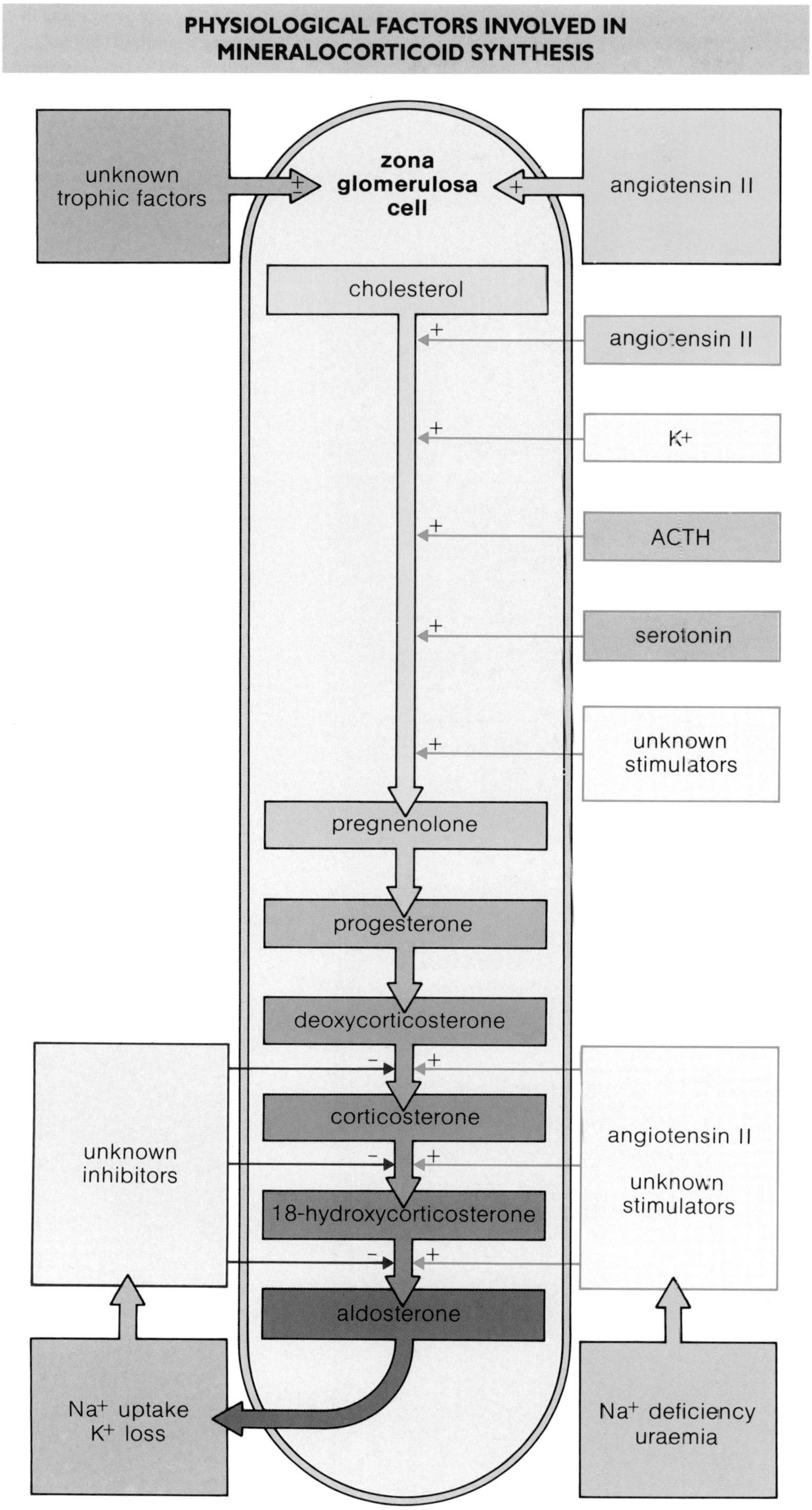

PHYSIOLOGICAL FACTORS INVOLVED IN MINERALOCORTICOID SYNTHESIS

Fig. 7.5 Physiological factors believed to be important in the control of mineralocorticoid synthesis. Angiotensin II appears to be the major stimulus of mineralocorticoid synthesis and secretion. Other factors play a minor role.

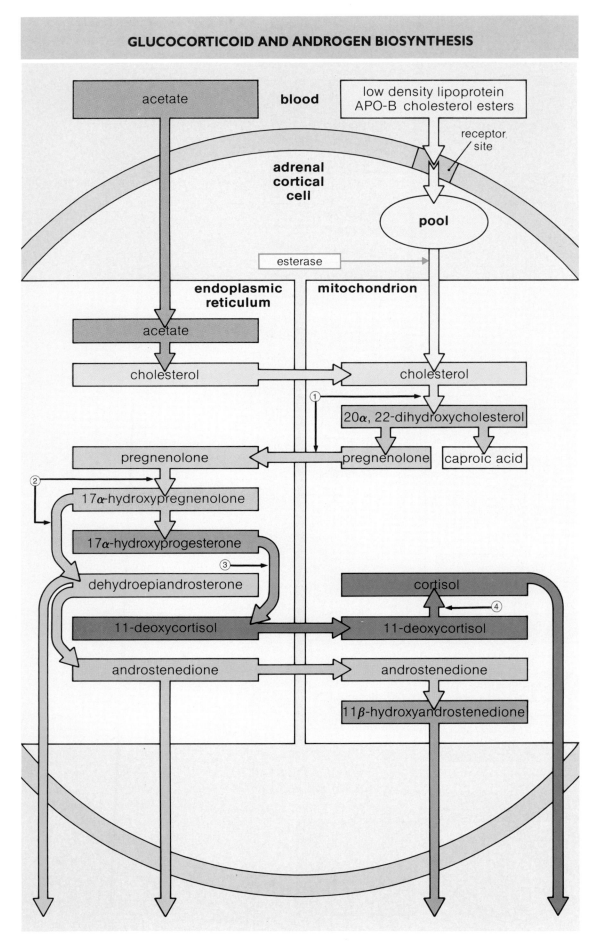

GLUCOCORTICOID AND ANDROGEN BIOSYNTHESIS

Fig. 7.6 An adrenocortical cell showing the intracellular organelles in which biosynthesis of glucocorticoid and androgen occurs from a cholesterol precursor. LDL is the major cholesterol-transport lipoprotein in human blood, and most of this cholesterol is located in the central core and is esterified. The core is surrounded by a small amount of free cholesterol, phospholipids, and a protein known as Apo B. This is specifically bound to the cell surface receptor site. It is this mechanism that is postulated as the major route of cholesterol entry to the adrenocortical cells. The sites of action of the cytochrome P_{450} enzymes that are involved in steroidogenesis are shown:

(1) P_{450} scc (cholesterol side-chain cleavage);
(2) P_{450} C17α (17α-hydroxylation);
(3) P_{450} C21 (21-hydroxylation);
(4) P_{450} C11β (11β-hydroxylation)

HYDROXYLATION OF STEROIDS

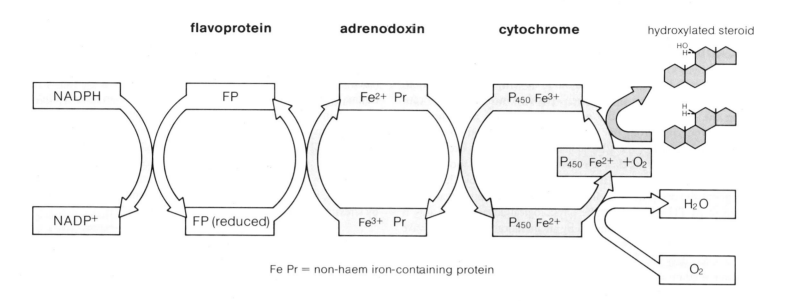

Fe Pr = non-haem iron-containing protein

Fig. 7.7 The role of NADPH, a flavoprotein, and cytochrome P_{450} in the hydroxylation of steroids. All hydroxylation steps share this common pathway.

SECRETION OF ADRENAL ANDROGENS

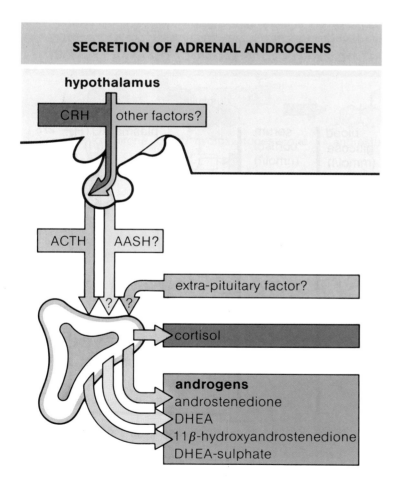

Fig. 7.8 The possible control mechanisms involved in the secretion of adrenal androgens. Although ACTH seems to be an important physiological regulator of adrenal androgen production, there is evidence supporting the existence of another separate hormone, AASH (as yet unidentified), which stimulates DHEA-sulphate production.

EPISODIC NATURE OF ADRENAL STEROID SECRETION

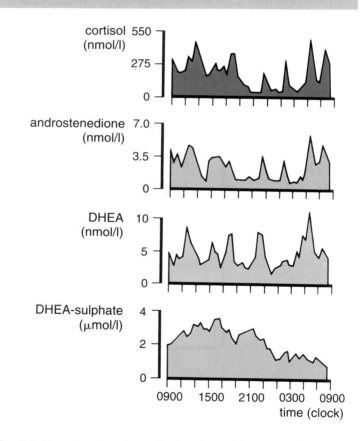

Fig. 7.9 The episodic nature of adrenal steroid secretion in plasma.

A small amount of cortisol (up to 150µg/d) is excreted unchanged and represents the unbound cortisol in plasma which is filtered through the kidney.

The average secretion rate of aldosterone is 100–200µg/d (Fig. 7.14). It is only weakly bound to plasma proteins and thus has a relatively short half-life (twenty minutes) and a high metabolic clearance rate (1500l/d). Both the liver and kidney are sites of metabolic clearance, and only a small percentage of aldosterone is excreted unchanged in the urine. A measurement of plasma aldosterone levels, or an estimation of the levels of the metabolite 18-glucuronoside, is commonly used in clinical situations. Diet, posture, and time of day affect aldosterone secretion and must be adequately controlled to permit interpretation of results.

The major androgens produced by the adrenal cortex are DHEA-sulphate, androstenedione, DHEA, 11β-hydroxyandrostenedione, and small amounts of testosterone (Fig. 7.15). Androstenedione and testosterone are also secreted by the ovary and the testis, and a small amount of DHEA arises from the ovary. Androgen metabolism is therefore complex because of these dual sources and also because androgens undergo extensive interconversion and metabolism. The major metabolic pathway proceeds via the reduction of ring A, and the resulting metabolites are conjugated and excreted into the urine as sulphates and glucuronosides. Formerly, the conjugated urinary metabolites DHEA, aetiocholanolone, and androsterone were measured collectively as 'urinary 17-oxosteroids'. Although this assay has been used extensively in the past, it is now little employed because of the difficulty of interpretation. Currently, clinical investigations of androgen metabolism are predominantly based on the measurement of plasma androgen levels rather than urinary excretion products.

The peripheral interconversion of androgens has important physiological consequences. Androstenedione is a major precursor of testosterone and, in the female, is a major source of this steroid. It is also converted to oestrone, and in older women, when ovarian secretion of oestrogen is less important, the production of oestrone from androstenedione contributes significantly to the total production of oestrogen.

INHIBITORS OF STEROID BIOSYNTHESIS

Steroid biosynthesis can be blocked by a number of compounds that inhibit the activity of one or more of the enzyme systems involved in the pathway. These agents have been found to have clinical use in the investigation of pituitary–adrenal function, as an adjunct to the treatment of Cushing's syndrome, and as a method of reducing oestrogen synthesis in the treatment of women with breast cancer.

Metyrapone acts by interfering with the cytochrome P_{450} system and mainly affects 11β-hydroxylation. This causes a relative increase in the production of the immediate precursor steroid, 11-deoxycortisol, with a concomitant decrease in cortisol synthesis. These actions have been exploited in the development of a test of pituitary–adrenal function which has been used clinically. In a subject with intact pituitary–adrenal function, following administration of metyrapone, a fall in cortisol production is seen, with a subsequent fall in plasma cortisol levels (Fig. 7.16). This causes a compensatory release of ACTH for as long as the drug is administered. ACTH, acting on the adrenal cortex, accelerates the early stages of steroid biosynthesis and therefore increases the production of all of the steroids up to the step that is blocked by metyrapone. The increased production of 11-deoxycortisol can be measured directly in the blood,

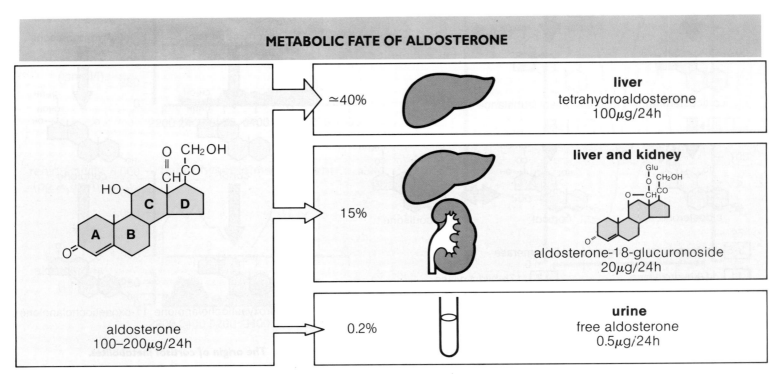

METABOLIC FATE OF ALDOSTERONE

Fig. 7.14 The metabolic fate of aldosterone. Only 0.2 per cent of the daily amount of aldosterone that is produced is directly excreted in the urine, while approximately forty per cent is converted to tetrahydro-aldosterone within the liver. The remaining aldosterone is converted into many other metabolites.

or by measuring the metabolite tetrahydro-11-deoxycortisol in urine where it appears as a 17-hydroxy-corticosteroid. A patient with hypothalamic, pituitary, or adrenal insufficiency will show a diminished or absent response.

Aminoglutethimide also interferes with several of the biosynthetic steps involved in steroid biosynthesis, exerting its effects on the C20-, C22-, 11β-, 18-, 19- and 21-hydroxylases, and also on aromatase. Since it inhibits biosynthesis early in the pathway, it is useful as a blocking agent when alleviating the effects of excessive steroid production, as in the treatment of patients with Cushing's syndrome that has resulted from adrenal carcinoma. The action of aminoglutethimide on aromatase is useful in the treatment of breast cancer since it inhibits peripheral formation of oestrogens; however, it has now been superseded for this purpose by more selective aromatase inhibitors such as 4-hydroxyandrostenedione, which do not cause the problem of cortisol deficiency (as seen with aminoglutethimide).

Ketoconazole, an antifungal drug, inhibits several cytochrome P_{450}-dependent enzymes, including 11β-hydroxylase, thus interfering with cortisol synthesis (an unwanted effect in most cases). It is, however, being used increasingly to treat Cushing's syndrome, precocious puberty, and prostatic carcinoma.

Trilostane inhibits steroid hormone synthesis by acting on 3β-hydroxysteroid dehydrogenase; it has been used to reduce cortisol and aldosterone production in the treatment of Cushing's syndrome and Conn's syndrome, respectively, but its action is weak.

METABOLIC ERRORS

The major pathways of steroid biosynthesis within the human adrenal cortex (see Fig. 7.12) emphasise the crucial dependence upon the availability of specific enzyme systems. Given the vital role which adrenocortical steroids play in human metabolism, it is not surprising that even a partial deficiency in the activity of these enzymes

produces serious metabolic disturbance. Clinical syndromes corresponding to deficiencies of each of the enzymes that are involved have been described and are referred to as different forms of congenital adrenal hyperplasia.

The most common group of disorders of the type are due to C21-hydroxylase deficiency. This results in an inability to produce cortisol and in an increase in ACTH levels, which leads to adrenocortical hyperplasia and to excessive production of androgens.

This in turn results in virilisation of the external genitalia in the female fetus, and precocious pseudopuberty in male infants. If the deficiency extends to the zona glomerulosa P_{450} C21, deficiency of aldosterone production with salt loss will also occur. This can result in adrenocortical deficiency or crisis, neonatally or later in life. In this disorder, the substrate for the defective enzyme is 17-hydroxyprogesterone (see Fig. 7.12), and synthesis of this steroid, and its plasma levels, will increase.

11-hydroxylase deficiency is relatively less common and results in inadequate production of cortisol, an increase in ACTH levels and an increase in the production of the precursor steroids, 11-deoxycortisol and deoxycorticosterone. The latter is a powerful mineralocorticoid and produces hypertension and salt retention.

Deficiency of P_{450} scc results in a serious disorder since the biosynthesis of all of the steroid hormones is prevented, leading to lipid accumulation in the gland (lipoid adrenal hyperplasia) and differentiation disorders in the male fetus. The defect is rare, and few patients survive early infancy. Deficiency of 17-hydroxylase is also rare, but if it does occur, it will result in a decreased synthesis of cortisol (see Fig. 7.12) an overproduction of ACTH, and decreasing secretion of androgens because of the lyase deficiency.

Hydroxysteroid-isomerase deficiency leads to the inadequate production of cortisol, mineralocorticoids and androgens; an inadequate production of the latter causes developmental abnormalities in the male and female fetus. Cortisol and aldosterone deficiencies also produce metabolic disorders in this condition.

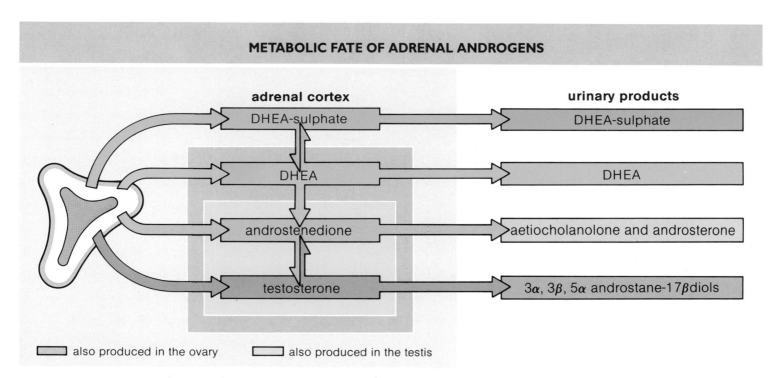

METABOLIC FATE OF ADRENAL ANDROGENS

adrenal cortex | urinary products

DHEA-sulphate → DHEA-sulphate

DHEA → DHEA

androstenedione → aetiocholanolone and androsterone

testosterone → 3α, 3β, 5α androstane-17βdiols

▢ also produced in the ovary   ▢ also produced in the testis

Fig. 7.15 The metabolic fate of adrenal androgens. DHEA, DHEA-sulphate, aetiocholanolone, androsterone and the androstanediols are all excreted in the urine.

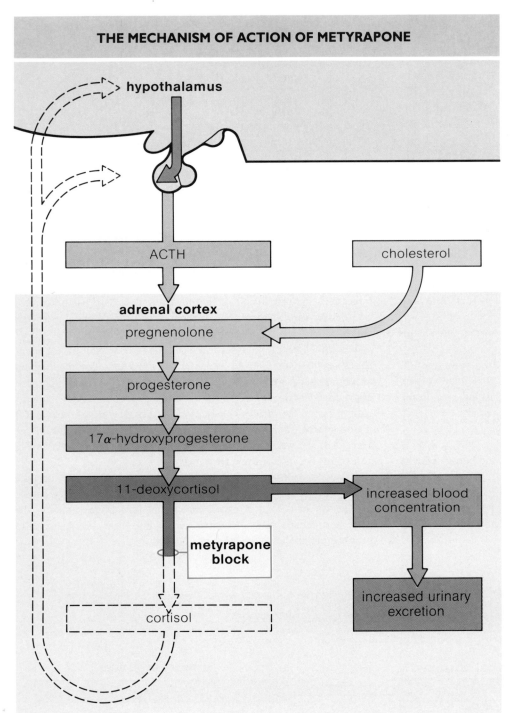

THE MECHANISM OF ACTION OF METYRAPONE

hypothalamus

ACTH

cholesterol

adrenal cortex

pregnenolone

progesterone

17α-hydroxyprogesterone

11-deoxycortisol

increased blood concentration

metyrapone block

increased urinary excretion

cortisol

Fig. 7.16 The mechanism of action of metyrapone. Metyrapone will cause an increase in the production of deoxycortisol and of its urinary metabolites, providing that the function of the hypothalamus, pituitary and adrenal is intact.

8

Cushing's Syndrome

Peter J Trainer, MB, ChB ,BSc, MRCP

Michael Besser, MD, DSc, FRCP

Cushing's syndrome is the clinical condition resulting from prolonged, excessive, inappropriate exposure to free (nonprotein-bound) circulating glucocorticoids. It was first fully described clinically by Harvey Cushing in 1932 before the isolation of either the adrenal or pituitary hormones, although many earlier cases, often referred to as 'diabetes of bearded women', had been recognised. Cushing's syndrome most commonly results from the therapeutic use of synthetic glucocorticoids or adrenocorticotrophic hormone (ACTH). Doses of corticosteroids greater than replacement requirements (for example, more than 7.5mg prednisolone, 0.75mg dexamethasone, or 30mg hydrocortisone, daily, in adults) may simulate the naturally occurring condition.

CLINICAL FEATURES

Virtually every system in the body is affected by exposure to excess glucocorticoids. A summary of the major clinical features in Cushing's syndrome is shown in Fig. 8.1. The most common presenting symptoms are weight gain and central obesity with muscle weakness. General symptoms of weakness are particularly common in proximal upper and lower limb muscle groups (Fig. 8.2). Lethargy and malaise, as well as hirsutism and acne (Fig. 8.3), skin-thinning, bruising, and striae (Fig. 8.4) are also common, as are oligomenorrhoea or amenorrhoea in the female and decreased libido and impo-

MAJOR CLINICAL FEATURES IN CUSHING'S SYNDROME

weight gain
central obesity
'moon face' with purpleish plethora
muscular weakness, especially proximal
backache and vertebral collapse
malaise
agitated depression and/or psychosis
hirsutism
purple striae
acne
skin–thinning
bruising
nocturia/polyuria
decreased libido and impotence in men
oligomenorrhoea or amenorrhoea
  in females
hypertension
diabetes mellitus or impaired
  glucose tolerance
infection

Fig. 8.1 The major clinical features in Cushing's syndrome. Patients with Cushing's syndrome gain weight but suffer muscular disability, malaise, and depression. In addition, they are susceptible to various skin disorders such as acne and bruising; decreased fertility and libido may also be present.

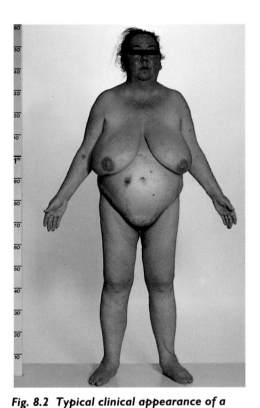

Fig. 8.2 Typical clinical appearance of a patient with Cushing's syndrome. Central obesity with proximal muscle wasting can be seen.

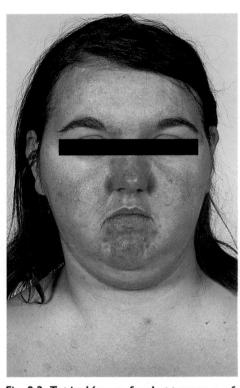

Fig. 8.3 Typical 'moon face' appearance of a patient with Cushing's syndrome. A plethoric face with acne and hirsutism is characteristic, and there is evidence of temporal hair recession.

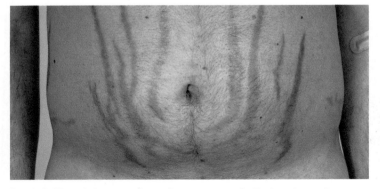

Fig. 8.4 The abdomen of a male patient with Cushing's syndrome. The skin is stretched by underlying adipose tissue to such an extent that streaks of capillaries, or striae, can be seen.

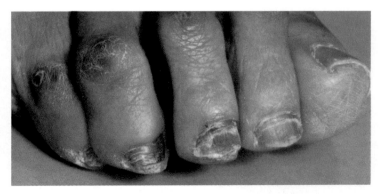

Fig. 8.5 The nails in a patient with ectopic ACTH syndrome. The nails are grossly pigmented compared with those of a normal subject.

tence in the male. Bony features include osteopenia and vertebral collapse, rib fractures (see Chapter 18), kyphosis, and avascular bone necrosis. Depression, often with associated anxiety, occurs in approximately sixty per cent of patients, and frank psychosis may also occur. Symptoms relating to hypertension and diabetes mellitus may develop, and patients show an increased susceptibility to infection which may be hidden or suddenly become overwhelming as the body's defence mechanisms are suppressed. In ACTH-dependent disease, pigmentation may be present (Fig. 8.5) and, with pituitary-dependent disease, headaches and visual-field defects are occasionally found if a pituitary macroadenoma is present. All disease forms may be cyclical or intermittent, and pituitary-dependent disease may occasionally undergo spontaneous remission.

When the clinical features are unclear, examination of previous photographs of the subject may be valuable. Rapid onset of the disease is more likely to result from an adrenal tumour or ectopic ACTH production than from pituitary-dependent disease, but even in the former two cases, a slow progression and prolonged course may be found. Overt pigmentation is more common with the ectopic ACTH syndrome, while marked virilisation is usually associated with malignant adrenal tumours. The histological appearance of the adrenal gland in ACTH-dependent Cushing's syndrome reveals hyperplasia of the reticularis and fasciculata layers when compared with the normal gland (Fig. 8.6).

AETIOLOGY

Apart from corticosteroids or ACTH therapy, other factors are implicated in the cause of Cushing's syndrome (Fig. 8.7); the effects of various factors on the hypothalamic–pituitary–adrenal axis are shown in Fig. 8.8.

Pituitary-dependent disease (i.e. Cushing's disease) is four times more common in women than in men and occurs most often between the ages of twenty and forty years.

Ectopic ACTH production may be associated with a large number of tumours, most commonly small (oat) cell bronchial carcinomas (see Chapter 7), or bronchial and thymic neuroendocrine tumours of the carcinoid type (Fig. 8.9), other gastrointestinal carcinoid tumours, and neuroendocrine tumours of the pancreatic islets. When ectopic ACTH production is associated with a rapidly advancing tumour, a severe wasting syndrome is seen in which typical Cushingoid appearances are absent (Fig. 8.10), although more slowly growing lesions may produce a clinical picture identical to that of classic Cushing's syndrome.

Adrenal tumours may occur at any age, but predominate in children, particularly carcinomas. Their underlying aetiology is not known. Carcinomas are usually locally aggressive and large (over 6cm in diameter); they may be palpable abdominally and may disseminate widely via the blood. Adenomas are slower growing and are usually

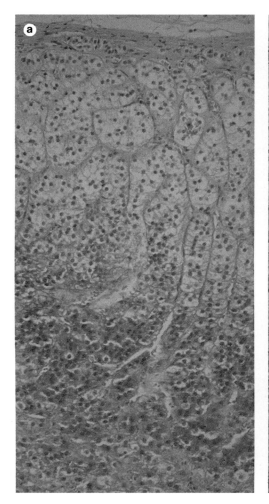

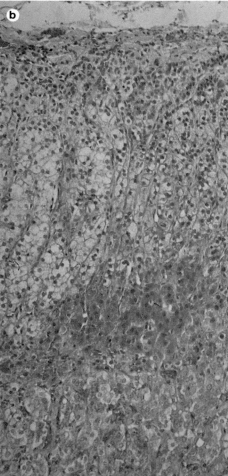

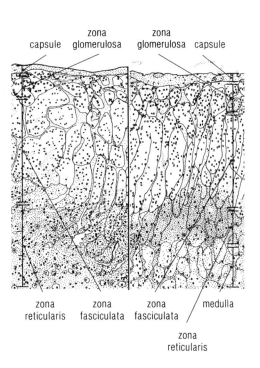

Fig. 8.6 A histological section of the adrenal cortex. (a) A section from a patient with Cushing's syndrome. Diffuse hyperplasia of the zona fasciculata with cords of cells can be seen, in contrast to section (b) where the less-organised appearance of the normal cortex is shown. By courtesy of Prof I Doniach.

of moderate size (1.5–6cm diameter) at presentation; rarely they are part of the multiple endocrine neoplasia (MEN) syndrome, type 1. Excess androgen production is common with adrenal tumours, but is usually only severe enough to cause virilisation with carcinomas. Occasionally, functioning or non-functioning adrenocortical adenomas are found unexpectedly during abdominal CT scanning for unconnected reasons ('incidentalomas').

The pathophysiology of alcohol-induced pseudo-Cushing's syndrome is poorly understood. It is clear, however, that it is not entirely ACTH-dependent in that ACTH levels are not as high as would be anticipated from the cortisol levels. Withdrawal of alcohol leads to remission of the biochemical abnormalities over a period of days, but the clinical signs may take longer to abate.

Adrenocortical macronodular hyperplasia is a rare cause of Cushing's syndrome. High-resolution computerised tomographic (CT) scanning typically demonstrates adrenal nodules that coexist with a variable degree of bilateral adrenal hyperplasia. Plasma ACTH levels tend to be low and intermittently undetectable.

AETIOLOGY OF SPONTANEOUS CUSHING'S SYNDROME

	Proportion of all causes
ACTH-dependent	83%
pituitary cushing's syndrome (79%)	66%
ectopic ACTH (14%)	12%
ACTH source unknown (6%)	4%
macronodular hyperplasia (1%)	1%
ACTH-independent	17%
adrenal adenoma (58%)	10%
adrenal carcinoma (42%)	7%

Fig. 8.7 The aetiology of spontaneous Cushing's syndrome in 225 patients seen at St Bartholomew's Hospital between 1969 and 1991. Eighty-three per cent of all causes are ACTH-dependent and seventeen per cent ACTH independent. Although the most common cause is pituitary-dependent disease (Cushing's disease: sixty-six per cent of all cases of Cushing's syndrome and seventy-nine per cent of ACTH-dependent cases), ectopic ACTH production is also important (twelve per cent of all cases of Cushing's syndrome and fourteen per cent of ACTH-dependent cases).

INVOLVEMENT OF ACTH AND CORTISOL IN THE HYPOTHALAMIC–PITUITARY–ADRENAL AXIS

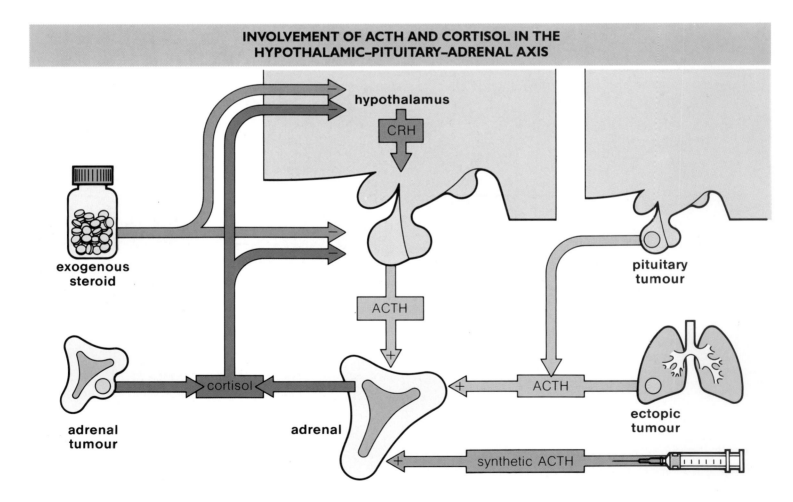

Fig. 8.8 The involvement of ACTH and cortisol in the hypothalamic–pituitary–adrenal axis. Cortisol produced in the adrenals or by an adrenal tumour has a negative feedback effect on ACTH production. Oral steroids have the same effect. Conversely, ACTH stimulates cortisol production and secretion, as do pituitary or ectopic tumours and intramuscular injections of ACTH.

Carney's syndrome is an autosomal dominant condition characterised by mesenchymal tumours, spotty skin pigmentation, peripheral nerve tumours, atrial myxomas and endocrine disorders. When associated with Cushing's syndrome, the adrenal glands are small or normal sized with multiple small, deeply pigmented nodules.

The association of pigmentation with an enlarging pituitary tumour following bilateral adrenalectomy in a patient with Cushing's disease is known as Nelson's syndrome (Fig. 8.11). It is estimated that approximately thirty per cent of patients who undergo bilateral adrenalectomy without prophylactic pituitary radiotherapy will develop this condition.

DIAGNOSIS OF CUSHING'S SYNDROME

When investigating a patient with suspected Cushing's syndrome, two stages are necessary: confirmation of the presence of Cushing's syndrome and, if present, differential diagnosis of the precise cause.

BIOCHEMICAL FEATURES

The biochemical hallmark of the condition is inappropriate cortisol secretion. The biochemical features, however, can also be associated with psychological or physical stress, alcoholism, coma, depression, and obesity, while Cushing's syndrome itself may also be intermittent or cyclical. The diagnosis of Cushing's syndrome relies upon the demonstration of excessive cortisol secretion and abnormal feedback regulation of the hypothalamic–pituitary–adrenal axis. Loss of the normal circadian pattern of cortisol secretion, and lack of dexamethasone suppressibility (0.5mg administered orally precisely every six hours for two days), is characteristic of the disease (Fig. 8.12), but can be mimicked by the conditions described above.

In normal individuals, serum cortisol levels should be less than 100nmol/l at midnight if the patient was asleep just before the blood was taken; after forty-eight hours of dexamethasone 2mg/d, 0900 serum cortisol levels should be less than 50nmol/l. Single-spot measurement of serum cortisol levels is of little diagnostic value. Twenty-four hour urinary-free cortisol excretion is a useful screening investigation for Cushing's syndrome. Failure of serum cortisol to increase after adequate insulin-induced hypoglycaemia (plasma glucose <2.2mmol/l), plus symptoms of sweating and palpitations, is a strong indication of the presence of Cushing's syndrome since this response is usually intact in depressed and obese subjects. Normal responsiveness, however, may be retained in intermittent Cushing's syndrome. To exclude the possibility of alcohol-induced pseudo-Cushing's syndrome, ethanol consumption should be rigorously banned during assessment as the biochemical abnormality may revert to normal within days of abstinence from alcohol.

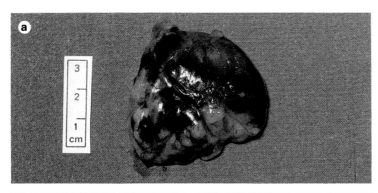
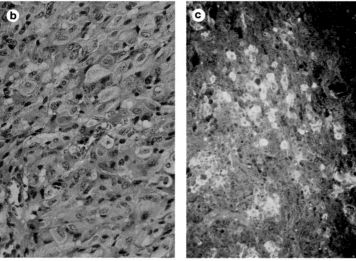
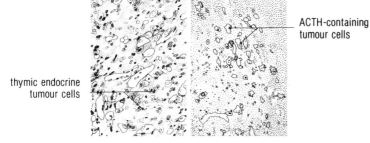

Fig. 8.9 Macroscopic and microscopic views of a thymic tumour. The whole tumour (a) is from a patient with Cushing's syndrome. The conventional histology of the tumour is shown in (b). The immunofluorescent staining in section (c) is used to reveal ACTH-containing tumour cells by staining them yellow with an anti-ACTH antibody. By courtesy of Mr GM Rees and Prof I Doniach.

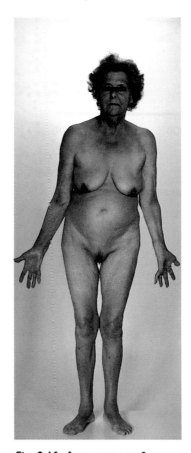

Fig. 8.10 Appearance of a patient with ectopic ACTH syndrome. Marked wasting and skin pigmentation are present.

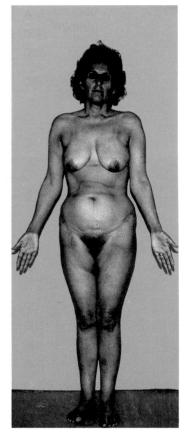

Fig. 8.11 Appearance of a patient with Nelson's syndrome. The gross pigmentation that occurs in this syndrome is best seen on the flexural surfaces of the body.

Most ACTH-secreting pituitary adenomas are less than 1cm in size and enhance with CT contrast in the same manner as normal pituitary tissue. High-resolution CT scanning identifies only a minority of adenomas; MRI with gadolinium enhancement is probably superior (Fig. 8.17). It must be noted, however, that incidental adenomas are present in twenty-five per cent of pituitaries at postmortem and therefore abnormalities identified on CT or MRI cannot automatically be assumed to be functional. The biochemical data must also be consistent with the imaging results.

Venous Catheterisation

Venous catheterisation may be of value in confirming a pituitary origin of ACTH and in locating some ectopic sources of the hormone. The most powerful investigation for the discrimination between an ectopic cause and a pituitary cause of Cushing's syndrome is the technique of bilateral inferior petrosal sinus sampling

(Fig. 8.18). Simultaneous samples for ACTH are obtained from a peripheral vein and the petrosal sinuses bilaterally, before and after the intravenous administration of 100μg CRH. If concentrations of ACTH are more than twice the values when peripheral and petrosal sinus levels are compared or between the petrosal sinuses before and after the administration of CRH, an ACTH-secreting pituitary adenoma is present and may indeed be localised with reasonable accuracy to one side of the fossa.

Whole-body venous sampling for ACTH is occasionally of value in a patient with suspected ectopic ACTH secretion, highlighting the source (Fig. 8.19). Though largely supplanted by CT scanning, catheterisation is still useful in the study of a peripheral ACTH-secreting or adrenal cortisol-secretory tumour where doubt exists as to the hormonal activity of a structural abnormality seen on a CT scan.

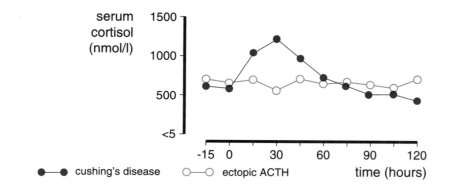

THE SERUM CORTISOL RESPONSE TO CRH IN TWO PATIENTS WITH CUSHING'S SYNDROME

Fig. 8.14 The serum cortisol response to CRH in two patients with Cushing's syndrome. In the patient with pituitary-dependent disease, the characteristic marked plasma cortisol rise after an intravenous bolus of 100μg of CRH is seen. Serum cortisol levels are unaltered in the patient with ectopic ACTH secretion.

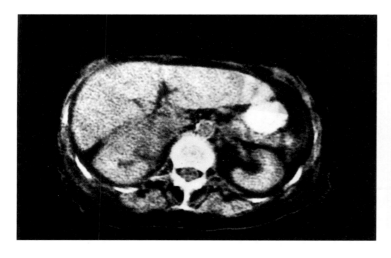

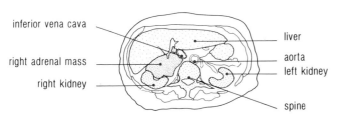

Fig. 8.15 CT scan of the abdomen in Cushing's syndrome. The irregular lobulated mass in the position of the right adrenal was confirmed at operation to be an adrenal carcinoma. By courtesy of Dr FE White.

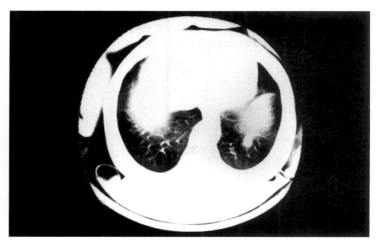

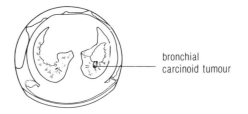

Fig. 8.16 CT scan of the chest in Cushing's syndrome. The small mass in the left lung was found to be a bronchial carcinoid tumour. The resultant hypercortisolaemia was cured on removal of the tumour. By courtesy of Dr FE White.

TREATMENT

If left untreated, the life expectancy of patients with Cushing's syndrome of moderate or severe degree is less than five years, death usually occurring from cardiovascular disease.

Where a benign adrenal tumour or ectopic source of ACTH is present, successful removal of the tumour will cure the patient (Fig. 8.20). This is almost always possible for adrenal adenomas and for some ectopic sources, but adrenal carcinomas are rarely curable by surgery, although the use of the adrenolytic drug *ortho-para*-diethyl-diphenyl-diethane (*o,p*-DDD) (see below) may improve the patient's condition.

Transsphenoidal surgery has become the treatment of choice for Cushing's disease. In specialist centres, remission rates following

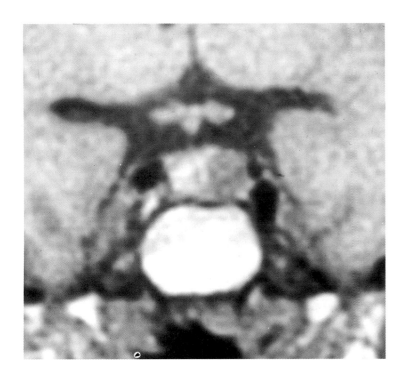

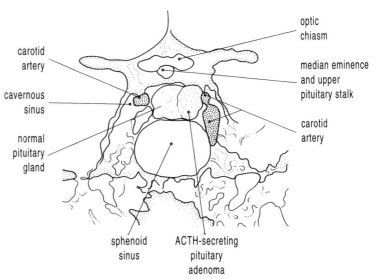

Fig. 8.17 MRI of the pituitary in Cushing's disease in coronal plane. A right-sided pituitary tumour can be seen.

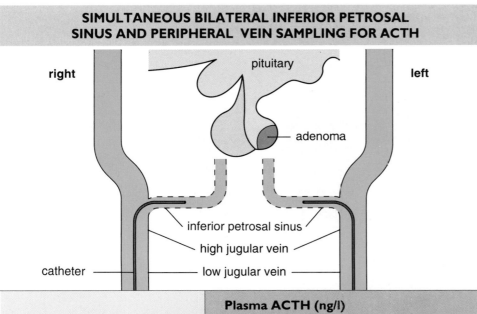

Fig. 8.18 The technique of simultaneous bilateral inferior petrosal sinus and peripheral vein sampling for ACTH with CRH stimulation. The positions from which samples are obtained are shown. The diagnosis of Cushing's disease is established by an ACTH ratio of more than two between simultaneous peripheral vein and petrosal sinus samples. A ratio of over two between the right and left petrosal sinuses indicates that the tumour is left-sided.

	Plasma ACTH (ng/l)			
	After i.v. CRH 100mg			
	0 min	5 min	10 min	15 min
left inferior petrosal sinus	14	477	280	123
right inferior petrosal sinus	16	23	28	54
simultaneous peripheral vein	17	19	25	32

transsphenoidal hypophysectomy of eighty per cent are being achieved. Immediate postoperative ACTH insufficiency (undetectable serum cortisol levels) is a valuable marker of successful removal of the pituitary lesion. This isolated ACTH deficiency of the pituitary is usually transient but may take months or years to remit. If postoperative cortisol levels are lower than preoperative levels and under 300nmol/l but not below 50nmol/l, the patient's condition will be improved although the patient will probably not be cured. Careful follow-up is then essential, and consideration should be given to further therapy such as pituitary radiotherapy or re-exploration of the pituitary fossa. Formerly, bilateral adrenalectomy was the most common definitive therapy: however, its significant mortality and morbidity have been greatly reduced by preoperative preparation with metyrapone or other medical therapy. Total adrenalectomy may still be required if other more definitive treatments fail. Following adrenalectomy, patients require lifelong steroid replacement therapy and must carry steroid cards and MedicAlert bracelets. Recurrent Cushing's syndrome from incomplete adrenalectomy or ectopic adrenal tissue is not uncommon. Adrenalectomised patients require prophylactic pituitary irradiation to prevent the development of Nelson's syndrome.

Radiotherapy as a definitive therapy may be given conventionally using a linear accelerator or a cobalt source. Conventional external

pituitary radiotherapy takes 2–10 years to achieve a cure, except in children who appear particularly sensitive to this form of treatment. This method of treatment is used in combination with medical therapy to control cortisol secretion unless the patient has had an adrenalectomy. Radiotherapy is now largely limited to patients in whom transsphenoidal hypophysectomy has been partially or completely unsuccessful, or if a total adrenalectomy has been performed.

Metyrapone (0.5–4g daily in two to four divided doses) is commonly used for short- and long-term control of excessive secretion of cortisol of any aetiology. It reversibly blocks the 11β-hydroxylase enzyme involved in the final step in cortisol synthesis. Metyapone should be taken with food and used to control the condition prior to adrenal or pituitary surgery or pending a final decision on definitive therapy. Hirsutism is a problem in some women. Ketoconazole inhibits cortisol synthesis by a direct action on the P_{450} cytochrome enzymes. It is generally well tolerated (400–800mg/d), although hepatotoxicity is an occasional problem. Disseminated adrenal carcinoma responds poorly to any therapy but can sometimes be controlled by large doses (4–10g/d) of *o,p*-DDD: at these doses, unpleasant side effects, such as nausea and ataxia, are common. In Cushing's disease, lower doses (1–3g/d) may be successfully used in the medical management without side effects. The drug takes six weeks to be fully effective and often raises circulating lipid levels. In pituitary-dependent disease, occasional patients respond to bromocriptine. In all types of medical management of the hypercortisolaemia of Cushing's syndrome, circulating cortisol levels must be reduced to normal. This is best monitored by obtaining six samples of blood for cortisol assay in one day, via an indwelling venous cannula. The average of these values for cortisol should be between 150 and 300nmol/l.

While most cases of Cushing's syndrome respond dramatically well to treatment, a few cases remain very difficult to diagnose precisely and can be difficult to treat satisfactorily. The management of this condition often still presents a most difficult clinical challenge.

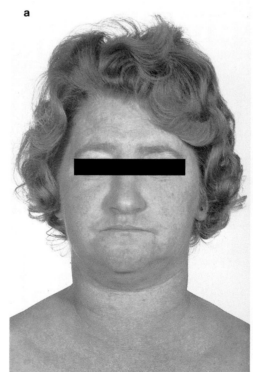

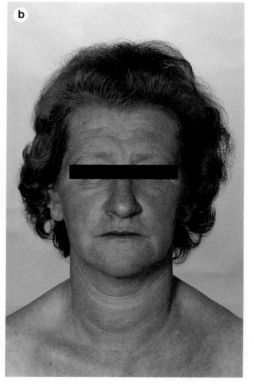

Fig. 8.19 Results of ACTH samples from whole-body venous sampling. The results obtained from a patient with the ectopic ACTH syndrome are shown. The peak ACTH (ng/l) levels that were found in the right adrenal vein were the result of an ACTH-secreting phaeochromocytoma which was later removed. Two independent samples were taken from this vein and both showed abnormally high levels of ACTH.

Fig. 8.20 Treatment of a patient with Cushing's syndrome. The facial appearance of the patient is seen before (a) and after (b) removal of an ectopic ACTH-secreting tumour.

9

Addison's Disease

Christopher R W Edwards, MA, MD, FRCP

Addison's disease results from primary adrenocortical failure. It was first described by Thomas Addison in his celebrated monograph published in 1855, which contains an illustrated description of eleven cases of the disease. After qualifying at Edinburgh University in 1813, Addison worked with a well-known dermatologist, Bateman, who was responsible for one of the first classifications of diseases of the skin; this probably stimulated his interest in the skin pigmentation that is so characteristic of Addison's disease.

AETIOLOGY

Addison's disease is a relatively rare condition with an incidence in the developed world of some 0.8 cases per one hundred thousand of the population. The causes of the disease are listed in Fig. 9.1. In Addison's original series, tuberculosis was the most common condition resulting in primary adrenal failure. With the decline in the prevalence of this infection, however, the incidence of tuberculous Addison's disease has fallen and autoimmune adrenalitis is now the most common cause, accounting for more than seventy per cent of cases. Congenital adrenal hyperplasia or hypoplasia are not normally included as causes of Addison's disease. Selective glucocorticoid deficiency can result from hereditary adrenocortical unresponsiveness to adrenocorticotrophic hormone (ACTH).

Several diseases are associated with autoimmune Addison's disease and may thus suggest the diagnosis. These are now classified as autoimmune polyglandular deficiency type I and type II (see Fig. 9.1). The human leucocyte antigens (HLA) DR3 and DR4 are strongly associated with autoimmune Addison's disease. The relative risks are 6 for DR3, 4.6 for DR4, and 26.5 for DR3/DR4 heterozygotes. These risks are similar to those of the HLA associations of type I diabetes mellitus. Interestingly, the HLA associations of patients with autoimmune polyglandular deficiency type I are not different to controls, thus suggesting that this condition has a different aetiology.

Adrenomyeloneuropathy is a rare disease in which neurological deficit is associated with Addison's disease. Patients may have both central and peripheral demyelination. The clinical picture may be one of a spastic paraparesis associated with a peripheral neuropathy, and diagnosis may be made by analysis of long-chain fatty acids in cultured skin fibroblasts. In contrast to adrenoleucodystrophy which begins in childhood, adrenomyeloneuropathy starts in adulthood. These conditions are inherited as sex-linked recessive states, and Addison's disease may precede the neurological deficit in both disorders. When adrenomyeloneuropathy develops, it may produce subtle changes such as lack of concentration, behavioural disturbance, or a compulsive disorder, before more obvious focal signs are found.

Another rare association of Addison's disease is with achalasia and alacrimation.

Fig. 9.1 The aetiology of Addison's disease. Some commonly associated conditions are also shown.

THE AETIOLOGY OF ADDISON'S DISEASE

tuberculosis

autoimmune:
autoimmune polyglandular deficiency type I
  Addison's disease
  chronic mucocutaneous candidiasis
  hypoparathyroidism
autoimmune polyglandular deficiency type II (Schmidt's syndrome)
  Addison's disease
  primary hypothyroidism
  primary hypogonadism
  insulin-dependent diabetes

metastatic tumour

lymphoma

amyloidosis

intra-adrenal haemorrhage (Waterhouse–Friedrichsen syndrome following meningococcal septicaemia)

haemochromatosis

bilateral adrenalectomy

adrenal infarction

adrenoleucodystrophy

adrenomyeloneuropathy

hereditary adrenocortical unresponsiveness to ACTH

aquired immunodeficiency syndrome

CLINICAL FEATURES

Unfortunately, because many of the symptoms of adrenocortical insufficiency are nonspecific, such as tiredness or weakness, the diagnosis of Addison's disease is often delayed until the patient is critically ill. It is therefore important to recognise that the presentation is most readily classified on the basis of the features associated with acute adrenocortical insufficiency and those seen in patients with the chronic condition.

In the acute stage, the most obvious feature is shock. Most patients presenting with an acute adrenocortical crisis will be known to have the primary adrenal condition. In this situation, the crisis will often have been precipitated by failure to take, or to absorb, glucocorticoids used in the treatment (for example when acute gastroenteritis occurs), or because the glucocorticoid dose was not increased to cover intercurrent stress (e.g. in pneumonia or major surgery). In acute adrenal failure occurring *de novo* (e.g. as with a septicaemia), the patient will not be pigmented and the symptoms will usually be weakness, malaise, nausea (often with vomiting), and non-specific

or vague epigastic abdominal pain associated with constipation or diarrhoea. A cardinal physical sign is postural hypotension. In chronic adrenal insufficiency, many of the same features are present, but the presentation is much more vague.

Pigmentation is present in more than ninety per cent of cases; this results from increased melanin in the skin and mucous membranes, and is more readily seen in areas exposed to light or pressure. Thus, the face (Fig. 9.2), the back of the hands (Fig. 9.3), elbows and knees, the buccal mucosa, conjunctivae, nails, axillae, and skin creases (Fig. 9.4) are commonly pigmented. Vitiligo, in which there is patchy and often symmetrical depigmentation of the skin, surrounded by areas of increased pigmentation (Fig. 9.5), occurs in ten to twenty per cent of cases of Addison's disease. Its presence is almost invariably an indication that the cause of the adrenal failure is autoimmune adrenalitis. One of the patients described by Addison in his 1855 monograph had extensive vitiligo; however, this was the only case in which permission for postmortem examination was refused.

The other clinical features of Addison's disease are less dramatic.

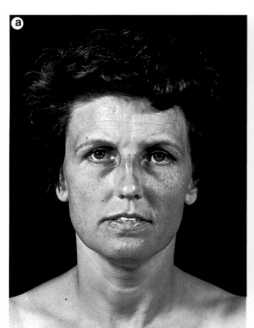
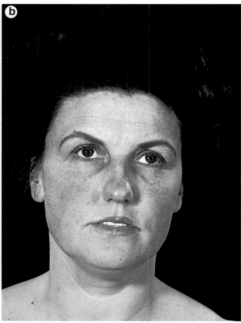

Fig. 9.2 A patient with Addison's disease.
(a) Before treatment. Note that the face is thin and pigmented. (b) During glucocorticoid replacement therapy.

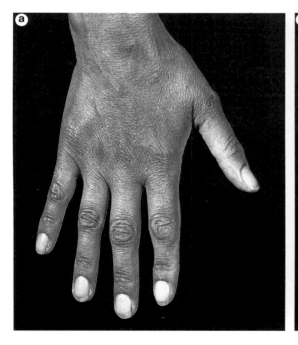
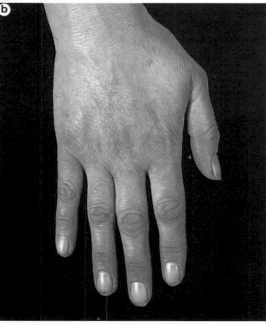

Fig. 9.3 Pigmentation of the dorsal surface of the hands in a patient with Addison's disease. (a) Before treatment. (b) During glucocorticoid therapy; the normal hand colour is now restored.

Weakness and weight loss are almost invariable. Anorexia, nausea, and vague abdominal symptoms including pain, diarrhoea, or constipation, are common. Symptoms suggestive of postural hypotension include dizziness and attacks of fainting on standing. It should be noted, however, that postural hypotension may only occur late in the course of the disease and therefore its absence does not preclude the diagnosis. Occasionally, hypoglycaemia may occur. The patient's ability to respond to stress is markedly impaired and thus the history may include a failure to recover normally after surgery or intercurrent illness.

DIAGNOSIS

In a patient with suspected adrenocortical insufficiency, the clinical sign of pigmentation will nearly always distinguish primary adrenocortical insufficiency from that which is secondary to either hypothalamic or pituitary disease (Fig. 9.6). Confirmation of the diagnosis of

Addison's disease is normally made either by measuring early morning plasma levels of cortisol and ACTH, or by determining the plasma cortisol responsiveness to ACTH stimulation. Measurement of early morning basal cortisol alone is not satisfactory as it is often in the normal 0900 reference range; however, in Addison's disease, this will be associated with an inappropriately high plasma ACTH level (i.e. above the normal 0900 reference range of 2.3–18pmol/l (10–80ng/l)).

ACTH is derived from a large precursor molecule, pro-opiomelanocortin (POMC) (Fig. 9.7). This precursor gives rise to three molecules that contain the melanocyte-stimulating hormone (MSH) sequence: the amino-terminal sequence containing the γ-MSH sequence; ACTH with α-MSH; and β-lipotrophin (β-LPH) with β-MSH peptide sequences. The relative importance of these molecules in the pigmentation that occurs in the disease is unclear. Assays have been developed for the amino-terminal sequence (N-POC) and for β-LPH. The levels of these molecules are high in Addison's disease and, since they are more stable in plasma than ACTH, they may

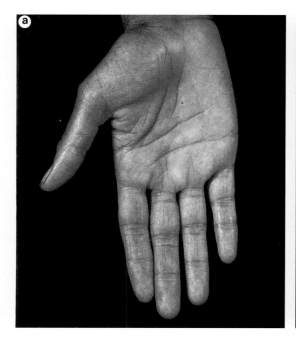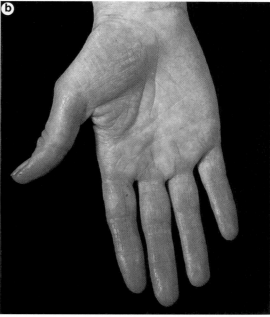

Fig. 9.4 Pigmentation of the palmar creases of the hands of a patient with Addison's disease. Pigmentation in Addison's disease commonly occurs in areas exposed to light and pressure. It is usually seen in the skin creases, as shown in (a). (b) During treatment, the normal colour returns.

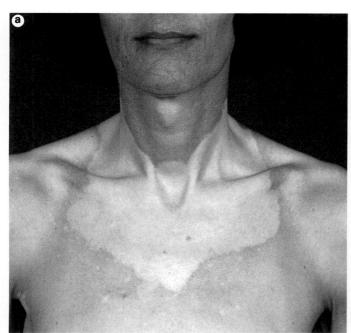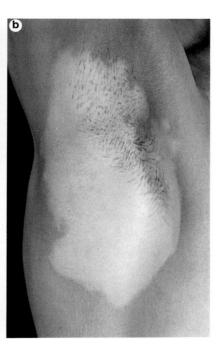

Fig. 9.5 Vitiligo in a patient with Addison's disease. Depigmentation can be seen on the neck and chest (a) and on the axilliary region (b). Increased pigmentation can be seen surrounding the areas of depigmentation.

prove to be useful in biochemical diagnosis, particularly where sample-handling facilities (e.g. cold centrifuge) are unavailable.

A variety of ACTH stimulation tests have been described in which either $ACTH_{1-39}$ or $ACTH_{1-24}$ is given. Only the first twenty-four amino acids of ACTH are required for full biological activity. Thus, synthetic preparations such as tetracosactrin ($ACTH_{1-24}$) are usually used.

In the 'short' tetracosactrin test, after taking a basal plasma cortisol sample, 250µg tetracosactrin (Synacthen) is administered either intramuscularly or intravenously. Further samples for cortisol assay are taken at thirty and sixty minutes following the injection. This test is best performed at 0900 and the patient does not need to be fasting. The normal increment in plasma cortisol is greater than 200nmol/l (Fig. 9.8). A lack of response to tetracosactrin (Synacthen Depot) does not distinguish between primary and secondary adrenocortical insufficiency; this can only be achieved by administering depot tetracosactrin – a zinc-adsorbed preparation with a prolonged action over approximately twenty-four hours. When this preparation is given

(1mg intramuscularly), the plasma cortisol levels at thirty and sixty minutes following the injection are virtually identical to those obtained with the short-acting preparation. With primary and secondary adrenocortical failure, there may be no rise in cortisol at these times. With secondary failure, when blood samples are also taken at eight and twenty-four hours, the cortisol level usually rises in contrast to the lack of response in primary failure. Further injections of depot tetracosactrin can be given at intervals of twenty-four or forty-eight hours to restore the adrenal response to normal in secondary hypoadrenalism. Where depot preparations are not available, continuous intravenous infusions of ACTH may be given.

Tetracosactrin tests in African patients with chronic pulmonary tuberculosis have shown that some thirty per cent have an impaired cortisol response. The significance of this is unclear.

Tests of adrenomedullary function are of no clinical relevance and are therefore not normally performed. Infusion of 2-deoxy-D-glucose has been shown to stimulate adrenalin output in idiopathic Addison's disease, but has minimal effect in tuberculous Addison's. This is in

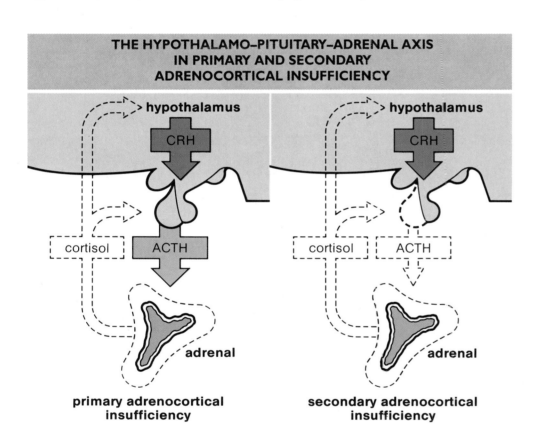

THE HYPOTHALAMO–PITUITARY–ADRENAL AXIS IN PRIMARY AND SECONDARY ADRENOCORTICAL INSUFFICIENCY

hypothalamus

CRH

cortisol   ACTH

adrenal

primary adrenocortical insufficiency

hypothalamus

CRH

cortisol   ACTH

adrenal

secondary adrenocortical insufficiency

Fig. 9.6 The hypothalamo–pituitary–adrenal axis in primary and secondary adrenocortical insufficiency. In primary adrenocortical insufficiency, circulating ACTH levels are elevated because of the negative feedback effects of low circulating cortisol. In secondary adrenocortical insufficiency, low circulating ACTH levels result from either hypothalamic or pituitary disease; as a consequence, cortisol levels are low.

STRUCTURE OF POMC

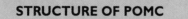

ACTH/β-LPH precursor

| 1 | 76 | 1 | 39 | 1 | 89 |

| N-terminal fragment | ACTH | β-LPH |

| 1 | 56 | 59 | 89 |

| γ-LPH | β-endorphin |

joining peptides lost in processing

Fig. 9.7 The structure of POMC. POMC is the ACTH/β-LPH precursor molecule, therefore its cleavage results in ACTH and β-LPH release. Precise residue lengths vary between species. Modified from Takahashi et al, 1981, and Whitfield et al, 1982.

keeping with the histology (Fig. 9.9) which shows that, in the tuberculous disease, the whole gland is often destroyed. Plasma electrolyte concentrations are not infrequently normal but may show the classical picture of hyponatraemia, hyperkalaemia, and elevated levels of urea. Serum aldosterone levels may be normal or low, but plasma

renin activity is elevated. Patients with Addison's disease have an increased basal level of plasma arginine vasopressin (AVP), together with a decreased osmotic threshold. This disturbance of osmoregulation of AVP is likely to play a major role in the failure to excrete a water load, which is a characteristic feature of Addison's disease.

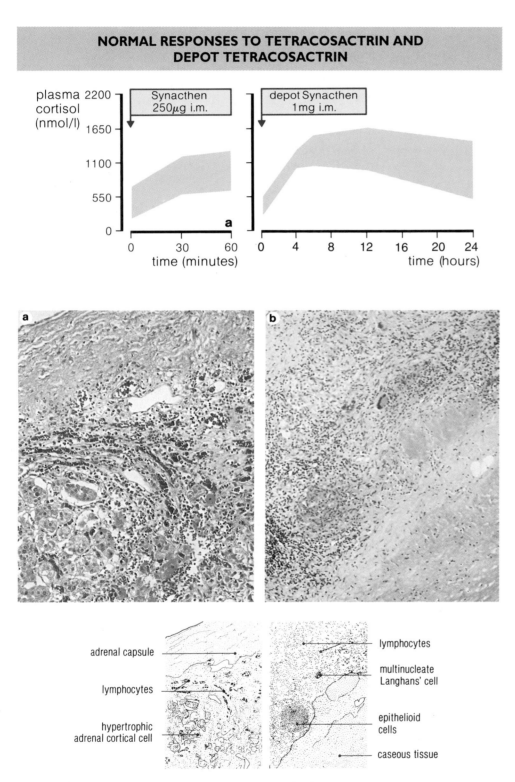

Fig. 9.8 The normal responses to (a) tetracosactrin (Synacthen) and (b) depot tetracosactrin. Tetracosactrin is administered intramuscularly in doses of 250µg, whereas depot tetracosactrin is given in doses of 1mg.

Fig. 9.9 Histological appearances in Addison's disease. The postmortem histology of (a) autoimmune acrenalitis and (b) tuberculosis adrenalitis in patients who died of Addison's disease is shown. (a) The adrenal capsule is markedly thickened, and the surviving cortex consists of scattered hypertrophied adrenocortical cells that are heavily infiltrated with lymphocytes. Haematoxylin and eosin (H&E) stain, magnification X 120. (b) Pink-staining amorphous, caseous necrosis can be seen in addition to tuberculous granulation tissue and a Langerhans' giant cell. H&E stain, magnification X 80. By courtesy of Prof I Doniach.

The differential diagnosis usually lies between autoimmune adrenalitis and tuberculosis. In a patient with suspected autoimmune adrenalitis, evidence for other organ involvement should be sought; thus, tests to determine the presence of thyroid, gastric parietal cell, and intrinsic factor antibodies should be carried out, in addition to tests for antibodies directed against adrenal tissue. Recent results have shown that measurement of adrenal antibodies by radioimmunoassay is more sensitive than measurement by the usual method using immunofluorescence.

Apart from destructive antibodies, there is some evidence to suggest that Addison's disease can be caused by antibodies that block the effect of ACTH. Such antibodies may be directed against the ACTH receptor. If adrenal antibodies are not found by sensitive methodology, then evidence of tuberculosis should be sought. Often, no active disease is found, but adrenal calcification usually indicates that tuberculosis was the cause of the adrenal failure. This is sometimes missed using conventional radiography and is most readily seen using computerised tomographic (CT) scanning of the adrenals (Fig. 9.10). In the acute phase of the tuberculous disease (i.e. less than two years' duration), CT scanning usually demonstrates that the adrenals are enlarged, whereas in patients with disease of longer duration, the adrenals are small. Fine-needle aspiration has been used to make the diagnosis of tuberculosis in patients with enlarged adrenals. In autoimmune adrenal failure, the glands are either small or undetectable. Both magnetic resonance imaging and CT scanning have

been used to diagnose intra-adrenal haemorrhage. It is worth screening patients with idiopathic Addison's disease for other associated diseases since approximately fifty per cent of them will have, or will develop, either autoimmune thyroid disease or insulin-dependent diabetes mellitus.

TREATMENT

All patients with Addison's disease require glucocorticoid replacement therapy, and the majority also need mineralocorticoid treatment. Hydrocortisone (cortisol) is now regarded as the drug of choice since, unlike cortisone acetate, it does not need to be metabolised before it is metabolically active; it is also more readily absorbed. In an acute adrenal crisis, hydrocortisone hemisuccinate should be administered (100mg intravenously), together with saline to correct sodium losses and dextrose to treat hypoglycaemia. Intramuscular hydrocortisone should also be given (100mg at six-hour intervals) until the patient is able to take oral therapy, at which time hydrocortisone is given (40mg on waking, 20mg at 1800). When the patient is well, the oral dose is halved. Since intercurrent infections often precipitate the crisis, evidence for any infections should be actively sought and the appropriate antibiotic treatment given. It is, however, important to recognise that a pyrexia *per se* may occur in adrenal insufficiency without any superadded infection.

For chronic adrenocortical failure, maintenance therapy with hydrocortisone is initiated, usually together with 9α-fludrocortisone to replace the mineralocorticoid deficiency. Most patients require 20mg oral hydrocortisone on waking and 10mg at 1800. Occasional patients feel better on hydrocortisone given three times daily rather than twice daily. Adequate replacement therapy should reverse the pigmentation (see Figs. 9.2–9.4) but should not produce Cushing's syndrome. Plasma cortisol levels should be measured during the day on replacement therapy to determine if the correct dose has been given (Fig. 9.11). Mineralocorticoid replacement with 9α-fludrocortisone is given either daily or on alternate days; the dose varies from 0.05mg on alternate days, to 0.2mg daily. If the dose is excessive, oedema and hypertension may result. Adequacy of mineralocorticoid replacement can be monitored by measurement of plasma renin activity. Elevated plasma renin activity usually signifcies that inadequate mineralocorticoid replacement has been given. In practice, twice-daily 9α-fludrocortisone may provide better suppression of renin than once-daily therapy.

Patients should be told to double their dose of hydrocortisone in the event of intercurrent stress or febrile illness. If they cannot take their steroid by mouth (e.g. in the event of surgery or gastroenteritis), it should be given parenterally. All patients should carry a steroid card, or preferably a bracelet or necklace, giving details of their condition. For minor operations (e.g. dental extraction), 100mg hydrocortisone hemisuccinate should be administered with the premedication. For major surgery, the steroid regime for acute adrenal crisis, outlined above, should be adopted. Other autoimmune diseases may be present in patients with autoimmune adrenalitis and these should be treated if necessary. Patients with tuberculous Addison's disease usually require antituberculous chemotherapy. It is important to recognise the problems that may ensue if rifampicin is used. The enzyme induction that is produced increases the metabolic clearance of cortisol and thus may precipitate an adrenal crisis. Higher-than-usual doses of replacement therapy are therefore required in patients on rifampicin, and also those on anticonvulsants (which induce the same enzymes). Measurement of plasma renin levels assists in tailoring the doses of 9α-fludrocortisone to suit the needs of individual patients.

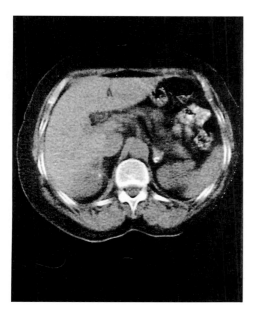
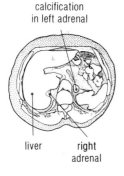

calcification in left adrenal

liver / right adrenal

Fig. 9.10 A computerised tomogram of the adrenal glands in a patient with tuberculous Addison's disease. Calcification of the left adrenal can be seen.

9

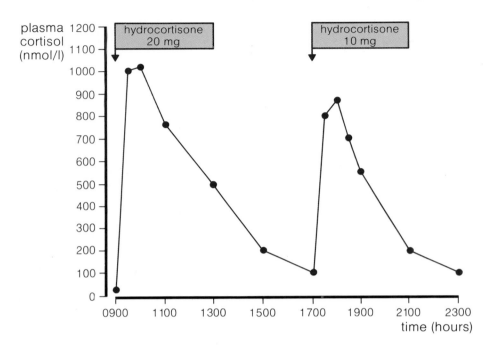

PLASMA CORTISOL PROFILE IN ADRENOCORTICAL INSUFFICIENCY FOLLOWING HYDROCORTISONE REPLACEMENT THERAPY

Fig 9.11 The plasma cortisol profile of a patient with adrenocortical insufficiency on hydrocortisone replacement therapy. Oral hydrocortisone (20mg) was administered at 0900, with a further dose of 10mg given at 1700.

10

Endocrine Hypertension

Christopher R W Edwards, MA, MD, FRCP

Hypertension is one of the major medical problems of the world since it affects approximately fifteen per cent of the population in Western countries. It is defined as a persistent increase in systemic blood pressure above an arbitrary limit, often set at 140mmHg systolic and 90mmHg diastolic (phaseV, i.e. disappearance of sound).

The lowering of blood pressure has now been shown to reduce the incidence of stroke and also renal failure, although it has very little effect on the incidence of coronary artery disease.

Since most patients with hypertension are symptomless for many years, population screening should be carried out. Moreover, since the diagnosis of hypertension may lead to lifelong drug therapy, secondary causes of hypertension, which may be remedied by surgery or respond to specific drug therapy, should be identified. A knowledge of the physiology and pathophysiology of the renin–angiotensin–aldosterone system, glucocorticoid hypersecretion or defective metabolism, and catecholamine excess is therefore essential.

AETIOLOGY OF HYPERTENSION

The prevalence of various conditions that result in hypertension is shown in Fig. 10.1. In the majority of patients with hypertension, no cause for the elevated blood pressure can be found and such individuals are defined as having 'essential' or primary hypertension. This is a familial condition, although the genetic basis for it is unknown; however, recent evidence suggests that the intrauterine environment may be important. Thus, blood pressure of adults in their fifties is significantly related to birth weight and placental weight: a small baby with a large placenta is more likely to have high blood pressure as an adult than is a large baby with a smaller placenta. Low birth weight is also a predictor of adult ischaemic heart disease and glucose intolerance.

A large number of secondary causes of hypertension have been described (Fig. 10.2). Although the prevalence of many of these conditions is debatable, it does, however, depend upon a variety of factors; primary hyperaldosteronism, for example, is approximately twice as common in non-Caucasian hypertensive patients as it is in Caucasian ones. The most common secondary cause is renal disease with activation of the renin–angiotensin system.

The mineralocorticoid excess associated with the ingestion of liquorice or carbenoxolone (the hemisuccinate derivative of glycyrrhetinic acid – the active component of liquorice) was once believed to result as a direct effect of either of these agents on the kidney; however, it is now known that this is not the case and that the condition is due to the inhibition of the enzyme 11β-hydroxysteroid dehydrogenase which converts cortisol to cortisone. This enzyme plays a critical role in aldosterone-selective tissues (such as the kidney) in preventing cortisol from gaining access to the non-specific mineralocorticoid receptor. If it is inhibited or congenitally absent, then the so-called syndrome of apparent mineralocorticoid excess ensues.

PHYSIOLOGY OF THE RENIN–ANGIOTENSIN–ALDOSTERONE SYSTEM

Renin is a proteolytic enzyme that is synthesised and stored by specialised cells in the wall of the afferent arteriole that is situated in the glomerulus of the kidney. These cells are anatomically and functionally associated with the cells in the wall of the distal convoluted tubules, which form the macula densa, and the whole structure is known as the juxtaglomerular apparatus. The release of renin activates a cascade system (Fig. 10.3) in which renin cleaves a leucine–valine bond in its specific substrate (angiotensinogen, an α_2-globulin that is produced by the liver). This, in turn, results in the production of the decapeptide angiotensin I, which is subsequently converted by angiotensin-converting enzyme (ACE) to the octapeptide angiotensin II (see Chapter 7). ACE is a dipeptidyl carboxypeptidase that is found in high concentrations in the pulmonary circulation; it is, however, also present in the systemic vasculature and the kidney. Angiotensin II is a potent vasoconstrictor and can thus elevate blood

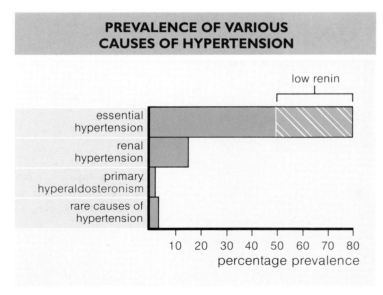

Fig. 10.1 The prevalence of various causes of hypertension. Eighty per cent of patients have primary or essential hypertension with no apparent cause. Many secondary causes of hypertension have been described, but their prevalence is limited to a minority of hypertensive patients.

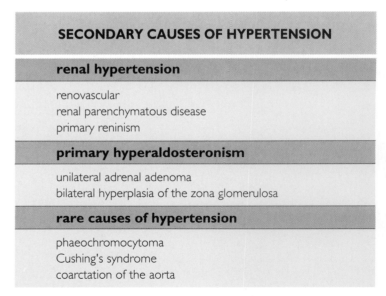

Fig. 10.2 Secondary causes of hypertension. These can be classified as primary hyperaldosteronism, renal causes, and rare causes.

pressure. It also directly stimulates aldosterone secretion, which leads to sodium retention and potassium loss. A seven amino-acid peptide, angiotensin III, is released by protease cleavage of angiotensin II. The role of angiotensin III in man is controversial; in many species, it has been shown to be at least as potent as angiotensin II in stimulating aldosterone secretion, although it has less pressor activity.

Renin is produced in both an active and inactive form. Various *in vitro* techniques have been used to activate the inactive enzyme, including treatment with trypsin, pepsin, or acid, or incubation at –4°C. The enzyme responsible for *in vivo* activation of renin is probably a serine protease, possibly kallikrein. The major trigger for renin release is a decrease in perfusion pressure, and this may result from haemorrhage, hypotension, or a reduction in the extracellular fluid volume after sodium depletion. The autonomic nervous system also plays a role in renin release, as do catecholamines which can directly stimulate renin secretion. Conversely, hyperkalaemia, angiotensin II,

and antidiuretic hormone (ADH or vasopressin) can all inhibit renin secretion.

Aldosterone is the principal mineralocorticoid that is secreted by the outermost zone of the adrenal cortex, the zona glomerulosa. The normal production rate is approximately 200μg daily; this is critically dependent on sodium intake being stimulated by sodium depletion and suppressed by salt loading. Plasma levels fall in the range of 140–420pmol/l (50–150ng/l) when normal subjects are recumbent and of 420–840pmol/l (150–300ng/l) when standing upright. In addition, there is a circadian rhythm of aldosterone secretion, with higher levels being present in the morning than at night. Thus, posture, sodium intake, and time of day all have to be taken into consideration when taking blood samples for aldosterone assay.

The three major factors that control the biosynthesis and release of aldosterone are angiotensin II, adrenocorticotrophic hormone (ACTH), and potassium. Of these, angiotensin II is almost certainly the most important; various factors can alter the adrenal responsiveness to this hormone. Thus, sodium depletion increases the adrenal sensitivity to angiotensin II and also stimulates the release of renin, which in turn leads to elevated angiotensin II levels. Although acute administration of ACTH stimulates aldosterone secretion, chronic ACTH excess is associated with normal or even low levels of aldosterone. Thus, when the renin–angiotensin system is suppressed, for example in patients with primary hyperaldosteronism, ACTH may play an important role. Aldosterone-secreting adrenal adenomas are extremely sensitive to ACTH stimulation and, as a result, plasma aldosterone has the same circadian rhythm as plasma cortisol in these patients. Hyperkalaemia can directly stimulate the zona glomerulosa. Conversely, hypokalaemia may inhibit aldosterone synthesis. Thus, in patients with Conn's syndrome, aldosterone secretion may be markedly stimulated by potassium replacement therapy.

The primary effect of aldosterone is to increase the resorption of sodium by the distal convoluted tubule of the kidney, in exchange for potassium and hydrogen ions. Therefore, if aldosterone levels are persistently elevated, hypokalaemia and alkalosis will ensue.

PATHOPHYSIOLOGY OF THE RENIN–ANGIOTENSIN–ALDOSTERONE SYSTEM

Hypertension may result from overactivity of one or more components of the renin–angiotensin–aldosterone system. Raised blood pressure may be associated with the excessive secretion of aldosterone due either to an adrenocortical abnormality (thus termed primary hyperaldosteronism) or secondary to the excessive secretion of renin (as in renovascular or renal parenchymatous disease). The latter is referred to as secondary hyperaldosteronism.

PRIMARY HYPERALDOSTERONISM (CONN'S SYNDROME)
The prevalence of primary hyperaldosteronism is not clear. Some have suggested that approximately two per cent of all subjects with hypertension have primary hyperaldosteronism and, of these, some seventy per cent have a unilateral adrenal adenoma (Fig. 10.4) and approximately thirty per cent have bilateral hyperplasia of the zona glomerulosa (Fig. 10.5).

Primary hyperaldosteronism is usually suspected when a hypertensive patient is found to be hypokalaemic. This diagnostic clue, however, may be missed unless blood samples are taken properly; sampling without occlusion or muscular exercise is essential, and the plasma must be rapidly separated from the red cells. In addition, the patient should have an adequate sodium intake since, with a low sodium diet, there will be little sodium for distal tubular sodium–potassium exchange and thus hypokalaemia will not persist.

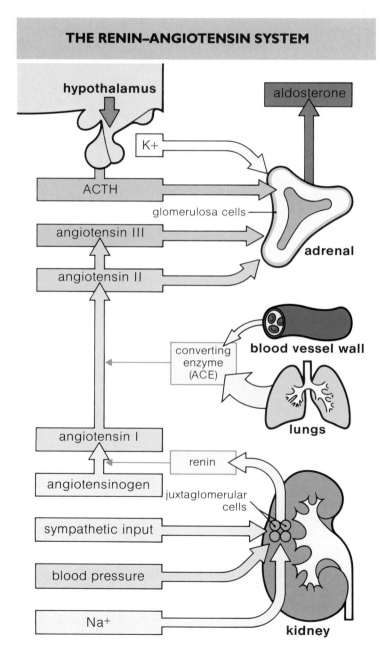

THE RENIN–ANGIOTENSIN SYSTEM

Fig. 10.3 The renin–angiotensin system. Following release, renin converts angiotensinogen to angiotensin I, which is subsequently converted to angiotensin II by ACE.

Once primary hyperaldosteronism is suspected, the diagnosis must be confirmed by demonstrating suppression of plasma renin activity and elevation of plasma aldosterone levels (Fig. 10.6).

Several methods are available to carry out the differential diagnosis between an adenoma and hyperplasia. The simplest test is to take blood at 0800, with the patient recumbent, in order to determine aldosterone levels, plasma renin activity, and cortisol levels, and then to repeat the blood sampling at 1200 after the patient has been standing upright for four hours. In patients with aldosterone-secreting adenomas, plasma renin activity is suppressed and plasma aldosterone levels decrease during the course of the morning as ACTH levels fall; the adenoma is sensitive to ACTH. Conversely, in patients with idiopathic bilateral hyperplasia, the hyperplastic adrenals are very sensitive to angiotensin II and hence the small amount of renin that is released on standing is sufficient to elevate aldosterone levels. The exception to this test is the rare condition of dexamethasone-suppressible hyperaldosteronism in which plasma aldosterone levels in the patient fall on standing. This diagnosis can be confirmed by demonstrating that the blood pressure is reduced to normal by ACTH suppression. If patients with adenomas are stressed by standing, then ACTH levels, and hence cortisol levels, will rise during the course of the morning. Furthermore, aldosterone levels will also rise. If this occurs, the test will need to be repeated.

The administration of radiolabelled cholesterol can also be used to distinguish between an adenoma and hyperplasia, since the labelled cholesterol is taken up only by the adenoma (Fig. 10.7). This is in contrast to the bilateral uptake found in patients with idiopathic hyperplasia. Scans may have to be performed after dexamethasone administration to suppress uptake by normal glucocorticoid-secreting cells. In some patients, misleading results can be obtained if spirono-lactone has been used as long-term therapy before the scan is performed. In such patients, adenomas can be missed as there may be bilateral uptake.

Adrenal vein sampling for aldosterone can be extremely useful in identifying whether there is a unilateral or bilateral source of aldosterone. Although cannulation of the left adrenal vein is relatively easy, it is difficult to enter the right adrenal vein. For this reason, blood samples should always be taken to determine cortisol levels, in addition to those for determining aldosterone levels, in order to confirm that the catheter tip is actually in the adrenal vein. A typical example of an adrenal vein catheterisation in a patient with an adenoma is shown in Fig. 10.8.

RENAL HYPERTENSION

Renal hypertension constitutes approximately fifteen per cent of all cases of hypertension. The causes can most readily be divided into three groups: renovascular, renal parenchymatous disease, and primary reninism (Fig. 10.9).

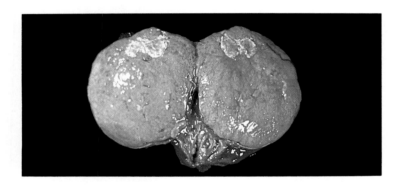

Fig. 10.4 An adrenal adenoma removed from a patient with primary hyperaldosteronism (Conn's syndrome). The canary-yellow colour of the adenoma is typical.

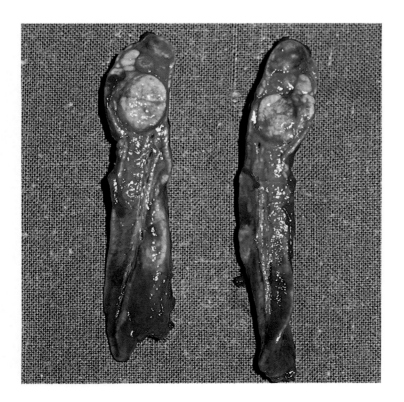

Fig. 10.5 Nodular hyperplasia associated with Conn's syndrome. Bilateral hyperplasia occurs in approximately thirty per cent of patients with hypertension that is caused by primary hyperaldosteronism.

MECHANISM OF PATHOPHYSIOLOGICAL CHANGES IN PRIMARY HYPERALDOSTERONISM

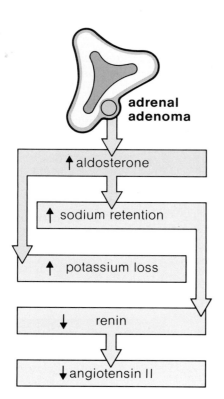

Fig. 10.6 The mechanism of pathophysiological changes that occur in primary hyperaldosteronism. The autonomous production and release of aldosterone from the tumour leads to excessive sodium retention and potassium wasting; these occur largely due to the effects of aldosterone on the distal tubule of the kidney. Renin release from the kidney is therefore inhibited and this leads to a fall in circulating levels of angiotensin II.

ADRENAL ¹³¹I-CHOLESTEROL UPTAKE IN CONN'S SYNDROME

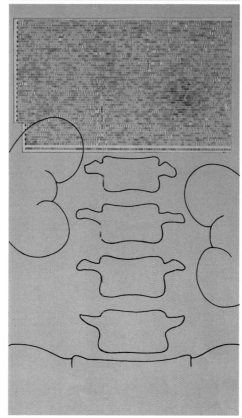

Fig. 10.7 An adrenal scan in a patient with Conn's syndrome. Selective uptake of ¹³¹I-cholesterol in a left adrenal adenoma is shown.

AN ADRENAL VEIN CATHETER STUDY

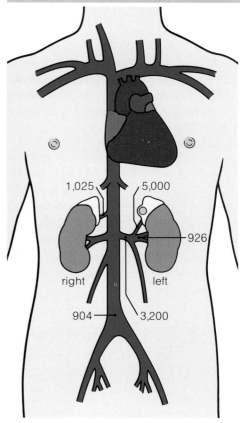

Fig. 10.8 An adrenal vein catheter study showing high levels of aldosterone in the left adrenal vein. The concentration of aldosterone (in picograms per millilitre) in the right adrenal vein is not significantly different from that found in the inferior vena cava. The patient illustrated had hypertension and hypokalaemia and was subsequently cured after removal of his left adrenal adenoma.

Fig. 10.9 Renal causes of hypertension. These can be classified into renovascular, renal parenchymatous disease, and primary reninism. Of these, renovascular hypertension is the most common.

RENAL CAUSES OF HYPERTENSION

renal parenchymatous disease	renovascular
acute and chronic glomerulonephritis	coarctation of the aorta
chronic pyelonephritis—especially if calculi or obstruction with hydronephrosis	renal artery stenosis e.g. with fibromuscular hyperplasia, atheromatous plaque, congenital
polycystic disease	malignant or accelerated phase hypertension
interstitial nephritis e.g. with gout, hypercalcaemia or excessive analgesics (analgesic nephropathy)	**primary reninism**
amyloidosis	reninomas (haemangiopericytoma)
connective tissue disease e.g. with polyarteritis, systemic lupus erythematosus and diabetes mellitus	some Wilms' tumours
	ectopic renin secretion

The two most common causes of unilateral renal artery stenosis are atheromatous plaques and fibromuscular hyperplasia. Atheromatous stenoses are most frequently found in the proximal third of the renal artery and present in the middle-aged and elderly. In contrast, fibromuscular hyperplasia involves the middle and distal thirds of the renal artery and is the most common cause of renal artery stenosis in young patients.

In patients with malignant hypertension, the elevated blood pressure leads to fibrinoid necrosis of the small vessels of the kidney; this, in turn, stimulates excessive renin release and thus further exacerbates the hypertension by activation of the renin–angiotensin–aldosterone system. Such patients therefore have secondary hyperaldosteronism (Fig. 10.10).

Renovascular hypertension may be suggested by finding a renal artery bruit. This is best heard over the long muscles of the back at the level of L1 or in the epigastrium. In many patients, however, there are no clinical clues. Isotope renography may reveal decreased uptake, and delayed excretion, of the isotope on the side of the lesion. Although this technique is less expensive than intravenous urography, it is also less widely available. On urography, a delayed nephrogram may be seen on the stenotic side in early films, with increased density and delayed excretion in later films (Fig. 10.11).

Plasma renin activity may be normal in patients with unilateral renal artery stenosis, but in some series, elevated peripheral venous levels of plasma renin activity have been found in up to sixty per cent of patients. Such patients may also have an exaggerated response of renin to dynamic function tests such as diuretic administration or sodium depletion.

The measurement of renal vein renin is important in the diagnosis of a haemodynamically significant renal artery stenosis (Fig. 10.12). The renin level in the renal vein that drains from the kidney on the opposite side to the stenosis should mimic the level in a peripheral blood sample taken simultaneously, thus indicating that the kidney is suppressed. There should be a gradient across the kidney on the affected side and, the ratio between the renal vein plasma renin activity on the affected side and the renal vein plasma renin activity on the normal side should be greater than 1.5:1. In patients with this pattern of renin secretion, renal artery surgery or transluminal balloon dilatation will probably reduce the blood pressure. In patients with suspected renal artery stenosis, renal arteriograms will need to be performed to define the site and nature of the lesion. In addition to midstream aortography, selective renal arteriography will be required (Fig. 10.13).

SEQUENCE OF EVENTS IN SECONDARY HYPERALDOSTERONISM

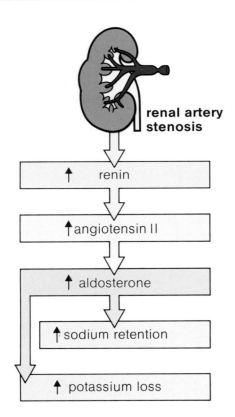

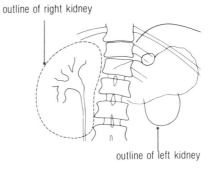

outline of right kidney

outline of left kidney

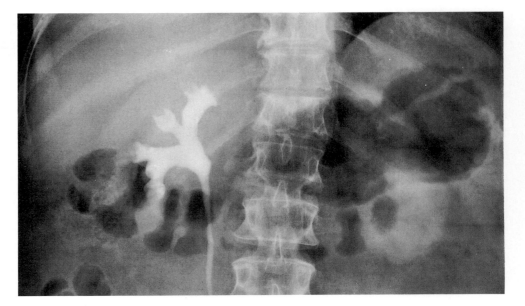

Fig. 10.10 The sequence of events that occur in secondary hyperaldosteronism. In secondary hyperaldosteronism, circulating renin levels are elevated as a consequence of renal artery stenosis, renal hypoperfusion, or volume depletion. High renin levels, in turn, lead to increased angiotensin II levels and hyperaldosteronism, with concomitant sodium retention and potassium wastage.

Fig. 10.11 A urogram in left renal artery stenosis, twenty minutes after an injection of contrast. Comparison of the left nephrogram with the right, where the contrast is in the calyceal system, demonstrates marked delay in excretion of contrast. This is caused by stenosis of the left renal artery.

Treatment of angiotensin-dependent hypertension has been revolutionised by the introduction of specific inhibitors of the renin–angiotensin–aldosterone system (Fig. 10.14). Of these, the most important have been captopril and enalapril, captopril being the first available effective and orally active inhibitor of ACE.

Transluminal angioplasty using a catheter with a balloon has been a major advance for treating patients with renal artery stenosis. Good results have been reported for both fibromuscular hyperplasia and atheromatous stenosis, with low morbidity.

HYPERTENSION ASSOCIATED WITH ABNORMALITIES OF THE HYPOTHALAMO-PITUITARY-ADRENOCORTICAL AXIS

GENETIC DEFECTS OF CORTISOL SYNTHESIS

Biglieri and colleagues have described a syndrome where defective 17α-hydroxylation is present in the adrenals and gonads. The resultant low levels of cortisol, acting via the negative feedback mechanism, stimulate ACTH release, with consequent bilateral hyperplasia and excessive secretion of corticosterone and deoxycorticosterone. These, in turn, cause sodium retention, potassium loss, hypertension, and a hypokalaemic alkalosis. The absence of normal androgen secretion in men causes male pseudohermaphroditism, while defective oestrogen secretion in women results in primary amenorrhoea. Renin levels are also suppressed. Replacement therapy with glucocorticoids rapidly suppresses ACTH levels and hence corticosterone and deoxycorticosterone levels. This results in correction of the hypertension and electrolyte abnormalities.

In the presence of 11β-hydroxylase deficiency, defective cortisol secretion leads to a secondary elevation of ACTH and to bilateral adrenal hyperplasia. In addition, there are high circulating levels of 11-deoxycortisol and deoxycorticosterone present. Hypertension ensues, as does virilism as a result of the elevated androgen levels. The process can be reversed by glucocorticoid replacement therapy.

RENAL VEIN PLASMA RENIN ACTIVITY IN RIGHT RENAL ARTERY STENOSIS

	renin activity (ng /l/h)	
	supine	standing (6 min)
high inferior vena cava	7,400	12,800
left renal vein	6,160 (7,740)	12,700 (7,240)
right renal vein	>36,000 (7,040)	>36,000 (12,300)
low inferior vena cava	7,060	10,000

Fig. 10.12 *Measurements of renal vein plasma renin activity in right renal artery stenosis.* The figures in brackets are the renin concentrations in peripheral blood samples taken simultaneously. For a diagnosis of haemodynamically significant right renal artery stenosis, the renin level in the right renal vein should be markedly higher than the level in a synchronous peripheral blood sample, and there should be no gradient on the left side. Additionally, the ratio between the left and right renal vein plasma renin activity should be greater than 1.5:1. See Appendix for normal values.

Fig. 10.13 *A selective renal arteriogram showing left renal artery stenosis in an 18-year-old boy with severe hypertension.*

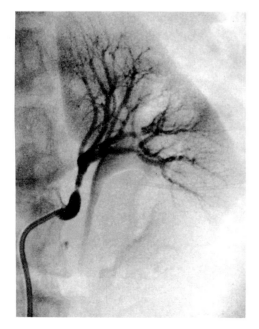
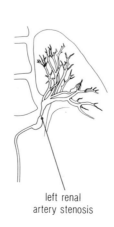

left renal
artery stenosis

CUSHING'S SYNDROME

Hypertension is commonly found in patients with Cushing's syndrome, although the aetiology of the high blood pressure is not well understood. Elevated levels of cortisol, which have mineralocorticoid and glucocorticoid effects, can increase the production of angiotensinogen. (For the investigation and treatment of patients with Cushing's syndrome, see Chapter 8.)

PHAEOCHROMOCYTOMA

Hypertension is the most common clinical feature in patients with phaeochromocytomas. Characteristically, the hypertension is labile and is often associated with a variety of symptoms. Patients may present complaining of attacks of palpitations, headache, excessive sweating, pallor, or flushing, which may be associated with anxiety. On examination, most will be found to have hypertension. There is a significant fall in blood pressure on standing in over sixty-five per cent of patients. In approximately ten to twenty per cent of cases, the phaeochromocytoma may be associated with other conditions such as

von Recklinghausen's disease and, in multiple endocrine adenomatosis, with medullary carcinoma of the thyroid and/or hyperparathyroidism. The typical neuromas found on the tongue and lips in a patient with medullary carcinoma of the thyroid and bilateral adrenal phaeochromocytomas are shown in Fig. 10.15. Patients with phaeochromocytomas not uncommonly present to psychiatrists with anxiety. In addition, glucose intolerance may be provoked by the excess catecholamine secretion, and such patients may therefore come under the care of the diabetologist. Some patients may have gastrointestinal complaints with abdominal pain, and constipation is common. It has been suggested, although not proved, that the constipation may be caused by very large amounts of metenkephalin that are produced by the tumours.

Most clinicians rely on the clinical history of the patient to suggest the diagnosis and do not routinely measure catecholamines in all patients with hypertension. In a patient suspected of having a phaeochromocytoma, the first investigative step is to measure the urinary excretion of vanillylmandelic acid (VMA); the excretion is

INHIBITORS OF THE RENIN–ANGIOTENSIN SYSTEM

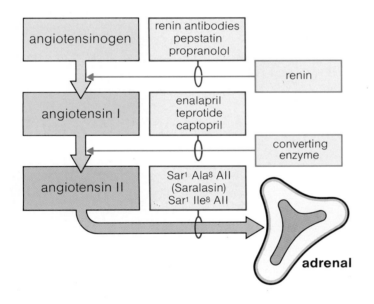

Fig. 10.14 Inhibitors of the renin–angiotensin system. Renin output may be reduced by β-blockade (using agents such as propranolol), or the activity of renin may be impaired by the presence of renin antibodies. ACE, present in the lungs and blood vessels, can be inhibited by captopril, teprotide, and enalapril. In addition, the drug saralasin is a competitive inhibitor of angiotensin II at its receptor site.

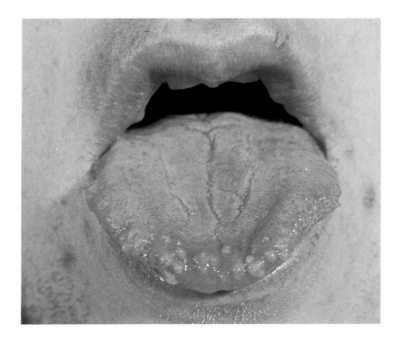

Fig. 10.15 Neuromas of the lips and tongue in a patient with medullary carcinoma of the thyroid and with adrenal phaeochromocytomas. This rare association is part of the multiple endocrine neoplasia (MEN) 2b syndrome.

elevated in ninety per cent of patients with phaeochromocytomas. Occasionally, however, the level of VMA is normal. In such instances, metanephrines should be measured in the urine; alternatively, and more reliably, plasma and urinary levels of adrenaline and noradrenaline should be measured. Adrenaline is particularly useful in making the diagnosis in patients with small adrenal phaeochromocytomas since the enzyme that converts noradrenaline to adrenaline is glucocorticoid dependent; hence, with the centripetal blood flow in the adrenal, the medulla is exposed to high levels of cortisol. A variety of pharmacological tests have been developed in an attempt to improve the diagnosis of patients with phaeochromocytomas. With advances in biochemical diagnosis, however, these have nearly all been discarded.

A test that was once commonly used involved the administration of phentolamine, an α-adrenergic blocking drug. With this technique, a positive response (Fig. 10.16) occurred within two to three minutes and resulted in a fall in blood pressure of at least 35/25mmHg. Other pharmacological tests involved the administration of tyramine or glucagon; however, as with phentolamine, these tests yielded false-positive and false-negative results.

A variety of methods have been used to locate phaeochromocytomas. Eighty-five to ninety per cent of these tumours arise from the adrenal medulla, and in ten per cent of cases, the tumours are bilateral. Non-adrenal tumours may arise from sympathetic ganglia, usually alongside the aorta or its branches or, rarely, in the wall of the

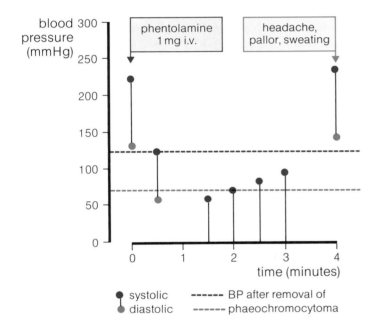

PHENTOLAMINE TEST IN A PATIENT WITH A PHAEOCHROMOCYTOMA

Fig. 10.16 A phentolamine test carried out in a patient with a phaeochromocytoma. A positive response occurs within 2–3 minutes and results in a transient fall in blood pressure of at least 35/25mmHg.

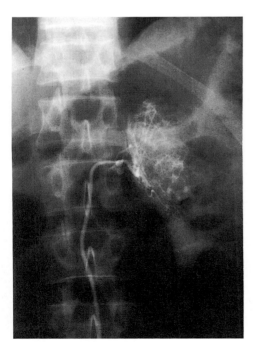
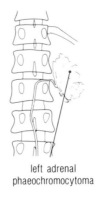

left adrenal
phaeochromocytoma

Fig. 10.17 A selective left adrenal arteriogram in a patient with a phaeochromocytoma. The abnormal vasculature and tumour blush are shown.

urinary bladder. Less than one per cent of phaeochromocytomas are found outside the abdominal cavity. Plain radiography of the abdomen may reveal displacement of the kidney by a suprarenal mass, whereas intravenous urography associated with tomography may delineate the tumour itself. Historically, adrenal arteriography (Fig. 10.17) was commonly performed but is not without risk. For this reason, computerised tomography (CT) of the adrenals is presently the method of choice (Fig. 10.18). In patients in whom a phaeochromocytoma cannot be localised by other means, it may be necessary to perform a venous catheter study and measure catecholamine levels in all the major veins to determine the source of catecholamine excess. Recently, however, a scanning agent, meta-iodobenzylguanidine (MIBG), was introduced. This compound is taken up by most benign and malignant phaeochromocytoma tissues and also by secondary deposits.

Surgery is the treatment of choice for all patients except those who are thought to be medically unfit, those in whom a tumour has not been localised, or those in whom there are multiple metastases. Prior to surgery or any major investigative procedure, including CT scanning with intravenous contrast, patients should be given a combination of α- and β-blockade. The most commonly used α-blocker is phenoxybenzamine, which is usually used in conjunction with the β-blocker propranolol. In one regimen, 0.5mg/kg/d of phenoxybenzamine is administered over a period of four hours by venous drip, for three days, with 40mg propranolol given three times daily following the first phenoxybenzamine infusion. If there is any delay in definitive surgery, the condition may be controlled by oral administration of 10mg phenoxybenzamine four times daily and 40mg propranolol three times daily. The author's own practice is to administer phenoxybenzamine orally for a minimum period of one month prior to surgery. This results in the restoration of the plasma volume to normal and a much smoother intra- and postoperative course. During surgery, sodium nitroprusside has proved to be extremely useful in controlling large swings in blood pressure that may occur even in patients who have been fully 'blocked' by α- and β-blockers.

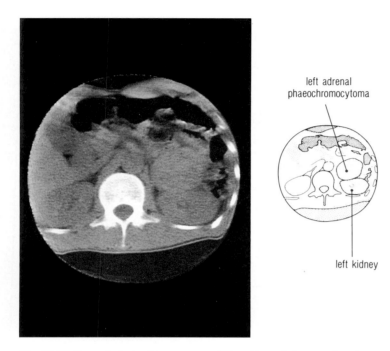

left adrenal phaeochromocytoma

left kidney

Fig. 10.18 A computerised tomogram of the upper abdomen, showing a left adrenal phaeochromocytoma.

11

The Testis

James E Griffin, MD

Jean D Wilson, MD

The testes produce sperm and the hormones that regulate male sexual function. Testicular hormones are responsible for the induction of male phenotype during embryogenesis and for maturation at puberty. As a consequence, abnormalities of testicular function cause different clinical effects during different periods of life.

STRUCTURE OF THE TESTES AND MALE REPRODUCTIVE TRACT

The testes contain two functional units: interstitial or Leydig cells that contain the enzymes for androgen synthesis; and a tubule network that is involved in the production and transport of sperm (Fig. 11.1).

The lipid droplets in Leydig cells contain esterified cholesterol that is derived from circulating lipoproteins and locally synthesised cholesterol (Fig. 11.2). Following hydrolysis, free cholesterol moves to mitochondria where the side chain is cleaved to form pregnenolone, which, in turn, is converted to testosterone in the endoplasmic reticulum. The amount of Leydig cell testosterone is small since newly synthesised hormone diffuses promptly into the plasma.

Spermatogenic tubules are composed of germ cells and Sertoli cells (Fig. 11.3). Tight junctions between the Sertoli cells form a diffusion barrier that divides the testis into two functional compartments. The basal compartment consists of Leydig cells and the outer portion of the tubules that contain the spermatogonia. The adluminal compartment contains the inner two-thirds of the tubules and includes primary and secondary spermatocytes and spermatids. The Sertoli cell lines the spermatogenic tubule, and the inner portion of the Sertoli cell consists of an arborised cytoplasm so that spermatogenesis takes place within a network of Sertoli cell cytoplasm.

The seminiferous tubules empty into the rete testes, a network of ducts that anastamose into the epididymis, which is 5–6m in length. The vas deferens is a 30–35cm tube that connects the epididymis to

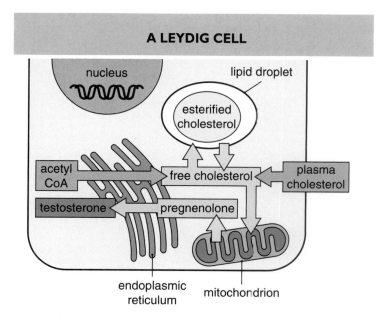

Fig. 11.2 A Leydig cell. The origin and storage of cholesterol, the conversion of cholesterol to pregnenolone in the mitochondrion, and the conversion of pregnenolone to testosterone in the endoplasmic reticulum are shown. Modified from JE Griffin and JD Wilson (1985) by courtesy of WB Saunders Company.

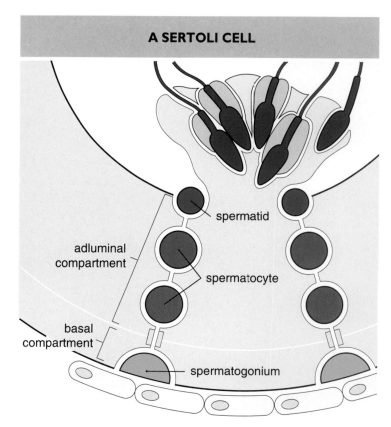

Fig. 11.3 A Sertoli cell. The relationship between Sertoli cell cytoplasm and developing spermatocytes is shown. Modified from Griffin and Wilson (1985) by courtesy of WB Saunders Company.

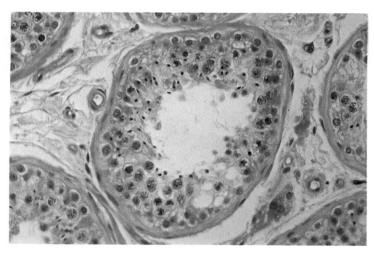

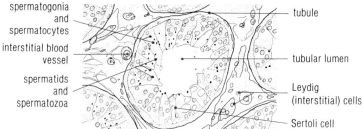

Fig. 11.1 A histological section of a normal testis. Spermatogenesis takes place between the Sertoli cells in the seminiferous tubules. Different stages of spermatogenesis may be seen in the same cross-section, a feature particular to man and different from most other mammals. In the normal mature testis, the Leydig cells appear in clumps between the seminiferous tubules. Haematoxylin & eosin (H&E) stain. By courtesy of Prof I Doniach.

the ejaculatory duct (which terminates in the prostatic urethra). The paired seminal vesicles are 4–5cm in length and empty into the ejaculatory ducts. The adult prostate, weighing some 20g, surrounds the urethra and contains a network of ductules that also terminate in the urethra.

HYPOTHALAMIC–PITUITARY–TESTICULAR AXIS

The hypothalamus communicates with the pituitary by neural pathways and by a portal vascular system that delivers regulatory hormones from the brain to the pituitary (Fig. 11.4). The preoptic and medial basal regions of the hypothalamus (particularly the arcuate nucleus) control gonadotrophin secretion. Peptidergic neurones in these regions secrete the decapeptide gonadotrophin-releasing hormone (GnRH), also known as luteinising hormone-releasing hormone (LHRH). Neurones from other regions of the brain terminate in this area and influence GnRH synthesis and release via catecholaminergic, dopaminergic, and β-endorphin-related mechanisms.

GnRH is widely distributed in the central nervous system and in other tissues, but a physiological role for GnRH outside the pituitary is not established.

The major hormones under GnRH control are luteinising hormone (LH) and follicle-stimulating hormone (FSH) (Fig. 11.4). GnRH

acts on pituitary gonadotrophs via cell-surface receptors to stimulate the release of LH and FSH by a calcium-dependent, cAMP-independent, mechanism. Diacylglycerols may amplify the calcium-mediated signal. In addition, GnRH probably has a long-term effect on LH and FSH synthesis. The episodic secretion of GnRH into the hypophysial portal system results, in turn, in episodic secretion of LH. In adult men, the secretory pulses of LH occur at a frequency of eight to fourteen per twenty-four hours. Pulsatile secretion of FSH also occurs but with a lower amplitude.

LH interacts with receptors on Leydig cells to stimulate a membrane-bound adenylate cyclase (Fig. 11.5). cAMP is subsequently released into the cytoplasm where it binds to a protein kinase.

REGULATION OF GONADOTROPHIN SECRETION

hypothalmus 'oscillator'

GnRH

inhibin   activin   FSH   LH   testosterone

dihydrotestosterone

spermatogenesis   virilisation

Fig. 11.4 The hypothalamic regulation of gonadotrophin secretion. Episodic release of GnRH stimulates the gonadotrophs, causing pulsatile release of LH and, to a lesser extent, FSH. LH acts on Leydig cells causing the production of testosterone which is responsible for virilisation (in some tissues through the production of dihydrotestosterone). LH release is suppressed by the negative feedback mechanism of the testosterone action on the hypothalamus and pituitary. FSH acts on Sertoli cells and this results in spermatogenesis. Inhibin has a negative feedback effect and activin has a positive effect on FSH production in the anterior pituitary.

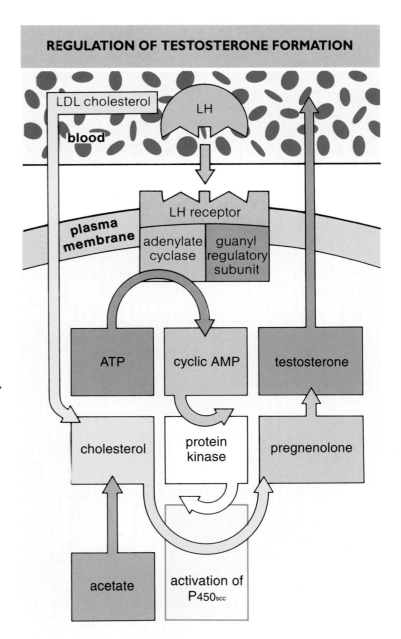

REGULATION OF TESTOSTERONE FORMATION

LDL cholesterol   LH

blood

plasma membrane   LH receptor

adenylate cyclase   guanyl regulatory subunit

ATP   cyclic AMP   testosterone

cholesterol   protein kinase   pregnenolone

acetate   activation of P450scc

Fig. 11.5 The regulation of testosterone formation in the Leydig cell. Testosterone is formed from cholesterol substrate by luteinising hormone (LH). This hormone occupies a receptor site on the plasma membrane of the Leydig cell to activate adenylate cyclase, which in turn catalyses the formation of cAMP from ATP. cAMP then binds to the regulatory subunit of protein kinase, leading to activation of the cholesterol side-chain cleavage enzyme (P450scc) which is responsible for the conversion of cholesterol to pregnenolone. Other enzymes subsequently complete the synthesis of testosterone.

Activation of the protein kinase, operating through unidentified intermediate steps, stimulates the conversion of cholesterol to pregnenolone. The control of LH operates primarily by negative feedback, and both testosterone and oestradiol can inhibit LH secretion. Testosterone can be converted to oestradiol in the brain, but the two hormones are believed to act independently on LH secretion. Testosterone slows the hypothalamic pulse generator in the hypothalamus and thus decreases the frequency of pulsatile LH release. It also exerts a negative feedback effect on LH secretion directly at the pituitary level.

The primary site of action of FSH is the Sertoli cell (Fig. 11.6). The biochemical events that follow the binding of FSH to its receptor on the cell surface are similar to those for LH. The elevation of Sertoli cell cAMP activates cAMP-dependent protein kinase and stimulates synthesis of mRNAs and proteins, including androgen-binding protein (ABP) (Fig. 11.6) and aromatase.

The control of FSH secretion involves peptide and steroid hormones. Serum FSH levels increase as germinal elements in the testis are lost, whereas there is a minimal change in LH levels. Inhibin, an

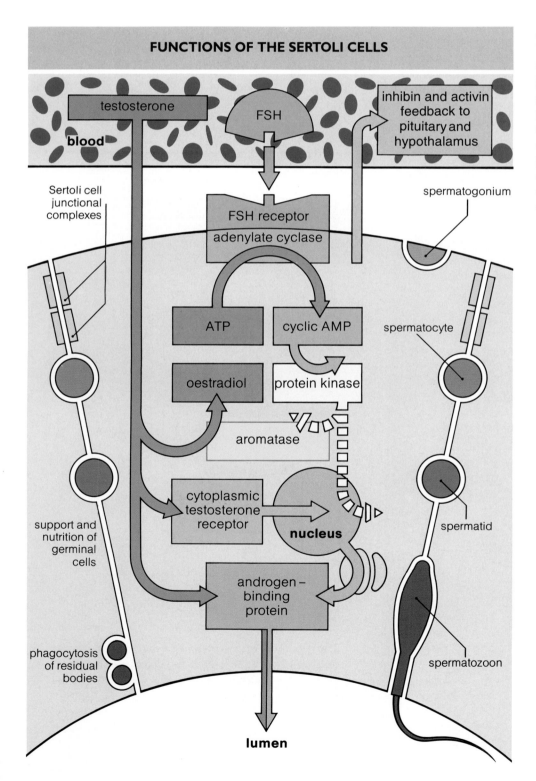

FUNCTIONS OF THE SERTOLI CELLS

Fig. 11.6 The functions of Sertoli cells.
These may be summarised as follows: maintenance of the blood–testis barrier by junctional complexes; nourishment of developing germ cells; phagocytosis of damaged germ cells; production of ABP, which is secreted by seminiferous tubules (ABP production is dependent upon FSH and testosterone action); production of tubular fluid to provide the major drive for flushing sperm from the testis to the epididymis; and production of inhibin and activin which control FSH secretion.

inhibitor of pituitary FSH secretion, is formed in Sertoli cells. It is a glycoprotein that consists of two disulphide-linked subunits – alpha combined with β_A or β_B. Both FSH and androgen control normal inhibin production. Combinations of the β-subunits of inhibin into homodimers or heterodimers, termed activins, in contrast to inhibin stimulate FSH release from the pituitary.

ANDROGEN PHYSIOLOGY

Five enzymatic processes are involved in the conversion of cholesterol to testosterone (Fig. 11.7): cholesterol side-chain cleavage ($P450_{scc}$), 3β-hydroxysteroid dehydrogenase/isomerase (3β-HSD), 17α-hydroxy-lase ($P450_{17\alpha}$), 17,20-lyase ($P450_{17\alpha}$), and 17β-hydroxy-steroid oxidoreductase (17β-HSOR). The initial step in testosterone synthesis involves the conversion of cholesterol to pregnenolone, controlled by LH, and is the rate-limiting step. The 3β-HSD complex oxidises the steroid A ring to the capital delta Δ^4-3-keto configuration. Both the 17α-hydroxylation and 17,20-lyase activities are controlled by a single enzyme known as $P450_{17\alpha}$. Testosterone is the principal steroid formed, but small amounts of its precursors are secreted in the pathway, as are small amounts of dihydrotestosterone and oestradiol. The majority of dihydrotestosterone and oestradiol is formed in androgen-target tissue and adipose tissue, respectively (see below).

Normal testes contain approximately 25μg of testosterone so that the testicular hormone turns over more than two hundred times to provide the average of 5–10mg secreted daily. In normal men, approximately two per cent of plasma testosterone is free (unbound), forty-four per cent is bound to testosterone-binding globulin (TeBG, also known as sex steroid hormone-binding globulin or SHBG), and fifty-four per cent is bound to albumin and other proteins. Since albumin-bound testosterone is available for tissue uptake, bioavailable testosterone (the free component plus the albumin-bound component) is equal to some fifty per cent of the total amount.

Testosterone serves as a circulating precursor or prohormone for two types of metabolites, which in turn mediate many androgen actions (Fig. 11.8). It can be converted to 5α-reduced steroids, principally dihydrotestosterone, which mediate many differentiative, growth-promoting, and functional actions. Alternatively, androgens can be aromatised in the extraglandular tissues to oestrogens that act independently or in concert with androgens to influence physiological processes. Thus, the actions of testosterone are the result of the combined effects of testosterone, dihydrotestosterone, and oestradiol. Dihydrotestosterone formation is mediated by two widely distributed membrane-bound 5α-reductase enzymes; the majority of dihydrotestosterone is produced in androgen-target tissues. Aromatisation also occurs in many tissues, perhaps the most important being the adipocyte.

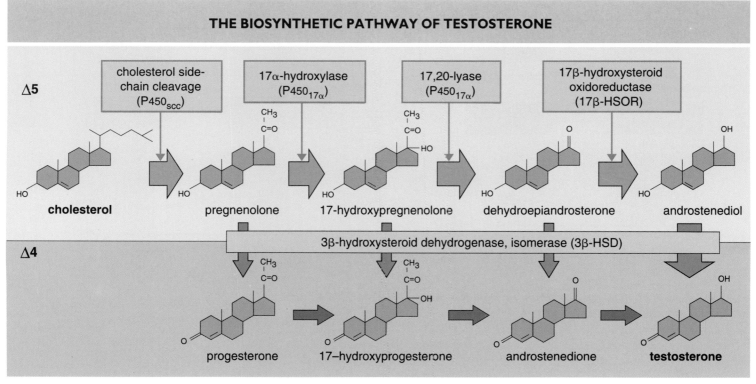

THE BIOSYNTHETIC PATHWAY OF TESTOSTERONE

Fig. 11.7 The major and minor routes of the biosynthetic pathway of testosterone. Partial or complete deficiencies of any of the enzymes involved cause inadequate testosterone synthesis and may lead to inadequate virilisation, resulting in male pseudohermaphroditism. The severity of the condition depends on the enzyme concerned. A deficiency of the enzymes $P450_{scc}$, or $P450_{17\alpha}$, or 3β-HSD is also associated with adrenal hyperplasia

STRUCTURE OF TESTOSTERONE, 5α-DIHYDROTESTOSTERONE AND OESTRADIOL

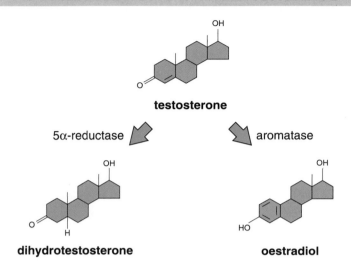

testosterone

5α-reductase   aromatase

dihydrotestosterone   **oestradiol**

Fig. 11.8 The structure of testosterone and of the two major active metabolites of testosterone, 5α-dihydrotestosterone and oestradiol.

In normal men, the production rates of testosterone and the adrenal androgen, androstenedione, average some 5 and 3mg/d, respectively, and the production rates of oestrone and oestradiol average approximately 66 and 45µg/d, respectively (Fig. 11.9a). All of the oestrone is formed from circulating precursors; thirty-five per cent of oestradiol is derived from circulating testosterone, fifty per cent from oestrone, and fifteen per cent is secreted by the testes. When gonadotrophin levels are elevated, oestradiol secretion by the testis increases.

Current concepts of androgen action are summarised in Fig. 11.10. Inside the cell, testosterone and dihydrotestosterone bind to the same intracellular androgen receptor, which is located primarily in the nucleus in the unbound state. The hormone–receptor complexes are believed to attach to specific DNA sequences to enhance gene transcription and mRNA synthesis. The androgen receptor (Fig. 11.11) contains DNA-binding and hormone-binding regions that share a high degree of homology with other members of the steroid/thyroid receptor family and an N-terminal region that has little homology with other receptors.

ANDROGEN AND OESTROGEN PRODUCTION IN NORMAL MEN AND IN PATIENTS WITH GYNAECOMASTIA

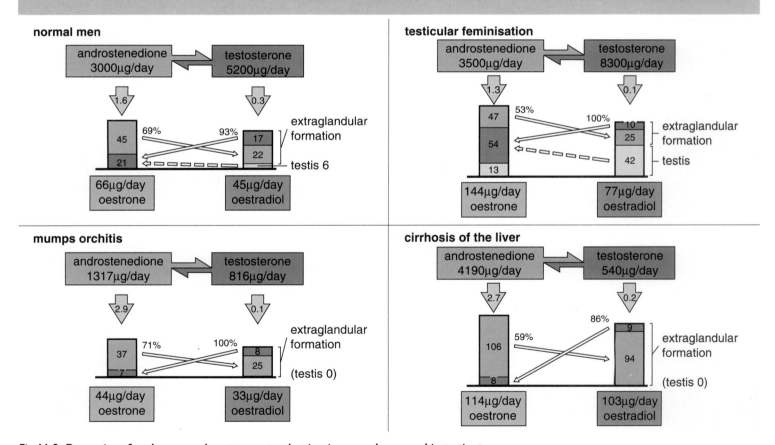

Fig.11.9 Dynamics of androgen and oestrogen production in normal men and in patients with gynaecomastia. Average production rates of androgen are indicated in the upper boxes, those of oestrogen in the lower boxes. The extent of conversion (per cent) of plasma testosterone and androstenedione to oestradiol and oestrone is shown by vertical arrows, and interconversions of oestradiol and oestrone, and of testosterone and androstenedione, are indicated by horizontal arrows. Sources of oestradiol and oestrone are indicated by vertical bars. Blue bars indicate oestrogen that is secreted directly by the testis. Thus, oestradiol arises from plasma testosterone, from oestrone, and from direct secretion by the testis; and oestrone arises from plasma androstenedione, from oestradiol, and, in some instances, by direct secretion from the testis. Modified from AG Frantz and JD Wilson (1992) by courtesy of WB Saunders.

ANDROGEN ACTION ON A TARGET CELL

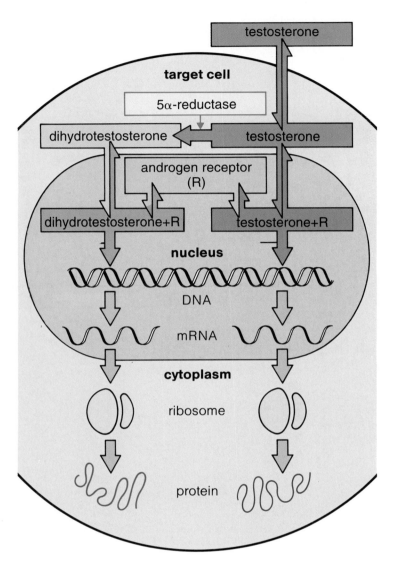

Fig. 11.10 Androgen action on a target cell. Testosterone exerts its effect on target tissues by binding to a specific androgen receptor. The testosterone–receptor complex leads to the synthesis of specific mRNA, and hence the translation of androgen-dependent proteins. In certain tissues, the active androgen is the 5α-reduced metabolite of testosterone – dihydrotestosterone – which is generated largely *in situ* and which acts by the same androgen receptor.

THE NORMAL ANDROGEN RECEPTOR AND MUTATIONS ASSOCIATED WITH ANDROGEN RESISTANCE

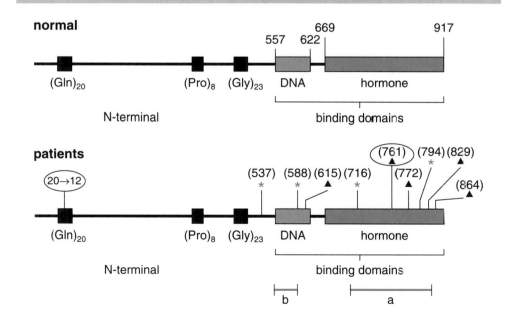

Fig. 11.11 The normal androgen receptor and some mutations associated with androgen resistance. The numbers in parentheses show the amino-acid position of the mutations. Triangles denote single amino-acid substitutions, asterisks termination codons. The two mutations marked in the colour ovals are both present in a single family. The segments indicated by A and B show the approximate positions of gene deletions in two families. Modified from JE Griffin (1992) by courtesy of *New England Journal of Medicine.*

The testosterone–receptor complex is responsible for gonadotrophin regulation, spermatogenesis, and virilisation of the Wolffian ducts during embryogenesis, whereas the dihydrotestosterone–receptor complex mediates external development during embryogenesis and most aspects of virilisation at puberty (Fig. 11.12). Analysis of single-gene mutations in man and animals indicates that a single-receptor protein mediates the action of both testosterone and dihydrotestosterone. The reason that dihydrotestosterone formation amplifies hormone action may be due to the fact that it binds to the receptor more tightly.

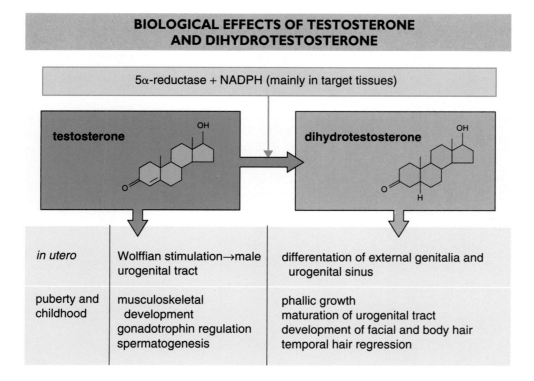

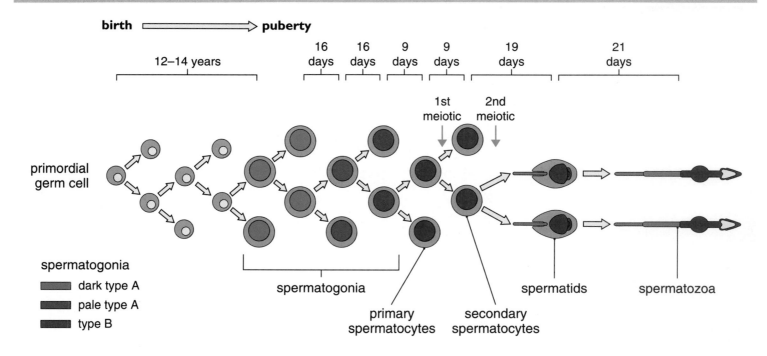

Fig. 11.12 The biological effects of testosterone and dihydrotestosterone in utero, early childhood, puberty, and adulthood.

Fig. 11.13 Cell divisions that occur during spermatogenesis. The overall number of cell divisions is higher than that in oogenesis.

SPERMATOGENESIS AND FERTILISATION

Approximately 3×10^5 germ cells migrate to each ridge during embryogenesis, and this number increases up to the time of puberty. After puberty, each spermatogonium that is undergoing differentiation gives rise to sixteen primary spermatocytes, each of which then enters meiosis and gives rise to four spermatids and ultimately four sperm (Fig. 11.13). In the adult male, approximately 10^8 sperm are formed each day. Transformation of the spermatid into the mature sperm involves reorganisation of the nucleus and cytoplasm, and development of the flagellum (Fig. 11.14). Sperm formation takes approximately seventy days, and transport through the epididymis to the ejaculatory duct requires an additional twelve to twenty-one days. Upon leaving the testes, sperm have a poor capacity to fertilise. During passage through the epididymis, the sperm mature, as evidenced by development of the capacity for sustained motility, modification of the nuclear chromatin and tail organelles, and loss of the cytoplasmic remnant.

The seminal fluid that reaches the ejaculatory ducts accounts for approximately twenty per cent of the ejaculate. The seminal vesicles contribute fructose and prostaglandins and account for some sixty per cent of the ejaculate volume. The remainder of the ejaculate is derived from the prostate which contributes spermine, citric acid, zinc, and acid phosphatase. Acquisition of the capacity of sperm to fertilise is poorly understood and may be completed in the female genital tract.

Spermatogenesis is controlled by both LH and FSH: FSH acts directly on the Sertoli cell, whereas LH influences spermatogenesis indirectly by its enhancement of testosterone synthesis. Testosterone interacts with androgen receptors in Sertoli cells to activate genes that are required for spermatogenesis.

PHASES OF NORMAL TESTICULAR FUNCTION

The phases of testicular function can be defined in terms of the levels plasma testosterone (Fig. 11.15). In men, testosterone production by the testis commences at approximately seven weeks of gestation (Fig. 11.16). Shortly thereafter, plasma testosterone reaches a high value; this level is maintained until late gestation when it falls, so that the level is only slightly higher in male newborns than in female newborns. Shortly after birth, plasma testosterone in the male newborn again rises and remains high for approximately three months, falling to low levels by the age of six months to one year. Plasma testosterone then remains low (but slightly higher in boys than in girls) until the onset of puberty, when it begins to rise in boys, reaching adult levels by the age of seventeen (see Chapter 13). During the adult phase, sperm production matures to allow reproduction to take place. The mean plasma testosterone level remains more or less constant in the adult until late middle age, and then declines slowly.

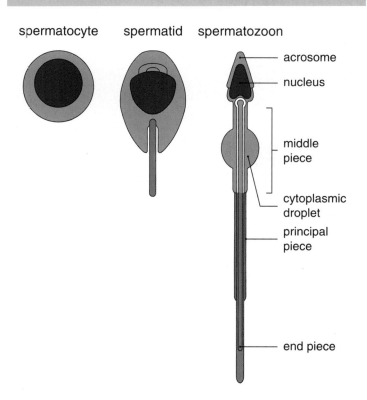

CONVERSION OF A SPERMATOCYTE TO A SPERMATOZOON

spermatocyte spermatid spermatozoon

- acrosome
- nucleus
- middle piece
- cytoplasmic droplet
- principal piece
- end piece

Fig. 11.14 The conversion of a spermatocyte to a spermatid and ultimately to a spermatozoon.

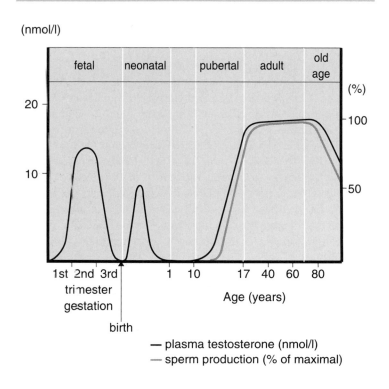

PHASES OF MALE SEXUAL FUNCTION

(nmol/l)

fetal | neonatal | pubertal | adult | old age

(%)

20

10

100

50

1st 2nd 3rd trimester gestation

birth

1 10 17 40 60 80

Age (years)

— plasma testosterone (nmol/l)
— sperm production (% of maximal)

Fig. 11.15 Phases of male sexual function, as indicated by mean plasma testosterone level and sperm production at different phases of life. Modified from JE Griffin and JD Wilson (1980) by courtesy of WB Saunders Company.

TIMING OF PRENATAL SEXUAL DIFFERENTIATION IN THE MALE

1st trimester   2nd trimester   3rd trimester

testosterone synthesis

Leydig cell development

germ cell migration

spermatogenic cords

growth of external genitalia

descent of testes

differentiation of external genitalia

Wolffian duct differentiation

Müllerian duct regression

40   56   70   84   91   168   250

day of gestation

Fig. 11.16 The timing of male prenatal sexual differentiation. Modified from JD Wilson et al. (1985) by courtesy of the AAAS.

ASSESSMENT OF TESTICULAR FUNCTION

Assessment of testicular function begins with the history and physical examination of a patient. Inadequate testosterone production or action during embryogenesis can cause hypospadias, cryptorchidism, or microphallus. Leydig cell failure prior to puberty prevents sexual maturation. Clinical features, termed eunuchoidism, include an infantile amount and distribution of body hair; poor development of skeletal muscles; and failure of closure of the epiphyses so that the arm span is more than 5cm greater than height, and the lower body segment (heel to pubis) is more than 5cm longer than the upper body segment (pubis to crown). Therefore, the assessment of androgen status should include an inquiry about developmental abnormalities at birth (e.g. hypospadias, microphallus, and/or cryptorchidism); sexual maturation and growth at puberty; rate of beard growth; and current libido, sexual function, strength, and energy. Long-standing hypogonadism of all causes can result in characteristic fine facial wrinkling (Fig. 11.17).

The prepubertal testis measures some 2cm in length and increases to 4.1–5.5cm in the normal adult. Testicular size can be assessed by use of a Prader's orchidometer (Fig. 11.18), which comprises a set of ellipsoids that can be related to testicular size (Fig. 11.19). When the seminiferous tubules are damaged before puberty, the testes are small and firm. Postpubertal damage characteristically causes small, soft testes. Considerable testicular damage may occur before overall size is below the lower limits of normal. Breast enlargement is a common feature of feminising states in men and may be an early sign of androgen deficiency.

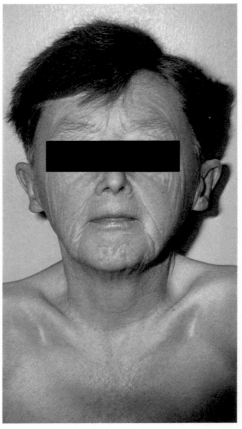

Fig. 11.17 The facial appearance in postpubertal hypogonadism. The very characteristic perioral wrinkling of the skin can be seen.

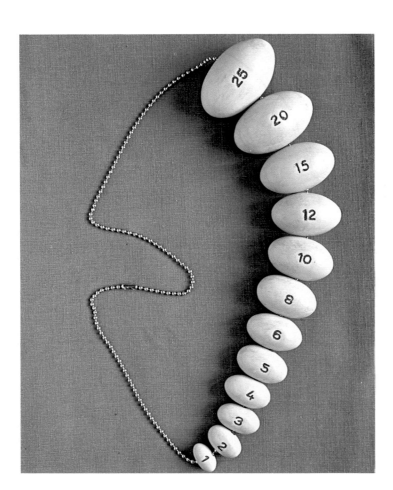

Fig. 11.18 A Prader's orchidometer. Testicular volume (in millilitres) may be estimated by direct comparison with the ellipsoids. During the assessment of testicular volume, the epididymis should not be included.

TESTICULAR SIZE AT DIFERENT STAGES OF DEVELOPMENT

Fig. 11.19 Testicular size and volume at three developmental stages, from infancy to puberty.

pre-pubertal

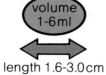

volume 1-6ml

width 1.0-1.9cm

length 1.6-3.0cm

pubertal

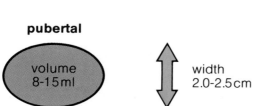

volume 8-15ml

width 2.0-2.5cm

length 3.1-4.0cm

adult

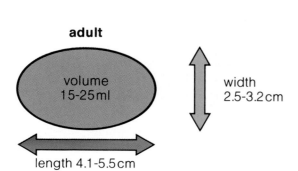

volume 15-25ml

width 2.5-3.2cm

length 4.1-5.5cm

Due to the pulsatile secretion of LH and testosterone (Fig. 11.20), and because of the effects of each on the synthesis of the other, gonadotrophins and testosterone may be measured in a pool that is formed by combining three to four samples of equal amounts of blood obtained at fifteen- to twenty-minute intervals. In this way, a single sample of serum is submitted to the laboratory, and the 'averaging' of values is accomplished prior to assay. In men, the normal range of plasma LH, determined by radioimmunoassay, is

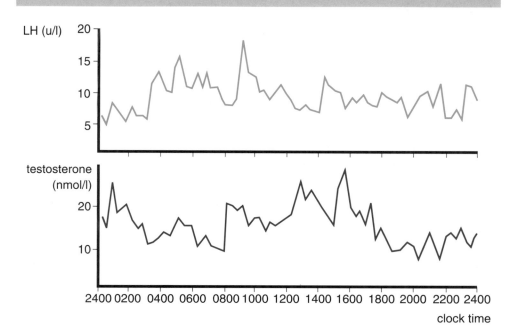

24–HOUR PATTERN OF PLASMA LH AND TESTOSTERONE LEVELS

Fig. 11.20 The 24-hour pattern of plasma LH and testosterone levels in a 21-year-old normal man, sampled every 20 minutes. Variations as great as three-fold were demonstrated in individual values of both LH and testosterone, depending on the time of sampling. Modified from JE Griffin and JD Wilson (1980) by courtesy of RM Boyar and WB Saunders Company.

PARAMETERS OF NORMAL SEMEN ANALYSIS

ejaculate volume	2–6ml
sperm density	>20 million/ml
total sperm per ejaculate	>60 million
motility	>60%
average motility grade	2.5 or more

Fig. 11.21 Parameters of normal semen analysis.

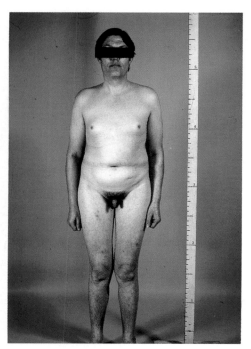

Fig. 11.22 The classical appearance of a patient with Klinefelter's syndrome. The patient is hypogonadal, has a female habitus, is poorly virilised with gynaecomastia and eunuchoidism, and has a small phallus. Body hair is sparse.

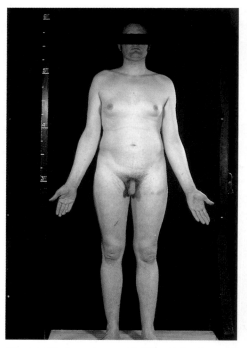

Fig. 11.23 A patient with Klinefelter's syndrome. The patient is eunuchoid but more virilised than the patient shown in Fig. 11.22. He has a normal phallus despite small testes, and gynaecomastia is present.

5–20iu/l, using the NIH reference standard LER-907. Bioactive LH may be detected when immunoreactive LH is immeasurable. Using LER-907 as the radioimmunoassay standard, normal FSH in adult men is also shown to range from 5 to 20iu/l. Pulsatile secretion is less pronounced for FSH. The normal range for plasma testosterone in adult men, determined by radioimmunoassay, is 10–35nmol/l (300–1,000ng/dl). Free testosterone concentrations can be measured by equilibrium dialysis. Dihydrotestosterone, as measured by radioimmunoassay, averages approximately ten per cent of the testosterone value.

Prior to puberty, Leydig cell function is assessed by measuring the response of plasma testosterone to gonadotrophin administration after three to five days of treatment with 1,000–2,000iu/d of human chorionic gonadotrophin (hCG); in prepubertal boys, plasma testosterone should increase to some 7nmol/l (200ng/dl). The response increases with the initiation of puberty and peaks in early puberty. In certain circumstances, the response of plasma LH to GnRH administration is utilised to assess the functional integrity of the hypothalamic–pituitary–Leydig cell axis. In general, the peak LH that follows a single GnRH injection correlates with the basal levels. A subnormal response indicates that an abnormality exists, but does not identify the site.

For routine evaluation of the seminal fluid, ejaculate should be analysed within one hour after masturbation into a clean glass or plastic container (Fig. 11.21). The normal volume is 2–6ml.

Sperm motility is assessed by examining a drop of undiluted seminal fluid and recording the percentage of motile forms. Sperm with grade 3 motility move rapidly across the field, those with grade 2 motility move aimlessly, and those with grade 1 motility have a beating tail but do not move. Normally, sixty per cent or more of sperm are motile, with an average grade of 2.5 or more.

Sperm density is determined by diluting seminal fluid with an appropriate solution and subsequently counting it in a haemocytometer or an electronic particle counter. The normal count is greater than twenty million per millilitre and more than sixty million per ejaculate. Sixty per cent or more of the spermatozoa should have a normal morphology. Random sampling of sperm density is complicated by variable extragonadal sperm reserves in the excretory ducts and by factors that influence sperm count, such as hot baths, acute febrile illness, and medications. Consequently, it is difficult to define the minimally adequate ejaculate. At least three ejaculates should be assessed to establish inadequacy of sperm number or cytology, and six or more estimates may be necessary if initial findings are equivocal.

Sperm structure can be defined by electron microscopy to identify specific abnormalities in immotile sperm. Testicular biopsy is useful in some men with oligospermia or azoospermia, both as an aid in diagnosis and as a guide to treatment, particularly in infertile men in whom the possibility of ductal obstruction is suggested by the finding of azoospermia and normal plasma FSH.

ABNORMALITIES OF TESTICULAR FUNCTION

Abnormalities of testicular function have different consequences – namely disorders of fetal development, puberty, adult life, and old age – depending on the phase of sexual life in which they first become manifest.

DISORDERS OF FETAL DEVELOPMENT
Klinefelter's Syndrome and its Variant
Klinefelter's syndrome is characterised by small, firm testes, azoospermia, gynaecomastia, and elevated plasma gonadotrophin levels in men with two or more X chromosomes. The common karyotype is either 47,XXY (the classic form) or 46,XY/47,XXY mosaicism. The incidence is approximately one in five hundred men. Prepubertally, the testes are small but otherwise appear normal. After puberty, the disorder is manifest as infertility, gynaecomastia, or underandrogenisation (Figs 11.22 & 11.23). Hyalinisation of the seminiferous tubules (Fig. 11.24), and azoospermia, are consistent features of the 47,XXY variety. The small, firm testes are usually less than 2cm in length and always less than 3.5cm (corresponding to a volume of 2 and 12ml, respectively). Mean body height is increased due to a larger lower body segment. Gynaecomastia ordinarily appears during adolescence and may progress to become disfiguring. The mosaic variant comprises some ten per cent of the total, as estimated by peripheral blood chromosomal karyotypes. In this variant the testes may be normal in size, endocrine abnormalities are usually less severe, and gynaecomastia and azoospermia are less common. Plasma FSH and LH levels are usually high; FSH shows the best discrimination, and little overlap occurs with normals due to the consistent damage to the seminiferous tubules. The plasma testosterone level averages fifty per cent of the normal value, but the range overlaps the normal.

A 46,XX karyotype in phenotypic males occurs in one in twenty to twenty-four thousand male births. Such men have an absence of all female urogenital structures and have male psychosexual identification. The findings and hormonal profile resemble those in the

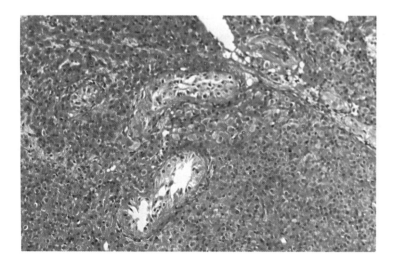

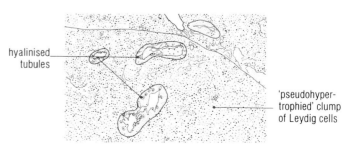

Fig. 11.24 A histological section of a testis of a patient with Klinefelter's syndrome. The dysgenetic seminiferous tubules are evident, and the clumps of Leydig cells give an illusory impression of hyperplasia. H&E stain. By courtesy of Prof I Doniach.

hyalinised tubules

'pseudohypertrophied' clump of Leydig cells

Klinefelter's syndrome: the testes are small and firm (generally less than 2cm in length), gynaecomastia is common, the penis is normal, and azoospermia and hyalinisation of the seminiferous tubules are usual. Such men differ from Klinefelter men in that average height is less than normal, the incidence of mental deficiency is not increased, and hypospadias is common. Many XX men are positive for the SRY gene that is normally found on the Y-chromosome and thought to be responsible for testis differentiation. Thus, interchange of a fragment of a Y-chromosome with another chromosome may be a common cause.

Embryonic Testicular Regression

A spectrum of phenotypes has been described in 46,XY males with absent testes but in whom endocrine function of the testis must have been present transiently during embryonic life (e.g. Müllerian duct regression and variable testosterone synthesis). The phenotypes vary from complete failure of virilisation to partial virilisation of the external genitalia, to otherwise normal men with bilateral anorchia. In the purest form of the vanishing testis syndrome, 46,XY phenotypic females have absent testes, sexual infantilism, and absence of Müllerian duct and Wolffian duct derivatives. By contrast, in 46,XY pure gonadal dysgenesis, streak gonads and a uterus are present. Testicular failure must have occurred after the onset of formation of Müllerian-inhibiting substance and before the initiation of testosterone synthesis; that is, after Sertoli cell development, but before the onset of Leydig cell function. In others, testicular failure must occur later in gestation, and these individuals may constitute problems in gender assignment. Some have incomplete Müllerian regression, but none has normal Müllerian development. At the final extreme is the syndrome of bilateral anorchia in which phenotypic men have an absence of Müllerian structures and gonads but a male Wolffian system and male external genitalia (Fig. 11.25). The pathogenesis is not understood. Management depends on the phenotype.

Male Pseudohermaphroditism due to Defective Testosterone Formation

Defective virilisation of the male embryo (male pseudohermaphroditism) can result from defects in androgen synthesis, in androgen action, and in Müllerian duct regression, and from uncertain causes (Fig. 11.26).

Rarely, the defect in androgen synthesis is postulated to be either Leydig cell hypoplasia or unresponsiveness to hCG/LH, but most defects in androgen biosynthesis are due to developmental defects of the testis or to single-gene defects that impair androgen synthesis. Defects in any of the enzymatic reactions in the pathway from cholesterol to testosterone can impair virilisation of the male embryo (see Fig. 11.7). Defects in $P450_{scc}$, $P450_{17\alpha}$, and 3β-HSD enzymes also result in congenital adrenal hyperplasia. In all of the enzymatic defects, Müllerian regression is usually normal. The masculinisation of the Wolffian ducts, urogenital sinus, and urogenital tubercle and virilisation at puberty vary from almost normal to absent and, therefore, the phenotype varies from men with mild hypospadias to

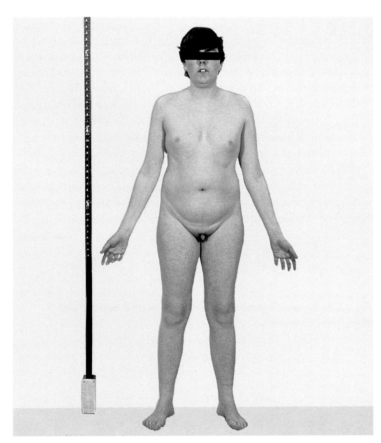

Fig. 11.25 A patient with the 'vanishing testis' syndrome. Such patients have evidence of hypogonadism, and no testicular tissue is found in the scrotum on surgical exploration. After hCG stimulation, testosterone levels do not rise. The term 'vanishing testis' derives from the presumption that testicular tissue was active in early fetal life in order to induce male phenotypic development. It is of unknown aetiology.

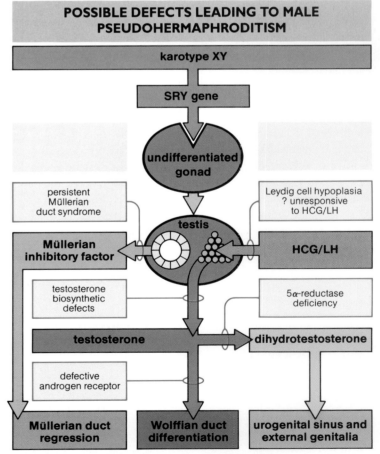

Fig. 11.26 The possible defects that lead to male pseudohermaphroditism. This condition is most commonly caused by failure of androgen action, leading to the 'androgen-resistance syndromes'.

women. This variability is due to the varying severity of the enzymatic defects and the varying effects of the steroids that accumulate proximal to the metabolic blocks. In subjects with partial defects, diagnosis may require measurement of the steroids that accumulate proximal to the metabolic block.

Each of these disorders is the result of rare autosomal recessive mutations. 3β-HSD deficiency usually results in salt wasting; variable

deficiency of the enzyme in the adrenal and liver may complicate diagnosis. 17α-hydroxylase and 17,20-lyase reactions are mediated by a single enzyme, $P450_{17\alpha}$, and it is not known why some patients have selective impairment of one enzymatic function. 17α-hydroxylase deficiency results in hypokalaemic alkalosis and hypertension, in addition to gonadal deficiency. 17β-HSOR deficiency is probably the most common of the defects. The external phenotype is usually female, but inguinal or abdominal testes and virilised Wolffian duct structures are present. At the time of expected puberty, both virilisation (phallic enlargement and facial hair growth) and some feminisation (appearance of gynaecomastia) take place.

Male Pseudohermaphroditism due to Androgen Resistance
Disorders of androgen action cause several types of male pseudohermaphroditism. In such disorders, testosterone formation and Müllerian regression are normal, and impairment of male development is a result of resistance to androgen action in the target cells.

5α-reductase deficiency is an autosomal recessive disorder characterised by:
• Severe perineoscrotal hypospadias.
• A blind vaginal pouch of variable size, opening either into the urogenital sinus or the urethra.
• Testes with normal epididymides, vasa deferentia, seminal vesicles, and ejaculatory ducts that terminate in the blind-ending vagina.
• A female habitus without female breast development but with normal axillary and pubic hair.
• Absence of female urogenital structures.
• Normal male plasma testosterone.
• Masculinisation to a variable degree at the time of puberty.

A failure of dihydrotestosterone formation in a male embryo is responsible for the phenotype (Figs 11.27 & 11.28). Since testos-

UROGENITAL TRACT IN NORMAL MALES AND 5α-REDUCTASE DEFICIENCY

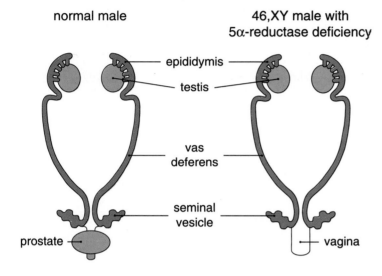

Fig. 11.27 The urogenital tract in a normal man and in a 46,XY male with 5α-reductase deficiency.

EFFECT OF DIHYDROTESTOSTERONE DEFICIENCY ON SEXUAL DEVELOPMENT

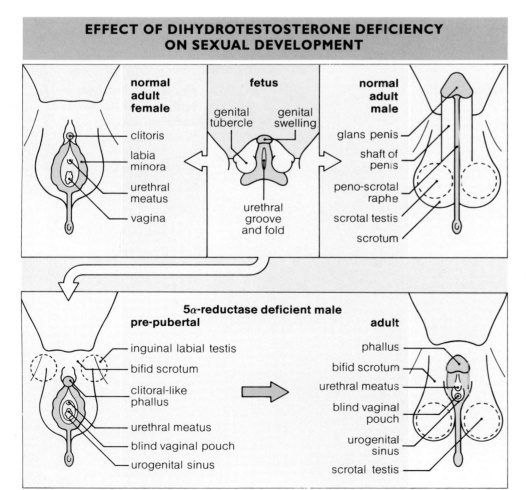

Fig. 11.28 The effect of dihydrotestosterone deficiency on sexual development. In the absence of 5α-reductase, dihydrotestosterone-dependent structures (prostate and external genitalia) fail to develop. Affected individuals have ambiguous genitalia, with a clitoral-like phallus and bifid scrotum. A blind vaginal pouch may be present, and testes may be found in the labia or in the inguinal canals. At puberty, limited development takes place, with some phallic enlargement and full testicular descent, but scrotal and urethral abnormalities remain.

terone itself regulates LH secretion, plasma LH levels are usually normal or minimally elevated. As a result, testosterone and oestrogen production rates are those of normal men, and gynaecomastia does not develop. Affected individuals have a defect in the 5α-reductase 2 gene.

Mutations in the androgen receptor gene are a more common cause of male pseudohermaphroditism. These mutations are inherited as X-linked defects and cause several syndromes that have similar pathophysiology and hormone profiles. Complete testicular feminisation, the most common form of male pseudohermaphroditism, is a common cause of primary amenorrhoea. The features are characteristic: the development of the breasts after puberty, the general habitus, and the distribution of body fat are female in character so that most subjects have a feminine appearance (Fig. 11.29). The disorder is ascertained either because of inguinal hernia (prepubertal) or primary amenorrhoea (postpubertal). Axillary and pubic hair are absent or scanty, but some vulval hair is usually present. Scalp hair is normal, and facial hair is absent. The external genitalia are unambiguously female, and the clitoris is normal. The vagina is short and blind-ending and may be absent or rudimentary. All internal genitalia are absent except for undescended testes that contain normal Leydig cells and seminiferous tubules without spermatogenesis (Fig. 11.30).

Incomplete testicular feminisation is some ten times less common than the complete form. In this variant, there is a minor virilisation of the external genitalia (partial fusion of the labioscrotal folds and some degree of clitoromegaly), normal pubic hair (Fig. 11.31), and a mixed pattern of virilisation and feminisation at the time of expected puberty. The vagina is short and blind-ending, and the Wolffian duct derivatives are partially virilised.

Reifenstein's syndrome is the term now applied to forms of incomplete male pseudohermaphroditism – Reifenstein's syndrome, Gilbert-Dreyfus syndrome, Lubs syndrome – that were originally assumed to be distinct entities. These syndromes constitute variable manifestations of mutations of the androgen-receptor gene. The most common phenotype is an undervirilised man with gynaecomastia (Fig. 11.32) and perineoscrotal hypospadias (Fig. 11.33), but the spectrum of defective virilisation ranges from men with azoospermia to phenotypic women with pseudovaginas. Axillary and pubic hair are normal, but chest and facial hair are minimal. Cryptorchidism is common, the testes are small, azoospermia is usual, and the vas deferens may be absent or hyperplastic.

The infertile male syndrome is not a form of male pseudohermaphroditism. Some cases are minimally affected men in families with Reifenstein's syndrome, who have azoospermia as the major manifestation of receptor abnormality. More commonly, men with uninformative family histories are ascertained because of infertility; indeed, a disorder of the androgen receptor may be present in twenty per cent or more of men with idiopathic azoospermia. The undervirilised fertile male is the least severe manifestation of an androgen-receptor defect. In such families, affected men have gynaecomastia and undervirilisation, and some are fertile.

Hormone dynamics are similar in all disorders of the androgen receptor. Plasma testosterone levels, and rates of testosterone production by the testes, are normal or high. The elevated testosterone production is caused by the high plasma level of LH, which in turn is due to defective feedback regulation caused by resistance to androgen action at the hypothalamic–pituitary level. Elevated LH levels cause increased oestrogen production by the testes (see Fig. 11.9b), and increased oestrogen production combined with variable androgen resistance leads to feminisation.

Each of these syndromes is the result of an abnormality of the androgen receptor. In some families, the fundamental defect is due to the point mutations which lead to premature termination codons that truncate the receptor. Other point mutations lead to single amino-acid

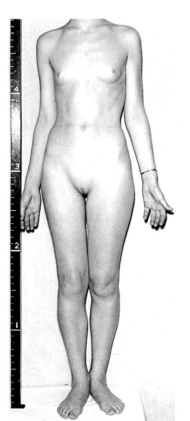

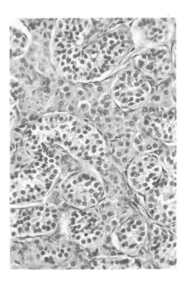

Fig. 11.29 Complete testicular feminisation. The female phenotype results from resistance to circulating androgens.

Fig. 11.30 A histological section of the labial testis in complete testicular feminisation. H&E stain.

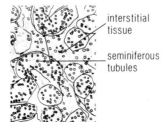

interstitial tissue

seminiferous tubules

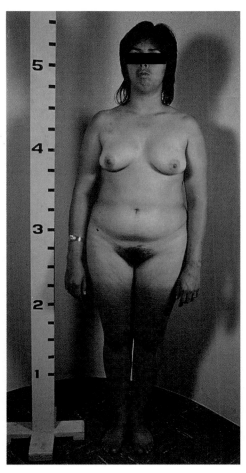

Fig. 11.31 A 46,XY patient with incomplete testicular feminisation.

substitutions that either interfere with hormone binding or DNA binding, selectively (see Fig. 11.11). In rare instances, deletions in the receptor gene may be present.

Male Pseudohermaphroditism due to Defective Müllerian Regression

Men with the persistent Müllerian duct syndrome have a normal male phenotype, testes, bilateral fallopian tubes, a uterus and upper vagina, and variable development of the vas deferens. Such men may have inguinal hernias that contain the uterus, and cryptorchidism is common. Most have uninformative family histories, but the condition can be inherited either as an autosomal recessive or X-linked recessive mutation. Since the external genitalia are well developed and the patients masculinise at puberty, it is assumed that during the critical stage of embryonic development, the fetal testes produce a normal amount of androgen. Müllerian regression, however, does not occur, either because of mutations that impair the formation of normal Müllerian inhibiting substance or its action.

PUBERTAL DISORDERS

Pubertal disorders of testicular function are discussed in Chapter 13. Isolated gonadotrophin deficiency may not be recognised until adulthood and is discussed below.

ADULT DISORDERS

The hypothalamic–pituitary–testicular axis is subject to a variety of influences. Spermatogenesis is sensitive to alterations in temperature, and brief increases either in systemic or local temperature can be

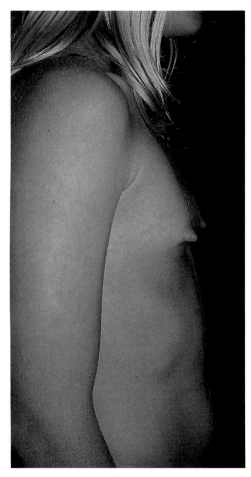

Fig. 11.32 A 17-year-old boy with Reifenstein's syndrome.

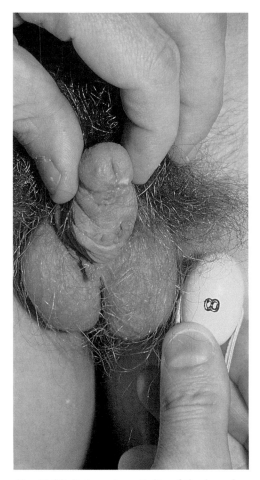

Fig. 11.33 External genitalia of the boy shown in Fig. 11.32 with Reifenstein's syndrome.

followed by temporary decreases in sperm production. Drugs, alcohol, environmental agents and psychological stress may also cause decreased sperm count.

Persistent abnormalities of testicular function after puberty can be due to hypothalamic–pituitary abnormalities, testicular defects, or abnormalities of sperm transport. Some of these conditions affect Leydig cell function or spermatogenesis selectively, but most cause both underandrogenisation and infertility (Fig. 11.34). Even partial decreases in testosterone production can cause infertility. Other dis-

orders (hyperprolactinaemia, radiation, cyclophosphamide therapy, autoimmunity, paraplegia, androgen resistance) can cause isolated infertility or combined defects in different subjects.

HYPOTHALAMIC–PITUITARY DISORDERS

Impairment of gonadotrophin secretion may be the consequence of generalised diseases that affect the hypothalamus and pituitary (e.g. craniopharyngioma, Fig. 11.35; see also Chapter 2), or it may be an isolated deficiency in which secretion of LH and FSH is impaired;

Fig. 11.34 Adult abnormalities of testicular function. Modified from JE Griffin and JD Wilson (1992) by courtesy of WB Saunders.

ADULT ABNORMALITIES OF TESTICULAR FUNCTION

type of defect	infertility with under-androgenisation	infertility with normal virilisation
hypothalamic–pituitary	panhypopituitarism isolated gonadotropin deficiency Cushing's syndrome hyperprolactinaemia haemochromatosis	isolated FSH deficiency congenital adrenal hyperplasia hyperprolactinaemia androgen adminstration

testicular	developmental and structural defects
	  Klinefelter's syndrome
	  XX male syndrome
	
	acquired defects
	  viral orchitis
	  trauma
	  radiation
	  drugs
	    (e.g.spironolactone
	    alcohol, ketoconazole,
	    cyclophosphamide)
	  environmental toxins
	  autoimmunity
	  granulomatous disease
	systemic disease
	  liver disease
	  renal failure
	  sickle cell disease
	  neurological disease
	  (myotonic dystrophy,
	  paraplegia)
	androgen resistance
		developmental and structural defects
		  germinal cell aplasia
		  cryptorchidism
		  varicocoele
		  immotile cilia syndrome
		  other structural defects
		acquired defects
		  mycoplasma infection
		
		  radiation
		  drugs such as
		    cycloposphamide
		    and sulfasalazine
		
		  environmental toxins
		  autoimmunity
		
		systemic diseases
		  febrile illness
		  coeliac disease
		
		  neurological disease
		  (paraplegia)
		
		androgen resistance

sperm transport		obstruction of epididymis or of vas deferens (cystic fibrosis, diethylstilboestrol exposure)

isolated hypogonadotrophic hypogonadism can be either congenital or, rarely, an acquired idiopathic defect. The manifestations of isolated gonadotrophin deficiency vary from infants with microphallus, to boys with eunuchoidal features and testes of prepubertal size, to men with partial LH and FSH deficiency and some testicular enlargement and pubertal development (Fig. 11.36). Anosmia or hyposmia, and cryptorchidism, are common. Histological examination of the testis reveals immature Leydig cells and germinal epithelium similar to that found in a normal prepubertal testis. The disorder is inherited as an X-linked recessive or autosomal dominant trait with variable expressivity. Serum FSH and LH levels are low or low–normal, and plasma testosterone levels are low for the age. The levels of other pituitary hormones are normal. The defect appears to be in the synthesis or release of GnRH and has a severity varying from the complete absence of pulsatile LH secretion, to impairment in amplitude and frequency of LH secretion. Distinction between this disorder and delayed puberty is difficult in boys of early or midpubertal age; the presence of microphallus, anosmia, or a positive family history may help in diagnosis. Sometimes, differentiation of the two states may require long observation.

Gonadotrophin secretion can be altered by additional factors. Elevation of plasma cortisol levels in Cushing's syndrome can depress LH secretion independent of a space-occupying lesion of the pituitary. Some patients with congenital adrenal hyperplasia have suppressed gonadotrophin secretion and infertility. Hyperprolactinaemia (as the consequence of either pituitary adenomas or drugs such as phenothiazines) can cause both Leydig cell and seminiferous tubule dysfunction, presumably due to inhibition of pulsatile LH and FSH secretion. Haemochromatosis impairs testicular function as the result of effects on the pituitary; less often, it affects the testis directly. The use of androgens for purposes other than replacement therapy is often associated with low plasma gonadotrophin levels and impaired sperm production (see below).

TESTICULAR DEFECTS

Abnormalities of testicular function in the adult can be grouped into several categories: developmental and structural defects of the testes, acquired testicular defects, disorders secondary to systemic and/or neurological disease, and androgen resistance.

Developmental Abnormalities

Klinefelter's syndrome (both the classic and mosaic forms) and the XX male may not be diagnosed until after the time of expected puberty (see above). Defects that cause infertility in the presence of normal androgen production include varicocoele, which occurs in ten to fifteen per cent of the general population and may be a contributory factor in one-third of cases of male infertility. It is caused by retrograde flow of blood into the internal spermatic vein, which eventuates in progressive, often palpable dilatation of the peritesticular plexus of veins (Fig. 11.37).

Some ten per cent of men with azoospermia and germinal cell aplasia (the Sertoli cell-only syndrome) have a positive family history and may constitute a specific entity; plasma testosterone and LH levels are normal, and the plasma FSH level is high. Other men with identical histological and clinical findings have androgen resistance or a history of viral orchitis or cryptorchidism so that diverse conditions may be grouped in this category.

Unilateral cryptorchidism, even when corrected prior to puberty, may be associated with abnormal semen, suggesting that the testicular abnormality is usually bilateral.

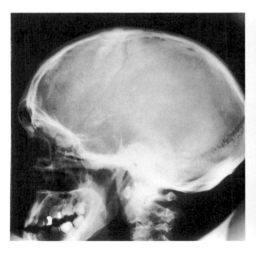
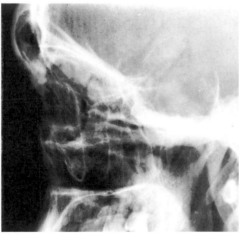
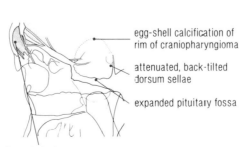

egg-shell calcification of rim of craniopharyngioma

attenuated, back-tilted dorsum sellae

expanded pituitary fossa

frontal air sinus

Fig. 11.35 A skull radiograph of a craniopharyngioma, showing egg-shell calcification in the suprasellar region. The sella turcica is grossly ballooned. An enlargement of the ballooned sella turcica is shown on the right.

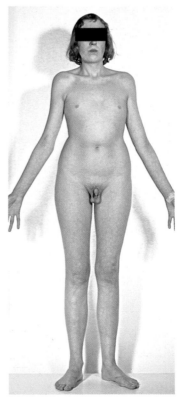

Fig. 11.36 A patient with hypo-gonadotrophic hypogonadism with anosmia (Kallmann's syndrome). This condition results from a deficiency of GnRH.

The immotile cilia syndrome is an autosomal recessive defect characterised by immotility or poor motility of the cilia of the respiratory epithelium and of sperm. Kartagener's syndrome is a subgroup of the immotile cilia syndrome associated with situs inversus, chronic sinusitis, and bronchiectasis. The specific defects of the cilia can usually be defined by the electron-microscopic appearance and include abnormalities in the dynein arms, spokes, or microtubule doublets (Fig. 11.38). Cilia from epithelia, and sperm from the same individual, usually exhibit the same defects, but the pulmonary manifestations may be minor. Less well-understood structural defects of sperm can lead to immotile sperm without involvement of cilia in the lung.

Acquired Testicular Defects

The most common cause of acquired testicular failure is viral orchitis. Responsible viruses include mumps, echovirus, lymphocytic choriomeningitis, and group B arboviruses. Orchitis is due to viral invasion of the tissue, occurs in as many as twenty-five per cent of adult men with mumps, and is unilateral in over sixty-five per cent of the cases. The testis may return to normal size and function or undergo atrophy. Bilateral atrophy, which occurs in approximately ten per cent of subjects with bilateral orchitis, may cause decreased testosterone production (see Fig. 11.9).

The exposed position in the scrotum renders the testis susceptible to both thermal and physical trauma, the second most common cause of acquired testicular failure. The seminiferous tubules and the Leydig cells are also sensitive to radiation damage; decreased secretion of

testosterone is the result of diminished testicular blood flow. Fractionated radiation may have a more profound effect than single-dose radiation. Recovery of sperm density depends on radiation dosage, and the complete recovery of sperm density may take as long as five years. Permanent infertility can occur after radiation therapy of a malignant lymphoma, despite the fact that the testes are shielded. Permanent androgen deficiency is uncommon after radiation in adults, but boys who receive direct testicular radiation for acute lymphoblastic leukaemia may have permanently low plasma testosterone levels.

Spironolactone and ketoconazole block the synthesis of androgen, and spironolactone and cimetidine interfere with androgen action by competing with androgen for binding to the androgen receptor. Testosterone may be low and oestradiol may be high in abusers of marijuana, heroin, or methadone, although the exact reasons are unclear. Alcohol can cause plasma testosterone levels to fall, independent of liver disease or malnutrition.

Antineoplastic and chemotherapeutic agents can impair spermatogenesis. Cyclophosphamide causes azoospermia or oligospermia within a few weeks after the initiation of therapy. Combination chemotherapy for acute leukaemia, Hodgkin's disease, and other malignancies may also impair Leydig cell function. Environmental hazards for the testis include microwaves, ultrasound, and chemicals such as the nematocide dibromochloropropane, cadmium, and lead.

Testicular failure due to circulating antibodies to the testis can be part of a generalised disorder of autoimmunity in which multiple primary endocrine deficiencies coexist (Schmidt's syndrome). Alternatively,

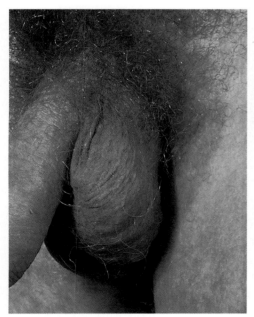
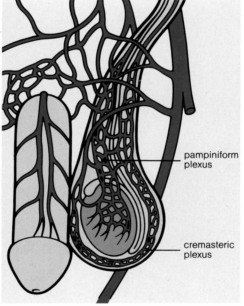

Fig. 11.37 A varicocoele and a diagram showing the venous drainage of the testis. Varicocoele of the testis, shown on the left, may impair fertility since the abdominoscrotal temperature gradient is reduced and spermatogenesis is affected. The abnormality in the varicocoele is thought to involve primarily the cremasteric venous plexus rather than the pampiniform plexus. Varicocoeles appear during or after puberty.

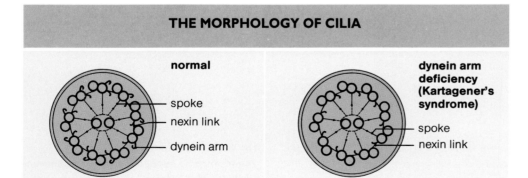

Fig. 11.38 The morphology of cilia. Transverse sections of the morphology of (a) normal spermatozoa and (b) spermatozoa from patients with Kartagener's syndrome are shown.

sperm antibodies can be a cause of isolated male infertility. In some instances, such antibodies develop secondary to duct obstruction or vasectomy. Granulomatous diseases such as leprosy can also destroy the testes.

Testicular Abnormalities Associated with Systemic Disease

In cases of cirrhosis of the liver, a combined testicular and pituitary abnormality causes decreased testosterone production, independent of the direct toxic effects of ethanol (see Fig. 11.9). Testicular atrophy and gynaecomastia are present in some fifty per cent of men with cirrhosis, and many such men are impotent. Although plasma LH is elevated, the level may be inappropriate for the degree of androgen deficiency, probably because of inhibition of LH secretion by oestrogen in patients with chronic liver disease. Increased oestrogen production results from impaired hepatic extraction and consequent increased extraglandular aromatisation of the adrenal androgen androstenedione (see Fig. 11.9). In effect, oestrogen precursors are shunted to sites of extraglandular aromatisation.

In chronic renal failure, decreased androgen synthesis and impairment of sperm production are associated with elevated plasma gonadotrophins. The elevated LH level is due to increased production, as well as reduced clearance, but is incapable of effecting normal testosterone production. Approximately twenty-five per cent of men with chronic renal failure also have hyperprolactinaemia.

Men with sickle cell disease usually have incomplete secondary sexual development, and testicular atrophy is present in one-third. The defect may either be at the testicular level or at the hypothalamic–pituitary level. Decreased Leydig cell function, with or without decreased sperm density, occurs in a variety of chronic systemic diseases; the lowered plasma testosterone level is coupled with a minimal increase in the plasma LH level, suggesting combined hypothalamic–pituitary and testicular defects.

Infertility in men with coeliac disease is associated with elevated testosterone and LH levels. In myotonic dystrophy, small testes may be associated with abnormalities of both spermatogenesis and Leydig cell function. Spinal cord lesions associated with paraplegia lead to persistent defects in spermatogenesis and to temporary decreases in testosterone levels that tend to return to normal; some patients retain the capacity to obtain an erection and to ejaculate.

Androgen Resistance

Defects of the androgen receptor cause resistance to the action of androgen usually associated with defective male phenotypic development, infertility, and underandrogenisation (see above). Less severe forms of androgen resistance can cause oligo- or azoospermia in phenotypically normal men or, rarely, under-androgenisation despite fertility.

Impairment of Sperm Transport

Disorders of sperm transport may cause six per cent of the cases of infertility with normal virilisation. Ductal obstruction may be unilateral or bilateral and may also be congenital or acquired. Congenital defects of the vas deferens can occur as an isolated abnormality that is associated with an absence of the seminal vesicles (and consequently an absence of fructose in the ejaculate), in patients with cystic fibrosis, or in men whose mothers received diethylstilboestrol during pregnancy.

In at least forty per cent of infertile men (Fig. 11.39), the cause is unknown. Biopsy of the testis in these individuals and those with a suspected cause may show a variety of nonspecific findings (Figs 11.40–11.44). Therapy in male infertility, except surgically correctable varicocoele, vas deferens obstruction, or treatable endocrinopathy, is unsatisfactory.

CAUSES AND ASSOCIATED CONDITIONS IN INFERTILE MEN	
cause or condition	**approximate %**
hypogonadotropic hypogonadism	0.8
Klinefelter's syndrome	2.0
cryptorchidism	6.0
varicocoele	39.0
immotile sperm	0.6
viral orchitis	2.0
radiation chemotherapy	0.2
obstruction of epididymis or vas deferens	5.0
coital disorders	2.0
idiopathic disorders	42.0

Fig. 11.39 *Relative frequency of causes and associated conditions in infertile men.*

DISORDERS OF OLD AGE

The major androgen-dependent disorder in the elderly is benign prostatic hyperplasia. In the fifth decade of life, the prostate resumes growth in most men, commencing in the periurethral region with proliferation of glandular and stromal elements. This growth spurt requires a functioning testis and is thought to be mediated by dihydrotestosterone that is synthesised within the gland. Inhibition of dihydrotestosterone formation in animals causes involution of the

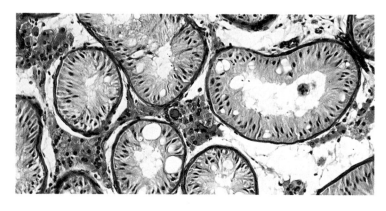

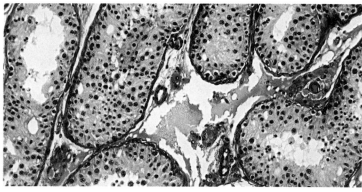

Fig. 11.40 Case 1: 'Sertoli-cells only' appearance. Bladder rupture and bilateral testicular haematomas were caused by a road-traffic accident. The patient presented with infertility some years later, when a left varicocoele and an abnormally small left testis were found, together with elevated FSH and LH levels. On biopsy, only Sertoli cells were found in the tubules; these extended from the basement membrane to the lumen. H&E stain. By courtesy of Dr WE Kenyon.

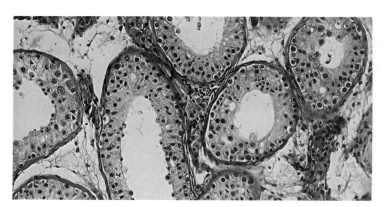

Fig. 11.41 Case 2: Focal atrophy. The patient presented with primary infertility, azoospermia, and small testes. Testicular biopsy revealed marked focal atrophy. There is heterogeneity of the histological appearance from area to area in the field shown. Much of this biopsy (not shown in the photograph) did, however, appear normal. H&E stain. By courtesy of Dr WE Kenyon.

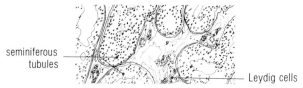

Fig. 11.42 Case 3: Maturation arrest. The patient had a history of right testicular maldescent and left herniorrhaphy. The right testicular size was normal, but the left testis was small and soft. A grade III left varicocoele was present and the patient was azoospermic. The arrest of sperm maturation can be seen in the biopsy. H&E stain. By courtesy of Dr WE Kenyon.

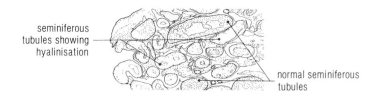

Fig. 11.43 Case 4: Maturation arrest. The patient had four years of infertility with his right testis in an inguinal canal. Seminal analysis showed very occasional spermatozoa (<10⁵/ml), although obstruction was excluded. Testicular biopsy revealed maturation arrest. Although more spermatozoa were present when compared with Case 3 (Fig. 11.42), none can be seen in this field. H&E stain. By courtesy of Dr WE Kenyon.

prostate, despite an elevated concentration of testosterone in the tissue. Furthermore, in elderly men, prostate dihydrotestosterone content remains high. In canine prostatic hyperplasia, oestrogen acts synergistically with androgen to facilitate prostate growth by increasing the amount of androgen receptor in the tissue. It is not known whether oestrogens act similarly in human prostatic hyperplasia. In men, however, plasma oestradiol levels increase slightly with age. The current treatment is surgical, but the availability of finasteride, a specific 5α-reductase inhibitor, offers the prospect that medical therapy may arrest or reverse the process.

DISORDERS OF ALL AGES

Testicular tumours and gynaecomastia may develop at any stage of life. The classification of testicular tumours is shown in Fig. 11.45. Only the endocrinological aspects of such tumours are considered in this chapter. hCG is present in normal testes, and it is therefore not surprising that plasma hCG levels may be elevated in men with testicular tumours. Indeed, an elevated plasma level of the β-subunit of hCG (hCG-β) is a sensitive and specific marker of tumour activity in some types of germ-cell tumours. Plasma levels of hCG-β are high in all patients with choriocarcinoma, in one-third of the cases of embryonal carcinomas and teratocarcinomas, and rarely in seminomas. Changes in plasma hCG-β levels correlate with response to therapy.

Elevated oestradiol and testosterone production in patients with testicular tumours can arise by at least two mechanisms. In trophoblastic tumours and in tumours of Leydig and Sertoli cells, the hormones are produced autonomously in the tumour tissue; plasma gonadotrophin levels and hormone production by the uninvolved portions of the testes are depressed, and azoospermia is common. Secretion of hCG by tumours, however, causes increased oestradiol and testosterone production in the unaffected areas of the testes, and azoospermia is uncommon. When oestrogens and androgens are formed (directly or indirectly) by tumours, feminisation, virilisation, or no obvious change may result, depending on the pattern of hor-

mones produced and the age of the patient. Other cellular markers of testicular tumour activity have been described in individual cases, including α-fetoprotein.

The predominant manifestation of feminisation in men is enlargement of the breasts. The incidence of gynaecomastia in autopsy studies is five to nine per cent, whereas some observers have reported that forty per cent of normal men and seventy per cent of hospitalised men have palpable breast tissue. The reasons for this discrepancy are not clear. It may be difficult to distinguish masses of adipose tissue without true breast enlargement (lipomastia) from true breast enlargement. In such cases, gynaecomastia must be diagnosed by mammography or by sonography. In this discussion, it is assumed that any palpable breast tissue in men (except for the three so-called physiologic states) may reflect an underlying endocrinopathy and deserves at least a limited evaluation.

Growth of the breast in men, as in women, is mediated by oestrogen and results from disturbances of the normal ratio of androgen to oestrogen in plasma or within the breast itself. The normal ratio of testosterone to oestradiol production in adult men is approximately 100:1 (5mg versus 45μg), and the normal ratio of the two hormones in plasma is approximately 300:1. Feminisation occurs when there is a significant decrease in this ratio as a result of diminished testosterone production or action, or enhanced oestrogen formation; it may, however, occur as a result of both processes.

Gynaecomastia can be classified as physiological or pathological. In the newborn, transient enlargement of the breast may be due to maternal and/or placental oestrogens. The enlargement ordinarily disappears in a few weeks but may persist. Adolescent gynaecomastia occurs in many boys. Although the origin of the excess oestrogen has not been identified, the onset of gynaecomastia correlates with transient elevations of plasma oestradiol prior to the completion of puberty, so that the androgen:oestrogen ratio is altered. Gynaecomastia of ageing also occurs in otherwise healthy men. This may be due to the increase in the conversion of androgens to oestrogens in

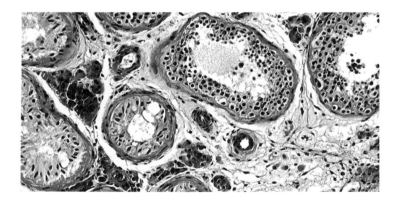

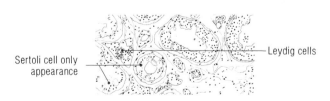

Fig. 11.44 Case 5: Hypospermatogenesis. The patient was obese, with small testes. He was found to be azoospermic with high FSH levels and also high LH and testosterone levels, suggesting possible androgen resistance. Hypospermatogenesis was revealed on biopsy. H&E stain. By courtesy of Dr WE Kenyon.

CLASSIFICATION OF TESTICULAR TUMOURS

I. germ-cell tumours (95%)
    A. single-cell-type tumours (60%)
        seminomas
        yolk sac tumours (embryonal cell tumours)
        teratomas
        choriocarcinoma
    B. combination tumours (40%)
II. tumours of gonadal stroma (1–2%)
        Leydig cell
        Sertoli cell
        primitive gonadal structures
III. gonadoblastomas
        germ cell+stromal cell

Fig. 11.45 Classification of testicular tumours. Data from FK Mostofi (1980) *Cancer* 45:1735.

extraglandular tissues with age. Abnormal liver function or drug therapy may be a contributory cause of breast enlargement in such men.

Pathological gynaecomastia can result from deficiency in testosterone production or action (with or without a secondary increase in oestrogen production), increase in oestrogen production, or drugs (Fig. 11.46). The causes of testosterone deficiency have been discussed above.

Increased testicular oestrogen secretion may result from elevations in plasma gonadotrophins (as in the aberrant production of hCG by testicular tumours or by bronchogenic carcinoma) or from the ovarian elements in the gonads of men with true hermaphroditism; it may, however, be a result of direct secretion by testicular tumours (particularly Leydig cell and Sertoli cell tumours). Increased conversion of androgen to oestrogens in extraglandular tissues can either be due to increased availability of substrate for oestrogen formation or to an increased amount of the enzymes involved in oestrogen formation in peripheral tissues. Increased substrate availability for extraglandular conversion can result from increased synthesis of androgens such as androstenedione (congenital adrenal hyperplasia, hyperthyroidism, adrenal tumours) or because of diminished catabolism of androstenedione by the usual pathways (liver disease). Increased extraglandular aromatase can result from a rare hereditary abnormality or from tumours of the liver or adrenal.

Drugs cause gynaecomastia by several mechanisms. Many drugs act as oestrogens or cause an increase in plasma oestrogen activity. An example of a direct oestrogen effect is diethylstilboestrol used for the treatment of prostate cancer. Gonadotrophin therapy causes enhanced testicular oestrogen secretion. Ketoconazole inhibits testosterone synthesis, whereas spironolactone and cimetidine act primarily to block androgen action at the receptor level. In many instances, the mechanisms by which drugs cause gynaecomastia have not been defined (Fig. 11.46).

Even when all known causes of gynaecomastia are considered, a satisfactory diagnosis is made in only some fifty per cent of patients, but fortunately, the idiopathic disorder is a benign condition. Gynaecomastia may resolve in men with treatable endocrinopathies or in whom an offending drug is discontinued. However, long-standing gynaecomastia may not resolve, even after correction of the cause. When the primary cause cannot be found and/or corrected, surgery is carried out.

HORMONAL THERAPY

ANDROGENS

Effective androgen therapy requires either the administration of testosterone in a slowly absorbed form (dermal patches or micronised oral preparation) or the oral or parenteral administration of chemically modified analogues. Such chemical modifications either retard the rate of absorption or catabolism so as to sustain effective blood levels, or enhance the androgenic potency of each molecule so that physiologic effects can be achieved at a lower blood level. Three types of modification have proved useful (Fig. 11.47): esterification of the 17β-hydroxyl group; alkylation at the 17α position; and modification of the ring structure, particularly substitutions at the 2, 9 and 11 positions. Most drugs contain combinations of ring-structure alterations and either 17α-alkylation or esterification of the 17-hydroxyl group.

The oral effectiveness of 17α-alkylated androgens (such as methyltestosterone and methandrostenolone) is due to slower hepatic catabolism so that the alkylated derivatives escape degradation by the liver and reach the systemic circulation. All 17α-alkylated steroids may cause abnormal liver function.

A transdermal therapeutic preparation of testosterone is under investigation, in which a testosterone-loaded patch is applied each day to skin making it possible to sustain serum levels in the normal male range throughout the day. This therapy avoids the wide swings in serum testosterone values that occur between injections of testosterone esters.

Esters such as testosterone cypionate and testosterone enanthate can be injected every one to three weeks. Since the esters are hydrolysed before the hormones act, the effectiveness of therapy can be monitored by measuring the plasma testosterone level following administration. At physiologic replacement doses, testosterone esters have no known side effects in mature men. At supraphysiologic doses, however, gonadotrophin secretion is inhibited, the testes decrease in volume, and the sperm count falls (indeed, low sperm counts may persist for as long as nine months after supraphysiologic doses are discontinued). The administration of testosterone esters results in an increase in plasma oestrogen levels and may, on occasion, cause gynaecomastia.

The aim of therapy in hypogonadal men is to restore, or bring to normal, male secondary sexual characteristics (beard, body hair, external genitalia) (Fig. 11.48) and male sexual behaviour, and to mimic the hormonal effects on somatic development (haemoglobin, muscle mass, nitrogen balance, and epiphysial closure). Since an assay for plasma testosterone is available for monitoring therapy, the treatment of androgen deficiency is almost universally successful. The parenteral administration of a long-acting testosterone ester, such as 100–200mg testosterone enanthate at one- to three-week intervals, results in a sustained increase in plasma testosterone levels to the normal male range.

CLASSIFICATION OF PATHOLOGICAL GYNAECOMASTIA

deficiency in testosterone synthesis or action

increased oestrogen production

increased testicular oestrogen secretion
  testicular tumours
  bronchogenic carcinoma and other tumours producing hCG
  true hermaphroditism
increased substrate for extraglandular aromatase
  adrenal and liver disease
  starvation
  thyrotoxicosis
increase in extraglandular aromatase

drug induced

oestrogens
drugs that enhance endogenous oestrogen formation
inhibitors of testosterone synthesis and/or action
drugs that act by unknown mechanisms

Fig. 11.46 Classification of pathological gynaecomastia.

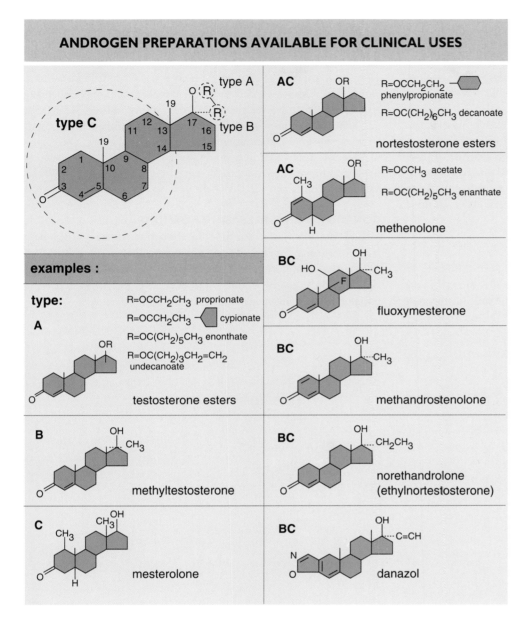

ANDROGEN PREPARATIONS AVAILABLE FOR CLINICAL USES

type C   type A   type B

AC R=OCCH$_2$CH$_2$— phenylpropionate
R=OC(CH$_2$)$_6$CH$_3$ decanoate

nortestosterone esters

AC R=OCCH$_3$ acetate
R=OC(CH$_2$)$_5$CH$_3$ enanthate

methenolone

BC **fluoxymesterone**

examples :

type:

A

R=OCCH$_2$CH$_3$ proprionate
R=OCCH$_2$CH$_3$— cypionate
R=OC(CH$_2$)$_5$CH$_3$ enonthate
R=OC(CH$_2$)$_3$CH$_2$=CH$_2$ undecanoate

testosterone esters

BC **methandrostenolone**

B **methyltestosterone**

BC **norethandrolone (ethylnortestosterone)**

C **mesterolone**

BC **danazol**

Fig. 11.47 Some of the androgen preparations available for clinical use, classified into three types. Type A derivatives are esterified in the 17β-position; type B steroids have alkyl groups in a 17α-position; and type C derivatives include a variety of additional alterations of ring structure that enhance activity or impede catabolism, or influence both functions. Most androgen preparations involve combinations of type AC or type BC changes. Modified from JE Griffin and JD Wilson (1991) by courtesy of WB Saunders.

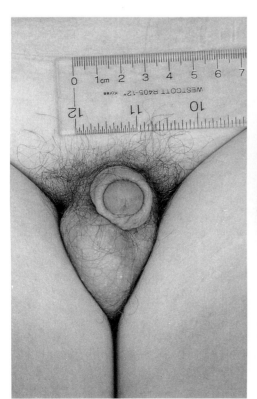
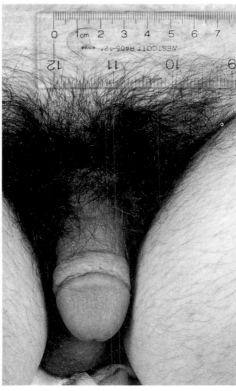

Fig. 11.48 The effect of testosterone cypionate therapy for 11 months in a 22-year-old man with hypogonadotrophin hypogonadism.

Androgens have been tried for a variety of disorders that are unassociated with hypogonadism, in the hope that potential benefits from the nonvirilising actions (such as an increase in nitrogen retention, muscle mass, and haemoglobin) would outweigh any deleterious actions of the drugs. The most common nonreplacement uses of androgen have been attempts to improve nitrogen balance in catabolic states; self-administration by athletes in the belief that muscle mass and/or athletic performance will be improved; attempts to enhance erythropoiesis in refractory anaemias, including the anaemia of renal failure; adjuvant therapy in carcinoma of the breast; and treatment of hereditary angioedema and endometriosis and of growth retardation of various aetiologies. Most expectations of beneficial effects in these disorders have been illusory.

GONADOTROPHINS

Gonadotrophin therapy is utilised to establish or restore fertility in patients with gonadotrophin deficiency of all causes. Two gonadotrophin preparations are available: human menopausal gonadotrophins (hMG) and hCG: hMG contains 75iu. FSH and 75iu LH per vial, while hCG has little FSH activity and resembles LH in its ability to stimulate testosterone production by Leydig cells. Due to the expense of hMG, treatment is usually initiated with hCG alone, and hMG is added later to stimulate the FSH-dependent stages of spermatid development. A high ratio of LH to FSH activity, and a long duration of treatment (three to six months), are necessary to bring about the maturation of the prepubertal testis. Once spermatogenesis is restored in hypophysectomised patients or initiated in hypogonadotrophic hypogonadal men by combined therapy, it can usually be maintained with hCG alone.

GONADOTROPHIN-RELEASING HORMONE

GnRH (gonadorelin) is available for endocrine testing and has been tried for chronic therapy of hypogonadotrophic hypogonadism. It is necessary to administer GnRH in frequent boluses (25–200ng/kg of body weight every two hours); however, it is unclear whether this regimen has any advantages over gonadotrophin therapy.

12

The Ovary

Eli Y Adashi, MD

The ovary, an ever changing tissue, is a multicompartmental organ with a broad range of distinct biological properties. Responding to cyclical pituitary gonadotrophin secretion, the various follicular compartments interact in a highly integrated manner, with a single central objective: the generation of a mature fertilisable ovum for the consequent preservation of the species. At the heart of the ovarian life cycle is the follicle, recognised as the fundamental functional unit of the ovary since the middle of the sixteenth century.

OVUM PRODUCTION AND MATURATION

GERM CELL ONTOGENY

Primordial germ cells originate in the wall of the yolk sac and the ventral wall of the hindgut near the origin of the allantoic evagination (Figs. 12.1 & 12.2) sometime towards the end of the third week of gestation. During weeks three to five of life these germ-cell elements migrate to the primitive gonadal folds. This migration, illustrated in Fig. 12.3, is accompanied by a steady increase in cell number through mitotic divisions. Locomotion is thought to be accomplished by amoeboid movements, the use of pseudopodia, and, most certainly, some form of chemotactic guidance.

Upon arrival at the genital ridge by the fifth week of gestation, the premeiotic germ cells, now referred to as oogonia, continue to multiply. During weeks five to seven of gestation, often referred to as the 'indifferent stage', the primordial gonadal structure constitutes no more than a bulge on the medial aspect of the urogenital ridge.

From this point on, the oogonial endowment is subject to three simultaneous ongoing processes: meiosis, mitosis, and atresia (degeneration). Those oogonia which enter the prophase of the first meiotic division become known as primary oocytes. From around sixteen weeks of gestation these become surrounded by a single layer of spindle-shaped (noncuboidal) primordial (pre)granulosa cells, giving rise to primordial follicles (Fig. 12.4).

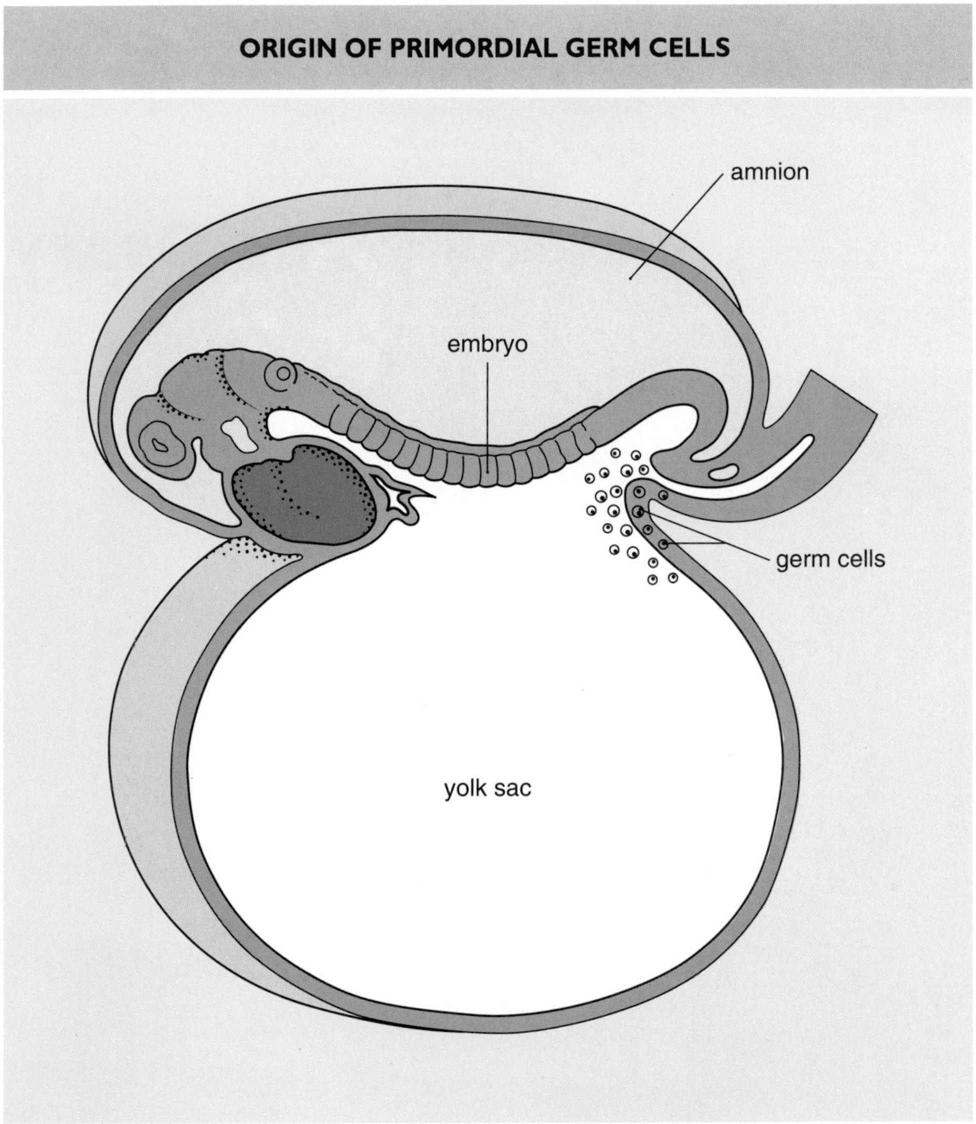

ORIGIN OF PRIMORDIAL GERM CELLS

Fig. 12.1 Origin of primordial germ cells.
Primordial germ cells originate either from or among the primitive endodermal cells in the wall of the yolk sac and the ventral wall of the hindgut near the origin of the allantoic evagination.

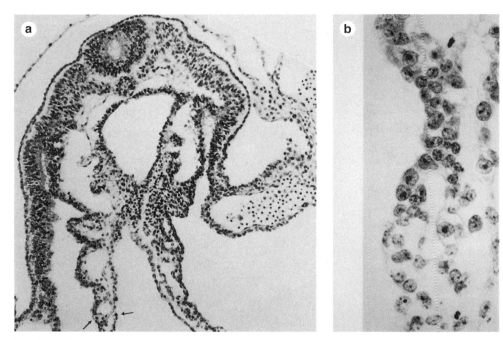
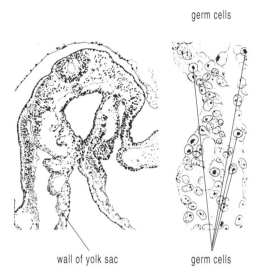

germ cells

wall of yolk sac   germ cells

Fig. 12.2 Germ cells in the early embryo. (a) A cross-section of the ventral wall of the hindgut below the level of attachment of the yolk sac reveals germ cells (magnification ×150), here indicated by arrows. (b) An enlarged view (magnification ×600) of the same is also provided.

MIGRATION OF PRIMORDIAL GERM CELLS

Fig. 12.3 A 4.5-week-old human tailbud embryo with 32 somites. The black dots on the lower gut, mesentery and mesonephros represent loci of primordial germ cells in the process of migration.

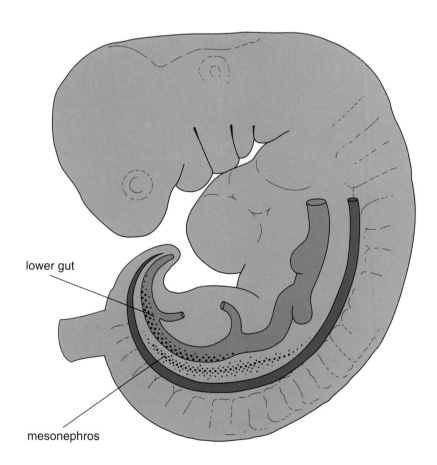

lower gut

mesonephros

The number of germ cells peaks at six to seven million by twenty weeks of gestation, at which time two-thirds of the total are intra-meiotic dictyate primary oocytes, while the remaining third are still oogonia (see Fig. 12.5). From around month six of gestation, attrition progressively diminishes the ovarian germ cell endowment by way of follicular (rather than oogonial) atresia. This continues throughout life (Fig. 12.5). Ultimately, some fifty years later, what has been referred to as the oocytic 'gene bank' is finally exhausted. Newborn female infants enter life having lost as much as eighty per cent of their germ cell endowment, and by the onset of puberty virtually ninety-five per cent of all follicles have been lost. Only four to five hundred follicles (i.e. less than one per cent of the total) will ovulate in the course of a reproductive life span.

FOLLICULOGENESIS

Little information exists at this time as regards the morphogenic principles responsible for follicular organisation. However, it is known that the first step in follicular development, the formation of primordial follicles, which ends no later than six months postpartum, is entirely gonadotrophin independent and that, although other factors are undoubtedly at play, even the earliest phases of follicular development beyond the primordial follicle stage are gonadotrophin dependent.

Primordial follicles migrate towards the medullary region of the ovary (Fig. 12.6) for the next phase in follicular development, the so-called slow growth phase (Fig. 12.7). In this phase, the spindle-shaped granulosa cell precursors which surround the primary oocyte

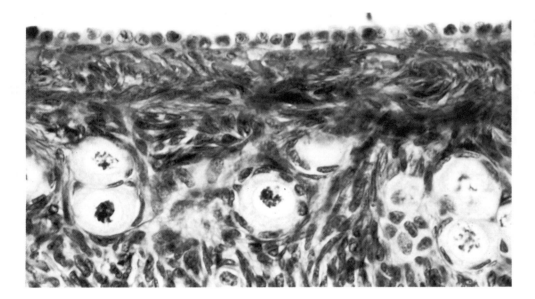

AVERAGE NUMBER OF GERM CELLS THROUGHOUT FEMALE LIFE

Fig. 12.4 Section of ovarian cortex showing developing primordial follicles. The primordial follicle consists of an oocyte surrounded by a single layer of spindle-shaped pregranulosa cells. By courtesy of the late Dr PR Wheater.

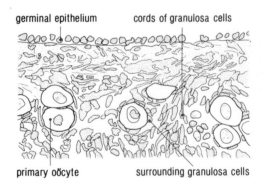

Fig. 12.5 Average number of germ cells throughout female life.

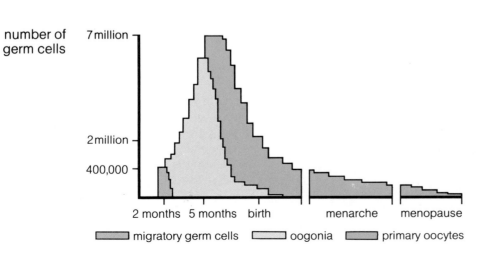

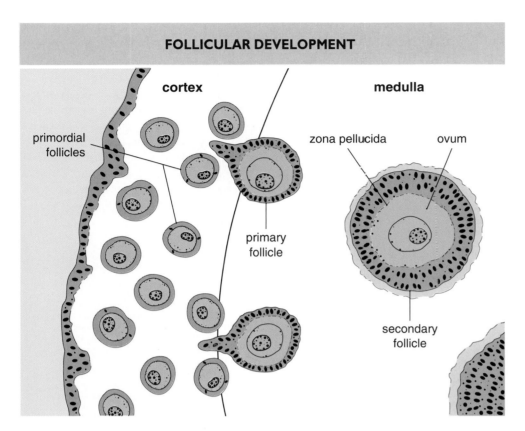

FOLLICULAR DEVELOPMENT

cortex

medulla

primordial
follicles

zona pellucida

ovum

primary
follicle

secondary
follicle

Fig. 12.6 Follicular development. Progressive follicular development from primordial to primary to secondary follicles is accompanied by a dramatic increase in oocyte size and differentiation. During oocyte growth the recruited follicles migrate out of the cortex into the medulla by actions presumed to involve the theca cone.

STAGES OF FOLLICULOGENESIS

	primordial follicle formation	**slow growth phase**	**accelerated growth phase**				**exponential growth phase**				
time		<-340 to -190 days	-70 days	-45 days	-25 days	-10 days	day 1 day 5		day 14		
							recruitment	selection	dominance		midcycle
class	primordial	primary	pre-antral class 1	early antral class 2	class 3	class 4	class 5	class 6	class 7	pre-ovulatory class 8	
diameter	0.06mm	0.12mm	0.2mm	0.4mm	0.9mm	2mm	5mm	10mm	16mm	20mm	ovulation
number of granulosa cells	1 layer	6×10^2 epitheloid cells in theca	$3-5\times10^3$	1.5×10^4	7.5×10^4	3.7×10^5	1.9×10^6	9.4×10^6	4.7×10^7	6.0×10^7	
atresia			24%	35%	15%	24%	58%	77%	50%		

Fig. 12.7 Stages of folliculogenesis in the adult human ovary. Classes are defined by the number of granulosa cells and the corresponding estimated follicular diameter (mm). Redrawn from Gougeon (1986) with permission.

in the primordial follicle differentiate into a single layer of cuboidal cells, thereby yielding primary follicles. Thereafter, proliferation of the granulosa cells of the primary follicule gives rise to multiple cellular layers, thereby yielding a preantral secondary follicle (Figs 12.8 & 12.9). The maximal granulosa cell endowment of the secondary follicle is estimated at six hundred.

At this point the granulosa cells become physiologically coupled by gap junctions, which results in an expanded yet integrated and functional syncytium concerned with metabolic exchange and the transport of diffusible low molecular weight substances, thus compensating for the otherwise avascular intrafollicular environment. Moreover, the granulosa cells extend cytoplasmic processes to form gap-junction-like

unions with the plasma membrane of the oocyte (Fig. 12.10). This latter communication system is largely responsible for the tight control exerted by the cumulus granulosa cells on the resumption of meiosis by the enclosed primary oocyte.

The early theca interna is acquired at the end of the primary follicle stage, with the cells of the theca interna assuming an epithelioid appearance and the characteristics of steroidogenic cells. The theca externa is a characteristic of the secondary follicle, forming only as the follicle expands and compresses surrounding stroma. The cells of the theca externa retain their spindle-shaped configuration, and thus merge with adjacent stromal cells (see Fig. 12.8).

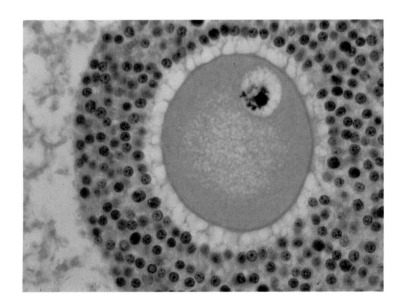

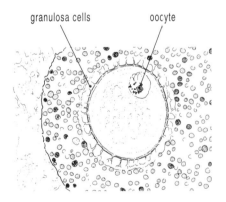

Fig. 12.8 Section through a secondary follicle composed of multiple layers of granulosa cells surrounding an oocyte.

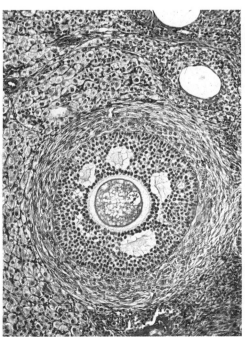
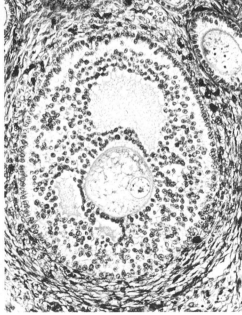

Fig. 12.9 Section showing secondary follicles. The cells surrounding the primary follicle divide to form a multilayered stratum granulosum. Fluid-filled antra, so-called Call–Exner bodies, develop within this layer, and later coalesce to form the antrum. By courtesy of the late Dr PR Wheater.

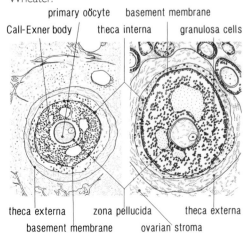

STRUCTURAL RELATIONSHIP BETWEEN GRANULOSA CELLS AND THE OOCYTE

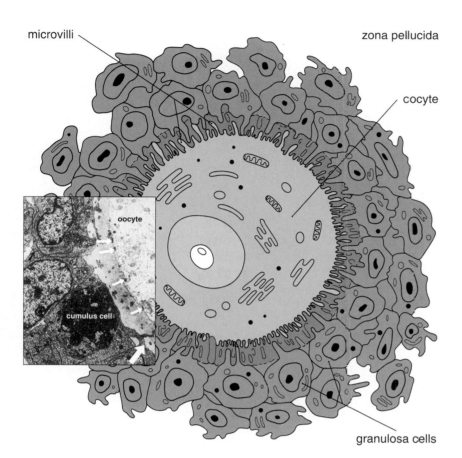

microvilli

zona pellucida

cocyte

granulosa cells

Fig. 12.10 Structural relationship between granulosa cells and the oocyte. Microvilli of the oocyte interdigitate with cytoplasmic extensions of granulosa cells, penetrating the zona pellucida. Inset: Small gap junctions (thin arrows) are observed between processes of the granulosa cell and the oocyte membrane. The thick arrow indicates a gap junction between granulosa cells. Modified from Erickson (1986) with permission.

The development of the preantral secondary follicle into the Graafian preovulatory follicle takes eighty-five days and spans three ovulatory cycles (Fig. 12.11). In the so-called accelerated growth phase (see Fig. 12.7), preantral secondary follicles of 120µm in diameter are converted into antral follicles of 2mm in diameter. This is accomplished by a six-hundred-fold increase in granulosa cell endowment and progressive enlargement of the central follicular fluid-filled cavity, the antrum.

Follicular Recruitment

Those follicles which are destined to ovulate in the next cycle are 'recruited' from the luteal pool of 2mm secondary antral follicles, i.e. they enter the terminal exponential growth phase (see Fig. 12.7) to become preovulatory (Graafian) follicles with a 20mm diameter. In the Graafian follicle the oocyte occupies an eccentric position, surrounded by several layers of cumulus granulosa cells (Fig. 12.12).

Follicular Selection

Importantly, it is during this last phase of folliculogenesis that follicular selection is completed, i.e. the number of follicles in the

maturing but not quite yet dominant follicular cohort is decreased by atresia to the species-characteristic ovulatory quota. In the human, follicular selection is presumed to occur during the first five days of the cycle at a time when the leading follicular diameter is 5–10mm.

Follicular Dominance

The term 'dominance' refers to the status of the follicle destined to ovulate, given its presumed key role in regulating the size of the ovulatory quota. In the human, a selected follicle becomes dominant about a week before ovulation, i.e. as early as days five to seven of the cycle, at a time when follicular diameter is around 10mm. Only the dominant follicle can at this point in time boast detectable levels of follicle stimulating hormone (FSH) in its follicular fluid (Fig. 12.13). This same follicle also displays significant follicular levels of oestradiol.

The dominant follicle, under the influence of the midcycle luteinising hormone (LH) surge, undergoes dramatic transformations designed to effect further oocyte maturation as well as follicular rupture (Fig. 12.14).

RATE OF FOLLICULAR GROWTH

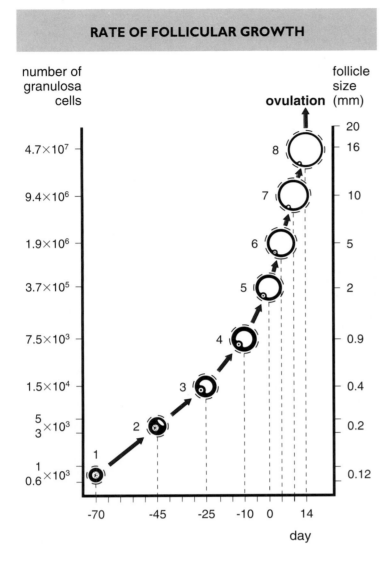

number of granulosa cells

ovulation

follicle size (mm)

4.7×10⁷	8	16 / 20
9.4×10⁶	7	10
1.9×10⁶	6	5
3.7×10⁵	5	2
7.5×10³	4	0.9
1.5×10⁴	3	0.4
5/3×10³	2	0.2
1/0.6×10³	1	0.12

day: -70 -45 -25 -10 0 14

Fig. 12.11 Rate of follicular growth (classes 1 through to 8) in the human ovary. Redrawn from Gougeon (1986) with permission.

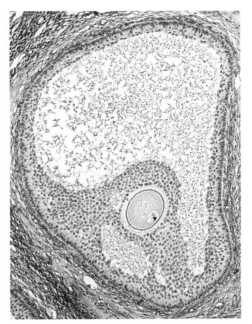

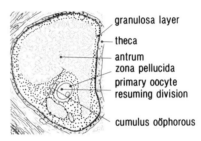

- granulosa layer
- theca
- antrum
- zona pellucida
- primary oocyte resuming division
- cumulus oöphorous

Fig. 12.12 Mature tertiary or Graafian follicle. The Call–Exner bodies have now coalesced and contain liquor folliculi. The ovum has been surrounded by a mound of cells known as the ciscus proligerus or the cumulus oophorus.

HORMONAL CHARACTERISTICS OF A DOMINANT FOLLICLE

	dominant	non-dominant
FSH level	2–4mu/ml	not detectable
oestradiol level	1000ng/ml	100ng/ml
Δ⁴ level	800ng/ml	800ng/ml
granulosa cell number	>1×10⁶ cells	<5×10⁵ cells
dihydrotestosterone	100ng/ml	100ng/ml

Fig. 12.13 Hormonal characteristics of a dominant follicle. High follicular concentrations of FSH and oestradiol are characteristic of the dominant follicle.

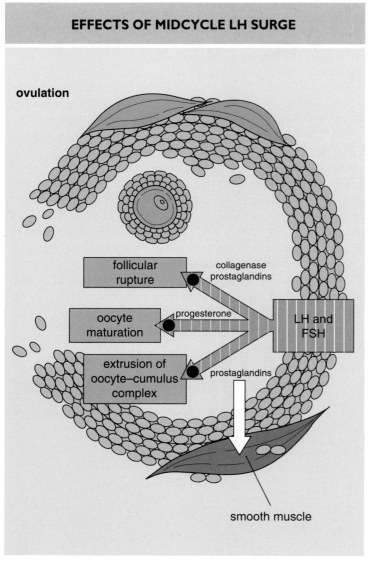

EFFECTS OF MIDCYCLE LH SURGE

ovulation

follicular rupture

collagenase prostaglandins

oocyte maturation

progesterone

LH and FSH

extrusion of oocyte–cumulus complex

prostaglandins

smooth muscle

Fig. 12.14 Effects of the midcycle LH surge. This leads to follicular rupture, oocyte maturation, and extrusion of the cumulus–oocyte complex.

OVULATION

As midcycle approaches, a dramatic rise is noted in the circulating levels of oestradiol, followed in turn by an LH (and to a lesser extent FSH) surge, which triggers follicular rupture (Fig. 12.15). This mid-cycle gonadotrophin surge marks the end of the follicular phase of the cycle and precedes actual rupture by as much as thirty-six hours. For reasons not well understood, but possibly because of unique microenvironmental circumstances, one (or rarely more than one) follicle ovulates and gives rise to a corpus luteum during each menstrual cycle.

Mechanically, ovulation consists of rapid follicular enlargement followed by protrusion of the follicle from the surface of the ovarian cortex. Rupture of the follicle results in the extrusion of an oocyte–cumulus complex. Endoscopic visualisation of the ovary around the time of ovulation reveals that elevation of a conical 'stigma' on the surface of the protruding follicle precedes rupture (Fig. 12.16). Rupture of this stigma is accompanied by gentle, rather than explosive, expulsion of the oocyte and antral fluid, suggesting that the latter is not under high pressure.

CORPUS LUTEUM FORMATION AND DEMISE

After ovulation, the dominant follicle reorganises to become the corpus luteum. Thus, following rupture of the follicle, capillaries and fibroblasts from the surrounding stroma proliferate and penetrate the basal lamina. This rapid vascularisation of the corpus luteum may be guided by angiogenic factors which are readily detected in the follicular fluid. Concurrently, the mural granulosa cells undergo structural changes collectively referred to as 'luteinisation'. These latter cells, the surrounding theca-interstitial cells, and the invading vasculature intermingle to give rise to a corpus luteum (Fig. 12.17).

Fig. 12.15 Hormonal events in the menstrual cycle.

HORMONAL EVENTS IN THE MENSTRUAL CYCLE

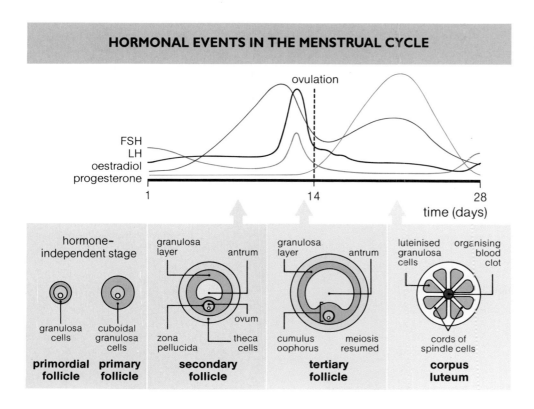

ovulation

FSH
LH
oestradiol
progesterone

1   14   28
time (days)

hormone-independent stage

granulosa cells

cuboidal granulosa cells

granulosa layer   antrum

zona pellucida   theca cells   ovum

granulosa layer   antrum

cumulus oophorus   meiosis resumed

luteinised granulosa cells   organising blood clot

cords of spindle cells

primordial follicle   **primary follicle**   **secondary follicle**   **tertiary follicle**   **corpus luteum**

The corpus luteum acts as an endocrine gland and is the major source of sex steroid hormones secreted by the ovary during the postovulatory phase of the cycle (see Fig. 12.15). An important aspect of this phenomenon is the penetration of the follicle basement membrane by blood vessels, thereby providing the granulosa/luteal cells with circulating levels of LDL.

Unless pregnancy occurs, the functional life span of the corpus luteum is twelve to sixteen days. Thereafter, the corpus luteum spontaneously regresses, to be replaced at least five cycles later by an avascular scar referred to as the corpus albicans (Fig. 12.18). The mechanisms underlying luteolysis remain unclear. However, LH plays a central role in the maintenance of corpus luteum function. Thus, withdrawal of LH support under a variety of experimental circumstances virtually invariably results in luteal demise.

In the event of an intervening pregnancy, human chorionic gonadotrophin (HCG) secreted by the fetal trophoblast maintains the ability of the corpus luteum to elaborate progesterone, thereby enabling the maintenance of early gestation until the luteo–placental shift.

SIGNALLING SYSTEMS

Preantral granulosa cells are predominantly targeted by FSH. Indeed, these cells contain a negligible number of LH receptors. At the preantral stage, the binding of LH is confined to theca-interstitial cells. Importantly, however, granulosa cells of antral follicles appear capable of binding both LH and FSH. Thus, although FSH receptors are present in granulosa cells from follicles of all sizes, LH receptors are found only in granulosa cells of large preovulatory follicles (Fig. 12.19). These observations are in keeping with the notion that the acquisition of LH receptors is under the influence of FSH.

As illustrated in Fig. 12.20, the action of both LH and FSH appears to require the intermediacy of the membrane-associated enzyme adenylate cyclase. Indeed, it is generally accepted that gonadotrophin-mediated stimulation of adenylate cyclase results in the conversion of intracellular ATP to cAMP. The latter, in turn, is thought to bind to the regulatory subunit of a protein kinase (commonly referred to as-A-kinase) whereupon the catalytic subunit of the enzyme is activated and dissociated. The latter, in turn, phosphorylates key intracellular proteins central to the signal transduction sequence. However, the exact nature of the proteins involved remains unknown at this time.

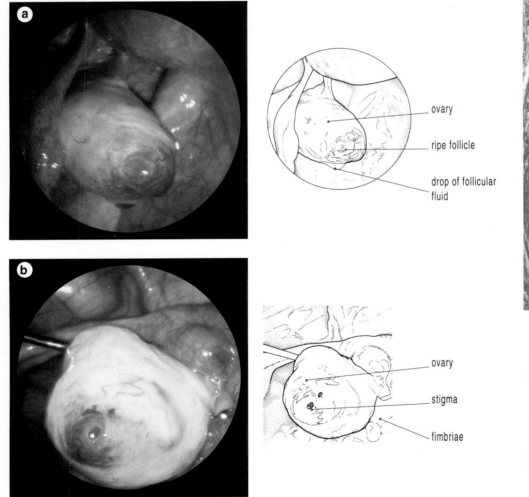

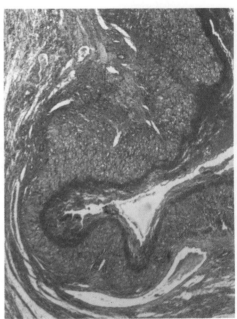

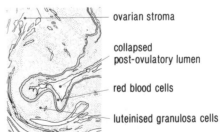

Fig. 12.16 Ovulation of the cumulus–oocyte complex. Endoscopic view of the ovary immediately prior to ovulation (a) and following ovulation (b). By courtesy of Prof H Frangenheim and Dr MR Darling.

Fig. 12.17 Section through the corpus luteum. Once ovulation has occurred the walls of the ruptured ovarian follicle collapse and become folded. Cells of the stratum granulosum increase in size and become luteinised. These cells form the major part of the corpus luteum. By courtesy of Prof I Doniach.

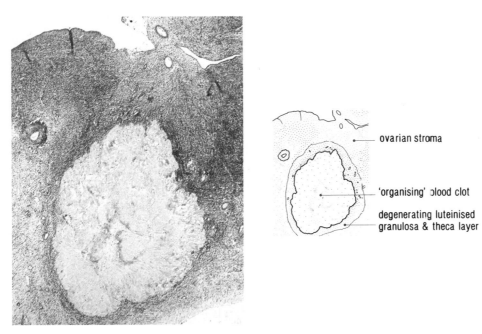

ovarian stroma

'organising' blood clot

degenerating luteinised
granulosa & theca layer

Fig. 12.18 Section through the corpus albicans. If fertilisation has not occurred, the corpus luteum degenerates over the succeeding months and the cells undergo colloid, then fatty, and finally hyaline degeneration to produce the corpus albicans.

RECEPTOR SITES ON SOMATIC OVARIAN CELLS

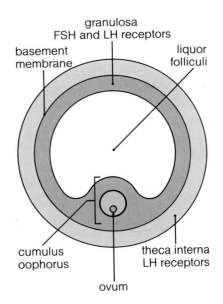

granulosa
FSH and LH receptors

basement
membrane

liquor
folliculi

cumulus
oophorus

theca interna
LH receptors

ovum

Fig. 12.19 Receptor sites on somatic ovarian cells. Note that LH receptors are found on both theca interna and granulosa cells whereas FSH receptors are found only on granulosa cells.

Fig. 12.20 The two cell/two gonadotrophin hypothesis of follicular oestrogen production.

TWO CELL/TWO GONADOTROPHIN HYPOTHESIS

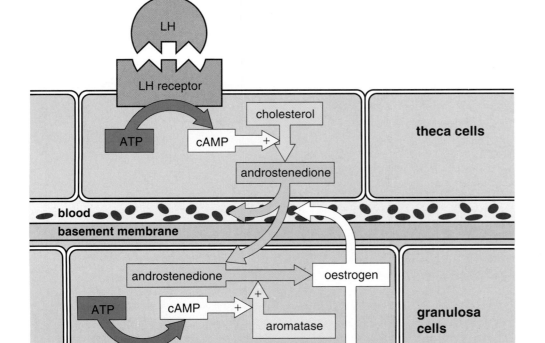

LH

LH receptor

ATP

cAMP

cholesterol

theca cells

androstenedione

blood

basement membrane

androstenedione

oestrogen

ATP

cAMP

aromatase

granulosa
cells

FSH receptor

FSH

follicular
fluid

CLINICAL ENDOCRINOLOGY

HORMONE PRODUCTION BY THE OVARY

OESTROGEN BIOSYNTHESIS

Granulosa cells are the cellular source of the two most important ovarian steroids, oestradiol and progesterone. Although the granulosa cells and their luteinised counterparts are capable of producing progesterone independently of other ovarian cell types, the biosynthesis of oestrogens requires cooperation between the granulosa cells and their thecal neighbours. The participation of these two cell types and of the two gonadotrophins (FSH and LH) in ovarian oestrogen biosynthesis underlies the concept of the two cell/two gonadotrophin hypothesis, an integrative processes required for ovarian oestrogen biosynthesis (see Fig. 12.20). According to this view, theca-derived, LH-dependent aromatisable androgens (androstenedione and testos-

terone) are acted upon by FSH-inducible granulosa cell aromatase activity. A broader view of this concept could and probably should allow its extension to include intercellular exchanges of other steroidogenic substrates (e.g. C^{21} progestins).

PROGESTIN BIOSYNTHESIS

The granulosa (like the theca-interstitial) cell has abundant supplies of cholesterol which serves as the starting material for the steroidogenic cascade. Recent studies have shown that cholesterol used for steroid hormone production is derived primarily from circulating serum LDL rather than from *de novo* cellular biosynthesis from acetate (Fig. 12.21). LDL particles are known to bind to specific membrane receptors, the LDL–receptor complexes entering the cell by receptor-mediated endocytosis. The resultant free cholesterol is

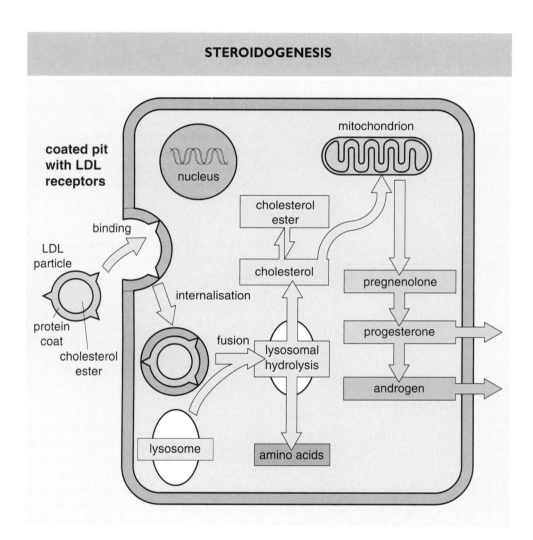

STEROIDOGENESIS

Fig. 12.21 Steroidogenesis. Circulating LDL constitutes the major source of cellular cholesterol substrate for steroidogenesis.
Circulating LDL particles, containing a cholesterol ester core surrounded by a protein coat, bind to specific cell membrane receptors.
The LDL–receptor complex is internalised and fuses to lysosomes; the cholesterol ester is hydrolysed to cholesterol and the protein coat to amino acids. Free cholesterol is either stored as re-esterified cholesterol or transferred to the mitochondria, where it is converted to pregnenolone by the cholesterol side-chain cleavage (CSCC) enzyme.

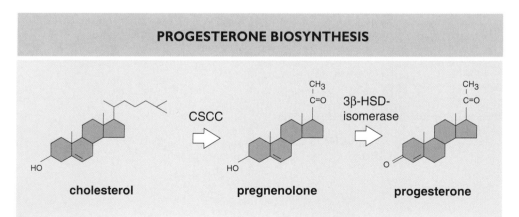

PROGESTERONE BIOSYNTHESIS

Fig. 12.22 Progesterone biosynthesis.
This involves two steroidogenic steps: conversion of cholesterol to pregnenolone as mediated by the steroidogenic CSCC enzyme and conversion of pregnenolone to progesterone mediated by the steroidogenic enzyme 3β-hydroxysteroid dehydrogenase (HSD)-isomerase.

re-esterified and is stored in the cytoplasm in lipid droplets. Faced with steroidogenic demands, the cholesterol ester is hydrolysed and the free cholesterol transported to mitochondria for standard steroidogenic processing. Cholesterol is converted to pregnenolone by way of the rate-limiting mitochondrial cholesterol side-chain cleavage (CSCC) enzyme. The subsequent conversion of pregnenolone to progesterone occurs relatively readily by virtue of the relative abundance of the cytoplasmic enzymes 3β-hydroxysteroid dehydrogenase and D^5 isomerase (3β-HSD-isomerase) (Fig. 12.22).

ANDROGEN BIOSYNTHESIS

The thecal layer is the major cellular source of follicular C^{19} androgens. LH, rather than FSH, stimulates thecal androgen production. Accordingly, this cell type is amply endowed with 17α-hydroxylase and 17,20-lyase activity (Fig. 12.23), capable of converting D^5 and D^4 (C^{21}) progestational precursors (i.e. pregnenolone and progesterone) to androgenic C^{19} products (dehydroepiandrosterone and androstenedione, respectively). These in turn are processed further as illustrated in Fig. 12.23.

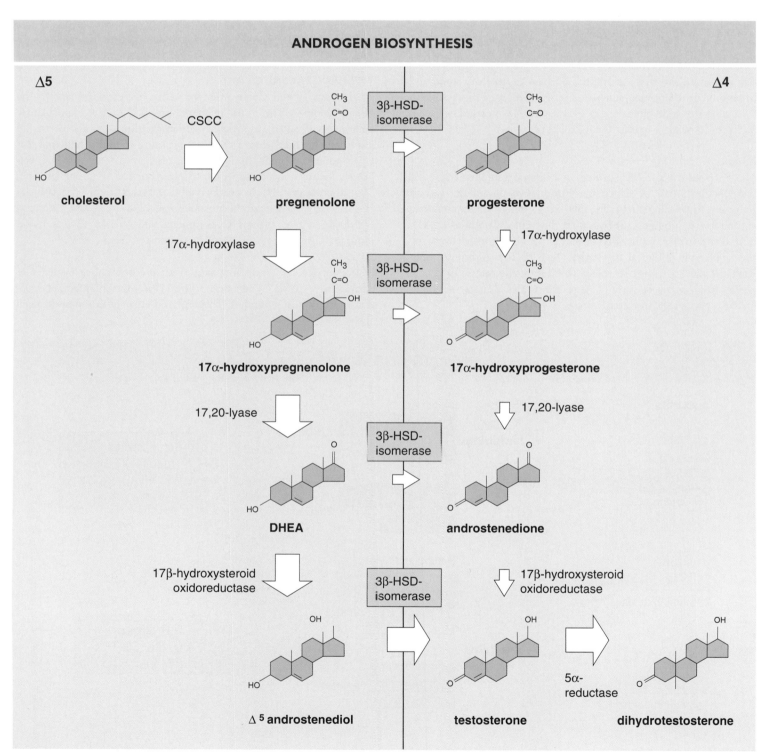

Fig. 12.23 Androgen biosynthesis. This involves conversion of the C^{21} progestins pregnenolone and progesterone to C^{19} androgens via Δ^5 and Δ^4 pathways, respectively. Testosterone can be further reduced to dihydrotestosterone, a transformation mediated by the steroidogenic enzyme 5α-reductase.

Aside from serving as substrates for the aromatase reaction, androgenic steroids exert a variety of receptor-mediated effects at the level of the granulosa cell. Paradoxically, androgens possess the capacity to promote gonadotrophin-stimulated granulosa cell aromatase activity. Thus, androgens augment FSH-stimulated aromatase activity not only by acting as a substrate but also by exerting a direct paracrine effect resulting in the upregulation of the activity of this steroidogenic enzyme. On the other hand, high follicular concentrations of reduced androgens (e.g. dihydrotestosterone) may act as competitive inhibitors of granulosa cell aromatase activity. Moreover, androgens have been shown to promote follicular atresia in the absence of gonadotrophins and to antagonise oestrogen-supported ovarian development. These findings are in keeping with the observation that an increased intraovarian androgen to oestrogen ratio is commonly associated with poorly developing follicular units.

PROTEIN BIOSYNTHESIS

The granulosa and theca-interstitial cells are capable of elaborating a large number of proteins, but the identity of most of these remains a mystery at this time. Some are steroidogenic enzymes and cell surface receptors; others are briefly discussed below.

Inhibin

This FSH-inducible, 32kDa protein, is a unique granulosa cell marker, the functional role of which in reproductive physiology is under active investigation. Structurally, inhibin is a hetero-dimer comprising a common α-subunit (18kDa) with different β-subunits (14kDa). Both forms (α/βA and α/βB) of inhibin (A and B, respectively) possess similar physiological properties (Fig. 12.24). Although inhibin seems to play an endocrine role by inhibiting the release of pituitary gonadotrophins, particularly FSH, recent studies indicate that inhibin may also play a local intraovarian role.

Activin

Activin comprises dimers of the β-subunits of inhibin (βA/βB or βA/βA). Although active at the level of the hypothalamic–pituitary unit, granulosa-cell-derived activin has also been shown to enhance the FSH-supported induction of granulosa cell LH receptors.

Follistatin

This recently isolated protein comprises a single chain polypeptide of 315 amino acids. Although structurally distinct from both inhibin and activin, this FSH-inducible granulosa-cell-derived polypeptide appears to suppress the release of pituitary FSH but not LH in a manner reminiscent of inhibin. The potential relevance, if any, of follistatin to ovarian physiology remains unknown at this time.

THE MENOPAUSE

THE MENOPAUSAL OVARY

At the time of the menopause, the ovary becomes resistant to the gonadotrophins. The initial resistance to FSH leads to anovulatory cycles, with elevated FSH. Later, as menstruation stops and oestradiol levels fall, LH levels rise. Despite its exposure to high circulating levels of gonadotrophins, the postmenopausal ovary is an atrophic, yellowish, lustreless structure with a wrinkled surface, weighing less than 10g. Microscopically, the cortex is thin and usually devoid of follicles (Fig. 12.25). However, the postmenopausal ovary is not a defunct endocrine organ; analysis of peripheral and ovarian venous blood indicates that androstenedione and testosterone are secreted (Fig. 12.26).

Occasionally, the postmenopausal ovarian cortex shows evidence of stromal hyperplasia. When this is florid, the ovary may be enlarged, consisting almost entirely of hyperplastic stromal nodules. In such

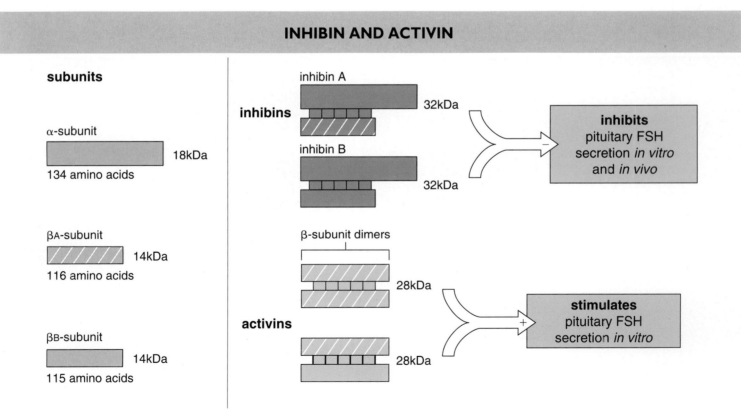

Fig. 12.24 Inhibin and activin. Heterodimers composed of a common α-subunit but different β-subunits give rise to inhibin A and B, which selectively suppress pituitary FSH release. Hetero- and homodimers of the βA- and βB-subunits give rise to activin, which may stimulate pituitary FSH release.

stromal hyperplasia. When this is florid, the ovary may be enlarged, consisting almost entirely of hyperplastic stromal nodules. In such cases, the lipid-rich luteinised cells of the hyperplastic stroma re- semble the theca interna cells of the follicle. Thus, ovaries with stromal hyperthecosis may produce enough androgens to result in circulating testosterone levels within the male range, leading to hirsutism and virilisation.

The medulla of the postmenopausal ovary is large in relation to the cortex, comprising of the corpora albicantia and corpora candicantia traversed by sclerosed blood vessels. Functionally, an important medullary component is the hilar cell. Groups of these large epithelioid cells are closely connected to bundles of nonmyelinated nerve fibres and small vessels. Histochemically, hilar cells are similar to the interstitial cells of the testes, and it is thought that they display considerable steroidogenic potential.

Rarely, hilar cells give rise to functional neoplasms, i.e. hilar cell tumours, which usually produce excess amounts of androgens, leading to the signs and symptoms of virilism. However, signs and symptoms of oestrogen excess may also be evident where there is significant peripheral aromatisation.

CLINICAL ASPECTS

Given the inevitable hypo-oestrogenic state consequent to the cessation of ovarian function, several key complications may ensue. These include urogenital atrophy, hot flushes, osteoporosis, and increased cardiovascular morbidity and mortality. These complications, most of which are partly if not fully traceable to oestrogen deficiency, are most appropriately managed by the provision of oestrogen replacement therapy; providing oestrogen for some or all of the calendar month, with supplemental progestin for women with an intact uterus in whom protection of the endometrial lining is essential. Persistent unopposed oestrogenic stimulation may, if unchecked, lead to endometrial hyperplasia and even endometrial cancer. Currently there is still controversy over the best type of hormone replacement therapy (HRT) and the best route of administration of sex steroids. However, although HRT is associated with small, albeit uncertain, risks, current consensus favours the notion that the benefits far outweigh whatever risks may be associated with this therapeutic approach.

Some of the consequences of oestrogen deprivation affect women's quality of life. These include the development of urogenital atrophy, which may lead to varying degrees of sexual dysfunction and urinary incontinence, and the development of hot flushes. This biophysically documented sequence of events, associated with real increments in skin temperature, may prove socially incapacitating if not addressed. Fortunately, both urogenital atrophy and hot flushes are readily manageable with conventional HRT regimens.

Of greater import is the impact of oestrogen deprivation on bone density and the virtual certainty of progressive postmenopausal osteoporosis. This potentially life-threatening complication, characterised by a one to three per cent loss of bone mass per year, requires immediate attention as soon as women enter the menopause. Fortunately,

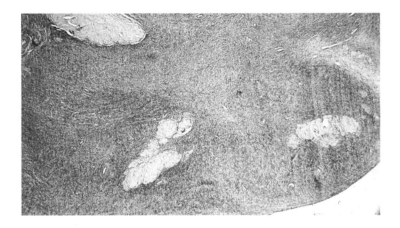

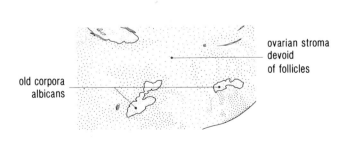

old corpora albicans

ovarian stroma devoid of follicles

Fig. 12.25 Section of postmenopausal ovary. By courtesy of Dr JW Keeling.

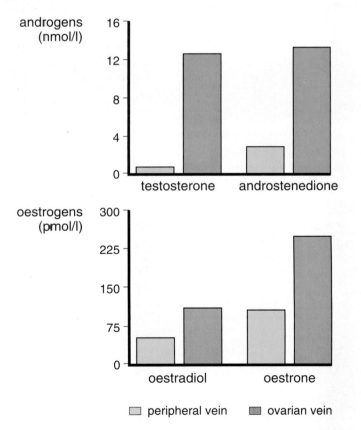

CIRCULATING ANDROGENS AND OESTROGENS IN POSTMENOPAUSAL WOMEN

androgens (nmol/l)

testosterone   androstenedione

oestrogens (pmol/l)

oestradiol   oestrone

☐ peripheral vein ▨ ovarian vein

Fig. 12.26 Circulating levels of key androgens and oestrogens in peripheral and ovarian venous blood of postmenopausal women. Redrawn from Judd *et al.* (1974) with permission.

HRT will prevent any bone loss, if initiated promptly; at the least HRT prevents further bone loss from the time of intervention.

Lastly, much attention is currently being paid to the cardiovascular consequences of oestrogen deprivation. The apparent cardioprotective edge which women seem to enjoy prior to the menopause is progressively lost following the menopause in a time-dependent fashion. It is currently estimated that more women die of cardiovascular disease than of any other causes. However, the provision of oestrogens has been shown to diminish the cardiovascular risk by about fifty per cent. Unfortunately, progestins may undermine this beneficial effect of oestrogens.

DISTURBANCES OF OVARIAN HORMONE PRODUCTION

POLYCYSTIC OVARY SYNDROME

Polycystic ovary syndrome (PCO) was first described by Stein and Leventhal in 1935; they also reported a successful outcome with bilateral ovarian wedge resection. The ovaries in PCO are two to four times the normal size (Fig. 12.27) and, although occasionally normal in configuration, are sometimes described as globular or fat and soft ('oyster ovaries'). The cortex is described as hypertrophic and the tunica is thick, fibrotic, and tough. Follicular cortical cysts lined with theca cells vary in size (Fig. 12.28).

The diagnosis of PCO is made on the basis of the clinical history, biochemical evidence, and, if available, histological evaluation of ovarian tissue. Obesity, amenorrhoea, enlarged ovaries and even hirsutism are not required.

Clinical Evaluation

PCO is characterised by a chronic anovulatory state with or without clinical evidence of hyperandrogenism. Consequent infertility is the rule. Accordingly, patients may present with one or more of the following: dysfunctional uterine bleeding, primary amenorrhoea, secondary amenorrhoea, hirsutism, acne (Fig. 12.29), or infertility. Both the chronic anovulatory syndrome and the hyperandrogenic state can be traced back to puberty, underscoring the fact that PCO is not likely to be acquired at a later date.

Biochemical Evidence

The most characteristic feature of PCO is the inappropriate secretion of pituitary gonadotrophins. Specifically, serum LH is significantly increased, secondary to increased amplitude or frequency of pulsation, whereas FSH levels are either normal or slightly decreased. Consequently, the LH to FSH ratio is often but not invariably

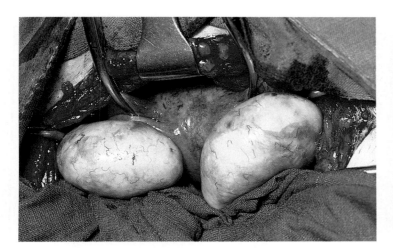

Fig. 12.27 Ovaries of a patient with PCO. The ovaries are enlarged and pearly white. The ovarian capsule is thickened.

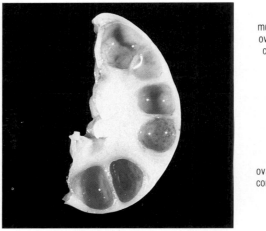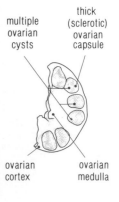

Fig. 12.28 Section through an ovary excised from a patient with PCO. The yellow coloration of the cyst is evidence of the luteinisation which has occurred. By courtesy of Dr JW Keeling.

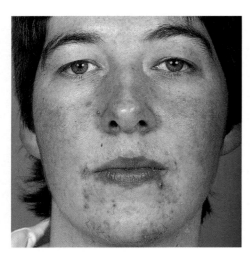

Fig. 12.29 Facial acne, greasy skin and hirsutism in a patient with PCO. The extent of hair growth in this patient is minimal.

BIOCHEMICAL ABNORMALITIES IN PCO

raised adrenal and ovarian androgens	normal or raised prolactin
raised testosterone	raised LH/FSH ratio
lowered sex-hormone-binding globulin (SHBG)	raised urinary oxosteroid excretion

Fig. 12.30 Biochemical events associated with PCO.

increased. Circulating levels of prolactin are elevated in some but not all patients (Fig. 12.30).

In addition to the inappropriate secretion of pituitary gonadotrophins, PCO is often (but not always) characterised by biochemical hyperandrogenism. Circulating levels of several Δ^5 and Δ^4 androgens may be elevated; an effect further compounded by a decrease in circulating levels of sex-hormone (androgen) binding globulin (SHBG).

Finally, PCO is characterised by a hyperoestrogenic state. Specifically, the total production rate of oestrone is increased secondary to extraglandular conversion from an enlarged pool of androstenedione. Although the limited ovarian secretion rate of oestradiol remains unchanged, the significant decrease in the binding capacity of SHBG results in a substantial increase in the free fraction of oestradiol and testosterone. Additional associated features may include insulin resistance and hyperlipidaemia.

Essentials of management

To a large extent, the management of individuals afflicted with PCO depends on the presenting symptomatology. Given isolated dysfunctional uterine bleeding as the main and only complaint, consideration may be given to the cyclical provision of combination oral contraceptives or of a representative progestin (such as medroxyprogesterone acetate). Under those circumstances, regular shedding of the endometrial lining is assured, thereby eliminating the unpredictable nature of dysfunctional uterine flow. The provision of combination oral contraceptives concurrently assures appropriate contraception should this be required. Although spontaneous ovulation and subsequent conception in patients with PCO is highly unlikely, this cannot be viewed as impossible. Consequently, the provision of contraception in this setting appears to enjoy a solid rationale. Given clinical hirsutism as the main and only symptom, treatment directed at the diminution of ovarian androgen production and/or action should be undertaken. Specifically, consideration should be given to suppressing ovarian androgen biosynthesis through the use of combination oral contraceptives or, in severe cases, a long-acting gonadotrophin-releasing-hormone (GnRH) agonist. Independently or concurrently, consideration might also be given to the provision of peripheral-androgen-receptor blockers such as cyproterone acetate or spironolactone. This gives a multipronged approach to the management of ovarian hyperandrogenism by addressing both androgen production and action. Lastly, given infertility as the presenting symptom, therapy should be directed at the reinitiation of ovulatory menstrual cycles. Under these circumstances, the agent of choice is clomiphene citrate, a nonsteroidal antioestrogen capable of restoring ovulatory menstrual cyclicity. Given resistance to clomiphene citrate, consideration must be given to the use of low-dose FSH, the efficacy of which in the context of PCO has been demonstrated. Use of GnRH delivered in a pulsatile fashion so as to mimic hypothalamic release patterns has proved largely disappointing. All told, the various symptoms associated with PCO are readily manageable, albeit not curable.

ANDROGEN-PRODUCING TUMOURS

Among the ovarian androgen-producing virilising tumours (Figs. 12.31 & 12.32), arrhenoblastoma (Sertoli–Leydig cell tumour) is the most common. However, even this tumour is extremely rare, accounting for less than one per cent of all solid ovarian tumours. Occurring in all age groups, some seventy per cent of cases are observed in women under forty, with the peak age of incidence being between twenty and forty years of age. Although variable in size, eighty-five per cent of these tumours are large enough to be palpable. The remainder, however, are rather small and may escape detection at the time of laparoscopy and even laparotomy. Bilateral occurrence of these tumours is rare. Malignant degeneration has been observed in twenty per cent of cases. Treatment (i.e. removal) results in a dramatic improvement in symptoms (Fig. 12.33).

Gonadoblastomas occur exclusively in phenotypically female individuals bearing the Y chromosome. The peak age of incidence is between ten and thirty years of age. Some forty per cent of these tumours are bilateral, and malignant degeneration is observed in some fifty per cent of cases. Tumour size at the time of diagnosis is highly variable.

Androgen-producing lipoid cell tumours of the ovary (Fig. 12.34) include the so-called adrenal rest tumours, formerly referred to as adrenal-like tumours (masculinovoblastoma, luteoma, hypernephroma, and androblastoma diffusum) and the so-called hilar cell tumours (Leydig cell tumours). Although the exact histological origin of these rare virilising ovarian tumours remains unknown, those resembling adrenal histology tend to be more malignant and palpable.

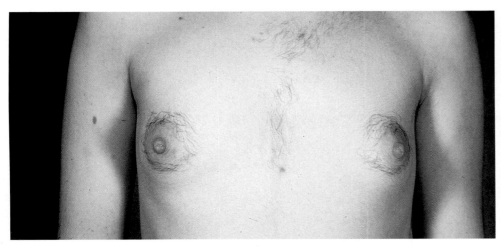

Fig. 12.31 Periareolar hirsuties and mammary hypoplasia in a patient suffering from an androgen-secreting ovarian tumour.

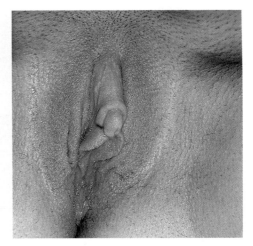

Fig. 12.32 Enlarged clitoris in a patient with an androgen-secreting tumour.

On occasion, virilising syndromes may be encountered in tumours not otherwise thought of as androgen producing, such as dysgerminoma, Brenner tumour, teratoma, simple cystadenomas, and cystadenocarcinomas. It is generally thought that these tumours, as well as some tumours that are metastatic to the ovary from sites such as the breast, stomach, and colon, stimulate androgen production by adjacent stromal androgen-producing cells.

Rarely, functional oestrogen-producing tumours will be encountered (Fig. 12.35). These so-called theca or granulosa cell neoplasms may lead to excessive endometrial stimulation and possibly towards the development of endometrial cancer.

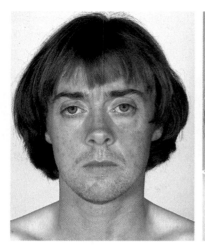
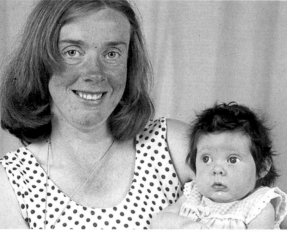

Fig. 12.33 A patient with an arrhenoblastoma with associated PCO before and after treatment. Before treatment (left), the patient had marked facial hirsutism. On the right the patient is shown successfully treated. The tumour was resected and ovulation ensued with clomiphene and HCG therapy.

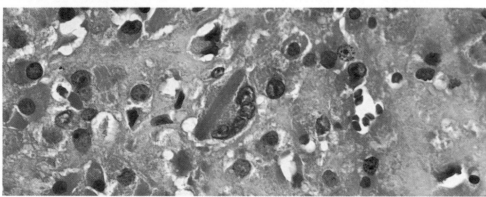

Fig. 12.34 Excised Leydig cell tumour (upper) with histological appearance (lower). Leydig cell tumours, as well as hilus cell tumours, secrete androgens, although the functional activity of tumours does not always correlate with their histological classification. By courtesy of Dr JW Keel ng and Prof I Doniach.

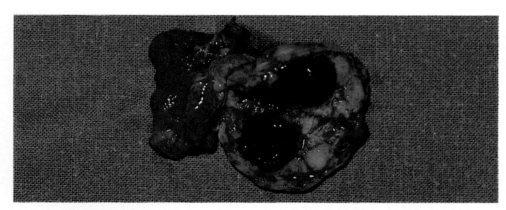

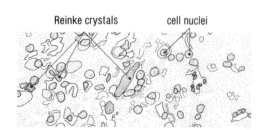

Reinke crystals   cell nuclei

Fig. 12.35 Section of an ovary showing a theca cell tumour. This tumour is oestrogen-secreting and is probably the most common type of functional ovarian tumour.

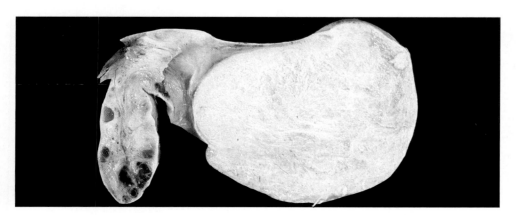

13

Normal and Abnormal Sexual Development and Puberty

Dennis M Styne, MD

Puberty is not an isolated event but rather one stage in the developmental continuum between conception and senescence. Although marked psychological changes occur during pubertal development, this chapter focuses on endocrine and physical changes of secondary sexual development.

Historical evidence indicates that the age of puberty today is younger than was true of past eras. During the last one hundred and fifty years, the average age of menarche (as an indication of the age of pubertal development) in industrialised European countries has decreased by two to three months per decade (Fig. 13.1). This secular trend of a progressively decreasing age of menarche has ceased in developed countries such as the USA in the last three decades, and was apparently due to improvements in nutrition and general standards of health in the developed world. In countries in which 'optimal socioeconomic status' has not been reached, the age of menarche remains later. The average age of menarche in the USA is 12.8 years.

Malnutrition occurs in modern society due to poverty, voluntary dieting or chronic disease, and delayed puberty occurs in association with any cause of malnutrition. Alternatively, moderate obesity can be associated with advanced pubertal development and advancement of bone age during childhood. Remarkably, pathological massive obesity may be associated with delayed puberty.

Increased physical activity, such as that found in female athletes, may arrest puberty in girls and is all the more likely to do so if the girl is thin and has a decreased percentage of body fat for age, such as is found in ballerinas. However, if a child is bedridden (especially when also developmentally delayed), menarche may occur at an early age and with a lower percentage of body fat than found in more active children with developmental delay.

Genetic factors play an important role in determining the age of onset of puberty. Girls within an ethnic population, and mother–daughter pairs, demonstrate a similar age of onset of puberty. In the USA, sexual development occurs earlier in Black girls than in White girls when socioeconomic factors are the same.

Thus, it appears that 'optimal' socioeconomic environmental factors and good health lead to an onset of puberty at an age determined largely by genetic factors. Negative environmental influences delay the age of onset of puberty over its genetic tendency, while certain disease states, which are discussed below, can advance the onset of puberty.

PHYSICAL CHANGES OF PUBERTY: SECONDARY SEXUAL CHARACTERISTICS

Observers must have a reproducible method of describing states of pubertal development so that observations may be standardised and conclusions may be drawn among populations. The internationally recognised Tanner method divides pubertal development into five stages (Figs. 13.2–13.5). In boys, pubic hair development should be rated separately from genital development, but the two changes are usually so closely linked that some observers combine them into a single descriptive stage. In girls, pubic hair development (a virilising process) emanates in large part from adrenal gland secretions and does not always occur in concert with breast development (a feminising process) caused by the secretion of oestrogen from the ovaries. Thus, it is best to separate pubic hair development from the breast developmental stage in girls.

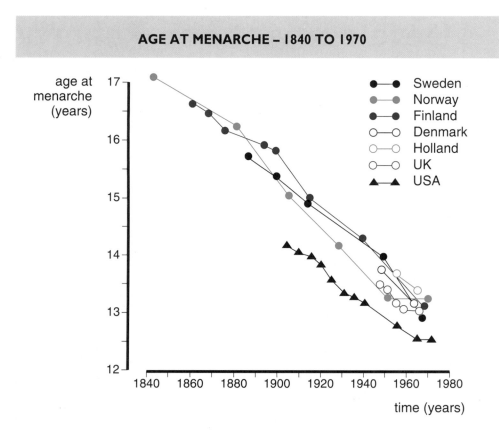

AGE AT MENARCHE – 1840 TO 1970

Sweden
Norway
Finland
Denmark
Holland
UK
USA

Fig. 13.1 The age of menarche during 1840 to 1970. Over the past century and a half, the age of menarche has decreased by three to four months per decade until approximately thirty years ago. Modified from Tanner (1975), by courtesy of WB Saunders Company.

GIRLS

The staging of breast development in girls (see Fig. 13.2) does not take into consideration the ultimate size or shape of the breasts, which is determined primarily by genetic and nutritional factors, but describes characteristics that are common to all girls. The earlier stages of breast development may be asymmetrical, with one breast developing more than six months before the other one starts to enlarge.

BOYS

Growth of the testes is usually the first sign of normal puberty in the male (see Fig. 13.4). In general, when the longitudinal axis of the testes (excluding the epididymis) is greater than 2.5cm, pubertal testicular enlargement has commenced. Most of the increase in size of the testes is due to seminiferous tubular enlargement since Leydig cell enlargement is minimal, even with active testosterone secretion.

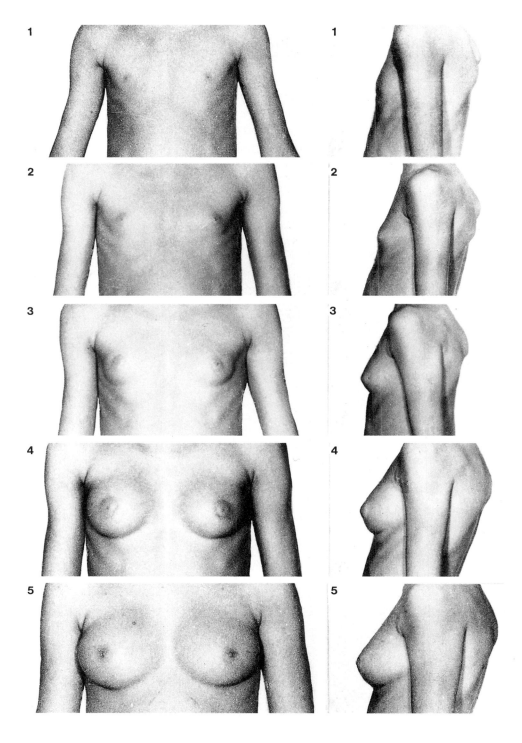

Fig. 13.2 Stages of pubertal breast development. Stage I: no discernible breast tissue – prepubertal. Stage 2: areolar widening and pigmentation, with some glandular tissue being palpable, with Montgomery gland development around the circumferance of the areola; this stage may be subtle. Stage 3: further unmistakable growth of breast and areolar tissue. Stage 4: further breast enlargement, with a secondary mound of areola protruding from the breast tissue. Stage 5: adult breast size has been achieved, and the areola has now receded into the contour of the breast. Reproduced from Tanner (1962), by courtesy of Blackwell Scientific Publications.

13

The phallus is best measured when in a flaccid state and stretched, without including either the foreskin or the fat pad at the base of the phallus. Obesity increases the fat pad, so the penis may falsely appear to be abnormally short in an obese boy. The length of the stretched penis (excluding the foreskin) increases from an average of 6.2cm in the prepubertal state to 13.2cm in adulthood.

OTHER DIMORPHIC CHANGES

OVARIAN DEVELOPMENT
Follicles appear during the fourth or fifth month of fetal development, and the number of follicles that are formed at this age constitutes the lifelong store of follicles for the individual throughout life. Postmortem or ultrasonographic studies demonstrate small antral follicles in the prepubertal ovary, but prior to menarche all follicles that develop antra ultimately undergo atresia. The ovaries in the prepubertal child have a volume of 0.7–0.9ml, but following the onset of puberty the volume increases to 2–10ml. In the prepubertal state the uterus is tubular and 2–3cm in length, but during puberty it becomes bulbous and 5–8cm in length.

SPERMATOGENESIS
Histological examination reveals the first evidence of spermatogenesis between eleven and fifteen years of age. Sperm can be found in early-morning voided urine specimens at a mean chronological age of 13.3 years, and the first conscious ejaculation occurs at a mean of 13.5 years of chronological age or bone age. Thus, the average age of onset of sperm formation occurs between stages 2 and 3 pubic hair or genital development, indicating that the achievement of fertility precedes the achievement of adult physical development.

PUBERTAL GROWTH SPURT
The rapid increase in growth noted during puberty is a striking physical change. Before the onset of puberty, growth velocities and heights (Fig. 13.6) are similar for boys and girls. Girls start their growth spurt just before the first physical evidence of breast development – on average two years before the male pubertal growth spurt.

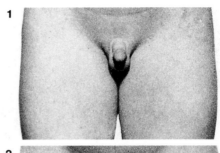
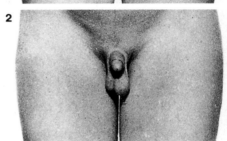
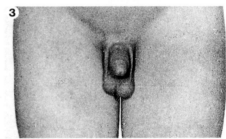
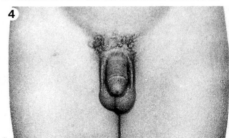
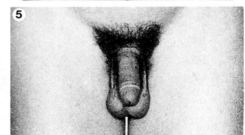

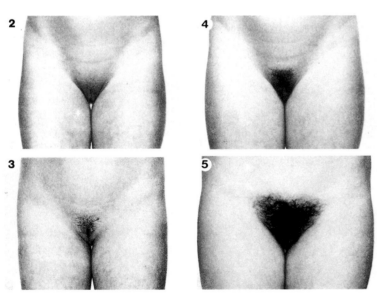

Fig. 13.3 Stages of pubic hair development in girls. Stage 1 (not shown): no pubic hair – prepubertal. Stage 2: sparse, long, dark, slightly curled hair on the labia; this stage may be subtle. Stage 3: hair is darker, coarser and curlier, and spreads over the mons pubis. Stage 4: hair is adult in type but does not spread to the thighs. Stage 5: the adult inverse triangle distribution is reached, with spread to the medial surface of the thighs occurring. Reproduced from Tanner (1962), by courtesy of Blackwell Scientific Publications.

Fig. 13.4 Stages of pubertal maturation of male genitalia. Stage 1: no pubic hair and no enlargement of penis or testes (testes <2.5cm in longest diameter). Stage 2: testicular enlargement to >2.5cm, and thinning and reddening of the scrotal skin occur; slightly dark and curly hair appears at the base of the penis. Stage 3: phallic enlargement in length and width occurs, with increasing testicular size; pubic hair is coarser, darker, and curlier, with spread. Stage 4: further darkening of the scrotum and enlargement of the testes and penis; hair is adult in type but does not spread to the thighs. Stage 5: adult genital appearance is achieved; hair is spread to the medial surface of the thighs. Reproduced from Tanner (1962), by courtesy of Blackwell Scientific Publications.

SECONDARY SEXUAL DEVELOPMENT

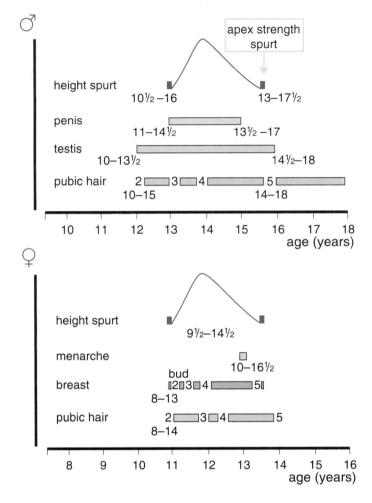

Fig. 13.5 Sequence of secondary sexual development in British boys and girls. The range of ages is indicated. Modified from Marshall and Tanner (1970).

HEIGHT VELOCITY CURVES

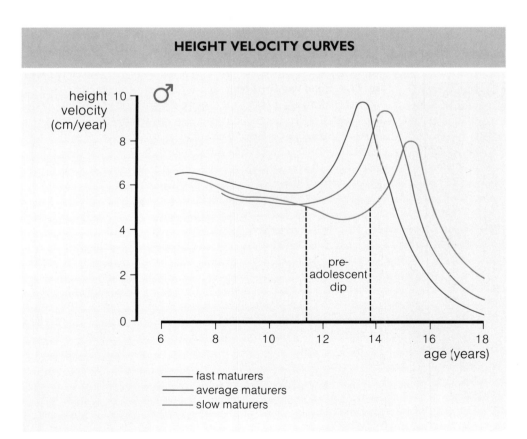

Fig. 13.6 Height velocity curves of normal boys with variable onset of pubertal maturation. These data show an example of the striking discrepancies between slow- and fast-maturing boys. Modified from Smith (1977), by courtesy of WB Saunders Company.

Thus, boys attain a greater height before beginning the pubertal growth spurt. In addition, boys achieve more growth during the pubertal growth spurt than do girls. The combination of these two factors leads to the differential heights between adult males and females. Peak height velocity occurs in stage 2 or 3 in girls but in stage 3 or 4 in boys. Thus, the pubertal growth spurt is effectively an premenarcheal event in girls. A short girl who has reached menarche is not likely to attain much greater height, while an early pubertal boy who demonstrates short stature can be expected to grow a considerable amount before completing his pubertal development.

For a normal child, the age of onset of the growth spurt is not a good predictor of adult height; the duration of pubertal growth is of greater importance in determining final height. Precocious puberty, however, causes an advanced bone age, which leads to the paradox of the tall child but the short adult. Similarly, delay in puberty due to constitutionally delayed puberty also has a tendency to decrease final height.

While stature is the most obvious change in growth during puberty, the ratio of the upper to lower segment also changes significantly (Fig. 13.7). The lower segment is measured from the surface on which the patient is standing to the pubic ramus, and the upper segment is measured from the pubic ramus to the top of the head. The mean upper to lower segment ratio of a newborn baby is 1.7, that of a one-year-old child is 1.4, and that of an eight-year-old child is 1. During puberty, growth of the legs exceeds that of the upper trunk and therefore the mean upper to lower segment ratio of White adults is 0.92 and that of Black adults is 0.85. Hypogonadal patients who lack the sex steroids that are necessary to fuse the epiphysial growth plates of the extremities continue to grow past the usual age of cessation, leading to eunuchoid proportions of a decreased upper to lower ratio and an increased arm span for height.

Numerous hormones are involved in the control of the pubertal growth spurt. Without secretion of growth hormone (GH) there can be no pubertal growth spurt; insulin-like growth factor-I (IGF-I) concentrations rise around the time of the pubertal growth spurt in normal individuals, and this GH-growth-dependent factor is believed to mediate the rapid growth that is involved in the process. GH pulse amplitude, but not frequency, increases during puberty, leading to increased GH secretion during the growth spurt. Sex steroids rise during the pubertal growth spurt, effecting the increased GH secretion and also directly stimulating epiphysial growth. Thyroid hormone is also necessary for a normal pubertal growth spurt.

BONE AGE

Determination of skeletal development by an X-ray of the left hand and wrist (Fig. 13.8) is a useful way of establishing the stage of the physiological development of a child, which may not be consonant with the chronological age. Thus, patients who are destined to undergo constitutionally delayed puberty will have a delayed bone

BODY PROPORTIONS AGAINST AGE

upper segment/ lower segment

- ±2SD
- ±1SD — mean

age (years)

Fig. 13.7 Body proportions (upper/lower segment) against age, for White and Black children (boys and girls). Modified from McKusick (1972), by courtesy of CV Mosby.

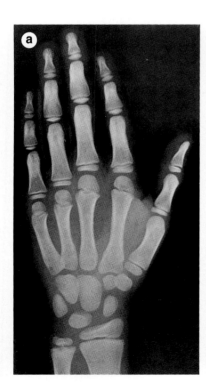
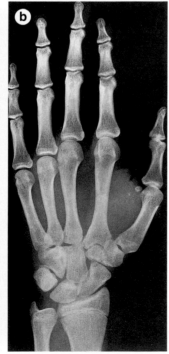

Fig. 13.8 Hand and wrist bone age. (a) 10-year-old prepubertal boy with open epiphyses. (b) Mature 17-year-old year boy in whom all epiphyses are closed. Reproduced from Greulich and Pyle (1959), by courtesy of Stanford University Press.

age at a given chronological age, while others who enter puberty early may have an advanced bone age for chronological age.

Skeletal maturation is more advanced in girls than boys at the same chronological age at any stage of puberty. In fact, a bone age of eleven years in girls is equivalent to a bone age of thirteen years in boys, with both being representative of an early stage of puberty. Standard deviations of the development of bone age are known for each chronological age, and any bone age that is delayed or advanced more than two standard deviations from the mean is considered to be abnormal. The finding of an advanced or delayed bone age cannot be used to make a diagnosis but may add to the evidence needed. Determinations of bone age can be matched with height, weight and chronological age to predict final adult height using the Bayley–Pinneau tables, or by using the RWT, Tanner–Whitehouse, or Walker methods.

ENDOCRINE CHANGES OF PUBERTY: GONADARCHE

Endocrine function similar to that of puberty occurs during the fetal period (Figs 13.9 & 13.10). The fetal hypothalamus and pituitary gland are connected via the pituitary portal system by twenty weeks of gestation, ten weeks after the formation of gonadotrophs in the pituitary gland and of gonadotrophin-releasing hormone (GnRH) in the hypothalamus. By midgestation, serum gonadotrophin levels are exceptionally high and, in midgestational males, testosterone is secreted by the fetal testes in large amounts. The fetal ovary responds to similar stimulation from the fetal pituitary gland. As fetal development proceeds, gonadotrophin secretion and sex steroid production decrease but do not disappear. With release from oestrogen-induced negative feedback inhibition, gonadotrophin concentrations once again rise in the newborn, as do sex steroid concentrations, for many months after birth. It is not unusual to measure a testosterone level in a male baby less than six months of age which is equal to or greater than that found in a fourteen-year-old pubertal boy.

HYPOTHALAMIC–PITUITARY–GONADAL AXIS

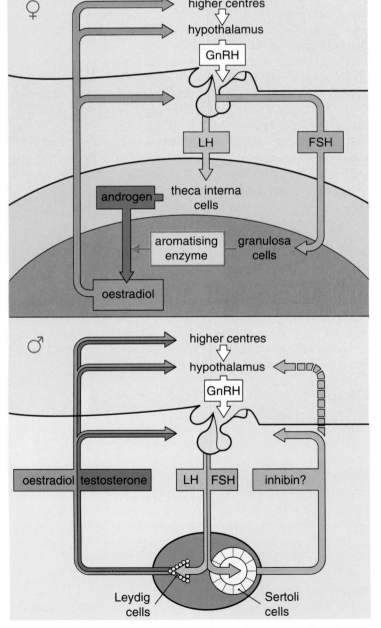

Fig. 13.9 The hypothalamic–pituitary–gonadal axis in a female (upper) and a male (lower).

LH, FSH AND OESTRADIOL/TESTOSTERONE AND PUBERTAL STAGE AND BONE AGE

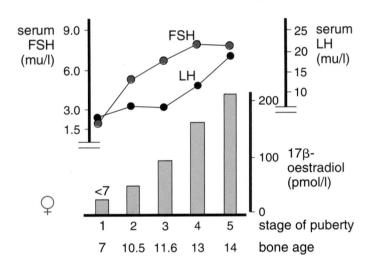

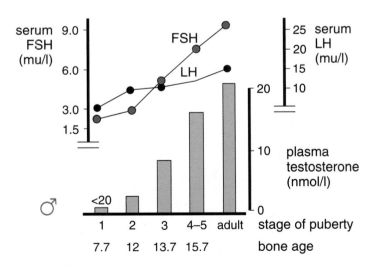

Fig. 13.10 Mean serum LH, FSH, and oestradiol (girls, upper) or testosterone (boys, lower) correlated with stage of puberty and bone age. Modified from Grumbach (1975), by courtesy of Martinus Nijhoff.

GONADOTROPHINS

Luteinising hormone (LH) stimulates the Leydig cells of the testes to produce testosterone but does not have a significant effect on the ovary until after ovulation first occurs. In contrast, follicle-stimulating hormone (FSH) stimulates ovarian oestrogen production in the female, but has little effect on the testes in males until the time of puberty, when seminiferous tubules enlarge under FSH stimulation and cause enlargement of the size of the testes. Sex steroids suppress LH secretion, primarily by means of negative feedback; FSH secretion is inhibited to a lesser degree. Inhibin, a protein that is produced by the Sertoli cells of the seminiferous tubules of the testes and by granulosa cells of the ovarian follicle, inhibits FSH secretion specifically and more strongly than sex steroids.

LH and FSH are released from the pituitary gland in episodic pulses throughout life, due to episodic stimulation by hypothalamic GnRH. The amplitude of the pulses in normal prepuberty is quite small and only detectable by ultrasensitive assays. At the time of puberty, the amplitude, and then the secretory frequency, increase, leading to an overall rise in LH and FSH concentrations. FSH is secreted in greater amounts than LH in girls at all stages of development, but LH is secreted in greater amounts in boys and girls after the onset of puberty than before the onset of puberty. The episodic nature of gonadotrophin secretion makes it very difficult to interpret individual serum gonadotrophin measurements. In fact, numerous determinations of GnRH-stimulated values are required to determine gonadotrophin reserve and readily releasable content.

Increased LH secretory amplitude occurs initially at night in early puberty. As puberty progresses, LH secretion increases during the day until finally, there is no diurnal variation of LH secretion between day and night.

The 'awakening' of the gonads due to increasing gonadotrophin secretion at the time of puberty is known as gonadarche.

GONADAL STEROIDS

Testosterone

Testosterone is produced by the Leydig cells of the testes, which also produce (in lesser amounts) androstenedione, Δ^5-androstenediol, dihydrotestosterone and oestradiol. While testosterone itself appears to produce development of the male body habitus and to change the male voice, 5α reduction of testosterone to form dihydro-testosterone within target cells is the factor that causes phallic development, prostate enlargement, temporal hair recession and beard growth in males. In females, testosterone is derived mainly from extraglandular conversion of ovarian androstenedione.

Testosterone concentrations are quite low in prepubertal boys but consistently increase after the onset of enhanced gonadotrophin secretion in early puberty, with exponential rises occurring during stages 2 and 3 of pubertal development.

Oestrogens

The major female oestrogen, oestradiol, is secreted mainly by the ovary, although a small amount arises from extraglandular conversion of testosterone and androstenedione. Oestradiol increases during pubertal development and then varies in association with the stage of the menstrual cycle.

Adrenal Androgens: Adrenarche

Levels of adrenal androgen, dihydroepiandrosterone (DHEA) and dihydroepiandrosterone sulphate (DHEAS) rise in plasma before pubertal development or before gonadotrophin secretion increases (Fig. 13.11). The driving force of this rise is unknown, but adrenocorticotrophic hormone (ACTH) is necessary. This process of increasing adrenal androgen concentrations is known as adrenarche. In premature adrenarche the rise occurs early, so that DHEAS and DHEA concentrations in a six- to eight-year-old boy may be equal to those found in normal boys at midpuberty.

Testosterone-binding Globulin

Almost all circulating testosterone and oestradiol are reversibly bound to testosterone-binding globulin (TEBG; also known as sex hormone-binding globulin: SHBG); however, only the free sex steroid is active, and TEBG appears to serve as a reservoir for storing and inactivating sex steroids. At puberty, levels of TEBG decrease slightly from prepubertal levels in girls, and a greater decrease occurs in boys. Thus, in adults, the plasma concentration of total testosterone is almost twenty times greater in men than in women, but the free testosterone is forty times greater in men.

Prolactin

Although prolactin levels rise in girls during puberty, they do not effectively change in boys; this is due to the increased oestradiol secretion that occurs in females compared to levels in males.

Inhibin

Inhibin, a protein product of the Sertoli cells of the testes and of the ovarian granulosa cells, exerts negative feedback inhibition on FSH secretion. The production of inhibin is stimulated by FSH, indicating the presence of a feedback loop. Immunoreactive inhibin-like activity rises in boys and girls during puberty.

Insulin-like Growth Factor-I

IGF-I rises during puberty to levels higher than ever again achieved in adults; it remains elevated after the time of peak height velocity and then falls to normal adult levels, decreasing further in the elderly.

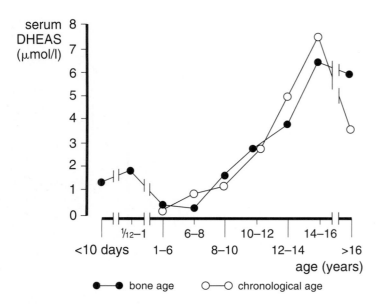

SERUM DHEAS CONCENTRATIONS DURING CHILDHOOD

Fig. 13.11 Serum DHEAS concentrations throughout childhood related to both chronological and skeletal age. Modified from Reiter *et al* (1977), by courtesy of CV Mosby.

DEVELOPMENTAL CONTROL OF PUBERTY

GnRH is first produced in the area of the primitive nose and migrates to the area of the basal hypothalamus by twenty weeks of gestation (Fig. 13.12). This process may be impaired by genetic factors: for example, a fetus with Kallmann's syndrome (isolated gonadotrophin deficiency and anosmia) demonstrated altered nasal development and absence of immunostainable GnRH in the basal medial and basal hypothalamus at twenty weeks of gestation, a time when normal male fetuses have ample GnRH in these areas.

GnRH is released in pulses to stimulate LH and FSH release, which ultimately stimulate sex steroid production and, in turn, will suppress gonadotrophin secretion, as well as cause the physical changes of puberty. This negative feedback loop remains sensitive to circulating sex steroids throughout prepuberty, but at the time of puberty becomes less sensitive, thereby allowing concentrations of sex steroids to increase without completely suppressing gonadotrophin secretion.

After midpuberty, positive feedback occurs in females where oestrogen secretion at midcycle increases gonadotrophin secretion, thereby further increasing oestrogen secretion and allowing ovulation. Thus, throughout pubertal development, other control mechanisms are superimposed upon basic episodic secretion of GnRH and gonadotrophins.

A major question which remains unanswered in the study of puberty is why gonadotrophin secretion decreases in midchildhood, with or without the presence of functioning gonads (Fig. 13.13). Children with Turner's syndrome have elevated gonadotrophin secretion in the newborn and pubertal period, but have less gonadotrophin secretion during midchildhood for unknown reasons. Factors that trigger the onset of puberty are likewise unknown, although the onset of puberty can be stimulated or delayed by certain destructive lesions: for example, anterior hypothalamic tumours or injuries can advance the onset of puberty, while posterior hypothalamic injuries or tumours can delay the onset of puberty or eliminate it. Thus, it appears that the onset of puberty is caused by a decrease in inhibition of the central nervous system – an inhibition that can be destroyed by certain disorders, leading to the early onset of puberty.

The earliest hormonal changes of puberty, found even before the onset of physical changes, is night-time episodic secretion of gonadotrophins (Fig. 13.14). This occurs at a time when levels of the readily releasable gonadotrophins in the pituitary gland are increased, as detected by the administration of GnRH. This is followed by increased episodic secretion of gonadotrophins during the day, until there no longer remains a diurnal variation in gonadotrophin secretion. Thus, administration of a dose of GnRH before puberty leads to a small rise in LH and FSH, while after puberty, a marked increase in LH secretion occurs (Figs 13.15 & 13.16).

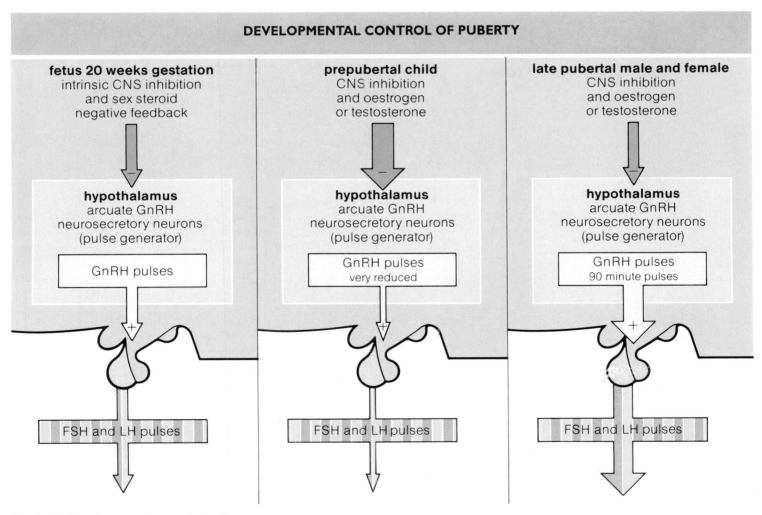

Fig. 13.12 Developmental control of puberty.

DISORDERS OF PUBERTY

DELAYED PUBERTY

Most authorities accept the definition of delayed puberty (Fig. 13.17) as the absence of secondary sexual development at an age two standard deviations above the mean age of onset of puberty – an age at which ninety-five per cent of normal children have already entered puberty. In the USA, this approximates to fourteen years of age for boys and thirteen years of age for girls, with similar ranges applying to European populations. Some children who have not gone through puberty at this age will do so within the few ensuing months and are simply classified as a variation from normal. Others, however, have a permanent disorder of the ovary, pituitary, or hypothalamus and will never go through pubertal development, leading to the diagnosis of primary, secondary or tertiary hypogonadism.

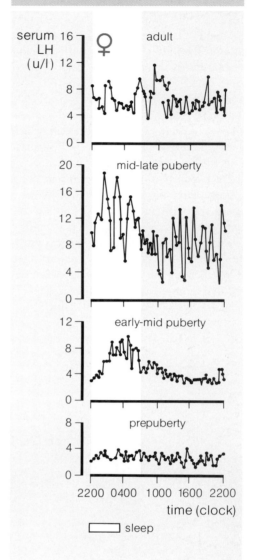

LH SECRETION DURING PUBERTAL DEVELOPMENT

Fig. 13.14 Patterns of LH secretion during pubertal development. Episodic pulses and circadian rhythms change in amplitude and frequency during development. Modified from Weitzman *et al* (1975), by courtesy of Academic Press.

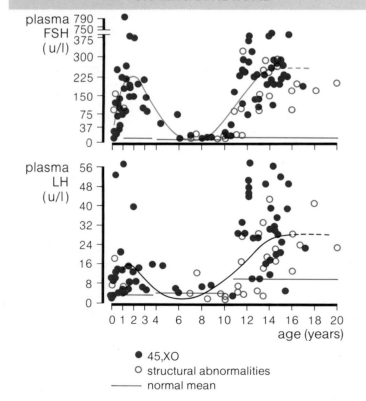

DIPHASIC PATTERN OF LH AND FSH IN TURNER'S SYNDROME

● 45,XO
○ structural abnormalities
— normal mean

Fig. 13.13 The diphasic pattern of serum LH and FSH levels in patients with Turner's syndrome. The pattern that is shown in normal subjects is similar to that in patients with agonadism, but the values are lower than in normals. Modified from Conte *et al* (1975), by courtesy of Williams and Wilkins Company.

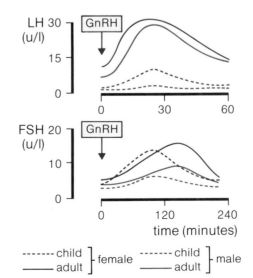

RESPONSE OF PITUITARY GONADOTROPHS TO EXOGENOUS GnRH

- - - - child ⎫ female   - - - - child ⎫ male
——— adult ⎭   ——— adult ⎭

Fig. 13.15 The response of pituitary gonadotrophs to exogenous administration of GnRH. The release of LH increases from prepubertal to pubertal levels, with a further rise seen during adulthood. The sex-related differences in GnRH-induced FSH release are seen.

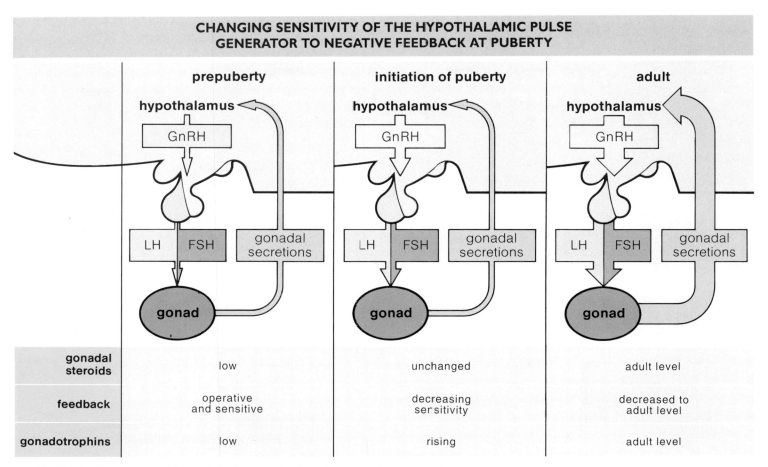

CHANGING SENSITIVITY OF THE HYPOTHALAMIC PULSE GENERATOR TO NEGATIVE FEEDBACK AT PUBERTY

	prepuberty	initiation of puberty	adult
gonadal steroids	low	unchanged	adult level
feedback	operative and sensitive	decreasing sensitivity	decreased to adult level
gonadotrophins	low	rising	adult level

Fig. 13.16 *The changing sensitivity of the hypothalamic pulse generator to negative feedback at puberty.*

Fig. 13.17 *Classification of delayed puberty.*

CLASSIFICATION OF DELAYED PUBERTY

Constitutional delay in growth and adolescence

Hypogonadotrophic hypogonadism

central nervous system disorders
  tumours
  other acquired disorders
  congenital disorders
isolated gonadotrophin deficiency
multiple pituitary hormonal deficiencies
miscellaneous
  Prader–Willi syndrome
  Laurence–Moon or Bardet–Biedl syndrome
  chronic disease
  weight loss
  anorexia nervosa
  increased physical activity in female athletes
  hypothyroidism

Hypergonadotrophic hypogonadism

Klinefelter's syndrome
other forms of primary testicular failure
anorchia or cryptorchidism
Turner's syndrome
other forms of primary ovarian failure
pseudo-Turner's syndrome
XX and XY gonadal dysgenesis

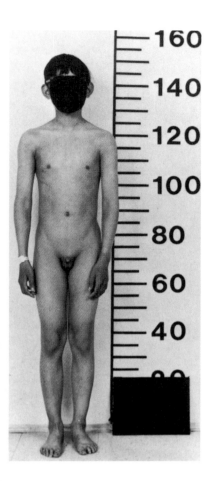

Fig. 13.18
A 16½-year-old boy with constitutional delay in growth and puberty. History revealed a normal growth rate for bone age but short stature at all chronological ages. Bone age was significantly delayed. Spontaneous pubertal development followed. Reproduced, with permission, from Styne and Grumbach (1991).

Fig. 13.19 A 13¾-year-old girl with constitutional delay in growth and puberty. History revealed a normal growth rate but short stature at all ages. Bone age was significantly delayed. Spontaneous puberty followed. Reproduced, with permission, from Styne and Kaplan (1979).

CONSITUTIONAL DELAY IN GROWTH AND PUBERTY

Children who are destined to go through puberty spontaneously only a few months or a few years after the upper limits of the normal range of puberty of thirteen years for girls and fourteen years for boys have constitutional delay in adolescence (Figs 13.18 & 13.19). They characteristically have been short throughout their childhood (probably two standard deviations below the mean values for height and for age) and have a bone age that is delayed more than two standard deviations for chronological age, but they have a normal growth rate for bone age. Their medical history often reveals that one of the parents had late puberty, manifested by delayed menarche for mothers or by delayed onset of shaving or of the growth spurt for fathers. These patients have a slow tempo of growth and maturation, and all aspects of their physical development are delayed. They may be considered to have a functional defect of the GnRH pulse generator. In such children adrenarche is characteristically late, as is gonadarche. This contrasts with patients with isolated gonadotrophin deficiency, in whom adrenarche usually occurs at a normal age.

When such patients reach a bone age of twelve to fourteen years for boys and eleven to thirteen years for girls, they begin to progress through puberty. At the time of presentation, these children rarely have any secondary sexual development, and their plasma gonadal steroids may likewise be prepubertal. However, as the bone age

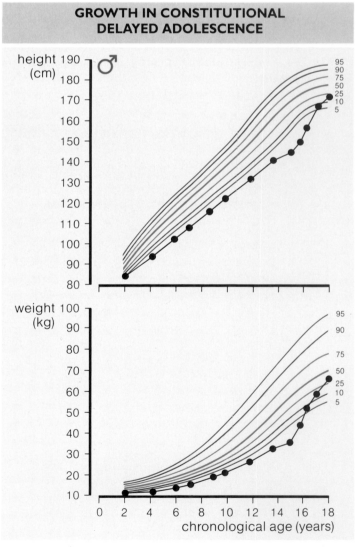

Fig. 13.20 Typical growth curve of a patient with constitutional delayed adolescence. The slow linear growth velocity in early teenage years is followed by the delayed growth spurt, so that adult height in the normal range is finally attained, but at an older than average age.

advances, levels of plasma gonadal steroids rise, increased LH secretion is noted (initially at night), and the entire pubertal process occurs.

Although it was expected that such patients with delayed puberty will ultimately reach average normal heights (Fig. 13.20), recent studies have suggested that height prediction in these children is overly optimistic and that the children ultimately achieve heights several centimetres shorter than expected. These patients are usually brought for evaluation because of the tendency to short stature due to genetic factors that are intensified by delayed puberty and lack of a pubertal growth spurt.

Growth rate in these children may decline prior to the onset of their pubertal growth spurt. Testing for GH secretion during this period may indicate reduced GH release; whether this represents permanent GH deficiency, or a temporary deficiency due to lack of gonadal steroids at an appropriate age, is not clear. Although some clinicians are presently treating such patients with androgen and GH, others simply feel it appropriate to wait until the phase of poor growth ceases and the pubertal growth spurt occurs (Fig. 13.20). Recent data indicate no increase in adult height with GH treatment of such subjects.

Hypogonadotrophic Hypogonadism
Decreased GnRH secretion, and subsequently decreased FSH and LH secretion, may arise due to congenital defects of GnRH production or secretion. It is often difficult to distinguish between patients with hypogonadotrophic hypogonadism, who will never progress through puberty, and those with constitutional delay of growth in adolescence who will develop, albeit at a late age. Patients with hypogonadotrophic hypogonadism tend to be of normal height until adolescent age when, because of their lack of a growth spurt, they become shorter than age-matched controls. Patients with idiopathic GnRH deficiency are physically and endocrinologically similar to normal

prepubertal children, even at their advanced chronological age.

At present there is no reliable method to determine which patient has constitutional delay in growth and which has total and complete gonadotrophin deficiency until several years of observation have passed. In general, if puberty has not started spontaneously by the age of eighteen years, the patient probably has GnRH deficiency, although there is at least one published case of a patient who spontaneously entered puberty at twenty-five years of age.

Isolated Gonadotrophin Deficiency
Patients with associated defects in olfaction have Kallmann's syndrome, the most common type of isolated gonadotrophin deficiency (Fig. 13.21). Within a given family that is afflicted with Kallmann's syndrome, some members lack a sense of olfaction and some have hypogonadotrophic hypogonadism, while some combine both features. Although some familial constellations have autosomal recessive or autosomal dominant patterns of inheritance, X-linked inheritance was suggested in the literature first, and an X-linkage has been proven by the demonstration of a contiguous gene deletion at Xp22.3 in affected patients. One affected male had an affected son, indicating autosomal dominant inheritance, and in another report, one identical twin had Kallmann's syndrome, while the other was normal.

Isolated LH deficiency (the fertile eunuch syndrome) is characterised by adequate FSH secretion and spermatogenesis but by reduced LH secretion and deficient testosterone production. Isolated FSH deficiency due to the deficient production of the β-subunit of FSH has also been documented.

Multiple Hormonal Deficiency
Gonadotrophin deficiency in association with GH deficiency is characterised by short stature and poor growth rate. Patients may also have associated corticotrophin-releasing factor and ACTH deficiency, and/or thyrotrophin-releasing hormone and thyroid-stimulating hormone (TSH) deficiency.

Central Nervous System Disorders Leading to Gonadotrophin Deficiency
Extrasellar masses may interfere with any aspect of gonadotrophin secretion or GnRH stimulation. Virtually all patients who have tumours in this area, however, have more than gonadotrophin deficiency; they may have any or all other pituitary deficiencies or, in the case of a prolactin-secreting adenoma, an increase in the secretion of prolactin. These deficiencies usually occur later in childhood than congenital defects and are characterised as acquired pituitary deficiencies – a more ominous sign than congenital pituitary deficiencies.

Craniopharyngioma is the most common central nervous system tumour during puberty which decreases pituitary function (Fig. 13.22). This is a tumour of the Rathke's pouch, emanating from the pituitary stalk and growing into the suprasellar area. Patients with craniopharyngioma may present with headaches, visual disturbance, short stature and symptoms of diabetes insipidus. These patients may have visual deficiency, including bilateral temporal field defects (due to pressure exerted by the enlarging tumour upon the optic chiasm), optic atrophy or papilloedema. They present with signs of GH deficiency, delayed puberty, glucocorticoid deficiency and/or hypothyroidism. Rarely, precocious puberty occurs with craniopharyngioma.

Calcification of the sella turcica or suprasellar area occurs in seventy to eighty per cent of cases with craniopharyngioma, and erosion of the sella turcica or clinoid processes is common. Smaller craniopharyngiomas can be resected by transsphenoidal microsurgery, but larger ones will require intracranial surgery. Radiotherapy is useful for incompletely removed tumours.

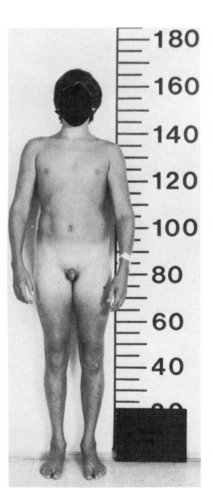

Fig. 13.21 A boy almost 16 years old with gonadotrophin deficiency and anosmia (Kallmann's syndrome). His testes were originally undescended, his stature low–normal, and his upper to lower segment ratio 0.86 (eunuchoid). Pubertal development did not occur in the absence of exogenous testosterone. Reproduced, with permission, from Styne and Grumbach (1991).

Germinomas are the next most common form of extrasellar tumours that cause hypogonadotrophic hypogonadism, but are rare overall; they may present in the teenage years (Fig. 13.23). Polydipsia and polyuria are frequent symptoms, as are abnormalities of growth and delayed puberty, but any type of anterior pituitary deficiency and posterior pituitary deficiency may be found.

Other tumours in the hypothalamopituitary area include hypothalamic or optic gliomas or astrocytomas. Chromophobe adenomas are rare in childhood compared to their frequency in adulthood, but are reported.

Langerhans' cell histiocytosis, also known as Hand–Schüller–Christian disease or histiocytosis X, may lead to pituitary deficiencies, including diabetes insipidus. Granulomatosis cyst-like areas in the flat bones of the skull, ribs, pelvis and scapula, in the long bones of the arms and legs, and in the dorsolumbar spine, are common. Infiltration of the orbit may lead to exophthalmos.

Radiation therapy of the head for treatment of central nervous system tumours, for prophylaxis of leukaemia, or for treatment of neoplasms of the head and face, may result within 1½–2 years in hypothalamopituitary deficiency. GH deficiency is the most common result of such radiation due to hypothalamic damage, but other disorders such as hypogonadotrophic hypogonadism may also occur. Congenital midline malformations (disraphism), such as septo-optic dysplasia or optic hypoplasia, may lead to any type of loss of hypothalamopituitary function, including hypogonadotrophic hypogonadism.

MISCELLANEOUS SYNDROMES
Prader–Willi Syndrome

Prader–Willi syndrome is characterised by massive obesity, short stature, small hands and feet, a distinctive face with almond-shaped eyes and postnatal hypotonia following poor fetal activity (Fig. 13.24).

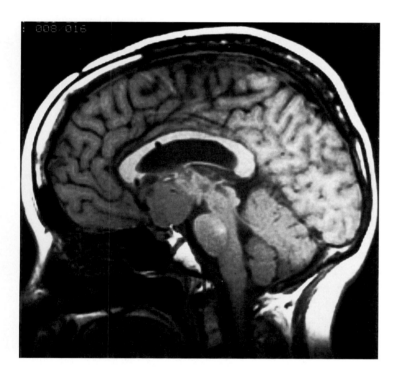

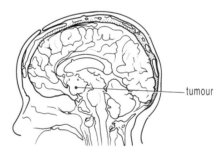

Fig. 13.22 An MRI scan of a craniopharyngioma in a 17-year-old boy. The calcification of the large tumour was evicent on a CAT scan. The patient ceased growing at 13 years of age and did not progress past stage 3 of puberty. By courtesy of Dr V Poirier, University of California, Davis, Medical Centre.

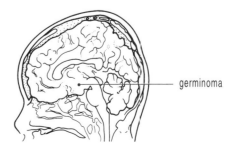

Fig. 13.23 An MRI scan of a germinoma of the pineal region in a 12-year-old boy. The patient has hypopituitarism, but germinomas may secrete human chorionic gonadotrophin (hCG) and actually cause incomplete sexual precocity in boys. By courtesy cf Dr V Poirier, University of California, Davis, Medical Centre.

Behavioural abnormalities in this syndrome include development delay and emotional instability. There is an association of Prader–Willi syndrome with delayed puberty due to hypothalamic dysfunction. Affected boys may appear to have a microphallus, partly due to the increased fat pad at the base of the phallus which 'buries' the penis, although hypogonadotrophic hypogonadism may also be present and cause decreased phallic size. Carbohydrate intolerance occurs in Prader–Willi syndrome, possibly related to the massive obesity. Up to fifty per cent of affected patients have an interstitial deletion of the long arm of chromosome 15 (Del 15) (Q11–Q12).

Laurence–Moon–Biedl Syndrome

Laurence–Moon–Biedl syndrome consists of polydactyly, obesity, mental retardation and retinitis pigmentosa. This autosomal recessive syndrome is often associated with delayed puberty due to hypothalamic deficiency, although primary hypogonadism has also been reported.

Chronic Disease

Most chronic diseases can lead to delayed puberty. In some cases, delay in puberty may be due to nutritional deficiency and is reversible with improved nutrition. Some chronic diseases exert direct destructive effects upon the endocrine system: for example, sickle cell anaemia causes testicular failure due to ischaemia. Other diseases are associated with endocrine disorders due to their therapy: for example, blood transfusions for thalassaemia cause haemosiderosis leading to hypothalamic dysfunction.

Endocrine Disorders

Various endocrine disorders can affect the onset of puberty. Moderate hypothyroidism delays the onset of puberty and menarche, but treatment with thyroxine causes the resumption of pubertal development. Uncontrolled diabetes mellitus can delay puberty and cause irregular menses. In its most severe form this is known as Mauriac's syndrome, which is associated with fatty infiltration of the liver, short stature, poor growth, and sexual infantilism. Untreated Cushing's disease can also delay the onset of puberty.

Anorexia Nervosa

Anorexia nervosa is characterised by a disordered body image, obsessive fear of obesity, and food avoidance, leading to weight loss that can be fatal (Fig. 13.25). Even after weight regain occurs, onset of menses and pubertal development may not occur for years. While uncomplicated weight loss can certainly lead to arrested puberty, amenorrhoea may occur even before the weight loss is severe in this condition, due to psychological factors inherent in anorexia nervosa. Psychological stress in other situations is also implicated in irregular menstruation.

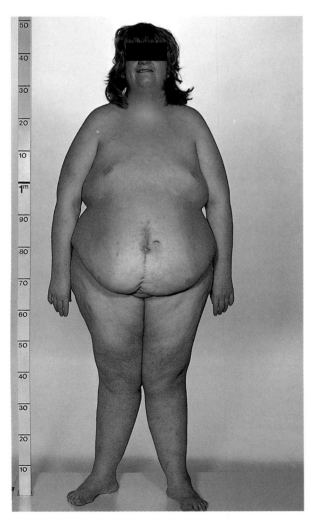

Fig. 13.24 A patient with the Prader–Willi syndrome. Massive obesity is present, as are short stature and delayed puberty. Developmental delay, insatiable appetite, and carbohydrate intolerance are characteristic of the syndrome.

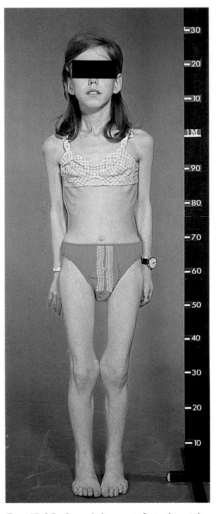

Fig. 13.25 An adolescent female with anorexia nervosa.
This life-threatening condition of disordered body image and avoidance of food is most common in young pubertal-aged girls. By courtesy of Dr D Grant.

Nutritional Deficiency

Any reason for decreased nutrient intake or loss of nutrients, which causes weight loss to less than eighty per cent of ideal weight for height (including chronic disease), can lead to reversion to the prepubertal state of decreased pulsatility of gonadotrophin secretion, causing effective hypogonadotrophic hypogonadism. When weight gain occurs, the subject passes through the stages of increased nocturnal gonadotrophin secretion, followed by increased gonadotrophin secretion throughout the twenty-four-hour period – the same sequence as found in a child going through normal puberty.

Increased Physical Activity

Female athletes may demonstrate impaired pubertal progression and delayed menarche. Although this can be related to weight loss, increased energy expenditure also plays a role. Ballet dancers are reported to cease menstruation when active, but when injured and confined to bed rest, menarche recurs.

Hypergonadotrophic Hypogonadism

Primary gonadal failure will lead to sexual infantilism (permanently delayed puberty). Some affected children have chromosomal abnormalities and characteristic physical features, while others manifest only the absence of pubertal progression.

Klinefelter's Syndrome

Hypergonadotrophic hypogonadism due to Klinefelter's syndrome does not usually lead to a delay in the onset of puberty but, due to decreased Leydig cell function, is associated with a failure to complete secondary sexual development. Klinefelter's syndrome is discussed in Chapters 11 and 14.

Turner's Syndrome

Turner's syndrome (the syndrome of gonadal dysgenesis) is the most common form of primary gonadal failure associated with a female phenotype (Fig. 13.26). The 45X karyotype occurs in one out of fif-

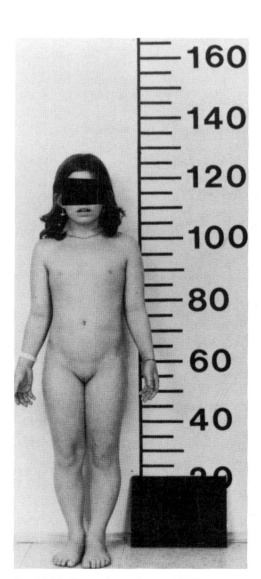

Fig. 13.26 Turner's syndrome (45X) in a 12½-year-old girl. She has downturned mouth, cubitus valgus (wide-carrying angle of arms), and an appearance of wide-spaced hypoplastic nipples. Reproduced, with permission, from Styne and Kaplan (1979).

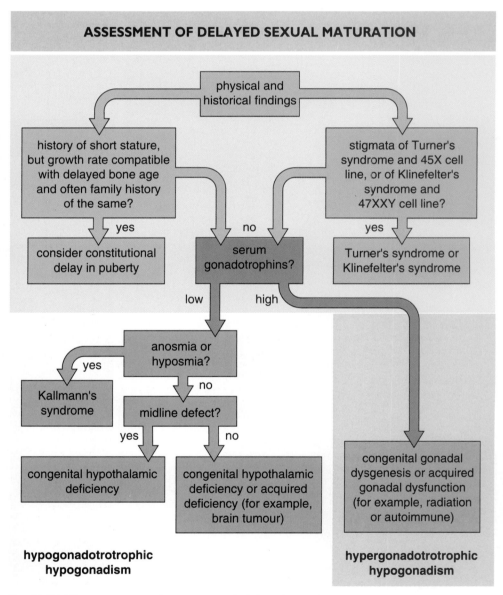

Fig. 13.27 The assessment of a patient with delayed sexual maturation.

teen spontaneous abortions; 99.9% of 45X fetuses do not survive to twenty-eight weeks of gestation; the incidence of Turner's syndrome is between 1:2,000 and 1:5,000 live phenotypic female births. Classic cases have a 45X karyotype, short stature, streak gonads, sexual infantilism, and a female phenotype. Other findings may include downturning of the corners of the mouth or 'fish-mouth' appearance, ptosis, low-set ears, a broad shield-like chest, the appearance of wide-spaced and hypoplastic nipples, short webbed neck with low hairline, short fourth metacarpals, wide-carrying angle of the arms, abnormalities in the shape of the kidneys (with or without functional impairment), multiple naevi, spoon-shaped (hyperconvex) hypoplastic nails, and left-sided heart anomalies (such as coarctation of the aorta). At birth, many patients have lymphoedema of the extremities and loose skin folds around the neck. Patients have normal intelligence but may perform poorly on tests of spatial perception. Frequent episodes of otitis media in childhood may lead to conductive hearing loss. Some girls may look quite normal except for short stature and delayed or absent puberty. Thus, any short girl with delayed puberty should have Turner's syndrome included in her differential diagnosis.

Variants of Turner's syndrome include XO/XX mosaicism. Such patients may have some gonadal function and a more normal female phenotype. Alternatively, patients with XO/XY mosaicism may have a phenotype ranging from infantile female to ambiguous genitalia or phenotypic male. These patients may have dysgenetic testes rather than streak gonads and are at risk of having malignant degeneration of the gonad; gonadectomy/orchidectomy is indicated.

Patients with gonadal dysgenesis may benefit from new developments in the treatment of their growth deficiency. Previously, oestrogen therapy was held until the late teenage years for fear of decreasing final height; presently, low-dose oestrogen therapy (5–10µg of ethinyloestradiol orally per day to begin) is started earlier, such as at thirteen years, to allow secondary sexual development at an appropriate age, to reduce psychosocial pressure, and to decrease the risk of osteoporosis. Recent studies with recombinant DNA-derived GH (hGH) indicate that growth rate can be increased in Turner's syndrome with administration of a twenty-five per cent larger than standard dose of GH. At present, these protocols are experimental, and while initial results look promising, the effect of GH therapy upon final height in Turner's syndrome is not yet clear.

Noonan's Syndrome

Noonan's syndrome, or pseudo-Turner's syndrome, is a dominantly inherited condition with features similar to Turner's syndrome (such as webbed neck, ptosis, short stature, wide-carrying angle, and lymphoedema), as well as features different from Turner's syndrome (such as normal karyotype, triangle-shaped face, pectus excavatum, right-sided heart disease and, commonly, mental retardation). Affected males may have undescended, often functionally impaired, testes.

XX and XY Gonadal Dysgenesis

XX and XY gonadal dysgenesis (not to be confused with Turner's syndrome) may be sporadic or familial. Stature is normal, and phenotype is sexually infantile female in the XX form or may be ambiguous in the XY form. Patients with an XY karyotype should undergo gonadectomy because of potential neoplastic degeneration of the dysgenetic testes (see Chapter 14).

Testicular Biosynthetic Defects

Testicular biosynthetic defects are congenital conditions (see Chapter 11). There are also acquired causes of hypergonadotrophic hypogonadism. Radiation therapy or chemo-therapy for tumours or leukaemia may cause primary gonadal failure. Autoimmune oophoritis can induce ovarian failure, leading to primary amenorrhoea or arrest of puberty.

Diagnosis of Delayed Puberty

The physician must decide whether a boy of fourteen years or a girl of thirteen years without signs of pubertal development might harbour an organic disorder or simply have a variation of the normal developmental pattern – constitutional delay in growth and adolescence. Historical factors may help to confirm the diagnosis of constitutional delay (Fig. 13.27). If the story is not characteristic for one condition or the other, however, and if the physical examination does not add to the diagnosis by the demonstration of some phenotypic anomaly, laboratory diagnosis is necessary. Unfortunately, in the absence of hyposmia, anosmia, a tumour or a midline defect, it is virtually impossible to separate a patient with isolated gonadotrophin deficiency from one with constitutional delay in growth. Patients with primary gonadal failure, however, will be easily diagnosed due to the elevation of gonadotrophin concentrations. The GnRH test may be useful in the diagnosis of subtle cases of gonadotrophin excess in primary gonadal failure and in the determination of endocrine onset of puberty in a patient with constitutional delay who is on the verge of physical development.

Treatment of Delayed Puberty

In most cases, brief treatment with sex steroids (Fig. 13.28) will be offered to a patient with constitutional delay in adolescence if severe psychosocial pressure leads to low self-esteem or worsening school performance. Every boy who is over fourteen years, and every girl who is over thirteen years, who has not gone into puberty does not necessarily require treatment. A three-month dose of low-dose sex steroids will cause some secondary sexual development to relieve the psychological pressure in selected patients. For boys, testosterone enanthate in a dose of 100mg given intramuscularly every month, or for girls ethinyloestradiol in a dose of 5–10µg given orally each day, may be administered over these three months. This temporising allows observation to determine whether the patient spontaneously enters puberty after the therapy has ended. The course of therapy can be repeated several months after the last doses if no spontaneous pubertal development or an increase in levels of plasma sex steroids is noted.

Patients with sexual infantilism due to permanent impairment of gonadotrophin secretion usually desire continuous therapy throughout adult life. Generally, sex steroid therapy is given. Gonadotrophin therapy or GnRH therapy may be offered to patients with pituitary or hypothalamic defects, respectively, although such therapies are more expensive and more complex than sex steroid therapy. If fertility is desired, these forms of therapy can lead to the onset of sperm

TREATMENT OF DELAYED PUBERTY

condition	treatment
constitutional delay	short-term low-dose sex steroid treatment
hypergonadotrophic	sex steroid replacement
hypogonadotrophic	sex steroid replacement GnRH administration

Fig. 13.28 Treatment of delayed puberty.

production or ovulation if the medications are administered on an appropriate schedule. In addition, studies have shown that the administration of human chorionic gonadotrophin (hCG) to boys with gonadotrophin deficiency, in addition to testosterone therapy, may produce more substantial pubic hair development than testosterone alone.

Patients with primary gonadal failure require sex steroid administration to replace the impaired gonadal secretion. Affected patients are, of course, infertile.

Patients with permanent defects in gonadotrophin secretion may receive sex steroids in slowly increasing doses up to a full replacement dose, taking care that maximal growth is obtained before sex steroid administration fuses the epiphysial growth plates. The dosage of testosterone enanthate may be increased from 100mg every four weeks to 200mg and then 300mg every four weeks over a period of six to twelve months. A large dose of testosterone offered immediately may cause priapism and psychological changes, but if offered in an increasing pattern, it is easier to tolerate. Girls starting with 10µg of ethinyl-oestradiol per day may have their dose increased to 20µg and up to 30µg per day for the first twenty-one days of the month over several years. After breakthrough bleeding occurs, medroxyprogesterone acetate is added in a dose of 10mg per day, given on days twelve through twenty-one of the month. In this way, a normal menstrual period is simulated by the administration of exogenous hormones.

In all cases of patients who have GH deficiency in addition to their hypogonadism, dosages of sex steroids should be kept low during GH therapy so that undue bone age advancement will not occur and height is not lost. Episodic administration of GnRH can be used to advance puberty in patients with hypothalamic GnRH deficiency and potentially functioning pituitary glands and gonads. This method is, however, cumbersome and, except to institute ovulation and spermatogenesis, is not usually used in patients with delayed puberty.

Delay in physical pubertal development during the adolescence age range, when personalities are particularly vulnerable to outside factors, can lead to significant psychological turmoil, and some patients may become suicidal. Patients should receive appropriate counselling by the treating physician, a psychiatrist, a social worker or a psychologist if depression is noted. Sometimes physical development that is induced by a three-month course of sex steroids (see above) may be adequate to support the child through this period of difficulty if temporary constitutional delay in adolescence is diagnosed.

SEXUAL PRECOCITY

The appearance of any sign of secondary sexual development at an age more than two standard deviations below the mean is defined as sexual precocity. Using data available from Britain and the USA, it may be stated that eight years in girls and nine years in boys are the lower limits of normal onset of pubertal development. Thus, any child who experiences pubertal development before these ages is precocious (Fig. 13.29). If the cause of the precocious sexual development is premature activation of the hypothalamic–pituitary–gonadal axis in the same pattern that occurs at a normal age in normal puberty, the diagnosis is central precocious puberty. If, however,

Fig. 13.29 Classification of precocious puberty.

CLASSIFICATION OF PRECOCIOUS PUBERTY
complete (true) precocious puberty
constitutional idiopathic central nervous system disorders severe hypothyroidism following androgen exposure
incomplete precocious puberty

males
  gonadotrophin-secreting tumours
  excessive androgen production
  premature maturation of Leydig and germinal cells
females
  ovarian cysts
  oestrogen-secreting neoplasms

sexual precocity due to exogenous gonadotrophin or exposure to sex steroids
variations in pubertal development
premature thelarche premature menarche premature adrenarche adolescent gynaecomastia

the aetiology is exogenous administration of sex steroids, autonomous production of sex steroids from the adrenal gland or gonad, or autonomous gonadotrophin production in boys, the diagnosis is incomplete sexual precocity. Girls who virilise and boys who feminise have contrasexual precocity.

All patients with sexual precocity experience the effects of increased sex steroids. Therefore, they grow in stature at a rate faster than is appropriate for their chronological age, and their bone age advances too quickly. In boys, muscle development and deepening of the voice occur, along with penile erections and increased aggressiveness, while in girls, breast development and menarche may be noted. Patients who are not treated for isosexual precocity will be tall during childhood, but due to premature epiphysial fusion will reach final heights below those determined by genetic factors in most cases. Only sparse data of untreated patients are available, but a mean final height of 151–152cm has been reported in girls and 161cm in boys with untreated sexual precocity.

Complete Precocious Puberty
Idiopathic Precocious Puberty
Some children will go onto puberty somewhat early, but not strikingly so. Thus, a girl between six and eight years of age, or a boy between

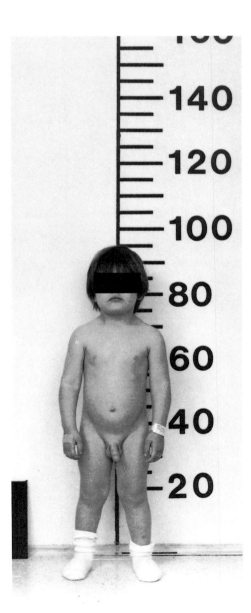

Fig. 13.30
A 4-year-old boy with idiopathic precocious puberty.
Reproduced, with permission, from Styne and Grumbach (1991).

seven and nine years of age, with isosexual precocity may simply be manifesting a family tendency. These children have constitutional precocious puberty and are the other side of the age curve of the onset of puberty from patients with constitutional delay of growth and development. There may be a history of early maturation in the families of these patients. True precocious puberty has been transmitted as an autosomal recessive trait in some children.

In boys with central precocious puberty, just as in boys with normal puberty, the first sign is the enlargement of the testes (Fig. 13.30). In girls, breast development usually appears first, followed by the normal changes of the vulva and labia minora and majora.

While some children rapidly progress through precocious puberty, some follow a waxing and waning course, and these more mild cases may not require treatment and may achieve acceptable final height. Nonetheless, the psychological stress of early sexual development and menarche in girls may mediate the decision towards therapy. It should be noted that fertility may be achieved early in boys and girls with central precocious puberty, and the possibility of sexual abuse is heightened. Furthermore, there is an increased risk of the development of carcinoma of the breast in girls in adulthood after central precocious puberty.

Patients with true precocious puberty have laboratory results that are equivalent to the results obtained in normal puberty. Thus, levels of alkaline phosphatase will be elevated, and nocturnal episodic gonadotrophin secretion and increased gonadotrophin response to the GnRH test are noted. Children with precocious puberty may have associated electroencephalographic abnormalities.

Central Nervous System Tumours
A central nervous system neoplasm must be considered in the differential diagnosis of any patient with central precocious puberty. Girls more frequently undergo central precocious puberty, but in boys the incidence of central nervous system tumours that cause true precocious puberty is higher than in girls. Such tumours may be anterior hypothalamic optic or hypothalamic gliomas, astrocytomas, ependymomas, and even occasionally craniopharyngiomas (although this tumour usually leads to delayed puberty). Precocious puberty occurs because the tumours exert their effects by destroying the central nervous system inhibitory pathways that restrain GnRH secretion during prepuberty.

Some patients have a combination of GH deficiency and central precocious puberty due to central nervous system tumours. These patients, while growing faster than their normal peers, do not grow as fast as patients with true precocious puberty with adequate GH secretion.

True precocious puberty may occur after cranial irradiation for local tumours or even for leukaemia.

Hamartomas of the Tuber Cinereum
Hamartomas of the tuber cinereum (Fig. 13.31) are congenital tumours that are composed of neurosecretory neurones and other neural tissue and which do not increase in size with time. They are frequently associated with true precocious puberty, often in patients younger than three years of age. These hamartomas are often connected with the posterior portion of the tuber cinereum or the mammillary body, or to the floor of the third ventricle by a stalk. In the past, a surgical approach has been used to excise them, but their location makes removal dangerous; furthermore, since they are so amenable to GnRH agonist therapy, surgical treatment is no longer appropriate. Immunohistochemical studies have shown that the hamartomas contain GnRH-containing neurones.

Other central nervous system conditions such as hydrocephalus, encephalitis, static cerebral encephalopathy, brain abscesses, sarcoid and tuberculous granulomas, arachnoid cysts, and head trauma have been associated with central precocious puberty.

Neurofibromatosis Type I

Neurofibromatosis type I (von Recklinghausen's disease) is characterised by café-au-lait spots and the development of neurofibromas. Central precocious puberty may often occur in association with optic gliomas or neurofibromas of the hypothalamopituitary area (Fig. 13.32). This disorder has an autosomal dominant pattern of inheritance, with an incidence of one in thirty-four thousand. Bone abnormalities such as cysts, hemihypertrophy, bowing, scoliosis, skull and facial defects, dumbbell-shaped neurogliomas of the spinal nerve roots, and Lesch nodules of the eyes, and an association with other neoplasms such as central nervous system astrocytomas, ependymomas, meningiomas, neurofibromas, neurofibrosarcomas, rhabdomyosarcomas and nonlymphocytic leukaemia, are also found. Phaeochromocytomas may

also develop in affected adults.

True precocious puberty that follows virilising disorders may occur in patients with congenital virilising adrenal hyperplasia who are initiated on glucocorticoid suppressive therapy after years of androgen exposure (such exposure causes maturation of the hypothalamic–pituitary–gonadal axis, along with skeletal maturation). Likewise, patients with virilising tumours, in whom the tumours have been removed after years of virilisation, can experience central true precocious puberty.

Treatment of Central Precocious Puberty

The field of therapy for central precocious puberty (Fig. 13.33) has been revolutionised by the development of superactive GnRH agonists. Episodic secretion of hypothalamic GnRH elicits pulsatile pituitary gonadotrophin release, but continuous infusion of GnRH downregulates GnRH receptors. The long-acting superagonists of GnRH have increased avidity for the GnRH receptors and are resistant

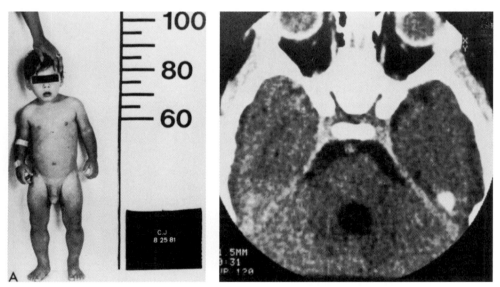 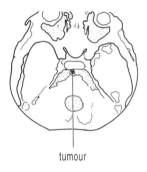

Fig. 13.31 A 17-month-old baby with a hamartoma of the tuber cinereum and true precocious puberty. The CT scan demonstrates a 1.5cm mass, posterior and rostral to the dorsum sella, which depresses the floor of the third ventricle. Reproduced, with permission, from Styne and Grumbach (1991).

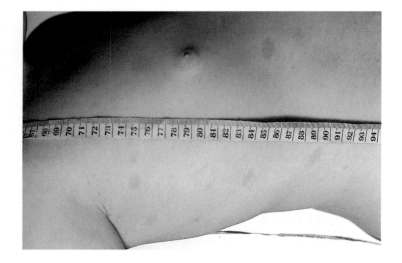

Fig. 13.32 Neurofibromatosis in a girl. Typical café-au-lait spots are shown. This patient also has breast enlargement as an indication of early pubertal development. By courtesy of Dr PHW Rayner.

to enzymatic degradation. These agents initially stimulate pituitary gonadotrophin secretion, but within days cause downregulation of the GnRH receptor, just as continuous GnRH infusion does, and gonadotrophin and gonadal steroid release decrease to the prepubertal level (Fig. 13.34). GnRH agonist is effective in organic and idiopathic forms of central precocious puberty and in patients with central precocious puberty following virilising disorders. Height prediction in patients with central precocious puberty who are successfully treated with GnRH agonists consistently improves with therapy; however, only a handful of patients have reached final height to confirm ultimately that GnRH agonists improve adult stature. Preparations of GnRH agonists are available which can be given every day or every month, and other delayed-release preparations are being developed. With such therapy, growth rate and bone age progression slow, pubertal advancement ceases, and the patient is returned to a prepubertal endocrine state as long as therapy continues. Patients who cease pubertal progression with GnRH agonist therapy resume their pubertal progression after cessation of therapy. It is appropriate to use GnRH in a patient who is shown to have progressive central precocious puberty that causes advancing bone age and physical development, or in girls who have started premature menstrual periods. Medroxyprogesterone acetate and cyproterone acetate were used in the past to treat central precocious puberty but have rarely been used since the advent of GnRH agonist therapy.

Psychosocial Aspects

Children who are taller than their peers and experience sexual advancement or, in the case of boys, demonstrate aggressive behaviour and possibly public masturbation due to elevated testosterone concentrations, are at risk of psychological disorders. While the majority of patients who fall into this category will physically benefit from GnRH agonist therapy, counselling from the treating physicians, psychological counsellors or psychiatrists will be of additional help. The risk of sexual abuse should not be underestimated – girls with precocious puberty have given birth to children. Furthermore, excessive expectations of intellectual and physical prowess may develop in parents or teachers of children who look older than their age, possibly leading to further stress. Intellectual function in precocious puberty is not related to the older-appearing physical appearance.

Fig. 13.33 Pharmacological therapy of sexual precocity.

TREATMENT OF SEXUAL PRECOCITY

disorder	treatment	action and rationale
GnRH-dependent true or central precocious puberty	GnRH agonists	desensitisation of gonadotrophs; blockade of action of endogenous GnRH
GnRH-independent incomplete sexual precocity		
girls autonomous ovarian cysts	medroxyprogesterone acetate	inhibition of ovarian streoidogenesis; regression of cyst (inhibition of FSH release)
McCune–Albright syndrome	medroxyprogesterone acetate	inhibition of ovarian steroidogenesis; regression of cyst (inhibition of FSH release)
	testolactone or fadrozole	inhibtion of P450 aromatase; blocks oestrogen synthesis
boys familial testotoxicosis	ketoconazole	inhibition of $P450_{C17}$ (mainly 17,20-lyase activity)
	spironolactone, cyprotone acetate or flutamide	antiandrogen
	testolactone or fadrozole	inhibition of aromatase; blocks oestrogen synthesis
	medroxyprogesterone acetate	inhibition of testicular steroidogenesis

Incomplete Isosexual Precocity

In disorders of incomplete isosexual precocity, boys will experience virilisation due to androgen production from their adrenal glands or testes, and girls will exhibit feminisation as a result of oestrogen secretion from their ovaries or adrenal glands. These patients will not respond to GnRH agonist therapy.

EFFECT OF A GnRH AGONIST ON IDIOPATHIC CENTRAL PRECOCIOUS PUBERTY

serum LH (u/l): 114, 76, 38, 0
serum FSH (u/l): 252, 168, 84, 0
serum oestradiol (pmol/l): 1095, 730, 365, 0

time (weeks): 0 2 3

☐ basal concentrations ☐ peak concentrations ↓ GnRH dose ☐ Trp₆Pro₉Net–GnRH

Fig. 13.34 The early effects of therapy with a GnRH agonist in a girl with idiopathic central precocious puberty. Basal and peak concentrations following an intravenous 100μg/kg dose of GnRH, before and after the indicated period of treatment with a GnRH agonist Trp₆Pro₉Net–GnRH, are shown. Decreased levels of serum LH, FSH, and oestradiol are seen by the second week of treatment. Modified from Kaplan and Grumbach (1990), by courtesy of Williams and Wilkins Company.

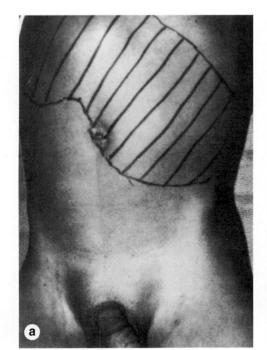 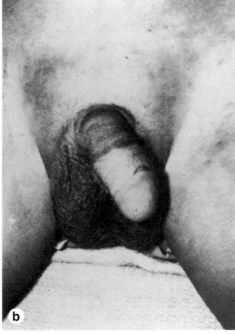

Fig. 13.35 A 1¾-year-old boy with an hCG-secreting hepatoblastoma. Note the outline of the large liver (a) and the penile enlargement (b). The testes were each 1cm, and pubic hair was at stage 2. The plasma hCG level was 30 miu/ml, plasma testosterone 168ng/dl, and plasma α-fetoprotein 160,000ng/ml. Metastatic lesions in both lungs were seen on the chest X-ray. Reproduced from Kaplan and Grumbach (1990), by courtesy of Williams and Wilkins.

Boys

Chorionic Gonadotrophin-secreting Tumours Many neoplasms secrete the embryonic protein hCG. hCG will crossreact in most immunoassays for LH and, due to its positive detection in hCG-β assays, causes a positive pregnancy test in boys. It stimulates the testes of affected boys to produce testosterone, and incomplete sexual precocity results. Young patients with incomplete precocious puberty may have hCG secreting hepatomas and hepatoblastomas which are often fatal within months of diagnosis (Fig. 13.35). Teratomas or chorioepitheliomas in the hypothalamic or pineal region can also produce hCG and cause incomplete sexual precocity. Such tumours are rare in girls, but even if they occur and produce hCG, no physical changes will result because of the elevated hCG levels. Boys with 47XXY Klinefelter's syndrome have an increased incidence of hCG-secreting mediastinal germ cell neoplasms.

Androgen Excess Disorders involving androgen excess due to congenital adrenal hyperplasia, virilising adrenal tumours or Leydig cell tumours, share the feature of incomplete sexual precocity. In congenital adrenal hyperplasia there will be no enlargement of the testes, since circulating androgens suppress endogenous gonadotrophin secretion. Adrenal rests in the testes, or Leydig cell tumours of the testes, will lead to irregular enlargement of the testes: the former are due to ACTH stimulation, and the latter to tumour formation.

Premature Maturation of Leydig and Germ Cells Boys with familial gonadotrophin-independent sexual precocity with premature maturation of Leydig and germ cells have enlargement of their penis and virilisation, but only minimal enlargement of their testes since there is predominant stimulation of Leydig cells and relatively less enlargement of the seminiferous tubules – the tissue most responsible for the pubertal enlargement of the testes. These patients have elevated testosterone levels but suppressed gonadotrophin levels. The condition is also known as testotoxicosis.

Preliminary reports suggest that these patients have circulating Leydig cell stimulatory factor, but the nature of this factor has not yet been determined. Remarkably, these children achieve only a small decrease in final height and, when they reach adulthood, fertility is achieved as demonstrated by the familial nature of this disorder (sex-limited autosomal dominant condition). Later in life the patients become responsive to GnRH administration, while they were not so during their childhood; this phenomenon appears to be related to hypothalamic–pituitary–gonadal maturation as found in patients with premature puberty after treatment of virilising disorders. Patients do not respond initially to GnRH agonists. Recently, spironolactone, an antimineralocorticoid and an antiandrogen agent, has been combined with testolactone, an inhibitor of P_{450} aromatase (a key enzyme in the conversion of androgens to oestrogens) as therapy for testotoxicosis. Alternatively, cyproterone acetate, a powerful antiandrogen that blocks the cytosolic androgen receptor, may be used on its own.

Girls

Ovarian Cysts Incomplete isosexual precocity in girls can be caused by autonomous ovarian follicular cysts – the most frequent type of oestrogen-secreting ovarian mass. Normal girls frequently have follicles up to 8mm in diameter, as proved by autopsy and ultrasound studies. Larger cysts, however, may be discovered because of an abdominal mass or pain, especially after torsion of the cyst. If these follicles secrete oestrogen, they may cause sexual precocity. Excessive FSH secretion is the aetiology in some girls. Such cysts can be monitored by ultrasonography and, while surgery is rarely indicated, the follicular fluid may be reduced by draining using laparoscopy. Characteristic findings in girls with recurrent cysts is the waxing and waning course of their feminisation. Granulosa cell tumours of the ovary are rare in childhood but may lead to a palpable tumour that secretes oestrogen and causes incomplete sexual precocity. Oestrogen-secreting adrenal neoplasms may less frequently cause this condition. Girls can also be exposed to oestrogens through ingestion of their mother's oral contraception or other preparations.

Oestrogen-secreting Neoplasms Gonadoblastoma or dysgerminoma, found in streak gonads, may secrete oestrogen and, if found in a patient with Turner's syndrome, may mistakenly suggest autonomous but minimal ovarian function.

Boys and Girls

McCune–Albright Syndrome Incomplete sexual precocity in boys and girls may occur with the McCune–Albright syndrome. This syndrome is characterised by the triad of irregularly edged hyperpigmented macules (café-au-lait spots), polyostotic fibrous dysplasia, and GnRH-independent sexual precocity (Figs 13.36 & 13.37). Patients may have autonomously functioning ovarian cysts but may also manifest autonomous hyperfunction of the thyroid, adrenal gland, pituitary gland (especially GH oversecretion), and parathyroid glands. Development of café-au-lait spots may occur after infancy and may not be apparent in the newborn period. The bone lesions, which may include cysts in the long bones and thickening of areas of the skull, likewise develop later and are not apparent at birth.

Initially, the precocious puberty of the McCune–Albright syndrome is autonomous, but exposure to oestrogens or androgens over a period of time may convert the patients to GnRH-dependent precocious puberty such as that which may occur after successful supression of androgen secretion in patients with virilising disorders. Testolactone has been effective as initial therapy in girls with McCune–Albright syndrome, as has medroxyprogesterone acetate or cyproterone acetate, while GnRH agonist has been effective later after maturation of the hypothalamic–pituitary–gonadal axis occurs.

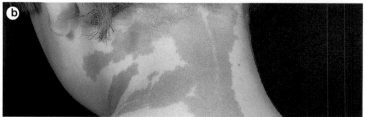

Fig. 13.36 A girl with the McCune–Albright syndrome.
Characteristic breast enlargement (a) and skin pigmentation over the neck (b) can be seen. By courtesy of Dr PHW Rayner.

Juvenile Hypothyroidism   Severe untreated hypothyroidism in boys and girls may be associated with incomplete sexual precocity. Levels of plasma prolactin are elevated in primary hypothyroidism, and galactorrhea may be demonstrable more commonly in girls than in boys. Growth is impaired in these patients as in any child with hypothyroidism so there is no pubertal growth spurt. Girls may manifest breast development, menstrual flow and oestrogen effects on the vaginal mucosa, while the size of the testes increases in boys due to enlargement of the seminiferous tubules. The pituitary gland may enlarge and erode the sella turcica due to increased TSH secretion and thyrotroph hyperplasia, thereby mimicking a tumour. Once the hypothyroidism is treated, sexual precocity reverts, and the sella turcica will decrease in size.

Diagnosis of Sexual Precocity

The goal in diagnosis of disorders associated with sexual precocity (Fig. 13.38) is to eliminate the possibility of life-threatening brain tumours or other central nervous system conditions and to therefore separate these patients from those with idiopathic precocious puberty. If the possibility of a central nervous system tumour has not been eliminated due to an alternative diagnosis, patients with precocious puberty should have a computerised tomography (CT) scan or an magnetic resonance imaging (MRI) evaluation of the brain.

Males with precocious puberty will usually manifest physical features that indicate the primary diagnosis. Symmetrical testicular enlargement is the first sign of central precocious puberty in males in most cases, while irregularly enlarged testes are found in Leydig cell tumours or adrenal rests. Elevated levels of hCG secreted from a tumour will only minimally enlarge the testes but will be associated with a positive pregnancy test. Small testes with virilisation lead to the possibility of congenital adrenal hyperplasia or an adrenal tumour.

Variations in Pubertal Development

Premature Thelarche

Breast enlargement in girls under eight years of age is relatively common and self-limited (Fig. 13.39). Premature thelarche most frequently occurs in girls by two years of age and almost always before four years of age. In most cases, the breast development will regress within six months of onset, but in some cases remains for

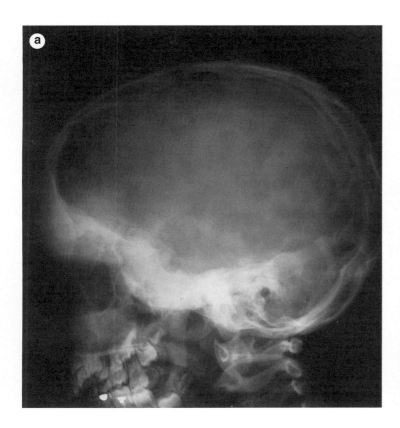 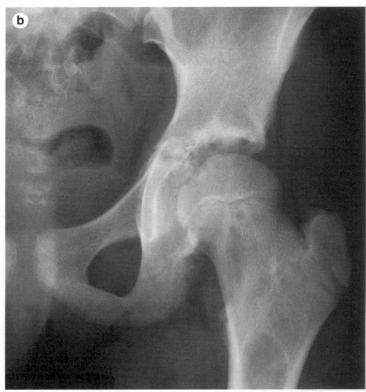

Fig. 13.37 *Lateral skull (a) and hip (b) radiographs of an 8-year-old girl with the McCune–Albright syndrome, showing the characteristic skeletal findings of polyostotic fibrous dysplasia.* (a) The lateral view of the skull demonstrates enlargement of the diploic space, bony enlargement, and some lucency in the frontal and sphenoid bones. (b) Changes in the long bones include the large area of lucency and ground-glass appearance in the proximal femur, with widening of the femoral neck and an altered trabecular pattern. Reproduced from Wheeler and Styne (1991), by courtesy of WB Saunders.

years after diagnosis. Long-term follow-up suggests that no untoward effects occur on later health. The cause of premature thelarche may be the development of a small ovarian cyst, but usually by the time the outward physical manifestations are noted, the cyst has regressed and no laboratory tests are indicated. Studies have shown elevation of FSH levels to be a potential cause of premature thelarche, but patients do not manifest a true pubertal GnRH test. This is a benign self-limited disorder and should be treated with reassurance.

Premature Isolated Menarche

There are rare reports of girls who have menarche at an early age with no breast development. This may occur as an isolated incident or over a period of years. These girls then go through normal pubertal development later in childhood. The aetiology of this condition is unknown.

Premature Adrenarche

Some children have elevated adrenal androgens years before the normal age of onset of adrenarche and experience pubic hair development, some axillary hair development, and even some acne years before the normal age of onset of normal puberty; this is apparently a normal variation of the normal onset of adrenarche (Fig. 13.40).

With the recent description of late-onset congenital adrenal hyperplasia, it is sometimes difficult to determine whether the patient has bona fide premature adrenarche or another genetic condition that is affecting the adrenal gland. Nonetheless, in premature adrenarche DHEAS is elevated to earlier midpubertal levels, and is useful for diagnosis of the condition.

Adolescent Gynaecomastia

Up to seventy-five per cent of normal boys in pubertal stages 2 to 3 have unilateral or bilateral breast development. No definitive endocrine test has indicated the cause of this breast development but it is self-limited and usually transient. It is intensified by obesity and minimised to some degree by weight loss. It may last in some children for years and cause significant psychological distress during adolescence. Only occasionally is plastic surgery indicated. Certain conditions, such as Klinefelter's syndrome and a variant of the androgen-resistance syndrome, are associated with gynaecomastia and respond best to surgical therapy. Thus, pathological conditions must be eliminated, usually by careful physical examination, before the diagnosis of adolescent gynaecomastia is made.

DIAGNOSIS AND ASSESSMENT OF SEXUAL PRECOCITY

Fig. 13.38 The differential diagnosis and assessment of children with sexual precocity.

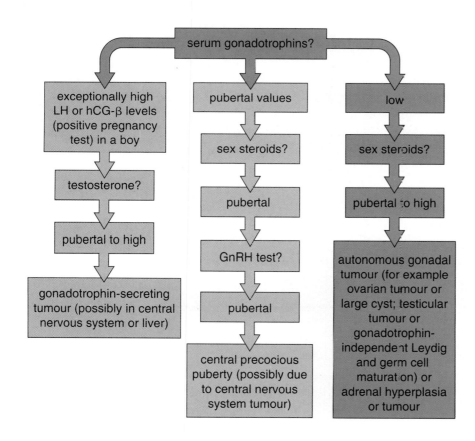

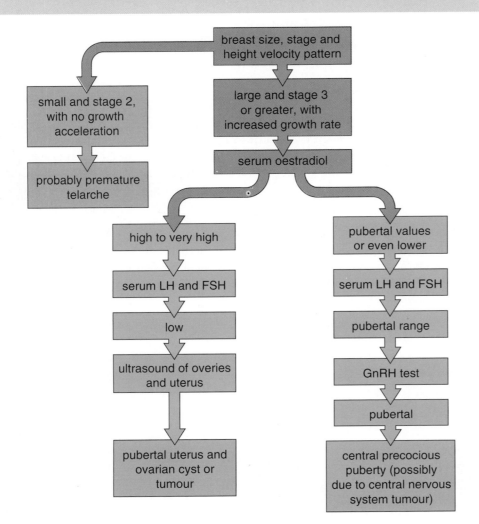

DIAGNOSIS OF THE CAUSES OF PREMATURE TELARCHE

breast size, stage and height velocity pattern

- small and stage 2, with no growth acceleration → probably premature telarche
- large and stage 3 or greater, with increased growth rate → serum oestradiol
  - high to very high → serum LH and FSH → low → ultrasound of overies and uterus → pubertal uterus and ovarian cyst or tumour
  - pubertal values or even lower → serum LH and FSH → pubertal range → GnRH test → pubertal → central precocious puberty (possibly due to central nervous system tumour)

Fig. 13.39 *The differential diagnosis of the causes of premature thelarche.*

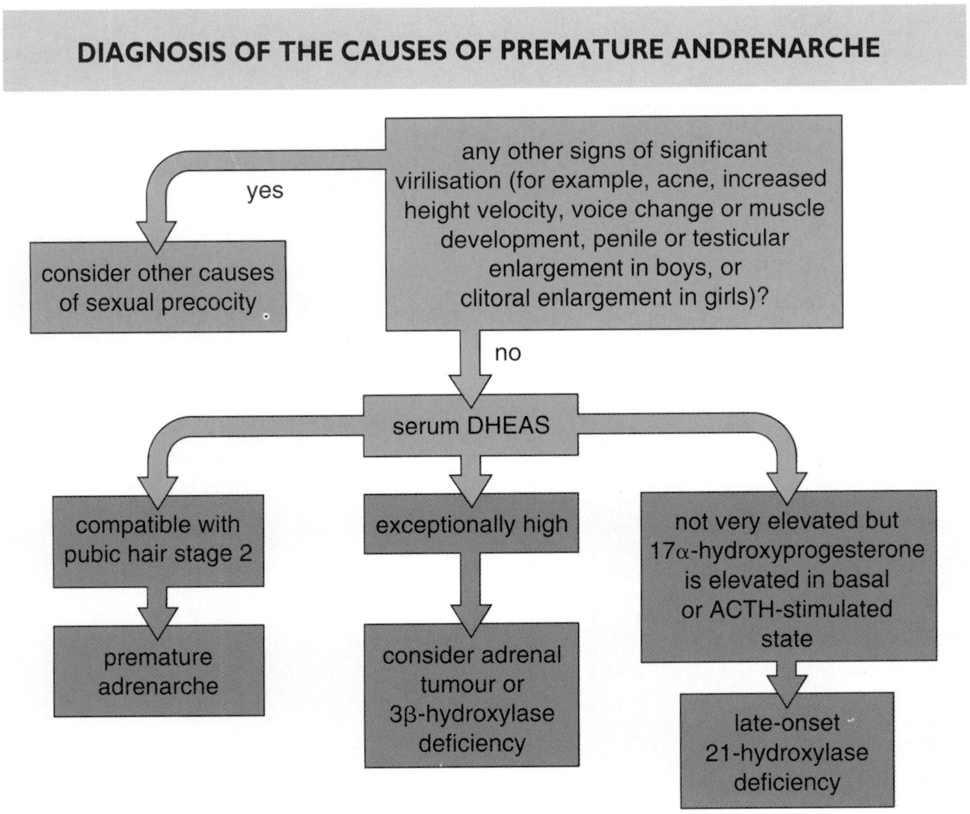

DIAGNOSIS OF THE CAUSES OF PREMATURE ANDRENARCHE

any other signs of significant virilisation (for example, acne, increased height velocity, voice change or muscle development, penile or testicular enlargement in boys, or clitoral enlargement in girls)?

- yes → consider other causes of sexual precocity
- no → serum DHEAS
  - compatible with pubic hair stage 2 → premature adrenarche
  - exceptionally high → consider adrenal tumour or 3β-hydroxylase deficiency
  - not very elevated but 17α-hydroxyprogesterone is elevated in basal or ACTH-stimulated state → late-onset 21-hydroxylase deficiency

Fig. 13.40 *The differential diagnosis of the causes of premature adrenarche.*

14

Growth Disorders

Charles G D Brook, MD, FRCP

Normal growth in height and size results from the complex interplay of many intrinsic and extrinsic factors on the innate, genetically determined capacity for growth of an individual. The ultimate height of a person is a function not only of the rate of linear growth of the bones, but also of its duration.

The growth of an individual from birth to adulthood may be pictorially represented in a height distance chart (Fig. 14.1). All normal children follow such a growth curve.

To determine the rate of growth of an individual child, a number of height measurements should be made at regular intervals: for instance, twice in one year. A height velocity curve (Fig. 14.2) is obtained by plotting the height gained during each year and yields

important information about the growth pattern of a child. The three phases of growth in childhood are easily recognised: initially, there is a period of rapid and rapidly decelerating growth in infancy, with a subsequent period of steady and slowly decelerating growth in middle childhood, followed by a rapid rise and fall of growth at adolescence. These phases of growth are primarily dependent on nutrition, growth hormone (GH), and sex steroids, respectively.

HEIGHT VELOCITY CHART FOR BOYS AND GIRLS IN THE UK

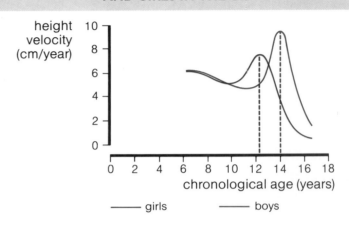

Fig. 14.3 Average height velocity chart for boys and girls in the UK. The earlier onset of the adolescent growth spurt of girls is shown together with the greater peak height velocity in boys.

HEIGHT DISTANCE CHART: BIRTH TO ADULTHOOD

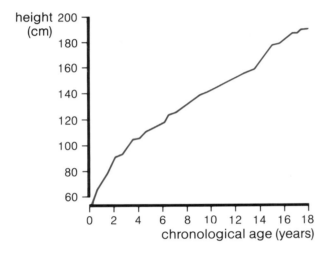

Fig. 14.1 Height distance chart showing the growth of an individual boy from birth to adulthood. All normal children follow a growth curve resembling this distance chart.

HEIGHT VELOCITY CHART: BIRTH TO ADULTHOOD

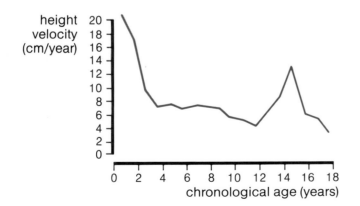

Fig. 14.2 Height velocity chart of the same boy as in Fig. 14.1. To produce such a chart, the annual gain in height is plotted against chronological age. The three phases of childhood – growth of rapid deceleration in infancy, slow deceleration in middle childhood, and rapid acceleration at adolescence – may be identified.

HEIGHT DISTANCE CENTILE CHART FOR GIRLS IN THE UK

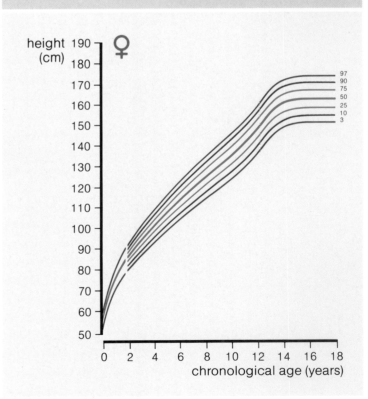

Fig. 14.4 Height distance centile chart for girls in the UK. This chart is no more than a description of the height of the female population. The fiftieth percentile is the median, so that fifty per cent of individuals are taller, and fifty per cent shorter, than this height.

prognosis (170cm) is well within normal limits for the centile position of his parental heights (shown on the right of the chart). Whether he will achieve this potential depends upon whether he is growing at a normal rate and on how long he continues to grow, which is defined by his bone age. To establish normal growth, a normal growth rate must be demonstrated.

To establish the growth rate of a child, height should be measured on two different occasions that are separated by a period of time. The length of time needed to establish a normal growth velocity depends upon the increment that might be expected and the accuracy of the equipment used. Instruments of the type shown in Fig. 14.7 would require approximately three years to establish normality because of the high error margin when using them. When measuring the height of children, it should be remembered that all individuals shrink slightly during the day. A child must therefore be drawn out to the maximum by traction under the mastoids.

MEASURING TECHNIQUE

Before measuring the standing height of children, they should remove their shoes and should stand with their heels and back in contact with an upright wall. The head should be held so that the

child looks straight ahead with the outer canthus of the eye socket being in the same horizontal plane as the external auditory meatuses, and not with the nose tipped upwards. A right-angled block is then slid down the wall until the bottom surface touches the child's head, and a scale that is fixed to the wall is read. During measurement, the child should be told to stretch the neck to be as tall as possible, although care must be taken to prevent the heels from coming off the ground. Gentle but firm traction should be applied by the measurer under the mastoid processes to keep the child stretched. In this way, the variation in height from morning to evening is minimised.

A stadiometer, as shown in Fig. 14.8, allows the height to be measured on successive occasions to within 1mm when the measurements are made with care by the same observer using the same technique. In a measurement of more than 1m, the accuracy of this instrument compares favourably with any other measurement made clinically or

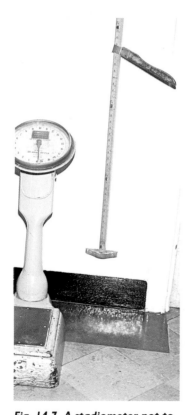

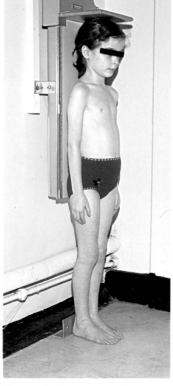

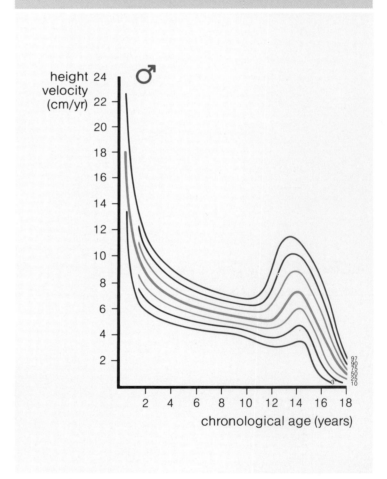

HEIGHT VELOCITY CHART FOR BOYS: BIRTH TO ADULTHOOD

Fig. 14.7 A stadiometer not to be recommended. This instrument should be avoided since it would take several years to produce a reliable growth curve because of the error margin involved.

Fig. 14.8 A recommended stadiometer in use. During measurement, the child should be told to stretch the neck while the measurer applies gentle traction under the mastoids to keep the child stretched. The outer canthus of the eye sockets of the child should be in the same horizontal plane as the external auditory meatuses, and the heels should be touching the ground.

Fig. 14.9 Height velocity chart for boys from birth to adulthood. Height velocity is the change in height over an interval of time. The length of time needed to establish a normal growth velocity depends upon the increment that might be expected and the accuracy of the equipment used. The child must maintain a height velocity at around the fiftieth percentile to maintain growth along the centile line on a distance chart.

in the laboratory. Nevertheless, measurement made over less than three to six months may produce considerable errors, and reliance should not be placed upon single estimates of height velocity made over a short period of time.

Height velocity measurements (Fig. 14.9) are converted into annual rates of growth by dividing the increment by the lapse of time. Such measurements are compared with centiles as before but, whereas a third centile position on a height distance chart may be, and probably is, normal, a velocity that is persistently on the third centile leads to progressive loss of height compared with children of the same age. The growth velocity of a given child must oscillate about the fiftieth percentile to maintain growth along a centile chart on a distance chart. Visual inspection on a distance chart is not a substitute for calculating the height velocity and plotting it on a centile chart.

SHORT STATURE

Short stature is a common cause of concern among children and adolescents, and their parents. Three per cent of the population has a height below the percentile and will be noticeably short; however, probably fewer than one per cent of the percentage will have a primary

endocrine defect. In order to detect such children, careful clinical assessment and measurements of the height velocity are needed to separate those who are small, but growing normally, from those who are failing to grow. For the latter, a diagnosis is needed in order for the appropriate treatment to be instituted without delay. The state of nutrition may help to point the diagnostic pathway, but any child who is growing slowly should have a diagnostic investigation to determine the cause. In assessing all short patients, a detailed history, physical examination, and urine analysis are required, together with a radiograph of the nondominant hand and wrist, allowing the bone age to be assessed and hence also the growth potential. Short stature that is out of keeping with the family background is likely to be significant. The midparental height (the mean of the parental centile heights) can be calculated in order to estimate height expectation. Information should also be obtained about the growth pattern in the parents, especially concerning the time of onset of the pubertal growth spurt. Physical examination may reveal an abnormal-looking child with either dysmorphic features of disproportionate short stature (short limbs or short back and limbs). The major causes of short stature in children with a normal appearance and those with disproportionate short stature are illustrated in Figs. 14.10 and 14.11, respectively.

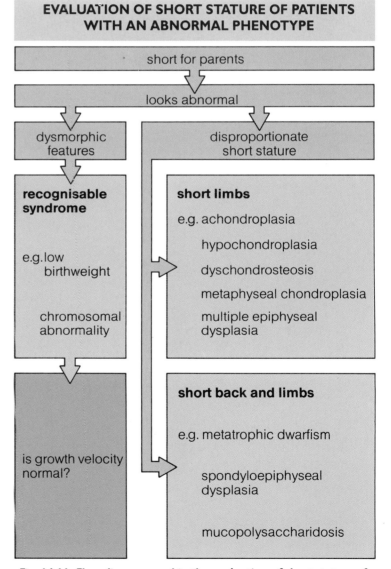

Fig. 14.10 Flow diagram used in the evaluation of short stature of patients who have a normal appearance.

Fig. 14.11 Flow diagram used in the evaluation of short stature of patients who have an abnormal phenotype.

A CHILD WITH OCCULT COELIAC DISEASE BEFORE AND AFTER TREATMENT

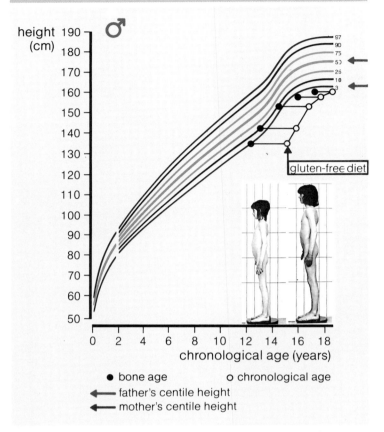

Fig. 14.16 *A child with occult coeliac disease with short stature, before and after treatment.* The effect on growth of introducing a gluten-free diet is shown. Note the delayed bone age at the start of treatment.

SYSTEMIC CAUSES OF SHORT STATURE

In systemic disease, there is often delayed skeletal maturation, but the potential for catch-up growth is present if the underlying systemic disorder can be successfully treated. A child with coeliac disease for example will continue to have stunted growth until gluten is removed from the diet, after which time, rapid growth and development may occur. Other chronic disorders which may also retard growth are Crohn's disease, respiratory disease (e.g. asthma), renal disease, cardiovascular causes, and nutritional causes (e.g. rickets; Fig. 14.15). In all such instances, the potential for catch-up growth remains if the disease is rapidly cured.

Occult coeliac disease is a common finding among children who grow slowly for no obvious reason. Most children with endocrine disease are obese; therefore, in a child who is not obese, a jejunal biopsy should be performed at an early stage to exclude villous atrophy. The effect of a gluten-free diet in a late-diagnosed asymptomatic coeliac patient, whose only complaint was short stature, is shown in Fig. 14.16.

PSYCHOSOCIAL AND EMOTIONAL DEPRIVATION

Psychosocial and emotional deprivation are commonly recognised in infancy and childhood. Infants suffering from maternal deprivation display behavioural abnormalities such as apathy, watchfulness, and autoerotic activity, as well as delayed developmental behaviour. There is often a history of maternal rejection or neglect, nonaccidental injury, or lack of physical handling. Emotional deprivation in childhood may lead to small stature (Figs. 14.17 & 14.18), retarded skeletal maturation and, in older children, delayed sexual maturation. Endocrine function may also be abnormal in affected patients, who may additionally have high levels of fasting GH and also cortisol nonresponsiveness with the insulin tolerance test.

EFFECT OF EMOTIONAL DEPRIVATION ON A CHILD

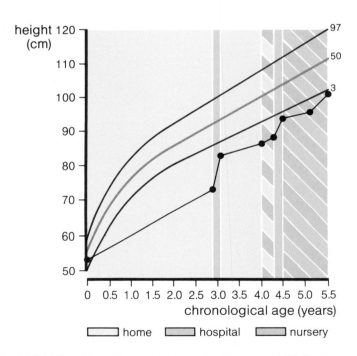

Fig. 14.17 *The effect of emotional deprivation on a child.* During hospitalisation, the growth rate of the child increased, but 'steadied off' during periods of emotional deprivation at home.

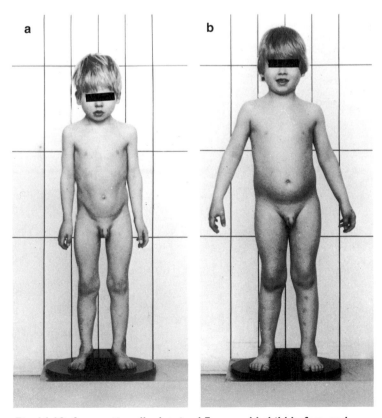

Fig. 14.18 *An emotionally deprived 7-year-old child before and after treatment (one year later).* Note the marked short stature (a) and the rapid growth following treatment (b).

NONENDOCRINE CAUSES OF SHORT STATURE
Constitutional Growth Delay
One of the most common causes of short stature is constitutional growth delay with delayed puberty: the bone age is retarded, but the growth velocity is normal. A normal growth spurt in puberty can be predicted, and eventual height will be normal (Fig. 14.29).

Although treatment is not essential, these patients are seriously disadvantaged by their condition, which is easily improved with small doses of sex steroids.

Turner's Syndrome
Chromosome analysis should be performed on any girl unexpectedly short for her family; signs of puberty should not inhibit this investigation since twenty per cent of girls with Turner's syndrome

have signs of spontaneous sexual development. The only constant feature is short stature.

The management of Turner's syndrome requires a growth-promoting regimen in childhood (GH or low-dose sex steroids) and phased introduction of oestrogen from the twelfth year of life. Unfortunately, although these treatments are beneficial to the child in the short term and promote normal secondary sexual characteristics, they have been unimpressive in terms of the final height that is achieved.

Skeletal Dysplasias
Patients who are short for their family in childhood, have a reduced height prediction, and are growing normally should be suspected of having a skeletal dysplasia. In hypochondroplasia for example, the

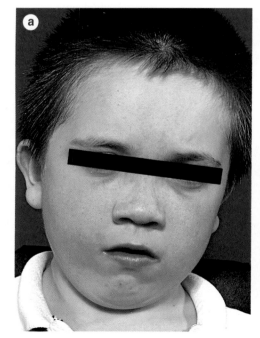
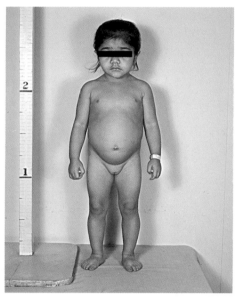
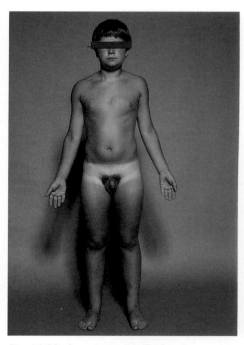
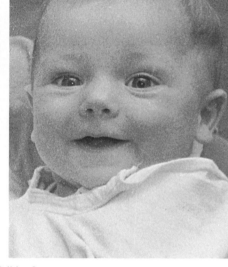
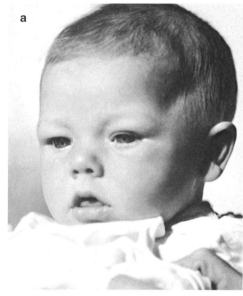
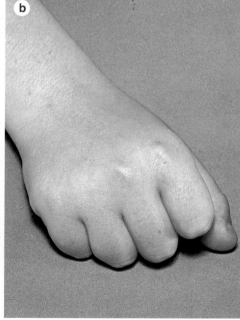

Fig. 14.25 A hypothyroid girl.

Fig. 14.26 A hypothyroid baby (a) before and (b) after treatment.

Fig. 14.27 A boy with pseudohypoparathyroidism. Note his round face and shortened neck (a) and his shortened metacarpals (b).

Fig. 14.28 A patient with Cushing's syndrome. This is uncommon in childhood. Short stature is a consequence of the suppression of GH secretion by corticosteroids. In addition to short stature, note the plethoric 'moon' face.

disproportionate short stature does not become manifest until adult life. Treatment with GH has been tried experimentally for these patients and for patients with familial short stature. The results in terms of final height have not been fully evaluated but do not appear impressive. Treatment with GH should be restricted at present to patients with GH insufficiency.

TALL STATURE

There are relatively few pathological cases of tall stature, with most children representing the upper end of normal distribution of height. Most often there is a family history of tallness in one or both parents.

Ultimate height can be predicted by assessment of bone age. A diagram showing the method of evaluation of tall stature is shown in Fig. 14.30.

TALL STATURE ASSOCIATED WITH NORMAL GROWTH VELOCITY

If a child looks normal and has a normal growth velocity, constitutional tall stature is usually present (Fig. 14.31). Obese children are often taller than average for their age, and if maturity is also advanced, then puberty may occasionally occur earlier. Tall stature may represent a considerable handicap and, if necessary, treatment to limit growth should be considered.

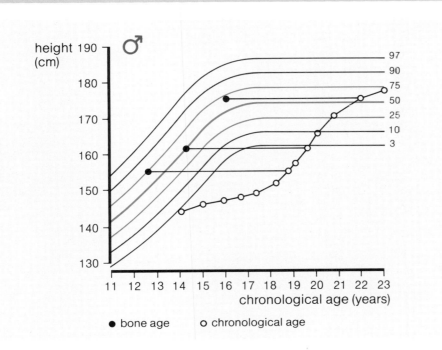

GROWTH CHART OF A BOY WITH CONSTITUTIONAL GROWTH DELAY

● bone age   ○ chronological age

Fig. 14.29 Growth chart of a boy with constitutional growth delay. The boy's short height during childhood would have been accompanied by a delayed bone age. When the average boys of his age started to grow rapidly in puberty, this boy was left behind. Thus, he was referred for short stature and delayed puberty. His pubertal stages were appropriate for his bone age and, due to previously normal growth velocity, a normal growth spurt in puberty was predicted and occurred as shown. It is difficult to determine whether there is a minor degree of GH deficiency if adequate previous growth records are not available.

Fig. 14.30 Flow diagram to evaluate tall stature.

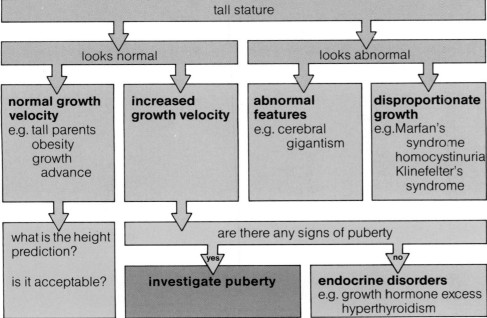

FLOW DIAGRAM TO EVALUATE TALL STATURE

GENERAL CONSIDERATIONS

Abnormalities of growth represent a frequent cause of referral to the endocrine clinic. The approach to the management of these patients is summarised in Fig. 14.37. The importance of accurate anthropometry cannot be overemphasised and, in the early assessment, it is mandatory to establish the parental pattern of growth and also the age at which puberty was entered. The midparental height, adjusted for the sex of the patient, enables the clinician to gain an estimate of the expected final height of the individual and, by using a height distance chart, to determine whether the child is on course to achieve this. The estimation of skeletal maturity, usually by radiography of the child's wrist, is essential in the assessment of growth prognosis of the likely final height.

Follow-up measurements should also be carried out at a minimum of six-monthly intervals, allowing the growth velocity to be calculated. The growth velocity is a very important clue as to the pattern of growth taking place. Abnormality of growth velocity requires systematic investigations directed at the diagnosis of systemic or endocrine pathology.

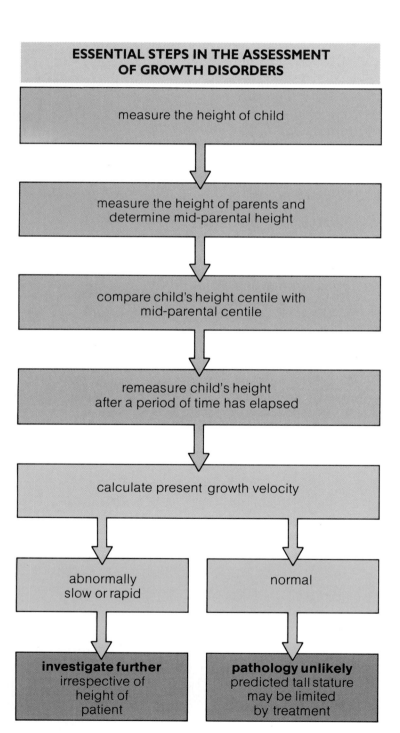

ESSENTIAL STEPS IN THE ASSESSMENT OF GROWTH DISORDERS

measure the height of child

measure the height of parents and determine mid-parental height

compare child's height centile with mid-parental centile

remeasure child's height after a period of time has elapsed

calculate present growth velocity

abnormally slow or rapid

normal

investigate further irrespective of height of patient

pathology unlikely predicted tall stature may be limited by treatment

Fig. 14.37 Summary of the essential steps in the assessment of growth disorders.

15

Thyroid Physiology and Hypothyroidism

Leslie J DeGroot, MD

follicular cells into the circulation. The steps involved in thyroid hormone synthesis are iodine concentration and transport; oxidation; coupling and secretion; colloid resorption; proteolysis; and deiodination.

Dietary iodine is wholly absorbed from the gut, 100–200µg being required daily. Inorganic iodide is concentrated in the follicles by active transport across the cell membrane, and then rapidly transferred across the cell into the colloid lumen. This 'trapped' iodide is oxidised by the thyroid peroxidase enzyme (TPO) and linked to tyrosine molecules in thyroglobulin to form monoiodotyrosines (MIT) and diiodotyrosines (DIT), neither of which are metabolically active. The iodotyrosines are formed within the thyroglobulin molecules (which are synthesised by the follicular cells and secreted into the lumen). Mono- and diiodotyrosines linked to thyroglobulin are then coupled by further TPO enzyme action to form the metabolically active T_3 and T_4 (Fig. 15.9) which are still contained within the thyroglobulin molecule which is secreted into the colloid. The

thyroglobulin containing T_4 and T_3 is then resorbed into the follicular cells in colloid drops by the process of endocytosis. T_4 and T_3 are subsequently released, by proteolysis, from the thyroglobulin in lysosomes that are rich in proteases and peptidases. Uncoupled mono-

SITES OF NORMAL AND ECTOPIC THYROID TISSUE

lingual

thyroglossal cyst

thyroglossal duct

pyramidal lobe

normal thyroid

retrosternal

Fig. 15.6 Sites of normal and ectopic thyroid tissue along the line of the thyroglossal duct. Remnants of the duct may persist as isolated nests of functioning thyroid tissue: for example, as a lingual thyroid, a pyramidal lobe, or simple thyroglossal cysts.

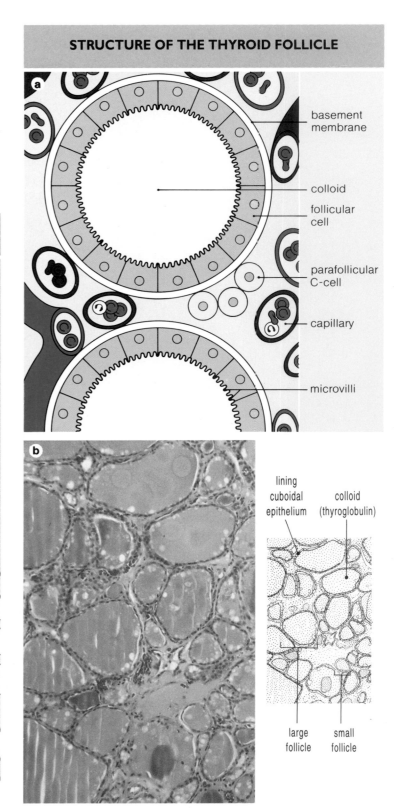

STRUCTURE OF THE THYROID FOLLICLE

basement membrane

colloid

follicular cell

parafollicular C-cell

capillary

microvilli

lining cuboidal epithelium

colloid (thyroglobulin)

large follicle

small follicle

Fig. 15.7 The structure of the thyroid follicle. (a) A schematic representation of a high-power view of thyroid follicles, showing their relationship with capillaries and parafollicular C-cells. (b) The histology of normal thyroid tissue. Thyroid follicles of variable sizes can be seen; they contain colloid and are lined by cuboidal epithelium. Haematoxylin and eosin (H and E) stain, magnification X 120. By courtesy of Prof I Doniach.

Measurement of circulating total thyroid hormone concentrations includes both protein-bound and free fractions of the hormones (Fig. 15.11), although the free fractions represent a tiny proportion (0.04% in the case of T_4) of the total. The normal concentration of the free fraction of T_4 lies between 9 and 24pmol/l (0.7 and 1.9ng/100ml), whereas the total T_4 concentration lies between 50

DEIODINATION OF T_4 TO T_3 OR TO rT_3

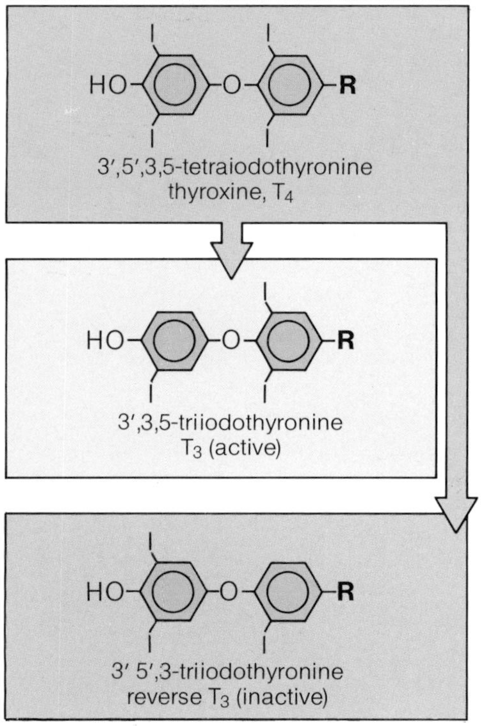

Fig. 15.10 Deiodination of T_4 to T_3 or to its inactive metabolite rT_3. Increased conversion of T_4 to rT_3 occurs during acute or chronic illness such as severe infection and starvation. Reduced metabolism of rT_3 in such patients leads to elevated blood levels of this iodothyronine.

THYROID HORMONE TRANSPORT

	percentage distribution		plasma concentration	
	T_4	T_3	T_4	T_3
free hormone	0.015	0.5	9–24 pmol/l	5–10 pmol/l
thyroxine binding globulin (TBG)	70	77	–	–
thyroxine binding prealbumin (TBPA)	10	8	–	–
albumin	20	15	–	–
total hormone	100	100	50–140 nmol/l	1–3 nmol/l

Fig. 15.11 Thyroid hormone transport. Nearly all T_4 and T_3 (more than ninety-nine per cent) are transported in a bound state, predominantly bound to TBG, but to a lesser extent to thyroxine-binding prealbumin (TBPA) and albumin.

MEASUREMENT OF THYROID HORMONES

direct methods

circulating levels of total hormones

total thyroxine (T_4)

total triiodothyronine (T_3)

protein bound iodine (PBI)

circulating levels of free hormones

free thyroxine (fT_4)

free triiodothyronine (fT_3)

thyroid hormone binding proteins

thyroxine binding globulin (TBG)

Fig. 15.12 The direct methods of measurement of thyroid hormones and binding proteins.

MEASUREMENT OF THYROID HORMONES

indirect methods

thyroid hormone binding tests

resin uptake of ^{125}I -T_3

free thyroxine index (FTI)

$$FTI = \frac{T_4 \times patient\ ^{125}I\text{ -}T_3\ resin\ uptake}{control\ ^{125}I\text{ -}T_3\ resin\ uptake}$$

Fig. 15.13 The indirect methods of measurement of thyroid hormones.

and 140nmol/l (4–11μg/100ml). The normal concentration of free T_3 lies between 5 and 10pmol/l (0.33 and 0.65ng/100ml), and that of total T_3 between 1 and 3nmol/l (65 and 195ng/100ml).

The level of free hormones governs the metabolic state and thyroid status of a patient.

MEASUREMENT OF THYROID HORMONES

TOTAL SERUM T_4, T_3, AND rT$_3$

Total serum T_4, T_3, and rT$_3$ (Fig. 15.12) are conveniently measured by widely available commercial radioimmunoassays (RIAs). Since serum T_4 is largely protein bound and does not correlate with free T_4 if there are binding protein abnormalities, T_4 is useful as a screening agent but is not reliable as a diagnostic test. Serum total T_3 is less affected by binding protein changes and is useful, particularly in diagnosis of thyrotoxicosis with borderline T_4 values. Serum rT$_3$ may be measured as an indicator of the 'euthyroid sick' syndrome in patients with low serum T_4 or T_3.

Measurement of protein-bound iodine (PBI) (used in past years) correlates with serum T_4 if no other organic iodine is present. It also can detect abnormal iodinated proteins. The test is not currently used in practice.

Indirect Methods for Assay of Free T_4 or Free T_3

Indirect methods of estimating free thyroid hormone levels are widely used (Fig. 15.13). These tests combine the determination of total serum T_4 or T_3 with an estimate of the free fraction to derive a free hormone index. Basically, the indirect methods 'correct' for the effect of altered binding proteins (primarily TBG), and have provided, for over three decades, a highly, although not perfectly, reliable estimate of free T_3 or free T_4.

Several different methods are used to estimate the free fraction of the total T_4 or T_3. Most commonly, the serum of patients is incubated with ^{125}I-labelled T_3 which occupies binding sites on the thyroid hormone binding proteins, mainly TBG, not already occupied by T_4, while the remainder is left in solution. The protein-bound and free fractions are separated by addition of a resin, to which the free hormone binds. The proportion of free to protein-bound ^{125}I-T$_3$ is inversely related to the residual unoccupied binding capacity of thyroid hormone binding proteins, and is directly related to free hormone fractions. The results are usually related to a standard reference serum and are used as a ratio of the results of the unknown serum to the reference serum for calculation of the free thyroxine index (FTI) (Fig. 15.13).

The FTI is calculated from the results of a total T_4 estimation and a thyroid hormone binding test. Depending upon the method used for the thyroid hormone binding test, the calculation is as shown in Fig. 15.13.

The FTI gives a value for T_4, which is corrected for alterations in TBG capacity and is of particular value in subjects taking oral contraceptive therapy, in pregnancy, and in hypoproteinaemic states. The index has been widely used for these reasons, but it involves the use of two tests and therefore may be superseded by the direct 'free' thyroid hormone assays, which effectively measure the same entity (see Fig. 15.12).

A summary of thyroid hormone concentrations and distribution is shown in Figs. 15.14 and 15.15.

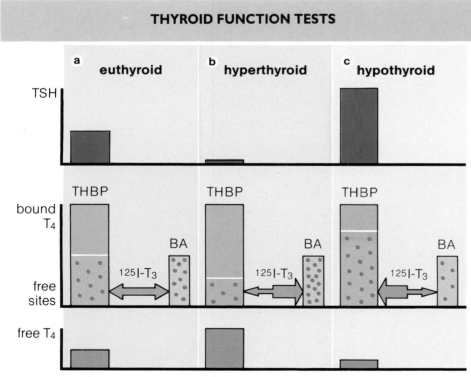

THYROID FUNCTION TESTS

a euthyroid   b hyperthyroid   c hypothyroid

TSH

THBP   THBP   THBP

bound T_4

BA   BA   BA

free sites   ^{125}I-T$_3$ ^{125}I-T$_3$ ^{125}I-T$_3$

free T_4

THBP = thyroid hormone binding proteins
BA = binding agent (resin or Sephadex)

Fig. 15.14 Thyroid function tests in various states. The distribution of isotope between binding agents (resin or Sephadex and the free sites on thyroid hormone binding proteins is shown. (a) In the euthyroid state, levels of free T_4, total T_4, and TSH are within the normal range. Using indirect testing, ^{125}I-T$_3$ attached to a binding agent (BA), normally resin or Sephadex, competes for free binding sites on the thyroid hormone binding proteins (THBP), mainly TBG, and competition between BA and THBP is approximately even. (b) In the hyperthyroid state, levels of free T_4 and total T_4 are increased, and TSH levels are suppressed. On indirect testing, few binding sites are unoccupied on THBP, and most ^{125}I-T$_3$ remains attached to the binding agent. (c) In primary hypothyroidism, levels of free T_4 and total T_4 are low, and TSH is increased. On indirect testing, many binding sites are unoccupied on THBP and will therefore take up ^{125}I-T$_3$, leaving only a small quantity on the BA.

Direct Methods
Assays that measure free T_4 or free T_3 directly are now available (see Fig. 15.12) and are useful in the assessment of the thyroid status of a patient. The single-step assays probably function effectively as a combined measure of T_4 and free hormone fraction (as does the FTI), and have the virtue of simplicity. Free thyroid hormone levels should not be affected by the concentration of normal thyroid hormone binding proteins.

Older Methods
PBI reflects the part of total serum iodine that is precipitated with serum proteins. Most of the organic iodine is in the form of T_4. Abnormal iodoproteins and large quantities of inorganic iodide will lead to artificially high PBI values. For these reasons, the measurement of PBI, although simple, cheap, and accurate, has been superseded.

DYNAMIC TESTS OF THYROID FUNCTION

One dynamic test of thyroid function used in clinical practice is that of radionuclide uptake using ^{123}I, or ^{99m}Tc as pertechnetate (Fig. 15.17). The proportion of a known tracer dose of such radionuclides present in the thyroid after a given time can be used as a test of thyroid function. The uptake is inversely related to the average iodine intake of a patient and is reduced by disorders of iodide trapping. Radioiodine uptake is increased in hyperthyroidism and decreased in hypothyroidism, but discrimination between normal and mildly disturbed thyroid function is poor. ^{123}I has a shorter half-life than ^{131}I and permits less exposure to radioactivity; technetium is trapped but not organified by the thyroid and is rarely used to assess uptake.

Radioiodine uptake tests have been largely superseded by more-precise direct hormone assays; however, they are still used in combination with thyroid scanners to provide a map of the thyroid. Scans are particularly useful when delineating areas of active and inactive tissue in the investigation of nodular goitre, toxic nodules, ectopic thyroid tissue, and thyroid carcinoma. ^{131}I remains the preferred isotope to use in twenty-four-hour uptake studies before ^{131}I therapy.

The T_3 suppression test was used in the past to demonstrate thyroid autonomy. A radioiodine uptake test is repeated after the patient has taken a suppressive dose of T_3 (at least $20\mu g$/tid for one week). In normal individuals, radioiodine uptake is suppressed to at least fifty per cent of the pretreatment value. Failure of suppression occurs in thyrotoxicosis and in patients with autonomous 'hot' nodules. The test is seldom necessary now, and the addition of T_3 can be dangerous to patients who are already hyperthyroid. The TSH stimulation test involves the administration of pharmacological doses of TSH (10 u/d intramuscularly, for three days) followed by a radioiodine uptake test. This test is rarely necessary since it has been superseded by more-sensitive direct measures of thyroid failure such as TSH estimation. It may, however, occasionally be useful for demonstrating the presence of suppressed thyroid tissue, and may be of more interest when recombinant human TSH becomes available.

TESTS OF THE THYROID–PITUITARY AXIS

Currently, two tests of the thyroid–pituitary axis are in use. One involves the measurement of basal serum TSH level, which provides most of the required information, and the other involves the measurement of the serum TSH response to exogenous TRH. A summary graph of basal TSH values and the TSH response to TRH is shown in Fig. 15.18.

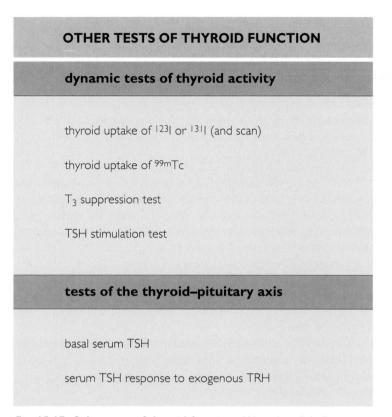

OTHER TESTS OF THYROID FUNCTION

dynamic tests of thyroid activity

thyroid uptake of ^{123}I or ^{131}I (and scan)

thyroid uptake of ^{99m}Tc

T_3 suppression test

TSH stimulation test

tests of the thyroid–pituitary axis

basal serum TSH

serum TSH response to exogenous TRH

Fig. 15.17 Other tests of thyroid function. Although radioiodine uptake tests have been largely superseded by more precise direct hormone assays, they are still used with thyroid scanners to provide a map of the thyroid (see Chapter 25).

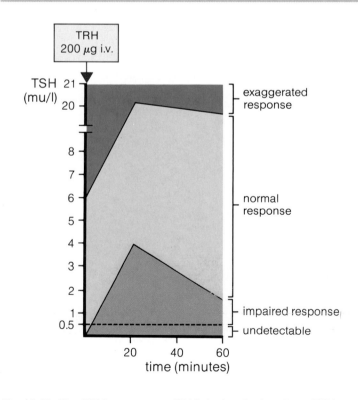

THE TSH RESPONSE TO TRH

Fig. 15.18 The TSH response to TRH. An impaired or absent TSH response to TRH is found in hyperthyroidism, while in hypothyroidism, an exaggerated response to TRH is characteristic. The lowest detectable level varies with the assay used.

Basal TSH Estimation

The lower limit of detection of serum TSH in most currently used sensitive RIAs is 0.05–0.1mu/l, while some assays can detect levels as low as 0.005mu/l. The range of basal TSH in the normal healthy population is 0.4–5mu/l, with a median of approximately 2mu/l. Basal TSH in always suppressed in hyperthyroidism, unless the hyperthyroidism is driven by the pituitary (pituitary adenomas or pituitary T_3 resistance) or an artifact is present in the assay. Suppression of TSH, usually to undetectable levels or 0.1mu/l, is currently considered the *sine qua non* for diagnosis of hyperthyroidism.

TSH is usually low in hypothyroidism secondary to pituitary disease, but in some patients, abnormally glycosylated and poorly active TSH is secreted and measured by RIA with levels up to 8 or even 10mu/l. Values above 5mu/l are usually indicative of some degree of thyroid failure, and in overt primary hypothyroidism, values may be in the range of 10–100mu/l or higher. A normal TSH value excludes primary hypothyroidism, provided that the hypothalamopituitary axis is intact.

TSH/TRH Test

Exogenous TRH, given intravenously in a pharmacological dose of 200–400µg, induces a rise in TSH which peaks approximately twenty minutes later and then declines, but not to basal levels, by sixty minutes in normal subjects.

The peak TSH response to TRH is proportional to basal TSH, and with current TSH assays, provides little added information in most cases. In hypothyroid subjects, the basal TSH is elevated and the TSH response is exaggerated. It is seldom necessary, however, to perform a TRH test in the diagnosis of hypothyroidism.

In hyperthyroidism, the TSH response to TRH is suppressed. Absent response to TRH may also be found in certain patients with nodular goitre and in patients with ophthalmic Graves' disease who are borderline toxic. An absent TSH response is thus consistent with, but not diagnostic of, hyperthyroidism. A normal TSH response to TRH excludes hyperthyroidism (except that due to TSH adenoma or pituitary T_4 resistance). Thyroid autonomy may result in a flat TSH response to TRH, but correlation with the T_3 suppression test is not as close as might be expected, perhaps because the two tests measure different aspects of the thyroid–pituitary axis.

CAUSES OF HYPOTHYROIDISM

Iodine deficiency is the most common cause of goitre and borderline hypothyroidism worldwide. In noniodine-deficient areas, however, autoimmunity is the most common cause of hypothyroidism (Fig. 15.19). Destructive therapy by surgery or radioiodine for thyrotoxicosis accounts for approximately one-third of all cases. Excessive iodine (e.g. as a result of chronic ingestion of proprietary cough medicines) may also cause hypothyroidism. Primary hypothyroidism due to failure of the thyroid gland itself is much more common than failure secondary to pituitary dysfunction, or tertiary hypothyroidism due to

CAUSES OF HYPOTHYROIDISM

primary		secondary
congenital	**acquired**	pituitary tumours
athyreosis	iodine deficiency	pituitary granulomas (e.g. sarcoid) or injury
	autoimmunity	
ectopic thyroid	post-radioactive iodine therapy	'empty sella' syndrome
dyshormonogenesis	post-thyroidectomy	**tertiary**
	antithyroid drugs: thionamides e.g. carbimazole	
iodide deficiency	iodine excess	hypothalamic disorders e.g. craniopharyngioma, sarcoidosis
antithyroid immunity	subacute thyroiditis	isolated TRH deficiency
(transient due to illness)	thyroid irradiation	

Fig. 15.19 Causes of hypothyroidism. These can be broadly classified into 'congenital' and 'acquired' categories.

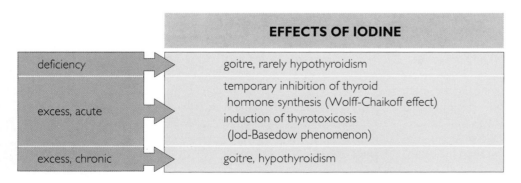

EFFECTS OF IODINE

deficiency	goitre, rarely hypothyroidism
excess, acute	temporary inhibition of thyroid hormone synthesis (Wolff-Chaikoff effect) induction of thyrotoxicosis (Jod-Basedow phenomenon)
excess, chronic	goitre, hypothyroidism

Fig. 15.20 Various effects of iodine on thyroid function. Whereas iodine deficiency will lead to goitre formation and rarely hypothyroidism, iodine excess can temporarily inhibit thyroid hormone synthesis (Wolff-Chaikoff effect) or induce thyrotoxicosis (Jod-Basedow phenomenon). Chronic iodine excess can also cause goitre formation and hypothyroidism.

hypothalamic disease. The effects of iodine on the thyroid gland are multiple and complex (Fig. 15.20).

Iodine deficiency today remains one of the world's most prevalent medical problems, despite years of effort to correct the problem through salt iodination or iodinated oil injections. Reduction of dietary iodine intake below the minimum daily requirement leads to reduced thyroid hormone production and a compensatory increase in TSH secretion. There is preferential secretion of T_3 rather than T_4. The frequency of goitre and of the occurrence of hypothyroidism is related to the degree of iodine deficiency. In areas of moderate endemic deficiency with urinary iodide excretion between 25 and $50\mu g/g$ creatinine, the prevalence of goitre is twenty to fifty per cent, but almost all individuals will be euthyroid. In areas with urinary iodide less than $25\mu g/g$ creatinine, as in the Andes, Himalayas, and Central Africa, goitre prevalence may be greater than fifty per cent, and some individuals in such communities are hypothyroid.

In excess iodine exposure, an acute increase in intracellular iodine concentration in normal glands interferes with iodination and temporarily inhibits thyroid hormone synthesis and release. The gland subsequently escapes from this effect perhaps by a reduction in the affinity of the iodide trap. Use has been made of this effect in preparing thyrotoxic patients for surgery by administration of iodide solution for several days prior to operation. This treatment blocks formation of hormone and also inhibits release of hormone from the thyroid gland.

The introduction of iodine therapy in areas of iodine deficiency has led to a temporary increase in the frequency of thyrotoxicosis (Jod-Basedow phenomenon) perhaps by unmasking thyroid autonomy that was previously protected by iodine deficiency. The phenomenon also occurs sporadically in patients given large doses of iodine (e.g. radiographic contrast media) in nonendemic areas.

Prolonged iodide ingestion (e.g. from proprietary cough medicines containing iodine) may lead to goitre formation and hypothyroidism in individuals with an underlying abnormality of thyroid hormone synthesis, such as occurs in patients with Hashimoto's thyroiditis. Congenital goitre and hypothyroidism may also be produced by maternal ingestion of excess iodides.

CONGENITAL HYPOTHYROIDISM

	TSH screening T_4 screening	1: ≃ 4,000 live births 1: ≃ 8,000 live births
	T_4	**TSH**
false positive	prematurity low TBG laboratory error	laboratory error
false negative	ectopic thyroid laboratory error	hypopituitarism laboratory error
recall rate	>1%	≃ 0.1%

Fig. 15.21 Incidence of congenital hypothyroidism using TSH or T_4 for screening. Neonates are screened five days after birth.

CONGENITAL HYPOTHYROIDISM

The incidence of congenital hypothyroidism in noniodine-deficient areas in Europe and North America is approximately one in four thousand live births. The condition usually results from absence of the thyroid or an ectopic thyroid and is often not recognisable clinically at birth. If not recognised and treated within three months, it leads to retarded physical and mental development.

Congenital hypothyroidism may be detected biochemically by screening all neonates five days after birth (Fig. 15.21). Persistent elevation of serum TSH at this stage will reveal hypothyroidism due to primary thyroid failure, but measurement of TSH will not detect the rare patient with hypothyroidism secondary to pituitary–hypothalamic disease. Low T_4 levels at this stage will also reveal secondary hypothyroidism, but false low T_4 levels may be found in premature infants, and misleading normal T_4 levels may occur with ectopic thyroids. Most screening is currently carried out using dried blood spots on filter paper and an assay of TSH. Replacement T_4 therapy should be commenced as soon as high TSH levels are detected.

HYPOTHYROIDISM AFTER RADIOIODINE THERAPY

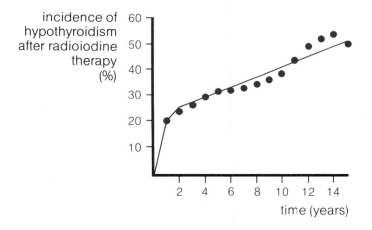

Fig. 15.22 Cumulative incidence of hypothyroidism after radioiodine therapy for thyrotoxicosis.

ACQUIRED HYPOTHYROIDISM

In noniodine-deficient communities, primary hypothyroidism is ten times more common in women than in men. The prevalence in women of all ages is two to four per cent of the population (with one-third of these cases presenting with iatrogenic hypothyroidism). The annual incidence of primary hypothyroidism in women of all ages is two per thousand population. It is most common in middle-aged women, but can occur at any age.

The incidence of hypothyroidism following radioiodine therapy is highest during the first year after treatment, regardless of the dose of ^{131}I, but continues to accumulate slowly and may reach fifty per cent after ten years (Fig. 15.22). The incidence of hypothyroidism after partial thyroidectomy, while less than that after radioiodine treatment, is also slowly cumulative and may reach twenty-five to thirty-five per cent after ten years. Hypothyroidism secondary to destructive therapy to the thyroid accounts for approximately one-third of all cases of hypothyroidism in the general population.

AUTOIMMUNE THYROID DISEASE AND HASHIMOTO'S THYROIDITIS

The term 'Hashimoto's thyroiditis' is probably best reserved for patients with a firm, diffuse goitre, often hypothyroidism, and evidence of an autoimmune process. Circulating autoantibodies are strongly positive. Histological examination of the thyroid shows diffuse lymphocytic infiltration, lymphoid follicles with germinal centres, and Askenazy cell change in the remnants of thyroid follicles (Fig. 15.23).

Focal lymphoid thyroiditis (Fig. 15.24) with normal follicles is a common finding at autopsy in patients without evidence of clinical thyroid disease during life. Such histological changes have been shown to correlate with the presence of thyroid antibodies in the circulation. Many patients with thyroid antibodies, while asymptomatic, can be shown to have minor biochemical disturbances of thyroid function, characterised by mild or moderately elevated TSH levels, while the serum T_4 is in the normal range. This is known as compensated or subclinical hypothyroidism.

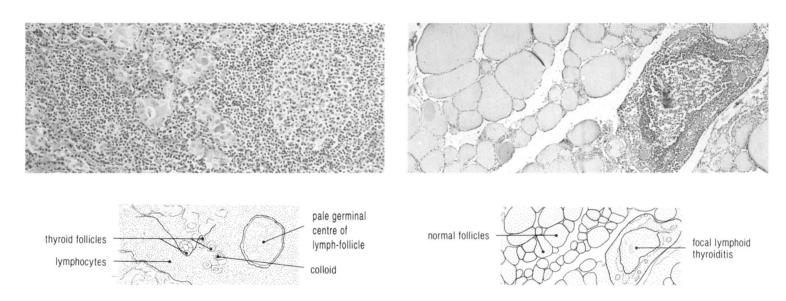

Fig. 15.23 *Histological appearance of the thyroid in a patient with Hashimoto's thyroiditis.* The parenchyma (comprising colloid-containing follicles) is almost totally replaced by oxyphil cells (Askenazy cell change). On the right of the field shown, a lymph follicle containing a large, pale, germinal centre can be seen. H and E stain, magnification × 80.

Fig. 15.24 *Focal lymphoid thyroiditis.* In this condition, most of the thyroid follicles are normal, but focal lymphoid infiltration is seen. The lymphocytes lie separately in a diffuse mass. H and E stain, magnification × 30.

THYROID ANTIBODIES AND RAISED TSH

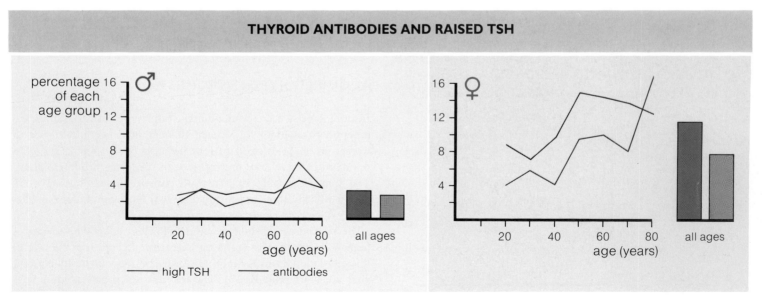

Fig. 15.25 *Prevalence of thyroid antibodies and raised TSH in a cross-section of a population in North East England.*

Thyroid microsomal and thyroglobulin antibodies are more common in women than in men at all ages and are most common in post-menopausal women (Fig. 15.25). Raised TSH values show a similar age and sex distribution, and there is a close correlation with thyroid antibodies.

Patients with thyroid antibodies may maintain normal thyroid function for their lifetime. Up to fifty per cent of people with thyroid antibodies, however, also have raised TSH levels, and such patients progress to overt hypothyroidism at the rate of approximately five per cent per annum. Prophylactic T₄ replacement therapy merits consideration in individuals with evidence of underlying autoimmune

thyroiditis and compensated hypothyroidism. Replacement therapy is used in patients with overt hypothyroidism and may also decrease goitre size.

SEVERE HYPOTHYROIDISM

In severe primary hypothyroidism, patients have thickened, dry, cool skin that does not pit as does the oedema of congestive cardiac failure, and thus is termed myxoedema (Fig. 15.26). The histology of the thyroid in a patient with severe myxoedema is shown in Fig. 15.27. The thyroid is replaced with fibrous tissue, there is minimal lymphocytic infiltration, and few follicles remain. This process is believed to be the end result of an autoimmune destructive process in most cases.

CLINICAL FEATURES IN HYPOTHYROIDISM

The symptoms of hypothyroidism (Fig. 15.28) are nonspecific and may be attributed by both patient and doctor to ageing, the onset usually being insidious. The diagnosis of hypothyroidism should be considered in the absence of other obvious explanations, particularly in older women with any of the above symptoms. These symptoms may be even less apparent in secondary hypothyroidism, depending upon the degree of failure of other pituitary hormones. Overt hypothyroidism with thickened, dry, cool skin, which led to the term myxoedema, is often well advanced before it is recognised clinically.

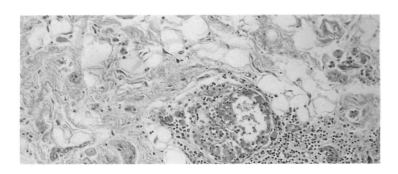

Fig. 15.26 A patient with myxoedema. A 'puffy' face, dry skin, diffuse capital hair loss, and skin pallor are characteristic of this condition.

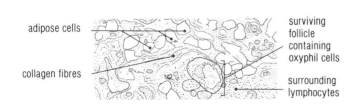

adipose cells

collagen fibres

surviving follicle containing oxyphil cells

surrounding lymphocytes

Fig. 15.27 Histology of the thyroid in a patient with severe myxoedema. There is severe destruction of the normal thyroid architecture, with much fibrous replacement. Some surviving parenchyma is present, and many lymphocytes can also be seen. H and E stain, magnification × 120. By courtesy of Prof I Doniach.

SYMPTOMS OF HYPOTHYROIDISM

usual	rare
lethargy	
increased sleep	
constipation	deafness
mild weight gain	
cold intolerance	psychosis
facial puffiness	
dry skin	cerebellar disturbance
hair loss	
hoarsensess	myotonia
abnormal menses	
acroparaesthesiae	
snoring	

Fig. 15.28 Symptoms of hypothyroidism.

PHYSICAL SIGNS OF HYPOTHYROIDISM

change in appearance
  e.g. face puffy and pale

periorbital oedema

dry, flaking, cool, pasty skin

diffuse hair loss

bradycardia

signs of median nerve
  compression
  (carpal tunnel syndrome)

effusions in body cavities
  e.g. ascites, pericardial effusion

delayed relaxation of reflexes

croaky voice

goitre

rarely stupor or coma

Fig. 15.29. Common physical signs of hypothyroidism.

The signs of hypothyroidism (Fig. 15.29) are nonspecific and are easily overlooked, especially if mild. These signs are usually even less apparent in secondary hypothyroidism when features of other pituitary hormone deficiencies tend to predominate.

CHANGES IN THE HYPOTHALAMO–PITUITARY–THYROID AXIS

In primary thyroid failure, the low circulating thyroid hormone levels stimulate the pituitary to increase TSH output (Fig. 15.30). The combination of low T_4 and a high basal TSH is therefore almost diagnostic of primary hypothyroidism. A normal basal TSH excludes primary hypothyroidism if the pituitary is intact. The TSH response to TRH is typically exaggerated, but the rise in TSH is proportional

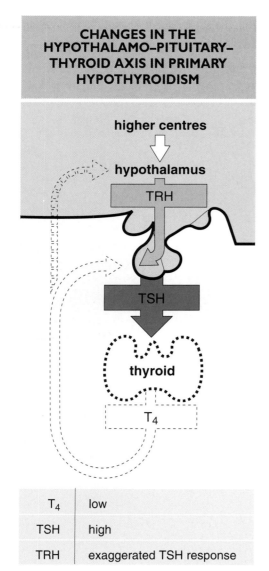

CHANGES IN THE HYPOTHALAMO–PITUITARY–THYROID AXIS IN PRIMARY HYPOTHYROIDISM

T_4	low
TSH	high
TRH	exaggerated TSH response

Fig. 15.30. Schematic representation of the changes in the hypothalamo–pituitary–thyroid axis in primary hypothyroidism. The TSH response is typically exaggerated.

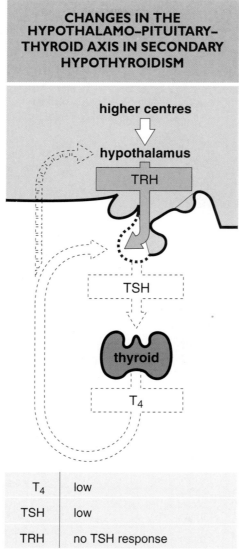

CHANGES IN THE HYPOTHALAMO–PITUITARY–THYROID AXIS IN SECONDARY HYPOTHYROIDISM

T_4	low
TSH	low
TRH	no TSH response

Fig. 15.31. Schematic representation of the changes in the hypothalamo–pituitary–thyroid axis in secondary hypothyroidism. In this situation, there is an absent TSH response to TRH because of pituitary disease.

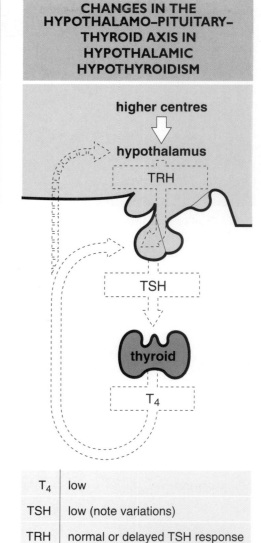

CHANGES IN THE HYPOTHALAMO–PITUITARY–THYROID AXIS IN HYPOTHALAMIC HYPOTHYROIDISM

T_4	low
TSH	low (note variations)
TRH	normal or delayed TSH response

Fig. 15.32. Schematic representation of the changes in the hypothalamo–pituitary–thyroid axis in hypothalamic hypothyroidism. In this form of 'tertiary' hypothyroidism, the sixty-minute TSH response in the TRH test is equal to or greater than the twenty-minute response. TSH measured by RIA may also be normal or increased in some patients (see text).

to the basal level, and the TRH test is seldom necessary. Serum T_3 levels may be normal, even though T_4 levels are low and TSH is raised. The preservation of normal T_3 levels may be interpreted as a compensatory mechanism of thyroid hormone production.

In secondary hypothyroidism, low circulating thyroid hormone levels are due to failure of TSH output as a result of pituitary disease (Fig. 15.31). The T_4 levels are low, as are the basal TSH levels. There is no TSH response to exogenous TRH in severe pituitary failure, but a blunted TSH response may still occur in less-severe pituitary disease. The T_3 levels may be normal despite low T_4 levels, as in primary hypothyroidism, therefore the measurement of T_3 is not a good diagnostic test for hypothyroidism of any origin. Some patients have mildly elevated TSH levels (6–10µu/ml). This paradox is explained by the finding that the TSH has low biological activity, since the normal thyrotrophs are not being stimulated by TRH, and the TSH is abnormally glycosylated.

Hypothalamic disease is a rare cause of thyroid failure. In such instances, circulating T_4 levels are low, T_3 may be normal or low, and basal TSH is normal or low (Fig. 15.32). The pituitary TSH response to exogenous TRH is usually sluggish and delayed, and values at sixty minutes are higher than at twenty minutes after TRH administration. A summary of the diagnostic tests for hypothyroidism is shown in Fig. 15.33. While a low T_4 is common to all causes of hypothyroidism, it is not absolutely diagnostic. This is because a variety of severe acute and chronic illnesses, together with interference of drugs in thyroid function tests, may also cause low T_4 values (Fig. 15.34). Thus, low TBG levels or competitive binding by drugs alters the binding capacity, and total T_4 levels are reduced, but free T_4 levels are usually normal. Even when TBG levels are not affected, severe illness may lower T_4 production and T_4 to T_3 conversion. rT_3 levels are usually increased, and TSH levels are normal. In asymptomatic autoimmune thyroiditis, total T_4 levels may be towards the lower limit of normal, but TSH levels are often mildly elevated.

TREATMENT

Hypothyroidism is treated with replacement T_4 therapy (Fig. 15.35). Replacement doses usually start at 50µg/d, being increased in a step-wise fashion at monthly intervals to 100–150µg/d as the response is assessed clinically and biochemically. When the patient is euthyroid, the TSH should be suppressed into the normal range and the T_4 levels also returned to normal. Typically, T_4 levels are just at top normal or above normal when patients are eumetabolic clinically on T_4 treatment, and TSH is normal. Maintenance therapy should be continued for life, and the patient should be rechecked annually. While most patients are replaced with 100–150µg/d of T_4, some patients may only require 75µg/d and others 200µg/d for full replacement therapy.

In patients with ischaemic heart disease, replacement therapy should be introduced cautiously, with starting doses of 25µg/d; increments should also be small. If an exacerbation of angina occurs, the dose of T_4 may need to be reduced and the patient also given a β–blocking agent (i.e. propranolol).

HYPOTHYROIDISM – SUMMARY OF DIAGNOSTIC TESTS			
	T_4	basal TSH	TRH response
primary hypothyroidism	low	raised	exaggerated
secondary hypothyroidism (pituitary)	low	low or normal	reduced or absent
tertiary hypothyroidism (hypothalamic)	low	low, normal or elevated	normal or delayed
non-thyroid illness	low	normal or low	normal or low

Fig. 15.33. A summary of diagnostic tests for hypothyroidism.

CAUSES OF A LOW SERUM T_4 IN CLINICALLY EUTHYROID PATIENTS

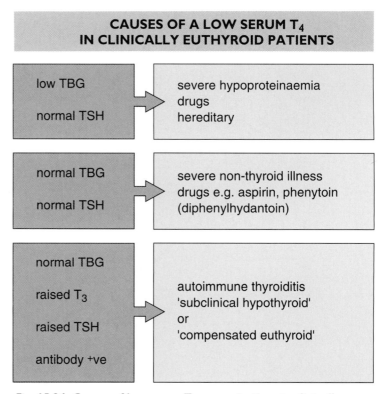

Fig. 15.34 Causes of low serum T_4 concentrations in clinically euthyroid patients.

Myxoedema coma is a rare complication of severe hypothyroidism but carries a mortality rate of over fifty per cent. It may be difficult to distinguish from hypothermia per se. Treatment is empirical, and the optimum form of management remains to be defined. One method is outlined in Fig. 15.36. As recovery proceeds, the dose of T_3 can be decreased over subsequent days and eventually changed to T_4 maintenance therapy. The dose of steroids can be reduced stepwise and 'tailed' off.

CHANGES IN TSH AND T_4 WITH T_4 REPLACEMENT THERAPY

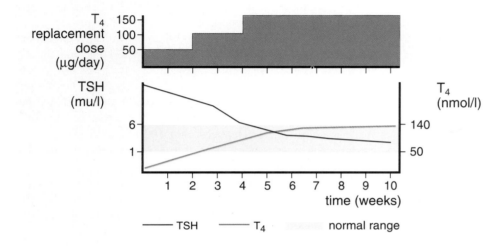

Fig. 15.35 Changes in serum TSH and T_4 with T_4 replacement therapy. With the gradual increase in T_4, the TSH slowly descends to the normal range.

PROTOCOL FOR THE MANAGEMENT OF MYXOEDEMA COMA

1   take blood for diagnostic tests: T_4, TSH and plasma cortisol

2   give 300µg T_4 i.v. and repeat approximately 100µg q.d; give via nasogastric tube if i.v. preparation is unaviable

3   maintain adequate ventilation

4   treat hypothermia with gradual rewarming using blankets

5   give i.m. hydrocortisone 75mg immediately and repeat 25–50mg 8-hourly

6   give T_3 20µg i.v, i.m. or by nasogastric tube 12-hourly, if possible

7   treat any heart failure with diuretics

8   correct any electrolyte disturbance

9   carefully exclude or treat infection

10   use sedative drugs and fluids sparingly

11   measure serum T_4, T_3 and TSH frequently

Fig. 15.36 A suggested plan for the management of myxoedema coma.

Carcinoma of the Thyroid

Israel Doniach, MD, FRCPath, FRCP

Carcinoma of the thyroid, which occurs worldwide (see Epidemiology – p. 16.10), is a rare cause of fatal malignant disease, accounting for some four hundred deaths each year in England and Wales, compared with thirty-five thousand from carcinoma of the lung and over thirteen thousand from carcinoma of the breast. The number of newly diagnosed cases of thyroid carcinoma reported annually averages seven hundred and fifty, the majority presenting as a solitary thyroid nodule that proves to be well differentiated and carries a good prognosis. Solitary nodules are comparatively common and must be investigated further, since approximately twelve per cent that are 'cold' on radioactive iodine or pertechnetate scan (i.e. take up less radioactivity than the surrounding normal thyroid) prove to be malignant. This percentage is higher still in children and young adults. Anaplastic thyroid carcinoma is rapidly fatal, but is much rarer

and occurs mostly in the elderly. A histopathological classification of thyroid malignancies is shown in Fig. 16.1. The follicular cell-differentiated carcinomas account for some eighty per cent of the total number of thyroid carcinomas, and the anaplastic carcinomas only fifteen per cent. The incidence of medullary carcinomas varies from five per cent to ten per cent, while that of malignant lymphomas is less than two per cent. Secondary tumours are often found at postmortem as microscopic deposits, sometimes within benign thyroid nodules.

Carcinoma of the thyroid is nearly three times more common in females than in males (Fig. 16.2). It occurs at all ages, and the standardised incidence per one hundred thousand women (Fig. 16. 3) rises steadily from the age of fifty-six years onwards. Although the clinical incidence in young people is high, mortality from thyroid

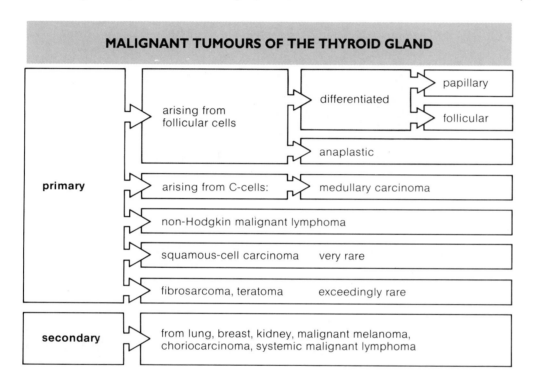

Fig. 16.1 A histopathological classification of malignant tumours of the thyroid gland.

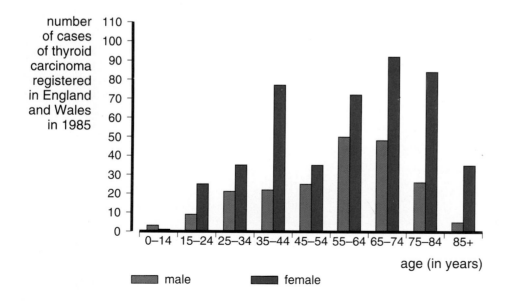

Fig. 16.2 The number of cases of thyroid carcinoma registered in England and Wales in 1985 for each age decade.

carcinoma occurs only in the middle-aged and the elderly (Fig. 16.4). Since the majority of differentiated carcinomas are either cured, cr allow the patient to live long enough to die of another cause, it follows that the prevalence of thyroid carcinoma far exceeds the number of patients who die annually from it.

The four major types of primary thyroid carcinoma (papillary, follicular, anaplastic, and medullary) are classified according to histology and clinical behaviour (Fig. 16.5). These are further divided into histopathological subtypes (Fig. 16.6) that correlate with prognosis.

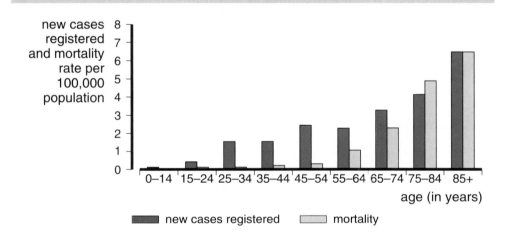

THE INCIDENCE OF THYROID CARCINOMA WITH AGE

Fig. 16.3 The incidence of thyroid carcinoma per 100,000 of the population in 1985. The greater incidence of this disease in middle-aged women and in the elderly of both sexes is shown.

NEW CASES OF THYROID CARCINOMA AND MORTALITY

Fig. 16.4 The number of new cases of thyroid carcinoma and the mortality per 100,000 of the population. There is negligible mortality in the younger age groups.

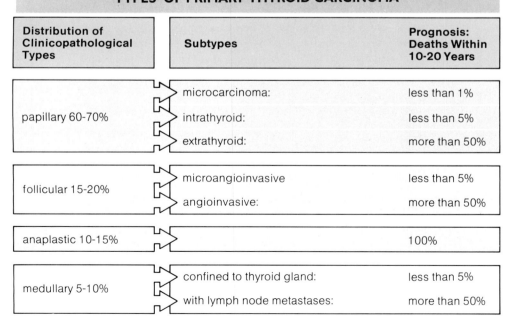

THE FOUR MAJOR CLINICOPATHOLOGICAL TYPES OF PRIMARY THYROID CARCINOMA

Fig. 16.5 Distribution and prognosis of the four major clinicopathological types of primary thyroid carcinoma.

Distribution of Clinicopathological Types	Subtypes	Prognosis: Deaths Within 10-20 Years
papillary 60-70%	microcarcinoma:	less than 1%
	intrathyroid:	less than 5%
	extrathyroid:	more than 50%
follicular 15-20%	microangioinvasive	less than 5%
	angioinvasive:	more than 50%
anaplastic 10-15%		100%
medullary 5-10%	confined to thyroid gland:	less than 5%
	with lymph node metastases:	more than 50%

PAPILLARY CARCINOMA

Papillary carcinoma is the most common type of thyroid carcinoma and occurs in all age groups. Since the majority of papillary carcinomas contain neoplastic follicles, in addition to neoplastic papillae, many authors classify mixed papillary and follicular carcinomas separately from pure papillary tumours. There is, however, no accepted evidence of any difference in clinical behaviour between the various types and the term 'papillary carcinomas' therefore includes all tumours that contain any neoplastic papillae. These tumours are predominantly lymphangioinvasive.

The three subtypes of papillary carcinoma are the microcarcinomas, the intrathyroid carcinomas, and the extrathyroid carcinomas. Microcarcinomas measure less than 1.5cm in diameter and are clinically occult. They are usually found unexpectedly in surgical thyroidectomy specimens: (for example, in patients with Graves' disease, colloid goitre, or Hashimoto's goitre, or in follicular adenomas). In these circumstances, follow-up has shown no evidence of either recurrence of the carcinoma or the development of metastases. Cervical lymph node metastases of papillary carcinomas are usually associated with a palpable primary tumour. Occasionally, however, an excision biopsy of a solitary enlarged cervical lymph node is found to contain a deposit of a papillary carcinoma, and the primary is subsequently demonstrated as an occult microcarcinoma of the ipsilateral lobe on thyroidectomy. Intrathyroid carcinoma presents as a palpable thyroid nodule, with or without enlarged cervical lymph nodes. On section, the tumour is seen to be confined within the thyroid, with no extension through the capsule of the gland. Extrathyroid carcinomas are usually larger and grow more rapidly than the other subtypes of papillary carcinomas. They are more common in older patients and

are found, at operation, to have penetrated the thyroid capsule and to have infiltrated adjacent tissues, including the strap-muscles.

Papillary carcinomas are made up of varying quantities of neoplastic papillae and follicles (Fig. 16.7). The papillae consist of elongated, branching fibrovascular cores covered by a single layer of epithelium. The follicles, however, may contain eosinophilic colloid or appear empty. The nuclei of the papillae and follicles in approximately sixty per cent of the tumours are characteristically empty-looking, with a prominent rim due to linear condensation of chromatin against the nuclear membrane. These nuclei are described as having a 'ground-glass' appearance and are large, misshapen, and overlapping. Two other characteristic appearances in occasional nuclei are the presence of a clearly circumscribed vacuole of intranuclear cytoplasmic invagination and nuclear grooving that resembles a coffee bean. Approximately fifty per cent of the tumours contain scattered, small, spherical, laminated, calcified bodies (psammoma bodies or calcospherites). These bodies are present in the fibrovascular core of the papillae, in the intervening connective tissue stroma, or even in the non-neoplastic thyroid stroma some distance from the tumour. In some cases there is an intense focal fibrous reaction, which may be seen as thick strands within the tumour, or as a pseudocapsule in which single or small clumps of atypical polygonal neoplastic cells lie embedded.

Occasionally, papillary carcinomas are grossly cystic – a change that can also be seen in the lymph node metastases. Over ninety per cent of papillary carcinomas, however, are nonencapsulated and discrete and vary in degree of local infiltration. On careful microscopy, other tumour foci may be found in both thyroid lobes; however, it is not possible to determine whether these are interstitial lymph-borne metastases or separate primaries including 'harmless' microcarcinomas.

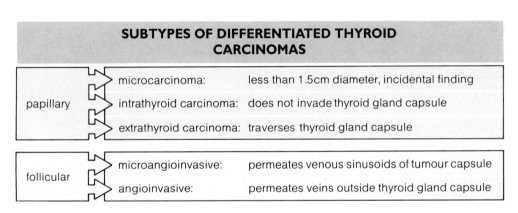

SUBTYPES OF DIFFERENTIATED THYROID CARCINOMAS		
papillary	microcarcinoma:	less than 1.5cm diameter, incidental finding
	intrathyroid carcinoma:	does not invade thyroid gland capsule
	extrathyroid carcinoma:	traverses thyroid gland capsule
follicular	microangioinvasive:	permeates venous sinusoids of tumour capsule
	angioinvasive:	permeates veins outside thyroid gland capsule

Fig. 16.6 The histopathological subtypes of differentiated carcinomas of the thyroid.

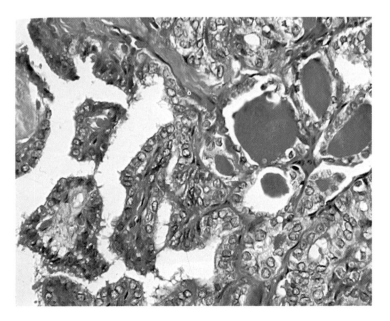

Fig. 16.7 Histology of papillary carcinoma. A typical mixture of neoplastic papillae and neoplastic colloid-containing follicles are shown. The nuclei are crowded, irregular in shape, and empty-looking. Haematoxylin and eosin (H&E) stain, magnification x 200.

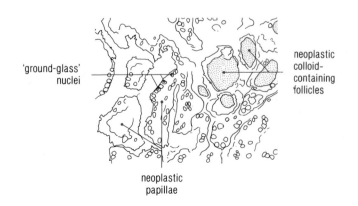

'ground-glass' nuclei

neoplastic colloid-containing follicles

neoplastic papillae

FOLLICULAR CARCINOMA

Follicular carcinomas are most common in middle-aged women and are comparatively rare in children and young adults. They predominantly invade blood vessels and are divided into two subtypes, microangioinvasive and angioinvasive. Microangioinvasive follicular carcinomas are well-differentiated encapsulated tumours whose major histological difference from adenomas is the presence of tumour tissue within the lumen of capsular venous sinusoids. The presence of bizarre giant nuclei within the tumour, and also of occasional mitoses and atypical differentiation, does not constitute malignancy in the absence of vascular invasion; such tumours are benign and are described as 'atypical adenomas'. Angioinvasive follicular carcinomas are less well differentiated, permeate veins outside the capsule of the thyroid gland, and may infiltrate through the tumour capsule into adjacent thyroid parenchyma and extrathyroid tissues.

Follicular carcinomas consist of a mixture of variably sized colloid-containing follicles, empty acini, and solid cords or alveoli of neoplastic cells (Fig. 16.8). They are surrounded by a well-defined capsule that is rich in arterioles, and also by venous sinusoids into which there are foci of capsular invasion extending into the venous sinusoid lumen. The less well-differentiated types of follicular carcinomas consist predominantly of trabeculae; they also show marked infiltration of the capsule and prominent invasion, not only of capsular venous sinusoids, but also of veins outside the capsule of the thyroid gland. A variant follicular carcinoma is the oxyphil (Hürthle or Askenazy) tumour in which most of the neoplastic cells are large with bizarre-shaped nuclei and voluminous cytoplasm and which contain abundant eosinophilic granules (mitochondria) (Fig. 16.9). Oxyphil change may also be seen in papillary carcinomas, adenomas and, focally, in non-neoplastic thyroid parenchyma – particularly in autoimmune thyroiditis (see Chapter 15). The major histological characteristics of the differentiated carcinomas are summarised in Fig. 16.10. Rare tumours of follicular and cell origin include columnar cell papillary carcinomas, diffuse sclerosing papillary carcinomas, clear cell carcinomas, and insular carcinomas. These variants tend to have a worse prognosis than the classical types.

ANAPLASTIC CARCINOMA

Anaplastic carcinomas occur in late middle age and in the elderly. Most tumours arise from a differentiated papillary or follicular carcinoma, sometimes with a long-standing history of goitre.

The tumours are undifferentiated (Fig. 16.11) with varying proportions of large spindle cells and giant cells, resembling a

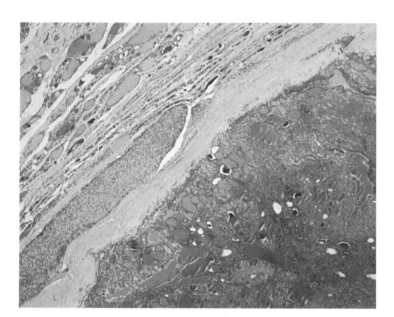

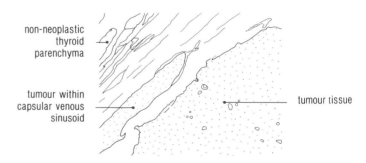

Fig. 16.8 Histology of follicular carcinoma. Follicular carcinomas consist of neoplastic colloid-containing follicles of varied sizes, separated by a thick fibrous capsule from normal thyroid parenchyma. The lumen of a large venous sinusoid in the capsule is almost filled by a plug of invasive tumour. H&E stain, magnification × 20.

Fig. 16.9 Histology of oxyphil follicular carcinoma. Large polygonal cells with an eosinophilic granular cytoplasm (due to proliferation of mitochondria) can be seen. H&E stain, magnification × 200.

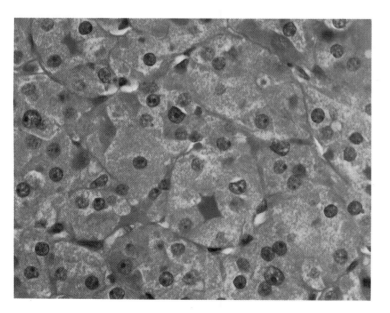

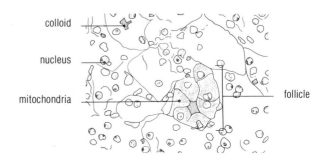

sarcoma. Mitoses are numerous, many being abnormal. Focal necrosis is often present. An undifferentiated small-cell type has also been found, although current opinion is that most tumours in this group are lymphomas.

MEDULLARY CARCINOMA

Medullary carcinomas are tumours of the calcitonin-secreting para-follicular C-cells and occur in males almost as frequently as in females. They represent a different entity from tumours of follicular cell origin since the parent C-cells are derived from neural crest cells that colonise the ultimobranchial bodies which fuse in early embryonic life with the thyroid anlage (which is itself derived from endodermal tissue).

Typically, these tumours are discrete and nonencapsulated and are made up of polygonal, round, or spindle-shaped cells arranged in sheets, nests or trabeculae, with prominent intervening collagenous stroma (Fig. 16.12). Amyloid is present in varying amounts, both within cell masses and in the stroma. The individual tumour cells show little variation in morphology, with stippled nuclei of regular shape and size and finely granulated cytoplasm. Surviving non-neoplastic thyroid follicles are incorporated into the periphery of the tumour. Occasionally, other patterns are seen, including glands and even mucin secretions.

HISTOLOGICAL CHARACTERISTICS OF THE DIFFERENTIATED CARCINOMAS

	papillary	follicular
capsule	–	+
papillae	+	–
follicles	+	+
'ground-glass' nuclei	+ (60%)	–
psammoma bodies	+ (50%)	–
additional tumour micro-foci	common	–
lymphatic spread	typical	rare
vascular spread	rare	typical

Fig. 16.10 Comparison of the histological characteristics of papillary and follicular carcinomas.

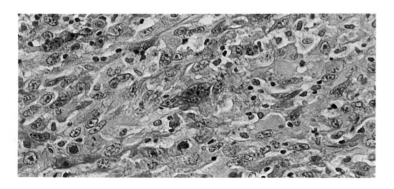

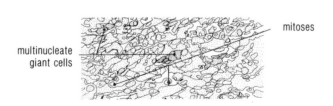

Fig. 16.11 Histology of anaplastic carcinoma. Large spindle and giant cells with bizarre-shaped nuclei are characteristic of this type of carcinoma. H&E stain, magnification × 200.

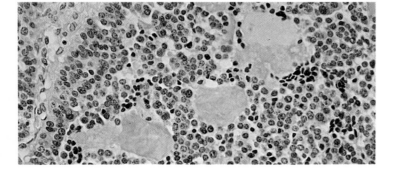

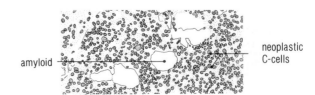

Fig. 16.12 Histology of medullary carcinoma. The tumour cells have round nuclei of regular appearance. Amorphous intercellular masses of pink, Congo-red positively stained amyloid deposits are also present. Haematoxylin and Congo-red stain, magnification × 200.

MALIGNANT LYMPHOMA

Malignant lymphomas are characterised by the replacement of large areas of thyroid parenchyma with lymphoma cells (Fig. 16.13). In the majority of cases the lesion is high grade, often immunoblastic, and the prognosis is poor. Most of the low-grade lymphomas are lymphoplasmacytoid. In over fifty per cent of the cases, surviving non-infiltrated parenchyma shows Hashimoto's thyroiditis.

IMMUNOSTAINING

Immunostaining of tumour sections with antithyroglobulin antibody is helpful in confirming the follicular cell origin of the differentiated carcinomas (Fig. 16.14), particularly in metastases of undetermined origin. Obtaining a positive reaction with anticalcitonin is now an essential step in the histological diagnosis of medullary carcinomas (Fig. 16.15). The majority of these tumours also give a positive immunoreaction with anticarcinoembryonic antigen. Other immunoreactive peptides that are occasionally demonstrable include somatostatin, gastrin-releasing peptide (or its fragment, known as bombesin), adrenocorticotrophic hormone (ACTH), and cortico-trophin-releasing hormone. During the past decade, case reports have indicated the existence of mixed follicular and medullary carcinomas: in one instance, positive immunostaining occurred with both antithyroglobulin and anticalcitonin in the same tumour cells. The identification of these mixed tumours has suggested that some follicular thyroid cells may have the capacity to differentiate into a C-cell phenotype or, alternatively, that some cells of ultimobranchial origin may differentiate to express a follicular phenotype.

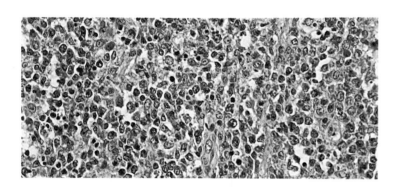

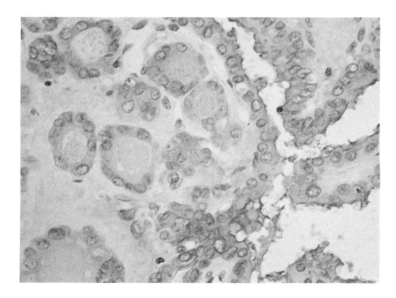

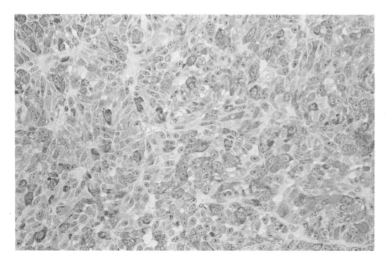

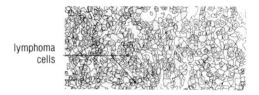

Fig. 16.13 Histology of non-Hodgkin's lymphoma. This consists of a diffuse proliferation of neoplastic lymphoid cells that have replaced normal thyroid parenchyma. The lymphoid cells are mixed lymphoplasmacytoid and immunoblastic in type. H&E stain, magnification × 200.

lymphoma cells

Fig. 16.14 Histological section of papillary carcinoma immunostained with antithyroglobulin. A positive brown reaction of varied intensity is present both in the tumour cells and the colloid.

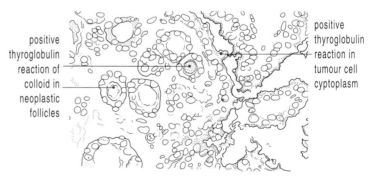

positive thyroglobulin reaction of colloid in neoplastic follicles

positive thyroglobulin reaction in tumour cell cyptoplasm

Fig. 16.15 Histological section of medullary carcinoma immunostained with anticalcitonin. A positive brown reaction of varied intensity is seen in the tumour cells.

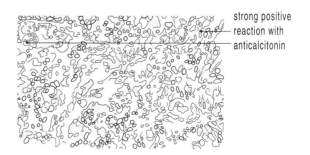

strong positive reaction with anticalcitonin

CLINICAL PRESENTATION OF MALIGNANT THYROID TUMOURS

A malignant thyroid tumour most commonly presents as a solitary nodule in one thyroid lobe or in the isthmus, often firm and indistinguishable from a colloid nodule or adenoma. The length of history is variable – in some patients the swelling is first noticed by a relative, while in other cases patients have been aware of the lump in the neck for some years. There are usually no systemic symptoms. Extrathyroid papillary carcinomas and angioinvasive follicular carcinomas present with more rapidly growing large tumours that may be associated with hoarseness, dysphagia, stridor, and dyspnoea. Enlarged cervical lymph nodes due to secondary deposits are found in approximately fifty per cent of the cases of papillary carcinoma and much less often in follicular carcinomas.

Intrathyroid papillary carcinomas and microangioinvasive follicular carcinomas are very slow-growing tumours in patients under the age of forty. This applies also to metastases, which may not become clinically apparent until five to ten or more years after the initial thyroidectomy; such metastases tend to occur either in the lymph nodes (papillary carcinomas) or in bones (follicular carcinomas). After the age of forty, previously diagnosed and newly diagnosed tumours show a tendency to grow and spread more rapidly, usually associated with less well-differentiated histopathology.

Papillary carcinomas may prove fatal as a result of lymphatic spread to the trachea, with resultant ulceration. More commonly, death occurs in papillary, follicular, and anaplastic carcinomas due to vascular spread to the lungs, brain, liver, and bones. Bone metastases usually involve the vertebrae, pelvis, and ribs; however, they may also occur in the long bones.

Anaplastic carcinomas give rise to a history of recent, very rapid enlargement of a normal or goitrous thyroid gland, with local pressure symptoms, particularly that of difficulty in breathing. On examination, the thyroid is markedly and asymmetrically enlarged by a large hard mass that is attached to adjacent structures. Vocal cord paralysis may also be present.

Malignant lymphoma of the thyroid may present as a thyroid nodule but more often causes gross symmetrical firm enlargement of the gland, and also dysphagia and dyspnoea, especially when the head is flexed. The condition may be mimicked by the fibrous variant of Hashimoto's goitre. The management, by a combination of radiotherapy and chemotherapy, is similar to that applied to lymphomas in other situations; thyroxine replacement is also indicated. Although the prognosis of high-grade lymphomas is very poor, it is better in low-grade tumours.

Diagnostic procedures vary between institutes. Following clinical examination, thyroid function tests and radiological examination of the neck, it is quite common to undertake a radioactive iodine or pertechnetate scan to determine whether the nodule is 'cold' (Fig. 16.16). In present times, however, increasing use is being made of fine-needle aspiration biopsy of thyroid nodules. Although cytopathologists can identify papillary (Fig. 16.17), anaplastic, and medullary carcinomas and lymphomas, it is not possible to differentiate between follicular adenomas and follicular carcinomas using cytological smears since the latter tumours require identification of vascular invasion for diagnosis. Additionally, it may be difficult to differentiate between colloid nodules and colloid-rich adenomas. Although false positives and false negatives have been reported to have occurred in a minority of cases, the procedure has proved to be extremely helpful (essential even) in the examination of a solitary

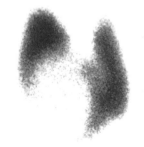

Fig. 16.16 A thyroid nodule: an area of decreased uptake on isotope scan. A 'cold' area in the lobe of the thyroid is shown. This appearance is due to a mass. Cysts, however, also display diminished uptake and an ultrasound scan is therefore needed in order to differentiate between a cyst and a solid lesion.

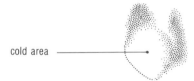

cold area ——————

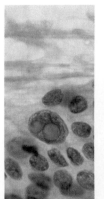
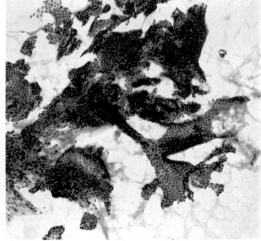

Fig. 16.17 Fine-needle aspiration biopsy of papillary carcinoma. (a) A high-power view showing a nucleus with a prominent, vacuolar, intranuclear, cytoplasmic invagination, typical of papillary carcinoma of the thyroid. (b) A low-power view showing branching solid clumps of cells. By courtesy of Drs Curling and Wells.

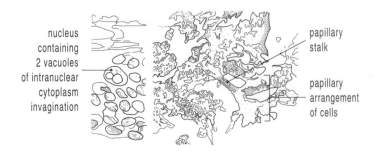

nucleus containing 2 vacuoles of intranuclear cytoplasm invagination

papillary stalk

papillary arrangement of cells

nodule. A clear-cut positive diagnosis of the carcinoma obviates the need for radioactive imaging.

Ultrasound scanning (Fig. 16.18) differentiates between cysts and solid lesions; differentiated carcinomas are only very occasionally cystic. A nodule that is 'cold' on scan may prove to be a benign cyst, a colloid nodule, an adenoma, part of an asymmetric Hashimoto's goitre, a differentiated carcinoma, or a medullary carcinoma. If a solitary intrathyroid tumour is found at operation, the surgeon may either carry out a lobectomy plus an isthmectomy and await the routine histology report, or send the lobe for frozen-section diagnosis. In the latter situation, the pathologist can usually rule out nonneoplastic lesions and positively recognise papillary carcinoma, provided that papillae are present in the sections taken. It is not necessarily possible with frozen sections to distinguish between adenomas and microangioinvasive follicular carcinomas but, with experience, medullary carcinomas can be recognised. Routine use of paraffin wax-embedded blocks allows much greater sampling of the tumour and more time for microscopy, and the histology of routine preparations is considerably easier to interpret than that of frozen sections. The more advanced thyroid carcinomas are usually recognisable macroscopically at operation and are radically dealt with if operable.

MANAGEMENT

The choice of an operative procedure for thyroid carcinomas varies with the surgeon's findings and predilections. In the more advanced cases, total thyroidectomy is performed with removal of macroscopically involved tissues and lymph nodes. The choice of three procedures for discrete, solitary, differentiated carcinomas is shown in Fig.16.19.

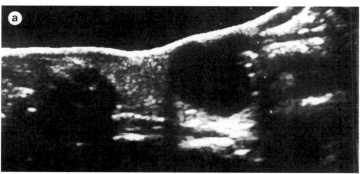

Fig. 16.18 Longitudinal ultrasound scans of thyroid lobes.
(a) A thyroid cyst. The right lobe of the thyroid is shown. The anechoic area in the lower pole and the increased through-transmission of sound behind it are characteristic of a simple thyroid cyst. (b) A thyroid tumour. The left lobe is shown containing a solid inhomogeneous mass. The reduced echogenicity around the mass suggests the presence of a capsule. It is not possible to differentiate between a benign tumour and a malignant tumour using ultrasound scans.

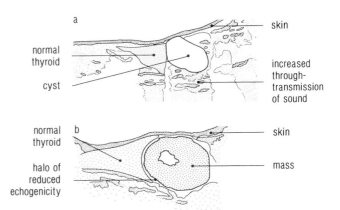

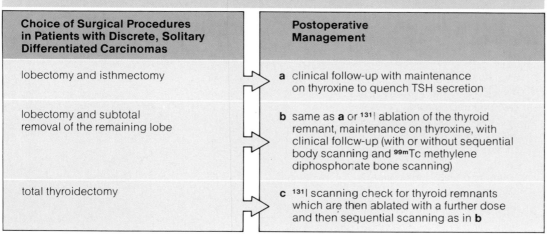

PROCEDURES FOR SURGERY AND POSTOPERATIVE MANAGEMENT OF DISCRETE SOLITARY DIFFERENTIATED CARCINOMAS

Choice of Surgical Procedures in Patients with Discrete, Solitary Differentiated Carcinomas	Postoperative Management
lobectomy and isthmectomy	a clinical follow-up with maintenance on thyroxine to quench TSH secretion
lobectomy and subtotal removal of the remaining lobe	b same as a or 131I ablation of the thyroid remnant, maintenance on thyroxine, with clinical follow-up (with or without sequential body scanning and 99mTc methylene diphosphonate bone scanning)
total thyroidectomy	c 131I scanning check for thyroid remnants which are then ablated with a further dose and then sequential scanning as in b

Fig. 16.19 The choice of procedures for surgery and postoperative management of discrete, solitary, differentiated carcinomas.

Lobectomy and subtotal removal of the remaining lobe is usually advocated in order to remove an occult carcinoma in the apparently normal lobe and to ensure preservation of parathyroid tissue. There is also a choice of postoperative management. Scanning is initially carried out at six-monthly intervals, and subsequently at longer intervals until the patient is deemed cured; the patient, however, should continue to attend for clinical follow-up.

During the six months before each scan, the patient is maintained on triiodothyronine (T_3). During the seven days preceding each scan, however, the patient should discontinue T_3. At other times, the patient is maintained on thyroxine (T_4).

The objections raised against simple lobectomy are the possibility of the presence of an occult tumour in the apparently normal lobe and the need to ablate the thyroid for follow-up scans and treatment of metastases that might arise. The arguments in favour of simple lobectomy are that recurrences or new primaries in the residual lobe do not occur after the operation in cases of microangioinvasive follicular carcinoma and are very rare in cases of intrathyroid papillary carcinoma. If metastases are subsequently found on clinical follow-up, it is possible to ablate the residual lobe and still treat these very slow-growing tumours. The more conservative approach in young patients, and the more radical approach in patients over forty years of age at the time of initial diagnosis, should be favoured.

Many now advocate undertaking follow-up measurements of serum thyroglobulin levels. Metastases from differentiated papillary and follicular thyroid carcinomas are associated with a raised serum thyroglobulin level of more than 10µg/ml in patients with an ablated thyroid that is maintained on T_4 replacement. Alternatively, provided that no normal thyroid tissue is present, serum thyroglobulin may be measured two weeks after withdrawal of maintenance T_3 or four to six weeks after withdrawal of T_4. A raised thyroglobulin level in the follow-up after initial treatment is an indication to determine the presence of metastatic disease. In general, a consecutive series of thyroglobulin assays, together with clinical assessment, can prove sufficient follow-up in many cases. Metastases, however, may rarely be present despite undetectable thyroglobulin levels.

TREATMENT OF ANAPLASTIC CARCINOMA

When anaplastic carcinomas are suspected, it is customary to carry out a needle biopsy for histological confirmation, followed by initiation of a course of radiotherapy to the neck, even in the presence of known metastases. Untreated anaplastic carcinomas infiltrate the trachea and may ulcerate through the skin.

CLINICAL ASPECTS OF MEDULLARY CARCINOMA

Approximately eighty per cent of medullary carcinomas are sporadic and twenty per cent familial, the latter showing an autosomal dominant inheritance with strong penetrance. In sporadic cases, the clinical presentation is usually that of a solitary hard thyroid nodule that is 'cold' on scan. Involvement of cervical lymph nodes at presentation is observed in some fifty per cent of cases, when chest radiography may show additional involvement of the upper mediastinum.

The clinical symptoms that may be associated with sporadic and familial cases are summarised in Figs. 16.20 and 16.21. The diarrhoea is severe and watery due to a combination of intestinal hurry and excessive secretion. It is relieved by removal of the tumour and recurs with metastases. The cause of the secretion has not been identified but calcitonin, a bradykinin-producing kallikrein, prostaglandins, and vasoactive intestinal peptide have all been implicated. The peptide hormones that have been identified in tumour tissue and in the blood are also listed in Fig. 16.20. The basal level of calcitonin is high and rises greatly after a provocative infusion of ionised calcium or following the oral administration of alcohol or pentagastrin. In all of the familial syndromes that lead to medullary carcinomas (see Fig. 16.21), the thyroid shows marked hyperplasia of C-cells plus two or more medullary carcinomas. In types 2 and 3, the adrenals show bilateral medullary hyperplasia and multiple phaeochromocytomas. These might present clinically before or after the thyroid tumours. In type 3, the mucosal neuromas are present on the eyelids, lips, and tongue of patients, and there may be ganglioneuromatosis of the small and large intestines. These patients have thick blubbery lips, marfanoid habitus, high arched palate, and pes cavus. In all types, relatives of clinically diagnosed patients must be screened routinely for the presence of raised calcitonin and, in types 2 and 3, for raised catecholamine secretions.

Sporadic and medullary carcinomas vary in their degree of malignancy. In some the condition is cured by thyroidectomy, while in others, especially in patients who present initially with lymph node metastases, the tumour may metastasise widely within one or two years to mediastinal nodes, lungs, bones, and the liver.

EPIDEMIOLOGY

The incidence of newly reported cases of thyroid carcinomas shows considerable geographical variation (Fig. 16.22) – from less than one per one hundred thousand women in Hamburg, to nine per one hundred thousand women in Hawaii. This is thought to be a result

Fig. 16.20 The associated clinical syndromes and peptide hormones secreted by medullary carcinomas.

MEDULLARY CARCINOMA

associated clinical syndromes		peptide hormones secreted	
intractable diarrhoea	in 20% of cases	calcitonin	always
		somatostatin	common
		carcinoembryonic antigen	common
		gastrin releasing peptide (bombesin)	common
		histaminase	common
carcinoid syndrome	rare	serotonin	rare
		ACTH	rare
		corticotrophin releasing activity	very rare
		prolactin stimulating activity	very rare
Cushing's syndrome	very rare	nerve growth factor	very rare

of ethnic and environmental factors. Geographical variation is also seen in the distribution of histological types that are associated with iodine content of the diet (Fig. 16.23). In areas of iodine deficiency (present or past), follicular carcinomas are more predominant than papillary carcinomas, and the converse is true where iodine is readily available. Reports from Switzerland have shown a decrease in percentage of follicular carcinomas and an increase in papillary carcinomas following the iodisation of salt. In Iceland, where the dietary intake of iodine is unusually large, the high incidence of thyroid malignancy is due mainly to papillary carcinomas. An interesting finding has been the variation in geographical incidence of microcarcinomas in step-sectioned postmortem glands in women – from seven per cent in Colombia, to twenty-eight per cent in Japanese residents in Hawaii. The equivalent figures for men were five per cent and twenty per cent, respectively.

TYPES OF FAMILIAL INHERITANCE OF MEDULLARY CARCINOMA

1 medullary carcinoma alone

2 medullary carcinoma and phaeochromocytoma

3 medullary carcinoma, phaeochromocytoma and mucosal neuromas

hyperparathyroidism due to parathyroid adenoma or hyperplasia may be associated with any of the three types, especially 2

Fig. 16.21 Types of familial inheritance of medullary carcinoma.

GEOGRAPHICAL INCIDENCE OF THYROID CARCINOMA

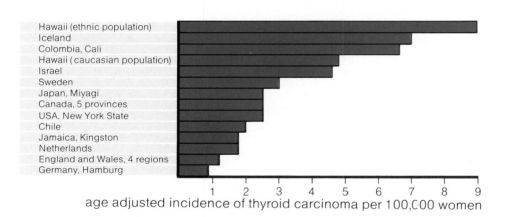

Hawaii (ethnic population)
Iceland
Colombia, Cali
Hawaii (caucasian population)
Israel
Sweden
Japan, Miyagi
Canada, 5 provinces
USA, New York State
Chile
Jamaica, Kingston
Netherlands
England and Wales, 4 regions
Germany, Hamburg

1 2 3 4 5 6 7 8 9
age adjusted incidence of thyroid carcinoma per 100,000 women

Fig. 16.22 The variation in incidence of thyroid carcinoma with geographical location.

author		number of cases		papillary/ follicular ratio	country
		papillary	follicular		
Woolner	1968	736	208	3.5:1	USA (Mayo clinic)
Russell	1973	552	124	4.5:1	USA (Texas)
Lindsay	1960	178	76	2.3:1	USA (San Francisco)
Correa	1969	105	169	0.6:1	Colombia (Cali)
Silink	1966	43	81	0.5:1	Czechoslovakia
Heitz	1976	145	225	0.6:1	Switzerland (Basel)

RATIO OF PAPILLARY TO FOLLICULAR THYROID CARCINOMA IN VARIOUS SERIES

normal dietary iodine

low dietary iodine

Fig. 16.23 The incidence of papillary carcinoma compared with that of follicular carcinoma. This rises with an increase in dietary iodine and varies geographically.

AETIOLOGICAL CONSIDERATIONS

The possible aetiological factors associated with thyroid carcinoma are listed in Fig. 16.24. In the past, the two major aetiological factors were thought to be iodine deficiency with its accompanying maintained stimulation of thyroid-stimulating hormone (TSH), and malignant change in a long-standing adenoma. Epidemiological surveys have not confirmed any excess incidence of thyroid malignancy in iodine-deficient areas. Current opinion is that malignant change in an adenoma must be a rare event since adenomas are common and follicular carcinomas are rare.

A major and definite aetiological factor that has been demonstrated is ionising radiation to the thyroid gland, given, in the past in some centres, in nonsterilising dosages to infants and children. Doses reported to have induced thyroid carcinoma vary from a few Gy (1Gy=100 rad) given to epilate the scalp in the treatment of ringworm, to 15Gy (1,500 rad) for the treatment of tuberculous glands in the neck. Other conditions include prophylactic irradiation of the thymus in infants and also therapeutic irradiation of acne, enlarged tonsils, skin tumours of the head and neck, and Hodgkin's and non-Hodgkin's lymphomas of the cervical lymph nodes. The carcinogenic risk factor has been calculated to be one per cent per 1Gy (100rad) in twenty years. The latent period is approximately ten to twenty years, or even longer. Occasional cases have been reported in irradiated adults. Therapeutic sterilising doses of radiation to the thyroid (for example radiological treatment of laryngeal carcinoma or ^{131}I treatment of Graves' disease) are not associated with cancer induction; in fact, such patients are liable to develop hypothyroidism.

Histology of the thyroid parenchyma in papillary carcinomas shows an increased incidence of focal lymphocytic thyroiditis, usually considered to be an effect rather than a cause. In view of the frequency of occult papillary microcarcinomas, it has been suggested that these might be *in situ* carcinomas that are sometimes promoted to invasive tumours by unknown endogenous factors or by environmental factors, or by both.

POSSIBLE AETIOLOGICAL FACTORS IN THYROID CARCINOMA	
iodine deficiency goitre	no clear evidence
precursor adenoma	possibly, rarely
precursor occult papillary microcarcinoma	possibly
ionising radiation	yes
dyshormonogenesis	yes, rarely
autoimmune thyroiditis	no
excessive iodine consumption	possibly
genetic	familial medullary carcinoma

Fig. 16.24 The possible aetiological factors implicated in thyroid carcinoma. Ionising radiation is a major cause.

17

Hyperthyroidism and Graves' Disease

Reginald Hall, CBE, MD, FRCP

Hyperthyroidism, the clinical condition that results from increased circulating levels of free (nonprotein-bound) thyroid hormones, is one of the most common endocrine disorders. It occurs in some 1.8 per cent of the adult population, but is much rarer in childhood. Women are affected more often than men (10:1), and the age of occurrence varies with the variety of hyperthyroidism.

Hyperthyroidism usually results from autoimmune thyroid disease (Fig. 17.1). Graves' disease (Fig. 17.2) is a useful term to describe a combination of eye signs, goitre, and hyperthyroidism (classical Graves' disease), and more rarely of localised myxoedema and thyroid acropachy. Variants of the Graves' disease syndrome (Fig. 17.3) include ophthalmic Graves' disease, where the eye signs of Graves' disease occur in the absence of hyperthyroidism or a history of past

hyperthyroidism; the patient is usually euthyroid but may be subclinically or clinically hypothyroid. Neonatal Graves' disease (Fig. 17.4) is transient and remits as the stimulating antibodies disappear from the circulation of the child.

Intrauterine fetal or neonatal hyperthyroidism can occur in cases in which a woman with previously treated Graves' disease has persisting stimulating antibodies to the thyroid-stimulating hormone (TSH) receptor (TSH-R). If stimulating [TSH-R(s)] and blocking [TSH-R(b)] antibodies are present in the maternal circulation, the onset of neonatal hyperthyroidism may be delayed, depending on the titre and affinity of the different antibodies that interact with the TSH-R. Graves' disease in children (Fig. 17.5) has a number of special features (Fig. 17.6).

CAUSES OF HYPERTHYROIDISM

most common causes

autoimmune thyroid diseases
  Graves' disease
  neonatal Graves' disease
  postpartum thyroiditis
  silent thyroiditis
toxic nodular goitre (including disseminated thyroid autonomy)
toxic adenoma

rarer causes

Jod–Basedow phenomenon
amiodarone-induced hyperthyroidism
de Quervain's subacute thyroiditis
factitious hyperthyroidism
  thyroid hormones
  hamburger-induced hyperthyroidism
hCG hyperthyroidism
  hyperemesis gravidarum
  hydatidiform mole
  choriocarcinoma
struma ovarii
thyroid carcinoma
  in situ
  metastatic
hypothalamopituitary
  selective pituitary resistance to thyroid hormones
  thyrotroph adenoma

Fig. 17.1 Causes of hyperthyroidism. Autoimmune thyroid disease is the most common cause of hyperthyroidism. Postpartum thyroiditis, although common, is usually biochemical, subclinical, and transient. Graves' disease is the most common cause of clinical hyperthyroidism worldwide, although in areas of iodine deficiency, toxic nodular goitre and toxic adenoma make up a greater proportion of cases. In North America, silent thyroiditis and de Quervain's thyroiditis are seen more frequently than in Europe.

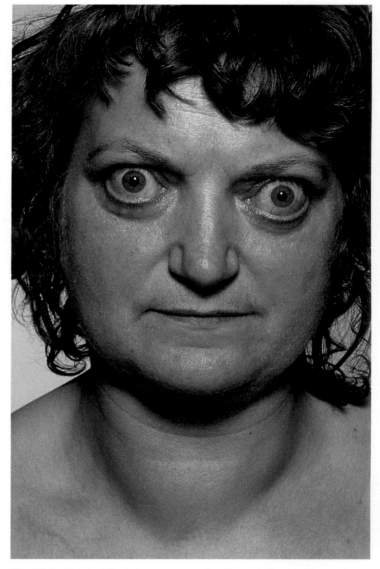

Fig. 17.2 Typical facial appearance in Graves' disease. The patient has a goitre, bilateral lid retraction, and exophthalmos.

GRAVES' DISEASE AND ITS VARIANTS

classical

ophthalmic

neonatal and its variants

potential

latent

Fig. 17.3 Graves' disease and its variants. Classical Graves' disease with hyperthyroidism, goitre, and eye signs is by far the most common. Ophthalmic Graves' disease is rarer and presents more often to the ophthalmologist or to the ear, nose and throat surgeon. It must be distinguished from a space-occupying lesion that affects the orbit. Neonatal Graves' disease is rare and results from the transplacental passage of TSH-R(s) antibodies from a mother with Graves' disease to her child; it is a self-limiting disease. The term potential Graves' disease can be applied to the unaffected identical twin of a patient with Graves' disease or siblings of such a patient who have identical HLA haplotypes. Latent Graves' disease can be used to describe patients in remission following treatment.

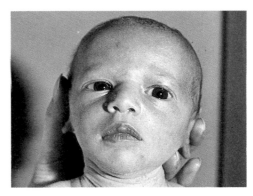

Fig. 17.4 Neonatal Graves' disease. The child shows features of hyperthyroidism and has a small goitre and minimal eye signs.

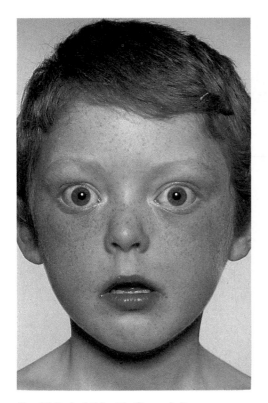

Fig. 17.5 A child with Graves' disease. Juvenile Graves' disease is rare and usually relapses after a course of antithyroid drugs.

GRAVES' DISEASE IN CHILDHOOD	
type	**particular features**
Graves' disease *in utero* neonatal Graves' disease	result from high maternal levels of TSH-R(s) antibodies crossing the placenta
delayed-onset neonatal Graves' disease	depends on relative titres and affinities of TSH-R(s) and TSH-R(b) antibodies
juvenile Graves' disease	may be complicated by cranial synostosis with premature fusion skull sutures there is a high tendency to relapse after courses of antithyroid drugs

Fig. 17.6 Graves' disease in childhood. Graves' disease is rare in children and shows a number of differences from the disease that occurs in adults.

COMMON CAUSES OF HYPERTHYROIDISM: AUTOIMMUNE THYROID DISEASES

Graves' disease is one of the autoimmune thyroid diseases (Fig. 17.7). Patients with Hashimoto's disease are predominantly female (5:1) and have a firm, finely nodular goitre. They are commonly euthyroid, but may be hypo- or hyperthyroid. Lymphocytic thyroiditis is the term used to describe a mild form of Hashimoto's disease, in which the patient is euthyroid, usually with a small firm goitre that histologically shows less-intense lymphocytic infiltration. Up to ten per cent of apparently normal adult women in the general population have this thyroid disorder and are asymptomatic.

Myxoedema refers to patients with overt hypothyroidism with an atrophic thyroid. Postpartum thyroiditis affects some five per cent of all women postpartum and may pass through hyperthyroid and then hypothyroid phases. The hypothyroidism, although usually temporary, may be permanent. Silent thyroiditis refers to a variety of self-limiting, painless and destructive hyperthyroidism, seen particularly in North America and related both to postpartum thyroiditis and Graves' disease.

The autoimmune thyroid diseases are members of the group of organ-specific autoimmune disorders that occur predominantly in women and may be associated in a single patient or in different members of an affected patient's family (Fig. 17.8). These disorders can be contrasted with the nonorgan-specific autoimmune disorders where antibodies arise to antigens that are not confined to a specific organ, as seen with the various antinuclear antibodies in systemic lupus erythematosus (SLE). Occasionally, the organ-specific and nonorgan-specific diseases occur in a given patient: for example, a woman may rarely show Hashimoto's disease and also SLE.

PATHOGENESIS OF GRAVES' DISEASE

Thyroid autoantibodies in Graves' disease react with three main autoantigens (Fig. 17.9): thyroglobulin; thyroid microsomes (now identified as the thyroid peroxidase (TPO) enzyme that is involved in the biosynthesis of thyroid hormones); and the TSH-R. All of these

---

AUTOIMMUNE THYROID DISEASES

Graves' disease and its variants

Hashimoto's disease

lymphocytic thyroiditis

myxoedema

postpartum thyroiditis

silent thyroiditis

Fig. 17.7 Autoimmune thyroid diseases. These are characterised by the presence of circulating antithyroid antibodies; a variable degree of lymphocytic infiltration of the thyroid, which is usually enlarged; differing levels of thyroid function, which may fluctuate spontaneously; and a strong female preponderance.

ORGAN-SPECIFIC AUTOIMMUNE DISEASES

endocrine	nonendocrine
Addison's disease	pernicious anaemia
premature ovarian failure	vitiligo
male infertility with antisperm antibodies	alopecia areata/totalis
	leucotrichia (white hair tufts)
primary hypoparathyroidism	premature greying of the hair
lymphocytic hypophysitis	halo naevi
insulin-dependent diabetes mellitus	allergic alveolitis
	chronic hepatitis
	primary biliary cirrhosis
	renal tubular acidosis
	myasthenia gravis
	Sjögren's syndrome

Fig. 17.8 Organ-specific autoimmune diseases. These may be endocrine or nonendocrine. Affected patients may exhibit circulating antibodies to an antigen in an affected organ that shows lymphocytic infiltration.

autoantigens have been cloned. The structure of the TSH-R, a glyco-protein, is shown in Fig. 17.10 in diagrammatic form, while Fig. 17.11 shows the mechanism of interaction of TSH with TSH-R(s) antibodies. The target autoantigen in patients with Graves' ophthal-mopathy remains controversial. The gene for a 64-kDa membrane protein of the eye muscle has recently been cloned. IgG antibodies to this antigen are found in many normal human sera, although increased concentrations are detected in the sera of Graves' ophthal-mopathy patients. The anti-64kDa antibodies may merely represent natural autoantibodies that react with recurrent autoepitopes.

The hyperthyroidism and goitre of Graves' disease result from the interaction of TSH-R(s) antibodies with the TSH-R, mimicking the action of TSH. In some patients, TSH-R antibodies bind to the TSH-R but fail to activate it; these blocking antibodies – TSH-R(b) – which are also found in some patients with Hashimoto's disease, myxoedema, and neonatal hypothyroidism, may contribute to the development of hypothyroidism and possibly to the remission of hyperthyroidism. Graves' disease is one of the receptor antibody diseases (Fig. 17.12).

AUTOANTIGENS IN AUTOIMMUNE THYROID DISEASE

	thyroglobulin	thyroid peroxidase	TSH-R
protein	iodinated glycoprotein	haemoprotein enzyme	G-binding protein-linked receptor
glycosylated	+	+	+
function	biosynthetic precursor of T3 and T4	catalyses iodination and coupling of tyrosine to yield T3 and T4	receptor for TSH
thyroid location	follicular lumen	membrane-bound cell surface (apical) exo-/endocytotic vesicles	membrane-bound cell surface (basal)
molecular weight	660,000	105,000 110,000	86,000
amino acids	2,748	TPO-1,933 TPO-2,876 alternatively spliced products	764 (excludes 20 amino-acid signal sequence)
region extracellular transmembrane		842(TPO-I) 29	418 265 (7 transmembrane domains)
intracellular		62	81
chromosome location	8	2	14
homologies	acetylcholinesterase receptors	myeloperoxidase	luteinising hormone/human chorionic gonadotrophin, follicle-stimulating hormone receptors

Fig. 17.9 Autoantigens in autoimmune thyroid disease. Modified from McGregor (1992) by courtesy of Oxford University Press.

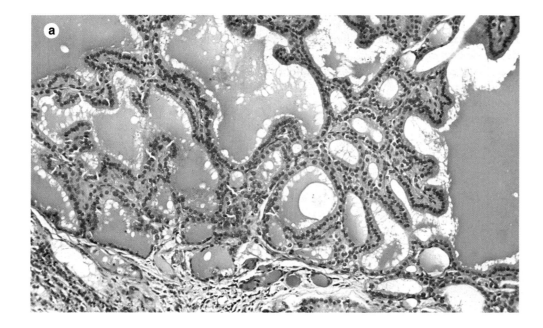

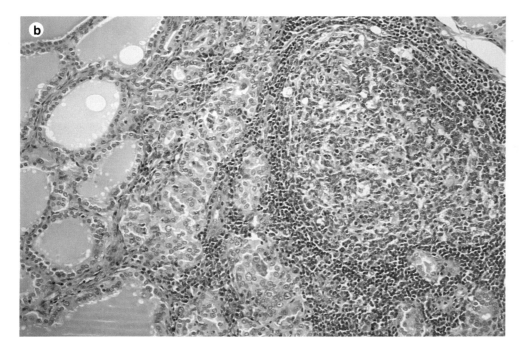

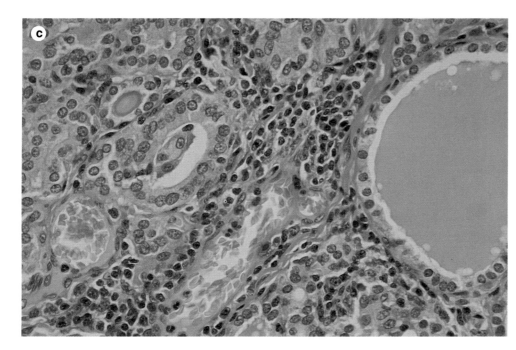

Fig. 17.23 Histology of thyroid tissue in Graves' disease. (a) A high-power view showing tall, unfolded columnar epithelium, together with scalloping of follicular colloid. (b) A low-power view of Graves' thyroid tissue showing a large lymphoid follicle with a well-formed germinal centre, immediately adjacent to which are hyperplastic thyroid follicles surrounded by a diffuse lymphoplasmacytic infiltrate. Further afield are partially suppressed thyroid follicles that are lined with tall cuboidal epithelium and contain colloid material showing the typical scalloping artefact. (c) A high-power view of hyperplastic thyroid follicles surrounded by a plasma cell-rich infiltrate. A profile of a single, partially suppressed thyroid follicle is included in the extreme right of the frame for comparison. (Haematoxylin and eosin staining of tissue sections that are 5μm in thickness, taken from a routinely formalin-fixed and paraffin-embedded subtotal thyroidectomy specimen.)

Exophthalmos

Protrusion of the globe from the lateral orbital margin (Fig. 17.24) can be measured using a Hertel exophthalmometer. If proptosis is present, the sclera is visible between the cornea and the lower lid, and the cornea protrudes by more than 18mm. Although exophthalmos is usually bilateral (Fig. 17.25), it may be unilateral (Fig. 17.26).

Asymmetry of more than 5mm is rare in Graves' disease and raises the suspicion of a space-occupying lesion that affects the orbit (Fig. 17.27).

A computerised tomography (CT) scan of the orbit, or magnetic resonance image (MRI) scanning (Fig. 17.28), can be used to demonstrate the characteristic extraocular muscle enlargement in Graves' disease.

Lid Retraction

In the relaxed position of forward gaze, the upper lid normally covers 3–4mm of the cornea. In Graves' disease, spasm of the striated levator palpebrae superioris results in elevation of the upper lid, with sclera

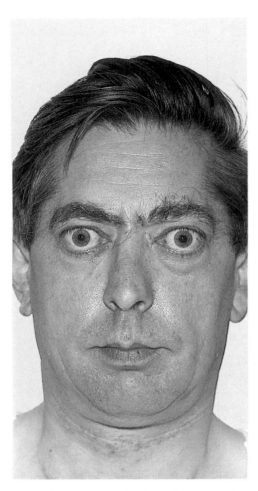

Fig. 17.24 Proptosis in Graves' disease. The eye protrudes from the lateral orbital margin by more than 18mm. In this case, sclera is visible both below the cornea (proptosis) and also above (lid retraction).

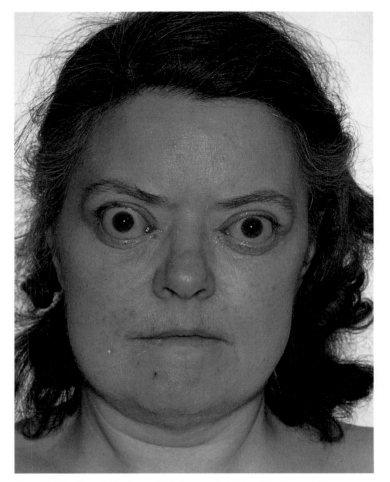

Fig. 17.25 Exophthalmos. This is usually bilateral in Graves' disease with hyperthyroidism.

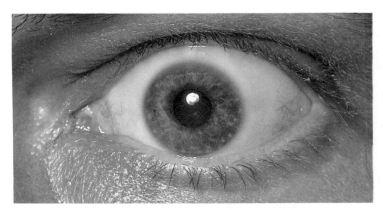

Fig. 17.26 Unilateral exophthalmos and lid retraction.

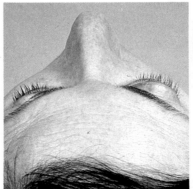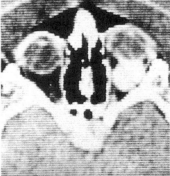

Fig. 17.27 Asymmetrical exophthalmos in excess of 5mm. This degree of asymmetry is unusual in Graves' disease, and its presence should raise the suspicion of a retro-orbital tumour.

visible above the cornea, and a stare (Fig. 17.29). Increased sympathetic tone due to hyperthyroidism from any cause may contribute to the lid elevation by stimulation of the sympathetically innervated Müller's muscle. Bilateral lid retraction (Fig. 17.30) is highly suggestive of Graves' disease but it can be seen, rarely, in lesions (usually vascular) that affect the upper brain stem. Ptosis is a rare eye sign of Graves' disease and may be unilateral or bilateral (Fig. 17.31). Its presence should always raise the possibility of myasthenia gravis, which can itself be associated with the autoimmune thyroid diseases.

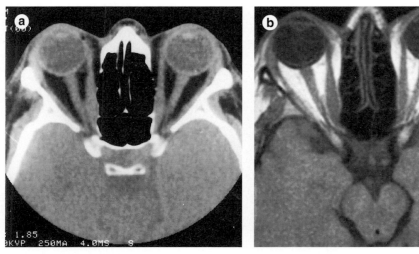

Fig. 17.28 CT and MRI scans in Graves' disease. (a) CT scan of the orbits in ophthalmic Graves' disease. The scan shows the characteristic enlargement of the medial rectus muscles bilaterally, and bilateral proptosis, in this patient with ophthalmic Graves' disease. (b) MRI scan of the orbits.

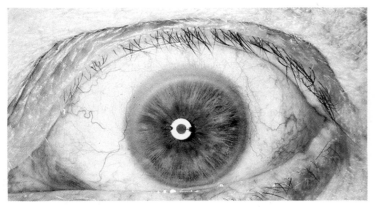

Fig. 17.29 Spasm of the levator palpebrae superiosis causing lid retraction. The sclera is visible between the upper lid margin and cornea when the head is vertical and the eye gaze is forward.

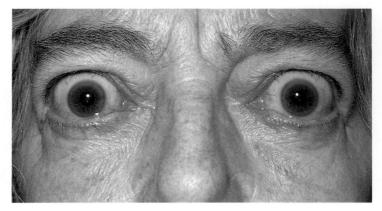

Fig. 17.30 Bilateral lid retraction in hyperthyroid Graves' disease.

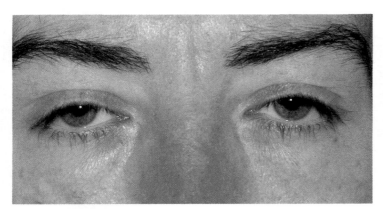

Fig. 17.31 Bilateral ptosis in Graves' disease. Ptosis is rare in Graves' disease, and care should be taken to exclude myasthenia gravis.

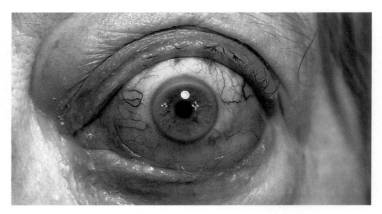

Fig. 17.32 Nonspecific periorbital swelling associated with proptosis.

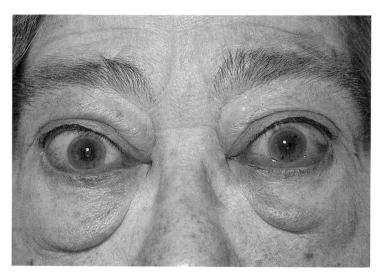

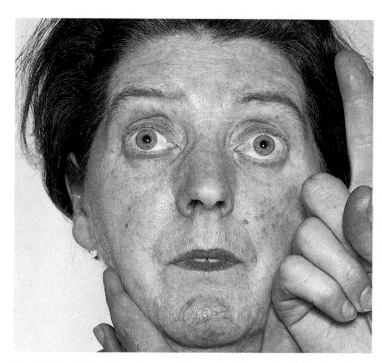

Periorbital Swelling

Periorbital swelling may be seen with any space-occupying lesion of the orbit which causes exophthalmos (Fig. 17.32) and as such is non-specific. Inflammatory swelling of one or both eyelids is characteristic of Graves' disease (Fig. 17.33); it is not dissimilar to the swelling of the lids seen in allergic conditions and in the rare condition of pseudotumour of the orbit.

Ophthalmoplegia

Ophthalmoplegia is a more severe eye sign in Graves' disease and first affects upward (Fig. 17.34) and outward gaze. Later, upward and inward gaze, and lateral, medial and downward gaze, are affected, in that order. Patients complain of double vision, particularly on looking upwards, which they find more unpleasant than normal. The defect in upward gaze is largely due to tethering of the muscles below the globe, particularly to fibrosis of the inferior rectus which may cause the globe to be deviated downwards (Fig. 17.35).

Conjunctival Changes

Conjunctival changes consist of oedema (chemosis); injection of the sclera (Fig. 17.36), particularly over the insertion of the lateral rectus; and swelling of the medial caruncles. These changes are most marked in congestive ophthalmopathy.

Fig. 17.33   Oedematous swelling of the eyelids in Graves' disease.

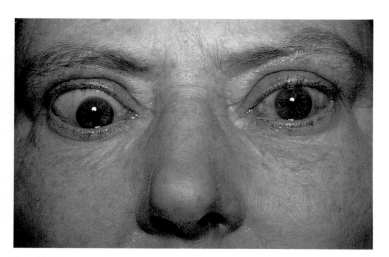

Fig. 17.34   Limitation of upward gaze. In this case, the limitation of movement is caused by tethering of the inferior rectus muscle.

Fig. 17.35   Deviation of the right globe downwards. This deviation is caused by fibrosis and contracture of the inferior rectus.

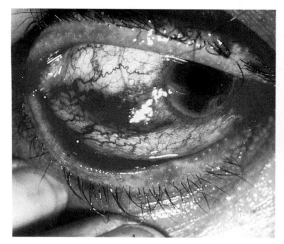

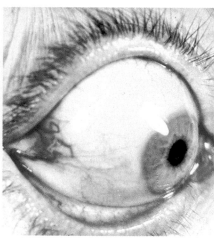

Fig. 17.36   Inflammation of the conjunctivae in Graves' disease.
The right-hand picture shows injection of the sclera over the insertion of the lateral rectus muscle.

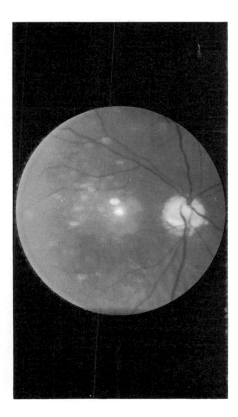

Fig. 17.37 Severe congestive ophthalmopathy. Optic atrophy is a late sign.

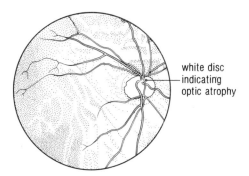

white disc indicating optic atrophy

Congestive Ophthalmopathy

Congestive ophthalmopathy (Fig. 17.37) refers to the severe sight-threatening condition where optic nerve compression can lead to failure of vision, loss of colour vision, and field defects. Papilloedema is not invariably present, and optic atrophy is a late sign. Blepharospasm and corneal ulceration may occur. The term congestive ophthalmopathy (Fig. 17.38) is preferable to that of 'malignant exophthalmos' since the condition is not malignant in the usual sense of the word and exophthalmos may not be present.

LOCALISED MYXOEDEMA

The term localised myxoedema is preferred to that of 'pretibial myxoedema' since the condition may affect other parts of the body, depending on local pressure or trauma. It may occur in several forms: a nodular form (Fig. 17.39), mimicking erythema nodosum (which differs by being tender to the touch); a sheet-like form with largely

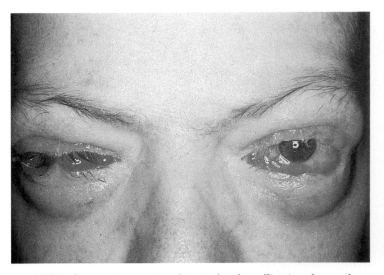

Fig. 17.38 Severe chemosis and periorbital swelling in advanced congestive ophthalmopathy.

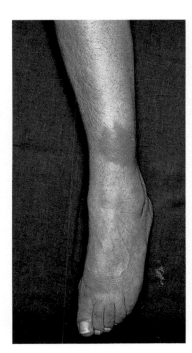

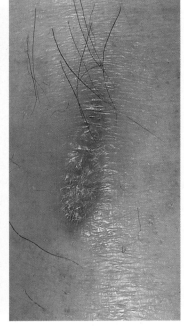

Fig. 17.39 Nodular localised myxoedema resembling erythema nodosum.

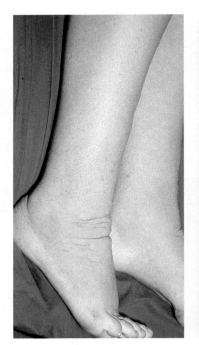

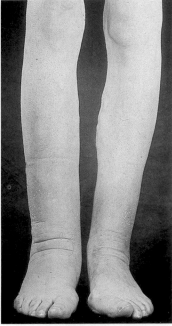

Fig. 17.40 Sheet-like localised myxoedema. This type gives rise to coarse violaceous skin, thickened hair, and nonpitting oedema.

nonpitting oedema, coarse thickening of the skin, a red-violaceous discoloration, and coarse hairs (Fig. 17.40); and a horny form with gross overgrowth of skin and subcutaneous tissue on the dorsum of the feet and toes (Fig. 17.41).

The affected areas are densely infiltrated by a hyaline mucopolysac-charide material. Very high circulating levels of TSH-R antibodies are usually present in patients with localised myxoedema.

THYROID ACROPACHY

Thyroid acropachy is one of the rarer signs of Graves' disease and is usualy associated with localised myxoedema. It resembles clubbing of the fingers (and toes), and the curving of the nails is most marked in the thumb and index fingers (Fig. 17.42). Patchy subperiosteal new bone formation may be apparent clinically or may be visible on X-ray (Fig. 17.43) and differs from the linear new bone formation seen in hypertrophic osteoarthropathy.

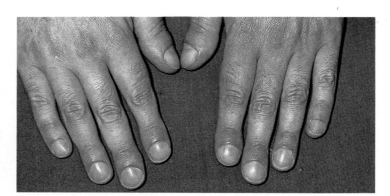
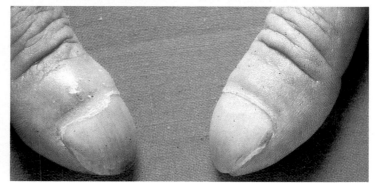

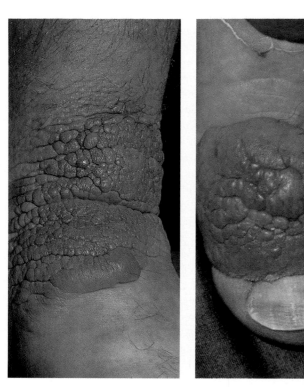

Fig. 17.41 Horny form of localised myxoedema. This type gives rise to gross papilliform overgrowth of skin and subcutaneous tissue, in this case involving the dorsum of the feet and toes.

Fig. 17.42 Thyroid acropachy. Thyroid acropachy (upper) closely resembles clubbing of the fingers (lower).

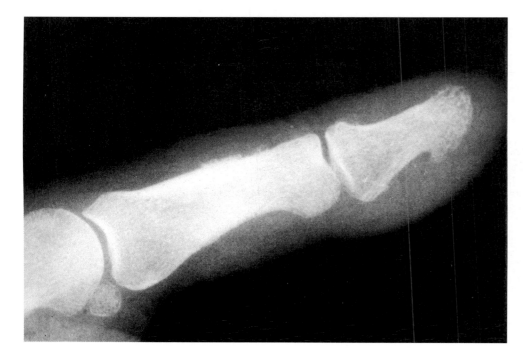

Fig. 17.43 Patchy subperiosteal new bone formation in thyroid acropachy.

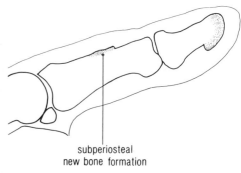

subperiosteal new bone formation

OTHER ASSOCIATED FEATURES

Onycholysis
Recession of the nails from the nail bed (Plummer's nails) (Fig. 17.44) may cause difficulty in keeping the nails clean and must be distinguished from the nail changes of psoriasis.

Vitiligo
The patchy, almost symmetrical depigmentation of the skin (Fig. 17.45), surrounded by an area of increased pigmentation, is associated with the organ-specific autoimmune diseases.

Leucotrichia
Leucotrichia (patches of white hair), premature greying of the hair, alopecia areata, alopecia totalis, and halo naevi are also associated with autoimmune thyroid diseases (Fig. 17.46).

TREATMENT OF HYPERTHYROIDISM

The general principles involved in the treatment of hyperthyroidism due to Graves' disease are shown in Fig. 17.47. The aim for the future is to develop a method of inducing a natural immunological remission, but as yet this remains a theoretical ideal.

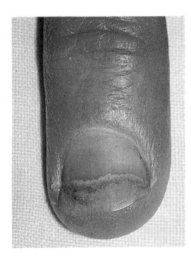

Fig. 17.44 Onycholysis (Plummer's nails). Separation of the nails from the nail beds makes it difficult to keep the nails clean. Onycholysis is also seen in psoriasis.

Immunosuppressive therapy with corticosteroids and other drugs such as azothioprine and cyclosporin A is not justified because of toxicity and the availability of other, safer forms of therapy.

The foundation of therapy lies in a reduction of thyroid hormone production using antithyroid drugs, partial thyroidectomy, or radioiodine therapy. Ancillary treatment, which reduces the peripheral manifestations of thyroid hormones, is sometimes employed using a β-adrenergic blocking drug such as propranolol, or drugs that impair the conversion of T_4 to the biologically active T_3, as well as blocking T_4/T_3 production (for example, propylthiouracil or ipodate).

ANTITHYROID DRUGS

The indications for antithyroid therapy are shown in Fig. 17.48. Absolute indications for drug therapy are pregnancy and thyrotoxic crisis. In North America, the dosage of antithyroid drugs required to control hyperthyroidism is generally higher than that required in Europe, and the relapse rate is greater, possibly because of the higher iodine intake in that part of the world. This results in a higher prevalence of drug side effects and favours the use of alternative treatment regimens such as radioiodine therapy.

In the UK and Europe, the drug of first choice is carbimazole, which blocks the organification of iodine in the thyroid and reduces the formation of new thyroid hormone, while having no effect on the release of preformed thyroid hormone. Two alternative regimens are used for antithyroid therapy. In both, treatment is commenced with a large dose – for example carbimazole 15mg three times daily – and when the patient is clinically euthyroid, usually within six to eight weeks, the strategies differ. In the traditional procedure, the dose is rapidly reduced to be titrated against the clinical and biochemical response, aiming to achieve a maintenance dose of 10–15mg given once daily. In the blocking-replacement regimen, the high initial dose is maintained, and T_4, 0.1mg or 0.15mg daily, is added. The advantages of this regimen are that control is smoother and that clinic visits are required only every three to four months. The duration of the course of antithyroid drugs remains empirical but is usually for 1–1½ years. Some, but not all, reports suggest that the use of a blocking-replacement regimen, followed by a maintenance dose of T_4 for a year or two, may enhance the likelihood of an immunological remission. In the UK, some sixty-five per cent of patients relapse within a year of antithyroid therapy, and even higher relapse rates are reported in North America. This result, combined with the greater frequency of drug side effects associated with higher drug dosage, has

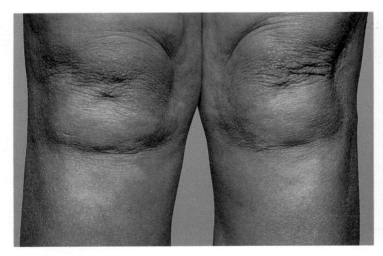

Fig. 17.45 Vitiligo. This patchy depigmentation of the skin is usually bilateral and almost symmetrical.

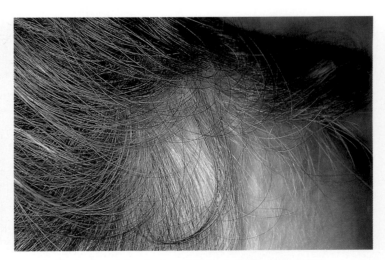

Fig. 17.46 Leucotrichia (tufts of depigmented, white hair).

led to disenchantment with antithyroid drugs as the primary therapy in North America and hence to a much more widespread use of radioiodine therapy.

The major and minor side effects of the antithyroid drugs are listed in Fig. 17.49. All patients treated with carbimazole, methimazole (carbimazole is rapidly converted to methimazole in the body), and propylthiouracil should be warned of the risks of leucopenia leading to agranulocytosis – presenting as a sore throat or ulcerated mouth. For medicolegal reasons, this warning should be conveyed to patients in writing, and should be noted in the patients' notes and in the letter to their general practitioner. Patients should be warned to discontinue the drug if these signs occur and to go to their doctor for a total and differential white blood cell count. When the drugs are discontinued, the blood picture rapidly returns to normal, providing that action is taken early.

Despite many studies, it has proved impossible to predict the outcome of a course of antithyroid drugs sufficiently reliably in an individual patient to achieve major clinical value. The results of different studies vary: Fig. 17.50 shows some of the factors that have been associated with remission or relapse; some of the problems associated with drug treatment are indicated in Fig. 17.51.

PARTIAL THYROIDECTOMY
The indications for partial thyroidectomy are shown in Fig. 17.52. The risks of surgery are minimised in the hands of an experienced surgeon. With the widespread use of radioiodine in North America such experienced surgeons are less readily available than in Europe, where some centres still regard partial thyroidectomy as the treatment of choice for young adults with a toxic diffuse goitre. Patients should be rendered euthyroid with antithyroid drugs prior to operation, and

GENERAL PRINCIPLES OF TREATMENT OF HYPERTHYROIDISM

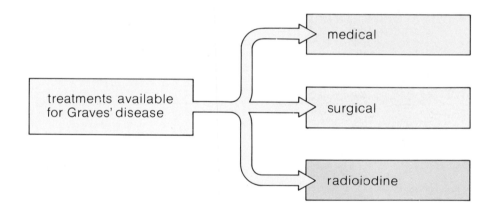

Fig. 17.47 General principles of treatment of hyperthyroidism. Most treatment regimens are directed at the thyroid, but there is a small place for peripherally acting drugs such as propranolol and ipodate.

INDICATIONS FOR MEDICAL TREATMENT

patient preference

small goitre

mild disease

other diseases

children

pregnancy

ophthalmopathy

preoperative

pre-radioiodine

thyrotoxic crisis

relapse after thyroidectomy

Fig. 17.48 Indications for medical treatment in Graves' disease.

SIDE EFFECTS OF ANTITHYROID DRUGS

nausea

vomiting

pruritus

leucopenia, leading to agranulocytosis, with carbimazole, methimazole, propylthiouracil (about 0.1%)

aplastic anaemia (perchlorate)

drug fever, lymphadenopathy, splenomegaly

cholestatic jaundice

Fig. 17.49 Side effects of antithyroid drugs. Drug treatment is relatively safe, but all patients should be warned of the signs of leucopenia and agranulocytosis.

there is now good evidence available that preoperative oral iodine administered for two weeks reduces vascularity of the gland and makes the operation easier: for example, potassium iodide 60mg three times daily may be given.

Complications of the operation should be rare (Fig. 17.53), and the only common problems are hypothyroidism (seen in fifteen per cent of cases) and recurrent hyperthyroidism. The frequency of hypothyroidism is less in areas of higher iodine intake, and that of recurrent hyperthyroidism greater than in less iodine-replete areas. The presence of recurrent upper pole nodules is a rare complication which may be associated with recurrent hyperthyroidism and which must be differentiated from malignancy.

RADIOIODINE THERAPY

The indications for, and the complications of, radioiodine therapy are shown in Fig. 17.54. This form of treatment, used widely in North America for all age groups, is now being used more freely in the UK and Europe, because, despite many years of follow-up, there is no convincing evidence of the development of thyroid carcinoma or leukaemia. Hypothyroidism is the only significant complication of radioiodine therapy, its prevalence being related to the dose. All patients treated with radioiodine must be followed up long term, as there is an increment of thyroid failure over many years. Administration of smaller doses of radioiodine does not avoid hypothyroidism and increases the need for additional courses of antithyroid treatment.

FACTORS THAT MAY INFLUENCE ANTITHYROID DRUG THERAPY

factors associated with remission

clinical	laboratory
small goitre	modest elevation of thyroid hormones
mild disease	low urinary iodine excretion
rapid response to antithyroid drugs	low or absent TSH-R(s) antibodies at end of therapy
small maintenance dose	
female sex	normal response to TRH at end of therapy
low iodine intake	normal suppression of thyroidal radioiodine uptake at end of therapy

factors associated with relapse

clinical	laboratory
large goitre	major elevation of thyroid hormones
vascular goitre	high urinary iodine excretion
severe disease	raised TSH-R(s) antibodies at end of therapy
slow response to antithyroid drugs	absent response to TRH at end of therapy
large maintenance dose	impaired or absent suppression of thyroidal radioiodine uptake at end of therapy
male sex	
high iodine intake	

Fig. 17.50 Factors that may influence the results of antithyroid drug therapy. Despite the variety of clinical and laboratory features associated with remission or relapse, none has proved sufficiently reliable or specific to be of clinical value in an individual patient.

PROBLEMS ASSOCIATED WITH DRUG TREATMENT

inconvenience and expense to patient of numerous visits to doctor

high relapse rate

long duration of therapy

difficulty in maintaining patient co-operation

Fig. 17.51 Problems associated with drug treatment. The great majority of patients can be controlled with a modest dose of antithyroid drugs. The frequency and expense of frequent visits to a doctor can be reduced by employing a blocking-replacement regime. The major problem of drug therapy is the high rate of relapse and its unpredictability.

INDICATIONS FOR PARTIAL THYROIDECTOMY

experienced thyroid surgeon available

patient preference

adults up to 40 years

severe disease

nodular goitre

large goitre

relapse after drug treatment

Fig. 17.52 Indications for partial thyroidectomy. Surgery, although now less widely used, is still a very effective treatment for Graves' disease, and, after operation, the immune process appears to remain quiescent in most cases.

COMPLICATIONS OF PARTIAL THYROIDECTOMY

early	late
recurrent laryngeal nerve palsy	cheloid scar
superior laryngeal nerve palsy	tethered scar
haemorrhage	hypothyroidism
hypoparathyroidism	recurrence of hyperthyroidism
pneumothorax	recurrent upper pole nodules
thyroid crisis	
infection	
damage to thoracic duct	
damage to carotid artery	
damage to jugular vein	

Fig. 17.53 Complications of partial thyroidectomy. The only common complications are hypothyroidism and recurrent hyperthyroidism.

INDICATIONS AND COMPLICATIONS OF RADIOIODINE THERAPY

indications	complications
patient preference	permanent hypothyroidism
poor-compliance with antithyroid drugs	transient hypothyroidism
side effects of antithyroid drugs	thyroiditis
patients over 40 years (many centres now treat younger patients)	sialadenitis
younger women who have been sterilised or had a hysterectomy	thyrotoxic crisis
recurrence after thyroidectomy	nodule formation
severe uncontrolled disease	
large goitre	
unco-operative patient	
presence of other disease(s)	

Fig. 17.54 Indications for, and complications of, radioiodine therapy. This form of therapy is being used more widely and requires a well-organised follow-up strategy to recognise late-onset hypothyroidism and lack of compliance (patients who have been treated for hypothyroidism but have stopped taking their medication).

Opinions vary as to the optimum dose schedule, but the author prefers to administer a large dose – 555mBq (15mCi) – to all patients, irrespective of gland size or the severity of hyperthyroidism. This renders some eighty per cent of patients hypothyroid within three months, but this is easily treated with replacement T_4. If the patient remains hyperthyroid at four months, a further similar dose of radioiodine can be given. When ablative doses of radioiodine are administered, it is mandatory that the patient is followed up at monthly intervals, otherwise severe hypothyroidism may develop.

Opinions also vary as to the need for antithyroid drug therapy prior to radioiodine administration. The author's policy is only to use antithyroid drugs to render patients euthyroid if they have some concomitant severe disease (such as heart failure), are markedly thyrotoxic, or are elderly. There is evidence that a higher dose of radioiodine is required to render a patient euthyroid after prior carbimazole treatment. If the toxic symptoms of the patient are troublesome, these can be alleviated by administration of propranolol.

TREATMENT OF THE EYE SIGNS OF GRAVES' DISEASE
In most patients with eye signs of Graves' disease (Fig. 17.55) no treatment is required other than reassurance and adequate control of the hyperthyroidism, being careful to avoid rendering the patient hypothyroid. For severe congestive ophthalmopathy, expert supervision is urgently required in a specialist endocrine unit to coordinate the expertise of the endocrinologist, ophthalmologist, radiotherapist, neurosurgeon, and ear, nose and throat surgeon.

OTHER COMMON CAUSES OF HYPERTHYROIDISM

TOXIC ADENOMA
One, or occasionally two, thyroid nodules may exhibit autonomy (Fig. 17.56). Such nodules are very rarely malignant. They occur more frequently in areas of iodine deficiency, such as southern Europe.

The development of hyperthyroidism from a hot nodule in the thyroid depends on the available iodine and the size of the nodule: the larger the nodule, the more likely is it to be toxic. Administration of iodine can induce the onset of hyperthyroidism. The size of a nodule can be assessed by ultrasound, and its functional capacity by a radioiodine or technetium scan. Some malignant tumours that present as solitary nodules can trap technetium but fail to organify iodine, so their true nature is best revealed by a radioiodine scan. It is not usually necessary to biopsy hot nodules since they are rarely malignant.

TREATMENT OF THE EYE SIGNS OF GRAVES' DISEASE

stage	management
mild	reassurance control of hyperthyroidism, avoiding overtreatment
moderate	diuretics elevation of head end of bed liquifilm artificial tear eyedrops dark glasses prismatic lenses to correct diplopia
severe	high-dose corticosteroids cyclosporin A azothioprine orbital radiation decompression of the orbits intravenous IgG (a preliminary report)

Fig. 17.55 Treatment of the eye signs of Graves' disease.

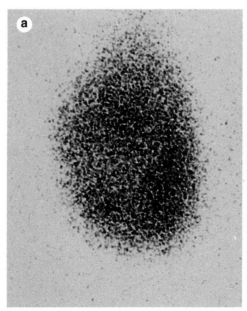 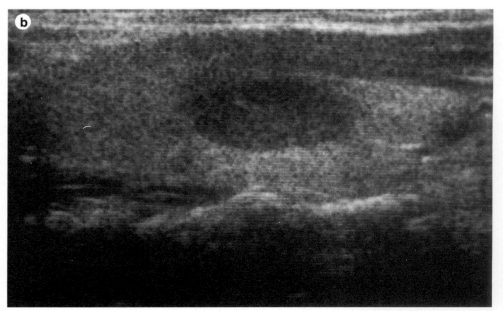

Fig. 17.56 A solitary hyperactive thyroid nodule. (a) The radioisotope (^{99m}Tc) scan shows a hot nodule in the right lobe. (b) Ultrasound demonstrates the thyroid nodule.

Toxic adenomas have a low intrathyroidal iodine pool and preferentially secrete T_3. Prior to the development of frank hyperthyroidism, the adenoma may secrete just enough thyroid hormone to lower TSH and suppress the TSH response to TRH – the so-called subclinical toxic adenoma.

Toxic adenoma may be treated by radioiodine therapy, or by surgical removal of the nodule and the affected lobe, after the patient has been rendered euthyroid with antithyroid drugs.

TOXIC MULTINODULAR GOITRE
Nodular goitres are more common in areas of iodine deficiency. In the UK, toxic multinodular goitre is more often seen in older patients and is associated with cardiac complications such as atrial fibrillation. The thyroid enlargement is often asymmetrical, and the nodules are easily palpable and sometimes visible (Fig. 17.57). The goitre may extend retrosternally and cause stridor, by compression of the trachea (Fig. 17.58), or dysphagia from oesophageal narrowing. When a large unilateral nodule is present, the displaced trachea may be mistaken for the other lobe of the thyroid which is erroneously

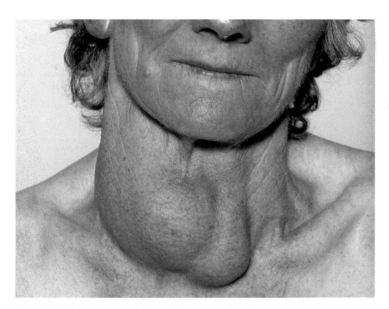

Fig. 17.57 Asymmetrical nodular thyroid enlargement.

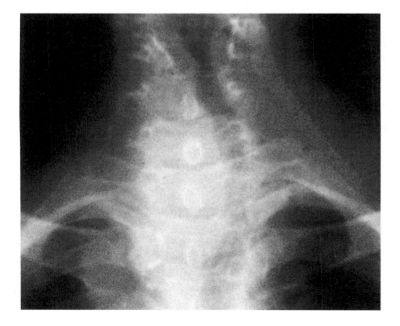

believed to be diffusely enlarged. The majority of apparently unilateral nodules are found at operation to be the largest nodules in a multinodular gland. The nodularity of a goitre is more easily demonstrated by ultrasound rather than by the patchy uptake on radioisotope scan.

Treatment of toxic multinodular goitre is preferably by radical partial thyroidectomy after administration of preoperative antithyroid medication to produce euthyroidism. There is still debate about the need for long-term postoperative T_4 administration to prevent recurrence of the nodules. If the patient is elderly or unwell, radioiodine can be used, but larger doses (for example, double) are required than those employed in the treatment of toxic diffuse goitre.

POSTPARTUM HYPERTHYROIDISM
Postpartum hyperthyroidism is usually due to postpartum thyroiditis, which affects some five per cent of all women during the year after pregnancy, particularly those with high titres of TPO antibodies. Postpartum thyroiditis is typically biphasic (Fig. 17.59) with an initial hyperthyroid state that occurs approximately three months after delivery. This is usually brief, biochemical and asymptomatic, and is followed by a hypothyroid phase four to five months postpartum, which may be symptomatic and is sometimes permanent. The differential diagnosis of postpartum hyperthyroidism is shown in Fig. 17.60.

SILENT THYROIDITIS
The silent thyroiditis variety of destructive hyperthyroidism is seen more frequently in North America than in Europe. It is usually mild and self-limiting and requires only symptomatic therapy. It may affect women who have previously had postpartum thyroiditis. Like hyperthyroidism due to postpartum thyroiditis, silent thyroiditis is differentiated from Graves' disease by a low thyroidal radioiodine uptake.

RARER CAUSES OF HYPERTHYROIDISM

JOD–BASEDOW PHENOMENON
The term Jod–Basedow is used to describe iodine-induced hyperthyroidism that is more common in subjects with pre-existing thyroid disease, such as the presence of a nodular goitre, but can also occur in individuals with an apparently normal thyroid. It should be suspected in any patient presenting with hyperthyroidism that is not due to Graves' disease, although the source of the iodine excess may

Fig. 17.58 Tracheal compression from a nodular goitre.

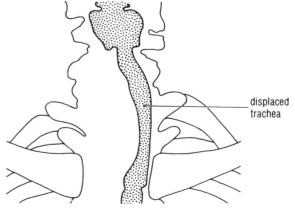

displaced trachea

be difficult to identify. The condition is more common in iodine-deficient areas where nodular goitre is frequent. It is difficult to treat because of the large stores of preformed hormone in the gland, and may require treatment with corticosteroids and perchlorate along with antithyroid drugs.

AMIODARONE-INDUCED HYPERTHYROIDISM

Amiodarone, a drug used in the treatment of resistant arrhythmias, contains a large amount of iodine and has multiple effects on thyroid function at the pituitary–thyroid–tissue levels. While most patients receiving amiodarone remain clinically euthyroid, there are clear alterations in thyroid function tests with slightly elevated FT_4 and TSH, elevated rT_3 and a low FT_3 level. Amiodarone may cause hyperthyroidism (more commonly in areas of iodine deficiency) or hypothyroidism (more frequently in iodine-replete regions). In patients with amiodarone-induced hyperthyroidism, the FT_3 level is characteristically raised, and levels of TSH are low or low–normal. The thyroid shows unusual histological features, with focal destructive changes against a background of inactive follicles. Amiodarone-induced thyrotoxicosis may be resistant to large doses of conventional antithyroid drugs and may require additional corticosteroid therapy.

De Quervain's Subacute Thyroiditis

De Quervain's subacute thyroiditis, a painful viral infection of the thyroid, causes temporary destructive hyperthyroidism, with low radioisotope uptake in the early phases of the disease. Treatment with simple analgesics is usually all that is required but in persistent cases, corticosteroids may be needed. Transient or, rarely, permanent hypothyroidism can develop.

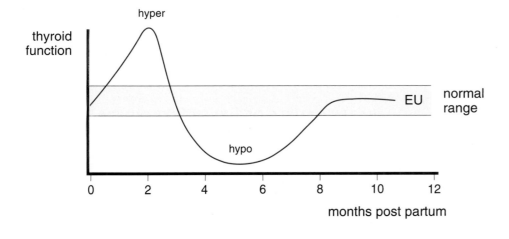

EVOLUTION OF POSTPARTUM THYROIDITIS SYNDROME

Fig. 17.59 Evolution of the postpartum thyroiditis syndrome. Postpartum thyroiditis is the most common cause of biochemical hyperthyroidism but is mild and usually asymptomatic. The pathogenesis of this transient destructive hyperthyroidism is unknown.

DIAGNOSIS OF POSTPARTUM HYPERTHYROIDISM

	^{123}I uptake	TSH-R antibodies
postpartum thyroiditis	low	−
prior Graves' disease and postpartum thyroiditis	low	+ −
prior Graves' disease and exacerbation	normal/raised	+ −
new Graves' disease	normal/raised	+ −

Fig. 17.60 Differential diagnosis of postpartum hyperthyroidism. Postpartum thyroiditis is the most common cause of postpartum hyperthyroidism, even in patients with previous Graves' disease. The key to diagnosis is measurement of the thyroidal ^{123}I uptake, which is low in the 'destructive hyperthyroidism' of postpartum thyroiditis and normal or raised in the 'stimulatory hyperthyroidism' of Graves' disease.

18

Calcium and Common Endocrine Bone Disorders

Gregory R Mundy, MD

CALCIUM HOMEOSTASIS

Extracellular fluid calcium or plasma calcium is very carefully controlled by fluxes of calcium which occur between the extracellular fluid and the skeleton, and between the gut and the kidney (Fig. 18.1). These fluxes are regulated by three systemic hormones, namely parathyroid hormone (PTH), 1,25-dihydroxyvitamin D, and calcitonin. In turn, the production of these hormones by their corresponding cells of origin is regulated either directly or indirectly by changes in the extracellular calcium, so that they all form long negative feedback loops (Fig. 18.2).

Calcium is one of the most carefully controlled variables in the body. Although the long negative feedback loops appear to overlap and are therefore redundant, they are probably necessary for such tight control of extracellular fluid calcium. Careful regulation of the latter is necessary for a whole range of cellular functions. Small changes in extracellular fluid calcium have major effects on neuromuscular function, and the symptoms and signs of hypercalcaemia and hypocalcaemia are accompanied by changes in both central and peripheral neuronal function.

The distribution of calcium in the body is important in considerations of calcium homeostasis. Ninety-nine percent of calcium is stored in the skeleton. Calcium, however, is also present in extracellular fluid and is located intracellularly. Small changes in intracellular calcium have major effects on cell function. Within cells, calcium is bound to a number of proteins. When calcium is bound to proteins it may change their conformation and, as a consequence, their function. Changes in protein conformation lead to changes in cell activation and subsequent cell function.

The extracellular fluid calcium is controlled not only by the homeostatic mechanisms that are mediated by long negative feedback loops, but also by a complex blood–bone exchange system that is still poorly understood. Bones contain a specialised fluid which has a different ionic composition to that of extracellular fluid. This specialised bone fluid, which can be considered to be similar to cerebrospinal fluid, is separated from extracellular fluid by a metabolically active membrane, probably comprised of the 'bone lining' cells that cover bone surfaces. The extracellular fluid is supersaturated with respect to the calcium concentration in the bone fluid and at the bone surface. Small changes in extracellular fluid calcium can be modified by the bone surface taking up this calcium. The bone membrane functions as a barrier to keep calcium out of the bone fluid and in the extracellular fluid.

PARATHYROID HORMONE

Parathyroid hormone (PTH) is a single-gene polypeptide of eighty-four amino acids and is synthesised by the chief cells of the parathyroid gland. Its synthesis and secretion are primarily controlled by the concentrations of ionised calcium in the extracellular fluid. An inverse relationship exists between the extracellular fluid calcium concentration and PTH synthesis and secretion (Fig. 18.3). As the extracellular fluid calcium concentration decreases, there is an increase in PTH synthesis and secretion. The first thirty-four amino acids from the amino-terminal part of the molecule are responsible for the biological effects of PTH and for the binding of PTH to its receptor. The overall effects of PTH are to increase the extracellular fluid calcium concentration and decrease the extracellular fluid phosphate concentration. It increases reabsorption of calcium in renal tubules, inhibits

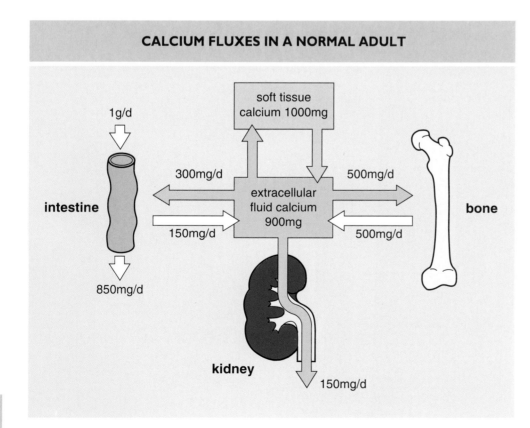

CALCIUM FLUXES IN A NORMAL ADULT

Fig. 18.1 Calcium fluxes between the extracellular fluid and gut, and between the kidney and bone, in a normal adult in zero calcium balance. Note that net calcium absorption (150mg/d) is equal to calcium losses in the urine.

phosphate reabsorption in renal tubules, and increases bone resorption. In addition, it indirectly increases the absorption of calcium and phosphate from the gastrointestinal tract by its effect of increasing the metabolism of vitamin D precursors – forming the highly active 1,25-dihydroxyvitamin D – in the proximal tubules of the kidney. PTH exerts its effects on its target cells both by increasing intracellular cyclic AMP, and by increasing intracellular calcium. The cell-surface receptor for PTH has recently been identified and molecularly cloned.

CALCITONIN
Calcitonin is a thirty-two amino-acid peptide that is synthesised and secreted by the parafollicular cells of the thyroid gland. Its synthesis and secretion are controlled by extracellular fluid calcium concentrations and also by hormones from the gastrointestinal tract, predominantly gastrin. The major biological effect of calcitonin is to inhibit transiently osteoclastic bone resorption, and it does this by inhibiting the formation and activity of bone-resorbing osteoclasts. Calcitonin mediates its effects on target cells by increasing intracellular cyclic

AMP. The cell-surface receptor for calcitonin has recently been identified and, surprisingly, seems to be closely related in structure to the PTH receptor.

1,25-DIHYDROXYVITAMIN D
1,25-dihydroxyvitamin D is the major biologically active metabolite of the vitamin D sterol family. Vitamin D precursor (7-dehydrocholesterol) is either ingested in the diet or synthesised in the skin to form hydroxylated metabolites which are hydroxylated in the liver and kidney to form 1,25-dihydroxyvitamin D. The renal 1-hydroxylase enzyme system is under the control of ambient phosphate concentrations, circulating PTH concentrations, calcium concentrations and other mechanisms, possibly including circulating sex hormones and prolactin levels. PTH and the ambient phosphate concentration appear to be the primary regulators. The 1-hydroxylase enzyme is present in the proximal tubules of the kidney and is a complex cytochrome P_{450} mitochondrial enzyme system.

HORMONAL REGULATION OF CALCIUM HOMEOSTASIS

hormone	effect	control
PTH	calcium↑ phosphate↓	calcium ions↓
calcitonin	calcium↓ phosphate↓	calcium ions↑ gastrin
vitamin D metabolites	calcium↑ phosphate↑	phosphate↓ PTH↑

Fig. 18.2 Hormonal regulation of calcium homeostasis.

RELATIONSHIP BETWEEN PTH AND CALCIUM

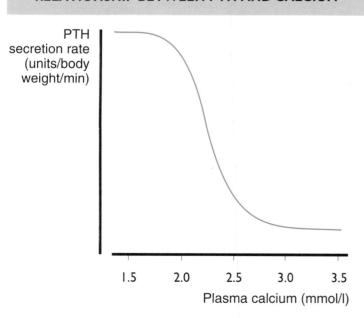

Fig. 18.3 Inverse relationship between PTH secretion rate and plasma calcium. Note that PTH secretion is not completely suppressible by extracellular calcium.

1,25-Dihydroxyvitamin D increases plasma calcium and phosphate concentrations by increasing the absorption of calcium and phosphate from the gastrointestinal tract. It also increases bone resorption and enhances the capacity for PTH to promote renal tubular calcium reabsorption in the renal tubules. It is a powerful differentiation agent for committed osteoclast precursors, causing their maturation to form multinucleated cells that are capable of resorbing bone. By these actions, 1,25-dihydroxyvitamin D provides a supply of calcium and phosphate available at bone surfaces for the formation of normal mineralised bone. Absence of 1,25-dihydroxyvitamin D leads to rickets or osteomalacia, bone disorders that are characterised by impaired mineralisation of the newly formed proteinous bone matrix.

DEFENCES AGAINST HYPERCALCAEMIA AND HYPOCALCAEMIA

The homeostatic response to increased plasma calcium concentration is controlled predominantly by PTH and 1,25-dihydroxyvitamin D. PTH is most important for short-term regulation of extracellular fluid calcium, and 1,25-dihydroxyvitamin D for more long-term responses. PTH has major effects on the kidney to promote renal tubular calcium reabsorption, and on bone to stimulate bone resorption. 1,25-Dihydroxyvitamin D works on the gastrointestinal tract to increase calcium absorption and thereby protect against hypocalcaemia. The defences against hypercalcaemia and hypocalcaemia are described in Fig. 18.4.

BONE REMODELLING AND CHANGES WITH AGE

TYPES OF BONE
There are two types of bone; cortical (or compact), and trabecular (or cancellous). Cortical bone is present in long bone shafts of the appendicular skeleton, while trabecular or cancellous bone is the flat plates of bone which crisscross the marrow cavity. The latter type of bone is in intimate contact with the cells of the marrow cavity and is probably metabolically regulated by these cells and their products. The axial skeleton, the vertebrae, and the proximal ends of long bones are rich in trabecular bone. The skeleton is comprised of eighty per cent cortical bone and twenty per cent trabecular bone.

BONE TURNOVER
Although bone is a mineralised tissue, it is cellular and metabolically active. The cells in bone are present on endosteal surfaces of cancellous bone adjacent to the marrow cavity, and within channels that tunnel through cortical bone known as the haversian systems. These cells are continually restructuring the skeleton. The bone restructuring or remodelling occurs in discrete packets known as bone-remodelling units. The cells involved in the remodelling of bone are osteoclasts and osteoblasts. Osteoclasts are large multinucleated cells that are responsible for breaking down bone, and osteoblasts are small cuboidal cells that are responsible for synthesising new bone and then mineralising it. Osteoclasts are unique cells that are the only cells in the body known to have the capability of resorbing bone. Bone is remodelled by a specific sequence of cellular events which always begins with osteoclastic bone resorption, followed by new bone formation (Fig. 18.5). This occurs both within the haversian systems and on trabecular bone surfaces. The cellular events are always the same, commencing with osteoclastic resorption and concluding with new bone formation. The bone that is removed by the activity of the osteoclasts is precisely replaced in normal health by the activity of osteoblasts. Thus, there is a balance in normal health between the processes of bone resorption and bone formation.

CONTROL OF BONE TURNOVER
The activity of osteoclasts and osteoblasts is under the control of systemic hormones and local factors. Systemic hormones that control osteoclastic activity are PTH, calcitonin, and 1,25-dihydroxyvitamin D. PTH and 1,25-dihydroxyvitamin D stimulate osteoclasts to resorb bone, whereas calcitonin inhibits the activity of osteoclasts. Local factors produced by bone cells and by immune cells in the marrow cavity are also capable of stimulating osteoclasts; these include cytokines such as interleukin-1 (IL-1), tumour necrosis factor (TNF), and interleukin-6 (IL-6). The activity of osteoblasts is also regulated by factors that stimulate the activity of osteoclasts. The major factors that stimulate osteoblasts to make new bone, however, may be peptide growth factors that are actually stored within the bone matrix and released as a consequence of bone resorption. These peptide growth factors include transforming growth factor β (TGF-β), the bone morphogenetic proteins and the insulin-like growth factors.

DEFENCES AGAINST HYPOCALCAEMIA AND HYPERCALCAEMIA	
protection against decreases in plasma calcium (for example, dietary deficiency, hormonal deficiency)	
glomerular filtration	filtration load of calcium decreases
renal tubules	hypocalcaemia stimulates PTH release, which increases calcium reabsorption
gastrointestinal tract	1,25-dihydroxyvitamin D increases fractional absorption of dietary calcium
skeletal system	increased osteoclastic activity leads to increased bone remodelling chronically, and the bone-exchange system prevents calcium in the extracellular fluid from entering the bone fluid
protection against increases in plasma calcium (caused by bone destruction, large dietary calcium load)	
glomerular filtration	filtered load of calcium increases
renal tubules	PTH suppressed, tubular reabsorption of calcium decreased
gastrointestinal tract	1,25-dihydroxyvitamin D suppressed, and calcium absorption decreased
possible diuretic effect of hypercalcaemia causing increased excretion	
skeletal system	decreased osteoblastic activity leads to suppressed bone remodelling chronically, and the bone-exchange system allows for extracellular fluid calcium to enter the bone fluid and to be incorporated into bone surfaces

Fig. 18.4 Defences against hypocalcaemia and hypercalcaemia.

The cellular events of bone remodelling are highly co-ordinated so that a balance usually exists between the processes of bone formation and bone resorption. When an imbalance occurs between bone formation and bone resorption, such as with ageing, there is usually more bone lost by the activity of osteoclasts than can be replaced by the activity of osteoblasts.

CHANGES WITH AGE

There are alterations in the rates of bone resorption and bone formation at different stages during life (Fig. 18.6). During adolescence, bone formation is relatively greater than bone resorption so that there is an increase in skeletal mass. In young adult life there is a perfect balance between bone resorption and bone formation, and skeletal mass

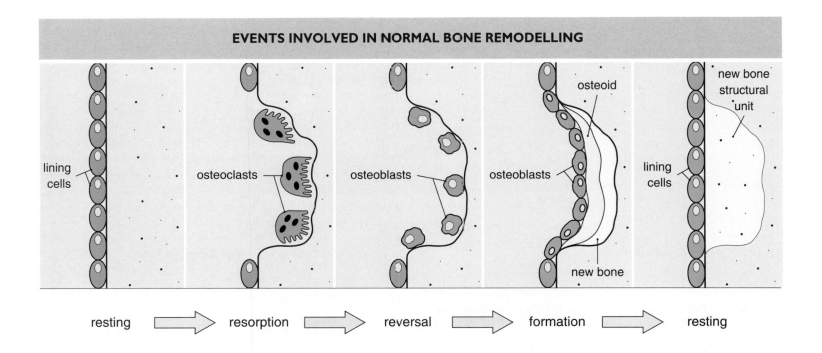

EVENTS INVOLVED IN NORMAL BONE REMODELLING

resting ⟹ resorption ⟹ reversal ⟹ formation ⟹ resting

Fig. 18.5 The sequence of events involved in normal bone remodelling on a trabecular bone surface. These remodelling events occur in discrete packets throughout the skeleton, known as bone-remodelling units.

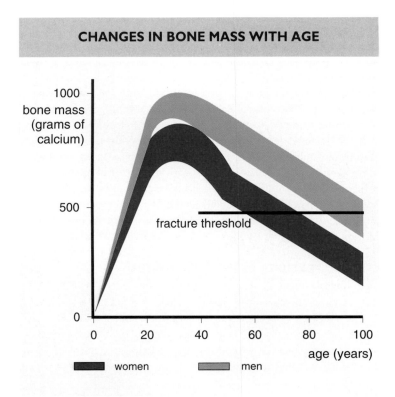

CHANGES IN BONE MASS WITH AGE

Fig. 18.6 Changes in bone mass with age. Note that bone mass increases during growth and adolescence and declines progressively after mid-adult life. Acceleration of bone loss occurs in women for ten years after menopause.

CAUSES OF HYPERCALCAEMIA

primary hyperparathyroidism

malignant diseases

  cancer with bone metastases

  cancer without bone metastases

  multiple myeloma

thyrotoxicosis

Paget's disease with immobilisation

fracture with immobilisation

vitamin A intoxication

vitamin D intoxication

milk–alkali syndrome

sarcoidosis and other granulomatous disease

  (tuberculosis, berylliosis)

idiopathic hypercalcaemia of infancy

familial hypercalcaemia

thiazide diuretics

diuretic phase of acute renal failure

Addison's disease

Fig. 18.7 Causes of hypercalcaemia.

CLINICAL MANIFESTATIONS OF HYPERCALCAEMIA

neurological

lethargy, confusion, irritability, stupor, coma

psychiatric

depression, hallucinations

gastrointestinal

anorexia, nausea, vomiting, constipation

cardiovascular

increased myocardial contractility, shortened ventricular systole

renal

nephrogenic diabetes insipidus, impaired glomerular filtration, nephrocalcinosis

Fig. 18.8 Clinical manifestations of hypercalcaemia.

remains constant. After the middle of the third decade, however, there is usually an increase in bone resorption relative to bone formation and bone is progressively lost. In women there is an additional marked acceleration of bone loss at the time of the menopause, which lasts for a period of ten years. This accelerated phase of bone loss is due to an increase in bone resorption and occurs as a consequence of the effects of withdrawal of oestrogen: oestrogen deficiency leads to increased bone resorption. In later life, decreased osteoblast activity occurs in men and women, and further progressive decrease in bone formation is seen in advanced age in both sexes. The decline in bone mass that occurs in men and women, but is more pronounced in women, makes the skeleton more fragile in the elderly and is the reason why older people develop fractures of susceptible bones following trivial injuries – a condition known as osteoporosis.

BONE REMODELLING

Bone physiologists have argued for many years over the primary function of bone remodelling; it may serve a number of purposes. Bone remodelling is presumably necessary to preserve structural integrity of the skeleton by continually replacing it. It also plays a minor role in calcium homeostasis, since the skeleton is the source of most of the calcium in the body, and bone resorption releases calcium into the extracellular fluid. The skeleton is also a storehouse for minerals and buffers which may be released when bone is resorbed. This may be important in the maintenance of the acid–base balance, and also in supplying minerals such as magnesium and phosphate to the extracellular fluid at times of need.

HYPERCALCAEMIA

Hypercalcaemia occurs when the total serum calcium, corrected for changes in plasma protein, is >2.55mmol/l (10.2mg/dl). This is now a very common clinical finding since measurements of total serum calcium have become routine in most patients in whom blood is drawn. Hypercalcaemia always indicates serious underlying pathology and should be evaluated carefully. The two most common causes are primary hyperparathyroidism and malignant disease (Fig. 18.7).

CAUSES OF HYPERCALCAEMIA

Hypercalcaemia occurs when the complex homeostatic mechanism that is responsible for maintaining normal extracellular fluid calcium concentrations is overwhelmed. It usually involves an increase in entry of calcium into the extracellular fluid from two of the major organ systems that control calcium homeostasis. In primary hyperparathyroidism there is an increase in renal tubular calcium reabsorption, an increase in bone resorption, and an increase in calcium absorption from the gastrointestinal tract. There is a marked increase in bone resorption in many patients with malignant disease, together with an increase in renal tubular calcium reabsorption. Since the homeostatic mechanism is so efficient under normal circumstances, hypercalcaemia occurs only when there are profound abnormalities in calcium fluxes, and always means severe underlying pathology.

CLINICAL FEATURES OF HYPERCALCAEMIA

The clinical features of hypercalcaemia are listed in Fig. 18.8; they vary considerably from patient to patient, and are related both to the absolute concentration of serum calcium and to the rate of rise in serum calcium. In patients who are older, symptoms of hypercalcaemia may be prominent with relatively small increases in serum calcium concentrations.

PRIMARY HYPERPARATHYROIDISM

Primary hyperparathyroidism is the most common cause of hypercalcaemia; it is responsible for more than fifty per cent of all cases, but is more common in the ambulant or outpatient population than it is in the hospitalised patient population. The annual incidence rate is between fifty and two hundred and fifty patients per million population per year. It is most common in elderly female patients, although it can occur at any age.

Pathology

There are three causes of primary hyperparathyroidism. Some eighty-five per cent of patients have a single benign adenoma of one of the four parathyroid glands. Most of the remainder have hyperplasia of four parathyroid glands. This occurs more commonly in patients with familial hyperparathyroidism syndromes, and particularly in patients with multiple endocrine neoplasia (MEN). Less than one per cent of all patients have a carcinoma of one of the four parathyroid glands. In rare cases, carcinoma seems to follow a previous adenoma.

Pathophysiology

In patients with primary hyperparathyroidism, the inverse relationship between serum PTH (and parathyroid cell number) and serum calcium still exists, although the relationship is altered and occurs at a different level of serum calcium. In other words, PTH secretion can be suppressed or kept constant by an increase in extracellular fluid calcium concentration above a critical level, although the sensitivity of the parathyroid glands to changes in serum calcium is altered and set at a different level. This occurs in the majority of patients with parathyroid gland adenomas. In patients with parathyroid hyperplasia, the set point for PTH release may be normal, but the mass of parathyroid tissue is increased and so the result is a relatively greater circulating PTH concentration for any serum calcium concentration.

Aetiology

The cause of primary hyperparathyroidism is unknown. Since this condition is not one pathological entity, but involves at least two and possibly more conditions, the heterogeneity of pathology probably means heterogeneity of causes. Recent data suggest that in most patients with parathyroid adenomas, there is a monoclonal disorder that arises from an abnormality within a single cell. However, four-gland

hyperplasia may be a polyclonal disorder caused by an external stimulus to parathyroid cell growth, as well as PTH synthesis and secretion. A parathyroid growth factor that is related to the fibroblast growth factor family has recently been identified and may be responsible, at least in some patients, for parathyroid hyperplasia related to the MEN type-I syndrome. Other growth factors that may be involved in parathyroid gland hyperplasia presumably exist, but have not yet been identified.

Another factor that has been implicated in the pathophysiology of primary hyperparathyroidism is external irradiation, since there is some evidence that patients with a history of neck irradiation may be predisposed to the condition.

Biochemical Effects

The biochemical effects of primary hyperparathyroidism are depicted in Fig. 18.9. These characteristics are due to the effects of PTH on target cells and on serum calcium and phosphate homeostasis. The characteristic abnormalities are an increase in serum calcium, a decrease in serum phosphate, and an increase in urine calcium.

Clinical Features

There has been a changing pattern of presentation of primary hyperparathyroidism in the past twenty years. Original descriptions of the disease suggested that it was a disease of 'bones and stones and abnormal groans associated with psychological moans'. Modern presentation has been influenced by the advent of the autoanalyser and by routine measurements of serum calcium. Most patients are now diagnosed when they are still asymptomatic, as measurement of serum calcium is routinely carried out in patients who have blood drawn for almost any reason. This has also meant a change in the age and sex incidence. Although primary hyperparathyroidism can occur at any age, it is now most commonly seen in elderly women, the same group of patients who are subject to postmenopausal osteoporosis.

In the past, primary hyperparathyroidism was characterised by presentation with recurrent renal stones due to hypercalciuria, associated with polyuria that occurred as a result of loss of the concentrating ability of the kidney. Some patients developed a peculiar type of bone disease known as osteitis fibrosa, characterised by increased generalised osteoclastic bone resorption, particularly involving the phalanges (causing subperiosteal resorption) (Fig. 18.10) and the skull (causing

BIOCHEMICAL EFFECTS OF PTH EXCESS	
serum	**urine**
calcium ↑	calcium ↑
phosphorus ↓	phosphorus ↑
alkaline phosphatase ↑	cyclic AMP ↑
chloride ↑	
bicarbonate ↓	
PTH ↑	

Fig. 18.9 Biochemical effects of PTH excess on calcium homeostasis.

the appearance known as salt and pepper skull) (see Chapter 23). This presentation is rarely seen nowadays. Some patients develop a form of muscle weakness, and many patients complain of anorexia, nausea and vomiting due to hypercalcaemia, associated with constipation. Acute pancreatitis is seen in some patients, and it has long been debated whether or not the disease is associated with peptic ulceration and with hypertension.

In a small number of patients, primary hyperparathyroidism is associated with other endocrine syndromes. This occurs in two familial syndromes, MEN type I and type II. The former type is associated with hypersecretion of hormones of the pituitary (growth hormone or prolactin, usually), islet cells of the pancreas (usually insulin or gastrin secreting), and the parathyroids. In MEN type II, patients develop medullary carcinoma of the thyroid associated with phaeochromocytoma. Primary hyperparathyroidism occurs in a minority of patients. Both of these MEN syndromes are inherited as autosomal dominant conditions, but hyperparathyroidism is not expressed in either before the age of ten.

Diagnosis

The diagnosis of primary hyperparathyroidism is best made by consideration of the natural history (most patients will be found to have been hypercalcaemic for more than one year if records are available) and by measurement of immunoreactive PTH. With improvements in the PTH assay and the availability of two-site assays (using antibodies directed at two different sites of the PTH molecule), intact PTH can be measured accurately and, in the majority of patients with primary hyperparathyroidism, the diagnosis can be

made with certainty as long as renal failure is not present. Other characteristic features of primary hyperparathyroidism which help distinguish it from other types of hypercalcaemia include: measurements of serum chloride (most patients have mild hyperchloraemic acidosis); serum phosphate (patients are hypophosphataemic due to renal phosphate wasting); urinary cyclic AMP (patients may have an increased urinary cyclic AMP due to the effects of PTH on the renal tubules); serum 1,25-dihydroxyvitamin D (often found to be normal or slightly elevated in patients); and urinary calcium excretion (calcium excretion is usually increased due to an increased filtered load of calcium, despite the effects of PTH to promote renal tubular calcium reabsorption).

Differential Diagnosis

The differential diagnosis of hypercalcaemia involves the consideration of all other causes of hypercalcaemia. In patients who are normocalcaemic but present with recurrent renal stones, other causes of recurrent renal stones (such as idiopathic hypercalciuria, oxaluria, urate stones or cystinuria) should be considered. In patients who present with osteopenia, osteoporosis, osteomalacia and malignant disease (most notably myeloma) should be excluded.

Management

Most patients with primary hyperparathyroidism are best treated by surgery. If the condition is due to a solitary adenoma, then this should be excised. If the condition is due to four-gland hyperplasia, then surgeons remove three-and-a-half parathyroid glands. In patients in whom surgery is contraindicated, medical therapy for hypercalcaemia may be necessary if the patient is symptomatic. In many patients who are asymptomatic, and whose serum calcium concentration is only marginally elevated, active therapy may not be indicated.

HYPERCALCAEMIA OF MALIGNANCY

Hypercalcaemia of malignancy is the most common cause of hypercalcaemia in hospitalised patients. It is one of the most common paraneoplastic syndromes associated with cancer, and is particularly

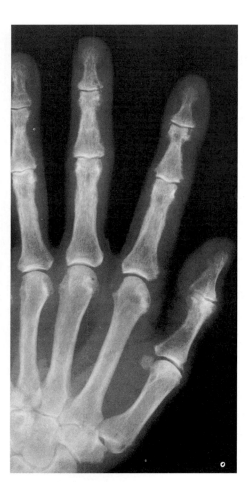
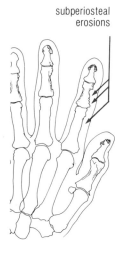

subperiosteal erosions

MALIGNANCIES ASSOCIATED WITH HYPERCALCAEMIA	
site	frequency (%)
lung	35
breast	25
blood (myeloma, lymphoma)	14
head and neck	6
renal	3
prostate	3
unknown primary	7
others	7

Fig. 18.10 A hand radiograph in primary hyperparathyroidism. Note the subperiosteal erosions, which are more prominent along the radial border of the phalanges.

Fig. 18.11 Relative frequencies of different malignancies as causes of hypercalcaemia of malignancy.

common in patients with breast cancer (thirty per cent), lung cancer (fifteen to twenty per cent) and myeloma (twenty-five per cent). The relative frequency of different types of malignancy associated with hypercalcaemia is shown in Fig. 18.11.

Several mechanisms are responsible for hypercalcaemia of malignancy, other than the condition being secondary to multiple lytic secondary deposits. In some patients, it is due to one or more factors that are secreted directly by the tumour cells, which are responsible for disrupted calcium homeostasis. One of the most commonly implicated factors is a peptide hormone related to PTH, which is secreted by many squamous cell carcinomas, binds to the PTH receptor, and shares all of the known effects of PTH, on its target organs. This factor is known as PTH-related protein (PTHrP). Its normal physiological role is unknown but may be related to maternal–fetal calcium fluxes during pregnancy. In some patients, hypercalcaemia is due to local factors that are produced by tumour cells in the bone environment which stimulate osteoclasts. These factors include IL-1, TGFs and TNF. In patients with myeloma, the myeloma cells secrete osteoclast-activating factors such as lymphotoxin, IL-6 and IL-1, which are responsible for osteoclast activation. In all patients with hypercalcaemia of malignancy, there is an increase in osteoclastic bone resorption, and in many there is also an increase in renal tubular calcium reabsorption. Medical therapy is therefore aimed at inhibiting bone resorption and promoting renal calcium excretion.

SARCOIDOSIS
In sarcoidosis, hypercalcaemia occurs together with hyperphosphataemia and impaired renal function, and is responsive to glucocorticoid therapy. Patients have increased plasma 1,25-dihydroxyvitamin D concentrations, but normal 25-hydroxyvitamin D concentrations. A likely explanation for these findings is increased 1-hydroxylase activity in the sarcoid granulomas.

FAMILIAL HYPOCALCIURIC HYPERCALCAEMIA
Familial hypocalciuric hypercalcaemia is an autosomal dominant condition that is frequently found in patients with a history of unsuccessful surgery for primary hyperparathyroidism. The characteristics of this condition are a family history in siblings or offspring, low renal excretion of calcium (<100mg/24h up to 2.5mmol/24h) and magnesium, and usually little or no symptomatology. This condition is also referred to as familial benign hypercalcaemia. Patients need to be identified since they have a very poor response to parathyroidectomy. Unlike familial forms of primary hyperparathyroidism, hypercalcaemia and hypocalciuria are present from the neonatal period. In contrast, primary hyperparathyroidism associated with MEN syndromes is rarely evident before the age of ten.

TREATMENT OF HYPERCALCAEMIA
Hypercalcaemia of malignancy should be treated by vigorous intravenous hydration with normal saline to ensure deficits in extracellular fluid volume are corrected. In addition, drug therapy to inhibit osteoclastic bone resorption should be instituted. Currently, the most effective forms of therapy are the new-generation bisphosphonates. These are very effective inhibitors of osteoclastic bone resorption and are successful in the majority of patients; however, since they are not rapidly acting, calcitonin should be instituted at the same time if a fast response is required. Other forms of calcium-lowering therapy include plicamycin (mithramycin), which is efficacious but more toxic than the bisphosphonates, corticosteroids (which are most likely to be effective in myeloma), and gallium nitrate. Therapies available for hypercalcaemia of malignancy are listed in Fig. 18.12.

THERAPY FOR HYPERCALCAEMIA OF MALIGNANCY

ablation of tumour

intravenous fluids

furosemide (frusemide)

bisphosphonates

calcitonin/glucocorticoids

plicamycin (mithramycin)

oral phosphate

indomethacin

gallium nitrate

Fig. 18.12 Therapy available for hypercalcaemia of malignancy.

CAUSES OF HYPOCALCAEMIA

primary hypoparathyroidism
　idiopathic
　postsurgical
pseudohypoparathyroidism
hypocalcaemia associated with malignant disease
hypomagnesaemia
toxic-shock syndrome
neonatal
acute pancreatitis
renal failure
vitamin D deficiency
　dietary
　malabsorption
　anticonvulsant therapy
　chronic liver disease
　chronic renal disease
　vitamin D-dependent rickets

Fig. 18.13 Causes of hypocalcaemia.

HYPOCALCAEMIA

CAUSES OF HYPOCALCAEMIA

The causes of hypocalcaemia are listed in Fig. 18.13; these include primary hypoparathyroidism, which is associated with decreased PTH secretion from the parathyroid glands due to disease or surgical damage to the parathyroids. Pseudohypoparathyroidism is an interesting condition in which there is decreased PTH effectiveness on peripheral tissues due to peripheral tissue resistance. One of the mechanisms for this increase in peripheral tissue resistance may be related to loss of an essential component of the PTH-receptor–adenylate-cyclase complex in the cell membrane (the G-protein or nucleotide regulatory unit). Patients with pseudohypoparathyroidism also have somatic features such as short stature, a short fourth metacarpal, and obesity (Fig. 18.14). They show no renal response to exogenous PTH administration, unlike normal individuals or patients with primary hypoparathyroidism, who respond to PTH with increased cyclic AMP excretion and phosphate excretion.

Hypocalcaemia also occurs in renal failure where it is due to vitamin D deficiency and to phosphate retention, both of which lower serum calcium. Hypocalcaemia occurs in magnesium depletion for several reasons; it can be due to the effects of magnesium deficiency impairing peripheral effects of PTH, and to a decrease in the release of PTH from the parathyroid glands, which may be the most important reason. Patients with hypocalcaemia due to magnesium depletion cannot be adequately treated until the magnesium deficiency is corrected.

Patients with acute pancreatitis become hypocalcaemic for multiple reasons, possibly because they are often in acute renal failure, because they may have increased circulating calcitonin levels which lower

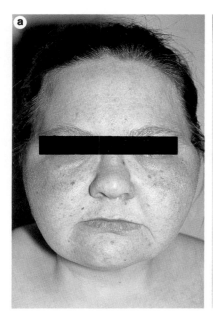

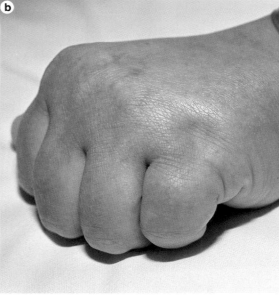

Fig. 18.14 A patient with pseudohypoparathyroidism. (a) Typical round facies characteristic of pseudohypoparathyroidism. (b) A dimpled knuckle as a result of a shortened fifth metacarpal.

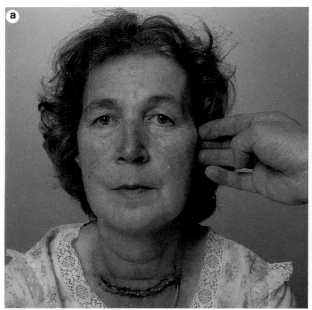

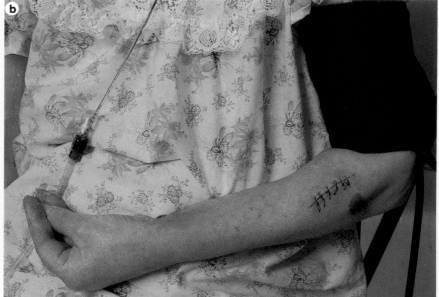

Fig. 18.15 The clinical signs of hypocalcaemia. (a) Chvostek's sign is elicited by tapping over the facial nerve and producing a contraction of the upper lip muscles. (b) Trousseau's sign is produced when a sphygmomanometer cuff is inflated to above systolic pressure for up to three minutes. This patient had four-gland hyperplasia and developed transient postoperative hypocalcaemia. All four glands were removed, and pieces from one were autotransplanted into the forearm. The site of the transplantation can be seen clearly.

serum calcium concentrations, or because they release enzymes from the pancreas which may cause the breakdown of lipids to form insoluble salts with serum calcium.

The vitamin D deficiency syndromes are considered later (p. 18.13). Vitamin D deficiency leads to decreased absorption of calcium from the gut, which is responsible for hypocalcaemia.

CLINICAL FEATURES OF HYPOCALCAEMIA

Hypocalcaemia is characterised by changes in neuromuscular function. The most common symptoms are paraesthesiae around the mouth and in the fingers, muscle cramps and seizures. Tetany (involuntary muscle contraction) may occur in the hands, producing the *main d'accoucheur* (obstetrician's hand) or carpopedal spasm. Chronic hypocalcaemia causes cataracts and calcification of the basal ganglia of the brain.

Incipient tetany can be predicted by Chvostek's sign. Chvostek's sign is elicited by tapping the facial nerve immediately after it exits from the auditory canal. Tetany can also be anticipated by Trousseau's sign. To perform this, a blood-pressure cuff is maintained for ten minutes at 3mm of mercury above the systolic pressure. Spasmodic contraction of the small muscles of the hand (carpopedal spasm) occurs in patients with Trousseau's sign. Chvostek and Trousseau's clinical signs are depicted in Fig. 18.15.

DIAGNOSIS OF HYPOCALCAEMIA

The diagnosis of hypocalcaemia is usually achieved by careful consideration of the clinical setting, and measurements of serum calcium and phosphate concentrations. In patients with suspected pseudohypoparathyroidism, measurement of plasma PTH is very useful and has, in most cases, replaced the measurement of responses of target organs to a PTH infusion or injection. Plasma PTH is elevated in pseudohyperparathyroidism.

TREATMENT OF HYPOCALCAEMIA

Successful treatment of hypocalcaemia (Fig. 18.16) usually requires calcium administered orally or intravenously, depending on the urgency for a rapid response, and by treatment with a short-acting vitamin D metabolite, most frequently 1,25-dihydroxyvitamin D.

OSTEOPOROSIS

Before discussing osteoporosis, this bone disease will be placed in context with other bone diseases in the ageing population which may be confused with osteoporosis and present a similar clinical picture. The generic term osteopenia may be used to cover the group of generalised diseases of bone which present with a radiological picture of a decreased amount of mineralised bone. This term is useful because it does not presuppose any particular bone pathology or disease from the radiological picture. In most cases, osteopenia will be due to osteoporosis. A similar radiological picture of osteopenia, however, can be produced by osteomalacia, osteitis fibrosa cystica (the bone disease sometimes associated with primary hyperparathyroidism), and the osteopenia associated with myeloma and other malignant diseases.

Osteoporosis is by far the most important of these conditions and affects between five and ten per cent of the population of Western countries. It is between five and eight times as common in women as it is in men, and represents a major public health problem. An estimated two hundred and fifty thousand hip fractures and five hundred thousand vertebral fractures in the USA each year are attributed to osteoporosis. Hip fracture is the most serious complication since it is a major cause of morbidity and often mortality in the elderly.

DEFINITION OF OSTEOPOROSIS

Osteoporosis is characterised by decreased trabecular bone mass in which both the mineral and the matrix are decreased to the same extent, but there is no gross abnormality of bone composition. Although cortical bone is also affected, trabecular bone loss is most striking. Subtle chemical defects in mineral or matrix (bone proteins such as type-I collagen) may exist in some patients. This disease accounts for more than ninety per cent of patients with osteopenia.

Fig. 18.16 Treatment of hypocalcaemia.

TREATMENT OF HYPOCALCAEMIA
chronic
vitamin D metabolite
oral calcium
parathyroid gland autotransplantation (postoperatively) in a patient with parathyroid gland hyperplasia
urgent
intravenous calcium
short-acting vitamin D metabolite

CLASSIFICATION OF OSTEOPOROSIS

There are several different classifications for osteoporosis. For many years it has been separated into primary osteoporosis, in which osteoporosis occurs without association with other diseases, and secondary osteoporosis, which occurs in association with other conditions (Fig. 18.17). A separate classification has been proposed in which primary osteoporosis is subdivided into type I (postmenopausal) and type II (senile). The type-I variant predominantly involves trabecular bone, occurs at an earlier age, is much more frequent in women, and is often complicated by vertebral fractures. The type-II variant occurs in men and women, is more common in the older age group, and is often complicated by hip fractures. Some workers have suggested that different pathogenetic events may be involved in these two forms. Type I may be due primarily to oestrogen deficiency, whereas type II may be due to a combination of impaired calcium absorption from the gut and impaired osteoblast function.

RISK FACTORS OF OSTEOPOROSIS

Since osteoporosis is of such slow onset and is difficult to treat once established, investigators have studied in some detail the risk factors that could predispose patients to later development of the disease. Factors that have been associated with increased risk of later development of osteoporosis are listed in Fig. 18.18.

CLINICAL FEATURES OF OSTEOPOROSIS

The clinical features of osteoporosis include pain, which occurs most frequently in association with crush or compression fractures of the lower thoracic, midthoracic or lumbar spine. Fractures frequently occur spontaneously or with minimal trauma. The most common fractures are those of the vertebral bodies, followed by fractures of the neck of femur. Femoral neck fractures are the most serious because they lead to considerable morbidity and mortality in the elderly population. Other fractures, such as those of the distal forearm following a fall on the outstretched hand, are less common.

The initial compression fractures usually occur in the midthoracic region. As bone is progressively lost, the patient loses height and develops a dorsal kyphosis (hunchback). Compression fractures occur at the lower dorsal–upper lumbar vertebrae. With further bone loss the kyphosis becomes more marked, the lower lumbar vertebrae become compressed as more height is lost, and the thoracic cage may eventually come to rest on the pelvic brim, producing a 'pot-belly' appearance. The radiological appearance of osteoporosis is shown in Fig. 18.19.

ABNORMALITIES IN CALCIUM HOMEOSTASIS

There are no detectable abnormalities in calcium or phosphate homeostasis in osteoporosis.

DIAGNOSIS OF OSTEOPOROSIS

There have been major advances recently in the development of techniques for monitoring changes in bone mass, and these have received widespread acceptance. The state-of-the-art technique is dual-beam X-ray absorptiometry, in which two X-ray sources are used to allow precise measurements of bone mass in specific and strategic areas of the skeleton, such as the lumbar spine, the neck of the femur, the forearm bones, or in the total skeleton. Other techniques include dual-beam photon absorptiometry, computerised tomography, neutron-activation analysis, and the previously used method of single-beam photon absorptiometry. These techniques may be used to follow treatment regimens and assess the risk of later development of osteoporosis. Their usefulness is, however, still somewhat controversial.

CLASSIFICATION OF OSTEOPOROSIS

primary: without associated diseases

senile or postmenopausal (involutional) (95% of all patients, most frequent in elderly white women)

idiopathic (occurring in middle age)

juvenile (occurring during adolescence or 20s)

secondary: associated with other conditions

Cushing's syndrome

chronic liver disease

Turner's syndrome

immobilisation

heparin therapy

alcoholism

diabetes mellitus

malabsorption

osteogenesis imperfecta

pregnancy and lactation

elite female athletes

anorexia nervosa

Fig. 18.17 Classification of osteoporosis.

RISK FACTORS FOR OSTEOPOROSIS

female sex

menopause

race – Blacks and Mexican Americans are protected

diet – calcium deficiency, phosphate and protein excess

smoking – smokers are leaner and have a lower bone mass

alcohol – alcoholics have less bone than corresponding non-drinking controls

inactivity

leanness

diseases associated with secondary osteoporosis, such as Cushing's syndrome, previous gastric surgery, and hypogonadism in males; the major risk factors in males may be cigarette smoking, alcohol consumption and leanness, which predisposes men to vertebral fractures

Fig. 18.18 Risk factors for osteoporosis.

TREATMENT OF OSTEOPOROSIS

The following approaches have been used in an attempt to increase bone mass in osteoporotic patients.

General Symptomatic Treatment

Patients with osteoporosis should be advised to avoid alcohol, smoking, caffeine and a sedentary lifestyle, since all of these factors have been associated with bone loss. Pain should be treated with analgesics. For vertebral fractures, orthopaedic support garments, heat and massage may be helpful. Bed rest should be avoided as far as possible, and patients should be advised to avoid situations where falls are most likely to occur.

Specific Medical Therapy

Treatment of osteoporosis can be prophylactic treatment or treatment of the established disease. The most useful prophylactic therapy is to avoid risk factors that are associated with osteoporosis where possible: patients at high risk should use oestrogen in the years following menopause unless contraindicated, or possibly an alternative inhibitor of bone resorption. In patients with established osteoporosis, therapies that are available include drugs that inhibit bone resorption, namely calcitonin, bisphosphonates and oestrogen. All of these drugs probably have similar efficacy, although this is still debated. Their effects on bone formation are probably much less prominent than their effects on bone resorption.

Attempts to stimulate bone formation over prolonged periods in patients with osteoporosis are still experimental. Fluoride increases bone mass, although it may also increase propensity to fracture. Low-dose PTH has an anabolic effect on the skeleton to increase bone mass, although this effect may not be maintained; this drug is still investigational.

OSTEOMALACIA

DEFINITION OF OSTEOMALACIA

Osteomalacia is the bone disease that results from impaired mineralisation of newly formed bone. The result is excess unmineralised bone matrix (known as osteoid tissue). Osteomalacia is due to a lack of vitamin D, impairment of vitamin D metabolism, or to a lack of calcium or phosphorus at the mineralising site. Before puberty the same condition is referred to as rickets and is characterised by failure of calcification of cartilage at the growth plate (that is, decreased endochondral ossification). The causes of osteomalacia are shown in Fig. 18.20

PATHOLOGY OF OSTEOMALACIA

The definitive diagnosis of osteomalacia is made by bone biopsy using undecalcified sections and labelling with tetracycline. A fluorescent antibiotic, tetracycline localises at sites of mineralisation so that when sequential courses of tetracycline are given before bone biopsy, rates of bone mineralisation can be assessed. Other histological parameters that are quantified in a bone biopsy include the volume of osteoid tissue (that is, the volume of tissue that is nonmineralised), the relative osteoid surface, and the osteoid seam thickness.

CAUSES OF OSTEOMALACIA

vitamin D deficiency

dietary lack – rare in developed countries because of supplementation of diet with vitamin D; however, may occur in elderly and alcoholics in association with other mechanisms

poor sunlight exposure

gut malabsorption (vitamin D is a fat-soluble vitamin) and fat malabsorption (steatorrhoea) leads to vitamin D deficiency

anticonvulsant therapy (these drugs stimulate liver metabolism of vitamin D to inactive metabolites and cause a decrease in serum 25-hydroxyvitamin D)

chronic liver disease, and particularly primary biliary cirrhosis

chronic renal disease due to impaired formation of 1,25-dihydroxyvitamin D by kidneys, and to circulating inhibitors of mineralisation found in uraemic state

vitamin D-dependent osteomalacia

type I – inherited deficiency of the 1-hydroxylase enzyme necessary for conversion of 25-hydroxyvitamin D to 1,25-dihydroxyvitamin D

type II – inherited inability of target organs to respond to vitamin D

hypophosphataemic

excess ingestion of aluminum hydroxide gels which decrease phosphate absorption

sex-linked hypophosphataemia (inherited phosphate transport abnormality, with renal phosphate wasting)

tumour osteomalacia (some tumours, particularly mesenchymal tumours, produce a humoral factor that causes renal phosphate wasting)

other renal tubular disorders, such as Fanconi's syndrome

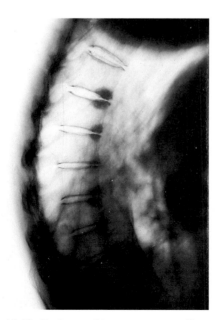
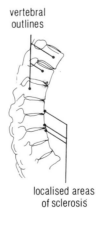

vertebral
outlines

localised areas
of sclerosis

Fig. 18.19 Radiographic appearance of osteoporosis. The vertebrae show decreased bone mineral density, and some are clearly compressed.

Fig. 18.20 Causes of osteomalacia.

ABNORMALITIES IN CALCIUM HOMEOSTASIS

In the majority of patients with osteomalacia the serum chemistry is abnormal (Fig. 18.21). When there is malabsorption or dietary lack of vitamin D, serum calcium is decreased or at the lower limit of normal, serum phosphorus is markedly decreased due to secondary hyperparathyroidism, and urine calcium excretion is also decreased. In patients with rickets or osteomalacia due to chronic renal disease, impairment of glomerular filtration leads to phosphate retention so that serum calcium is low because of impaired formation of 1,25-dihydroxyvitamin D and impaired gut absorption of calcium, but serum phosphorus is high. In patients with rickets or osteomalacia

due primarily to a renal phosphate leak, serum calcium concentrations may be normal but the serum phosphorus concentration is decreased.

The clinical features of rickets or osteomalacia are characterised by bone pain, occasional fracture, and sometimes deformity, particularly in patients with long-standing osteomalacia due to hereditary conditions or chronic renal disease (Fig. 18.22). This occurs particularly in children with renal rickets or sex-linked hypophosphataemic rickets who may have outward bowing of the lower extremities. Patients with osteomalacia also develop muscle weakness and tenderness, particularly affecting the proximal muscles of the lower extremities.

The diagnosis of rickets or osteomalacia may be suspected from the presence of a painful deforming bone disease that is associated with characteristic abnormalities of serum chemistry. In patients with malabsorption or dietary deficiency of vitamin D, serum 25-hydroxyvitamin D is an important measurement since it reflects the major transport form of vitamin D in the circulation. It is also a good parameter of gut absorption of vitamin D. X-Rays may be characteristic in children with rickets and in some adult patients with osteomalacia who develop pseudofractures. However, pseudofractures are uncommon, and in patients in whom osteomalacia is suspected on clinical or radiological grounds, it may be necessary to perform a definitive bone biopsy.

Rickets or osteomalacia due to lack of vitamin D is treated with oral calcium, and a form of vitamin D for patients with vitamin D deficiency. The form of vitamin D depends on the nature of defect in vitamin D metabolism. The available vitamin D preparations are shown in Fig. 18.23. Patients with rickets or osteomalacia due to hypophosphataemia require oral phosphate and a form of vitamin D, preferably 1,25-dihydroxyvitamin D.

HYPOPHOSPHATAEMIC RICKETS

Hypophosphataemic rickets is also known as sex-linked hypophosphataemia, phosphate diabetes, or vitamin D-resistant rickets. It is an inherited condition in which rickets develops in early life, and is associated with growth retardation and bowing deformities of the legs; it does not respond to vitamin D therapy. Patients have normal serum calcium concentrations with a low serum phosphate concentration due to increased urine phosphate excretion. Serum alkaline phosphatase is usually increased. The plasma 1,25-dihydroxyvitamin D concentration may be decreased or inappropriately normal. In the

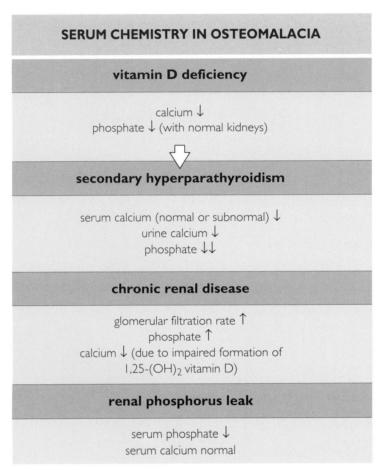

SERUM CHEMISTRY IN OSTEOMALACIA

vitamin D deficiency

calcium ↓
phosphate ↓ (with normal kidneys)

⇩

secondary hyperparathyroidism

serum calcium (normal or subnormal) ↓
urine calcium ↓
phosphate ↓↓

chronic renal disease

glomerular filtration rate ↑
phosphate ↑
calcium ↓ (due to impaired formation of
1,25-(OH)₂ vitamin D)

renal phosphorus leak

serum phosphate ↓
serum calcium normal

Fig. 18.21 Serum chemistry in different types of osteomalacia.

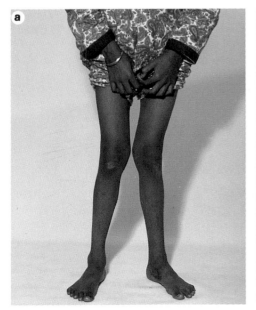
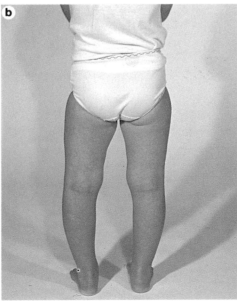

Fig. 18.22 Knock-knees, and bow legs in rickets. (a) The boy had simple nutritional vitamin D deficiency. (b) The girl had hypophosphataemic rickets.

presence of hypophosphataemia, it should be increased. The reason for this failure of increase in 1-hydroxylase activity in the renal tubular cells is unexplained. The basic defect is phosphate depletion due to renal tubular dysfunction, and therapy for this condition involves use of oral phosphate and a vitamin D metabolite. The clinical features of this condition are very similar to those of oncogenic osteomalacia described below.

ONCOGENIC OSTEOMALACIA
Rickets or osteomalacia develops in some patients with tumours. The tumour produces an unknown factor that causes phosphate wasting from the kidneys, due to an impairment of renal tubular phosphate reabsorption. The syndrome of oncogenic osteomalacia mimics hypophosphataemic rickets or osteomalacia very closely. Tumours are usually benign and slow growing, of the mesenchymal type. This syndrome is reversed when the tumour is successfully removed.

PAGET'S DISEASE OF BONE

Paget's disease of bone is a common disorder of the elderly, and is characterised by marked increases in bone resorption and bone formation. The consequence is disordered bone architecture. Although the aetiology is still unclear, it seems likely that the disease is related to a viral infection involving a virus in the measles family related to the parainfluenza viruses. In England, some researchers have linked Paget's disease to dog ownership and implicated canine distemper virus. The pathophysiology of Paget's disease, however, may also involve abnormal production of cytokines in the bone cell environment. Recently, IL-6 production by cells in the osteoclast lineage has been implicated as an autocrine/paracrine factor. There are often abnormal numbers of haemopoietic precursors in the bone marrow of patients with Paget's disease. This may reflect an increase in the precursors for the osteoclast, since the osteoclast shares its precursor with the mature cells of the blood.

PATHOGENESIS OF PAGET'S DISEASE
The primary abnormality is an increase in osteoclastic bone resorption. The osteoclasts are of enormous size and contain up to one hundred nuclei. The osteoclast nuclei contain inclusion bodies that resemble the those seen in viral diseases. The main reason for linking Paget's disease to a viral aetiology is the morphological observation of these inclusion bodies. There is also an increase in new bone formation which is probably secondary to the osteoclastic bone resorption. The

new bone that is formed is immature woven bone. It is disorganised in structure and of irregular pattern. There is also an increase in vascularity of the bone.

Lesions occur most frequently in the vertebrae, skull, pelvis and axial skeleton, and in the proximal ends of the long bones and the tibia. They usually occur as discrete but multiple lesions.

CLINICAL FEATURES OF PAGET'S DISEASE
The majority of patients with Paget's disease are asymptomatic. In patients who have symptoms, the most common is pain, which is usually localised to the area of pagetic bone disease. Occasionally, bone pain is due not to Paget's disease but rather to associated degenerative joint disease. Patients also develop characteristic deformities, most frequently an enlargement of the skull or outward bowing of the lower extremities. Furthermore, the disordered bone architecture may occasionally be associated with complications such as pathologic fracture, nerve entrapment syndromes due to increased bone formation, deafness (which may be due to compression of the eighth cranial nerve or to otosclerosis), cardiac failure due to increased cardiac output and increased blood flow through the highly vascularised Pagetic bones and, rarely, sarcomatous transformation. The latter condition is a complication that, although rare, is usually rapidly fatal. The tumours may be osteosarcomas, chondrosarcomas, fibrosarcomas or mixed mesenchymal tumours. The clinical features of Paget's disease are listed in Fig. 18.24, and bone deformities of the condition are shown in Figs 18.25 & 18.26.

LABORATORY EVALUATION OF PAGET'S DISEASE
There is no abnormality in calcium or phosphate homeostasis. There is, however, a marked increase in urinary hydroxyproline (hydroxyproline is an amino acid that is almost unique to collagen, and urinary excretion reflects increased bone turnover) and serum alkaline phosphatase. Alkaline phosphatase is an enzyme that is produced by osteoblasts and its increase reflects increased osteoblastic activity.

TREATMENT OF PAGET'S DISEASE
The main aim of treatment is to inhibit bone resorption. Three drugs that are effective inhibitors of bone resorption have been useful in Paget's disease: calcitonin, bisphosphonates and plicamycin (mithramycin). More than seventy per cent of patients respond to treatment, and the improvement in their wellbeing is dramatic. Current drugs of choice are the new bisphosphonates although, in the future, intranasal calcitonin or oral bisphosphonates may be preferable to therapies that are presently in use.

Fig. 18.23 *Vitamin D metabolites used in the treatment of hypocalcaemia.*

VITAMIN D METABOLITES USED FOR HYPOCALCAEMIA

nonproprietary name	abbreviation	effective daily dose	time for reversal of toxic effects (days)
ergocalciferol	vitamin D_3	1–10mg	17–60
calcifediol	25-(OH)D_3	0.05–0.5mg	7–30
dihydrotachysterol		0.1–1mg	3–14
alfacalcidol	1α-(OH)D_3	1–2μg	5–10
calcitriol	1,25-(OH)$_2D_2$	0.5–1μg	2–10

CLINICAL FEATURES OF PAGET'S DISEASE

pain

occurs over the area of bone disease

deformity

caused by the abnormal bone architecture

complications

fracture

nerve entrapment (due to increased bone formation)

deafness (due to compression of the VIIIth cranial nerve
and to otosclerosis)

cardiac failure (due to increased cardiac output)

sarcomatous tranformation (rarely, there may be development
of osteosarcomas, chondrosarcomas, or fibrosarcomas
in pagetic bones)

Fig. 18.24 Clinical features of Paget's disease. Most patients are
asymptomatic.

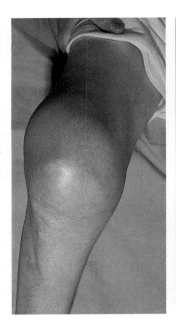
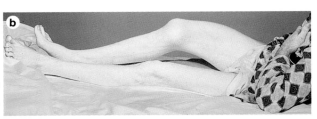
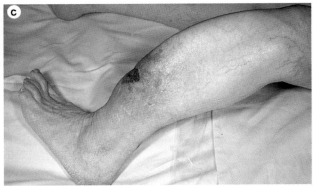

*Fig. 18.25 Bone deformity in Paget's
disease.* (a) Marked enlargement of the
cranium, with normalised facial bones – a hearing
aid can be seen. (b) Anterior bowing of the
femur. (c) Marked bowing of the tibia with
overlying ulceration.

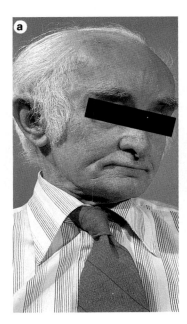
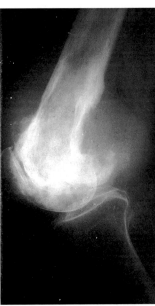
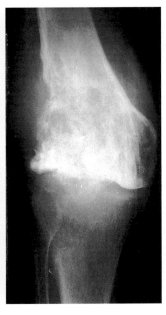

*Fig. 18.26 Development of osteogenic
sarcoma in Paget's disease.* Painful swelling
developed in the knee two years after the
diagnosis of Paget's disease. Marked bone
destruction and soft-tissue swelling can be seen
on the radiographs.

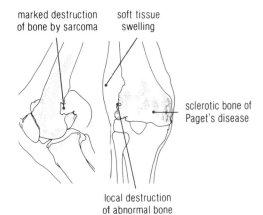

marked destruction   soft tissue
of bone by sarcoma   swelling

sclerotic bone of
Paget's disease

local destruction
of abnormal bone

19

Endocrinology of the Gastrointestinal Tract

Stephen Bloom, MA, MD, FRCP, DSc, FRCPath

Peter Hammond, MD, MA, MRCP

The endocrinology of the gastrointestinal tract is complex and incompletely understood. The first hormone described, secretin, was isolated from the gastrointestinal tract in 1902. Further advances in gastrointestinal endocrinology, however, were limited until recently, when reliable techniques for isolating regulatory peptides at extremely low concentrations became available.

In contrast to most endocrine tissues in which hormone-producing cells are grouped together into anatomically distinct glands, the endocrine cells of the gastrointestinal tract are scattered throughout its length, and hence peptide concentrations in any one area are very low – around 10pmol/l. The majority of the peptides that are isolated are found in one region of the gut (Fig. 19.1). Several have similar amino-acid sequences, such as vasoactive intestinal polypeptide (VIP) and glucagon which belong to the secretin family of peptides (Fig. 19.2), or are produced by different post-translational processing of the same mRNA and prohormone, such as glucagon in the pancreas and enteroglucagon and glucagon-like peptide-1 (GLP-1) in the gut (Fig. 19.3).

Once isolated peptides have been sequenced, pure synthetic peptide can be produced and administered by intravenous infusion to determine its physiological role as a circulating hormone. Gastrointestinal actions such as enzyme release or motility, or systemic effects such as vasodilatation, may be seen. Such effects are sometimes found only at markedly supraphysiological doses, suggesting that the peptides may be most important as paracrine agents, controlling gastrointestinal function locally where they will reach much higher concentrations than in the circulation.

A number of peptides are classed as neurotransmitters in the gastrointestinal tract (Fig. 19.4). These are released from enteric nerves and have a local role; they include calcitonin-gene-related peptide (CGRP), galanin, bombesin, and gastrin-releasing peptides, and do not have a clear physiological function in the gastrointestinal tract, nor do they produce a specific gastrointestinal syndrome when secreted in excess.

A variety of gastrointestinal pathologies are associated with significant alterations in circulating concentrations of gut peptides, and it is thought that, under these circumstances, they play a role in the adaptation of the gut: for example, in response to loss of absorptive or secretory surface by altering secretion and motility in unaffected regions. Neuroendocrine tumours of the gastrointestinal tract are rare, usually occurring in the pancreas or duodenum. They can secrete a variety of peptides, and each peptide is usually associated with a distinct clinical syndrome.

GASTROINTESTINAL HORMONES

GASTRIN–CHOLECYSTOKININ FAMILY

The gastrin–cholecystokinin (CCK) family of peptides is shown in Fig. 19.5.

Gastrin

Gastrin is produced by G cells in the gastric antrum (from which it was first isolated in 1905) and upper small intestine and exists in a variety of molecular forms. The principal ones are fourteen, seventeen, or thirty-four amino acids in length, the latter being described as 'big gastrin'. The bioactive part of the molecule is the four amino-acid carboxy terminal sequence, which is common to all. The predominant circulating forms of gastrin are G17 from the stomach and G34 from the small intestine. G17 has a half-life in the circulation of some five minutes, while G34 has a half-life of approximately forty minutes; the two forms, however, are almost equipotent.

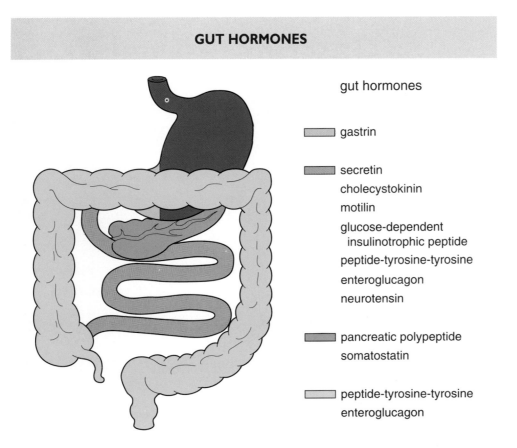

GUT HORMONES

gut hormones

gastrin

secretin
cholecystokinin
motilin
glucose-dependent
 insulinotrophic peptide
peptide-tyrosine-tyrosine
enteroglucagon
neurotensin

pancreatic polypeptide
somatostatin

peptide-tyrosine-tyrosine
enteroglucagon

Fig. 19.1 Hormone production in the gastrointestinal tract.

Gastrin stimulates the secretion of gastric acid from parietal cells and promotes growth of the gastric mucosa. These physiological effects are reflected in the classical features of the gastrinoma syndrome in which gastrin is hypersecreted. Infusions of gastrin provoke increased contractility of smooth muscle in the lower oesophagus and stomach, but the physiological significance of this action is unclear.

Gastrin secretion is stimulated by the presence of amino acids in the gastric antrum and upper small intestine, by local distension of the gastric antrum, and by increased vagal activity. Calcium, administered orally or intravenously, and intravenous infusions of adrenaline also stimulate gastrin release. A gastric pH of less than 3 inhibits antral gastrin secretion; this negative feedback effect prevents the excess secretion of gastric acid. Somatostatin, a peptide present in endocrine cells in the stomach, and peptides of the secretin family, can reduce gastrin release.

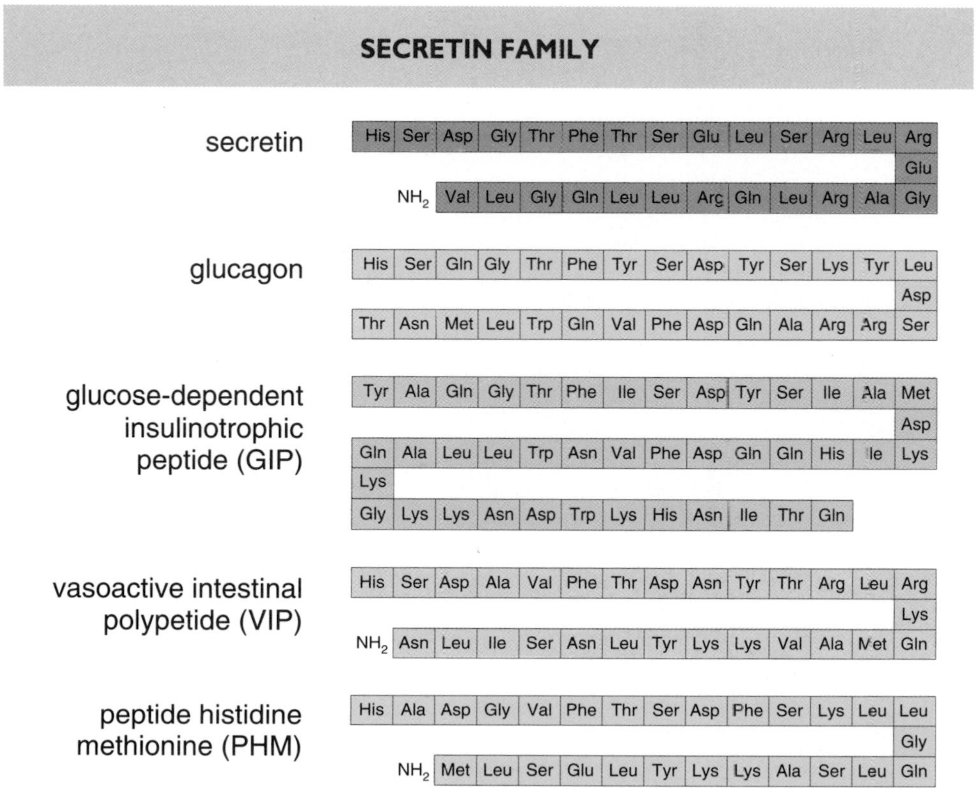

SECRETIN FAMILY
secretin
His Ser Asp Gly Thr Phe Thr Ser Glu Leu Ser Arg Leu Arg
Glu
NH_2 Val Leu Gly Gln Leu Leu Arg Gln Leu Arg Ala Gly
glucagon
His Ser Gln Gly Thr Phe Tyr Ser Asp Tyr Ser Lys Tyr Leu
Asp
Thr Asn Met Leu Trp Gln Val Phe Asp Gln Ala Arg Arg Ser
glucose-dependent insulinotrophic peptide (GIP)
Tyr Ala Gln Gly Thr Phe Ile Ser Asp Tyr Ser Ile Ala Met
Asp
Gln Ala Leu Leu Trp Asn Val Phe Asp Gln Gln His Ile Lys
Lys
Gly Lys Lys Asn Asp Trp Lys His Asn Ile Thr Gln
vasoactive intestinal polypetide (VIP)
His Ser Asp Ala Val Phe Thr Asp Asn Tyr Thr Arg Leu Arg
Lys
NH_2 Asn Leu Ile Ser Asn Leu Tyr Lys Lys Val Ala Met Gln
peptide histidine methionine (PHM)
His Ala Asp Gly Val Phe Thr Ser Asp Phe Ser Lys Leu Leu
Gly
NH_2 Met Leu Ser Glu Leu Tyr Lys Lys Ala Ser Leu Gln

Fig. 19.2 The secretin family of peptides.

PROCESSING OF PREPROGLUCAGON
preproglucagon
amino acids
20
30
29
37
35
enteroglucagon
GLP-1
GLP-2
small bowel processing
69
30
(7–36) NH_2
35
glucagon
GLP-1 + -2
pancreatic processing
29
88

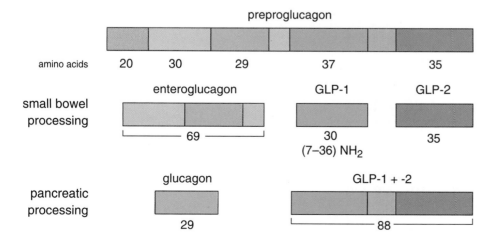

Fig. 19.3 Post-translational processing of preproglucagon.

Cholecystokinin

CCK has an identical five amino-acid carboxy terminal sequence to gastrin. Its specificity is conferred by the adjacent three amino acids, which include a sulphated tyrosine residue at position 7. CCK is found in the gut in predominantly thirty-three, thirty-nine, or fifty-eight amino-acid molecular forms, in contrast to the brain in which it is found at high concentrations in an eight amino-acid form. It is produced by the I cells of the duodenal and jejunal mucosa, which open onto the lumen. A small amount of CCK is found in specific enteric neurones of the upper gastrointestinal tract.

CCK stimulates the secretion of pancreatic enzymes, gallbladder contraction, and pancreatic growth, and may have a physiological role in inhibiting gastric emptying. Its secretion is stimulated by long-chain fatty acids and certain amino acids such as tryptophan and tyrosine, and it is inhibited by the secretion of bile salts into the small bowel lumen.

SECRETIN FAMILY

Secretin is one of a family of hormones (see Fig. 19.2) that share significant sequence homology: the hormones are glucagon, a catabolic hormone produced by the α-cells of the pancreas, which opposes the actions of insulin and raises levels of blood glucose; enteroglucagon (see opposite); VIP, a twenty-eight amino-acid neuropeptide that is found in the pancreas and gastrointestinal tract (see Fig. 19.4); peptide histidine methionine (PHM), a twenty-seven amino-acid neuropeptide with considerable sequence homology to VIP, which is derived from the adjacent exon of the preproVIP gene (see Fig. 19.4); growth-hormone releasing hormone (GHRH), a peptide with three immunoreactive forms of thirty-seven, forty, and forty-four amino acids which is released from the hypothalamus, principally in the forty-four amino-acid form, to stimulate growth hormone (GH) release, but is also found in significant concentrations, mainly in the forty amino-acid form, in the small intestinal mucosa where its function is unknown; and glucose-dependent insulinotrophic peptide (GIP).

GUT NEUROPEPTIDES

peptide	molecular size (amino acids)	distribution (nerves and commonest site)	actions
somatostatin	14	myenteric plexus gastrointestinal tract	multiple inhibitory effects (see Fig. 19.7)
vasoactive intestinal polypeptide (VIP)	28	myenteric and submucosal plexi mesenteric ganglia, blood vessels, gastrointestinal tract, gallbladder, pancreatic islets, salivary glands	inhibition of gastric acid secretion stimulation of bicarbonate secretion relaxation of vascular, biliary and intestinal smooth muscle stimulation of enterocyte secretion stimulation of insulin release
peptide histidine methionine (PHM)	27		
opioids enkephalin and dynorphin	5 17	myenteric and submucosal plexi gastrointestinal tract	inhibition of gastrointestinal secretion increased smooth-muscle contractility
substance P	11	myenteric and submucosal plexi	contraction of intestinal smooth muscle
neurokinins α and β	10	gastrointestinal tract, especially duodenum and jejunum	vasodilatation inhibition of intestinal absorption
calcitonin-gene-related peptide (CGRP)	37	extrinsic sensory nervous system blood vessels gastrointestinal tract, especially pylorus	inhibition of gastric acid secretion inihibition of pancreatic secretion relaxation of smooth muscle, especially vascular
galanin	29	myenteric and submucosal plexi gastrointestinal tract, pancreatic islets	contraction or relaxation of smooth muscle inhibition of postprandial insulin release
neuropeptide Y (NPY)	36	extrinsic adrenergic nerves to myenteric plexus proximal gastrointestinal tract and distal colon	vasoconstriction inhibition of stimulated intestinal secretion inihibition of intestinal muscle contraction
gastrin-releasing peptides	10, 23, 27	stomach and pancreas	stimulation of pancreatic enzyme and gastric acid secretion, motilin, gastrin and cholecystokinin release

Fig. 19.4 Gut neuropeptides.

Secretin

Secretin is a twenty-seven amino-acid peptide produced by S cells that are sparsely scattered throughout the duodenal and jejunal mucosa. Its main physiological function is to stimulate the secretion of watery alkaline juices from the pancreatic ducts. In common with other members of this family of peptides, secretin inhibits secretion of gastric acid and stimulates insulin release, although these effects occur only at pharmacological doses. The main stimulus to secretin secretion is a duodenal pH of less than 4. This occurs rarely, but the secretion of alkaline juices may protect the duodenum in the fasted state.

Glucose-dependent Insulinotrophic Peptide

GIP is a forty-two amino-acid peptide that is produced by K cells in the upper small intestinal mucosa. It was originally thought to inhibit gastric secretions (gastric inhibitory peptide), but this proved to be a pharmacological action. At physiological doses, GIP is a component of the enteroinsular axis, stimulating prandial insulin release. Such insulin-releasing factors are known as 'incretins'. Thus, food ingestion, particularly of carbohydrate and long-chain fatty acids, is the stimulus for GIP secretion.

ENTEROGLUCAGON AND GLUCAGON-LIKE PEPTIDES

Enteroglucagon and glucagon-like peptides are all derived from the preproglucagon gene. In the α-cells of the pancreas, post-translational cleavage of the preproglucagon mRNA produces glucagon and a large peptide that contains GLP-1 and -2 sequences. In the intestinal L cells, preproglucagon is cleaved into enteroglucagon (which contains the entire sequence of pancreatic glucagon and so is a member of the secretin family) and the two GLPs, GLP-1$_{7-36}$NH$_2$ and GLP-2 (see Fig. 19.3).

Enteroglucagon

Enteroglucagon is a sixty-nine amino-acid peptide. The L cells that secrete it are most abundant in the colonic mucosa, but are also present in the ileum. Enteroglucagon promotes gut growth and is important in gut adaptation, the amount of enteroglucagon secreted being proportional to the amount of unabsorbed food entering the colon. Enteroglucagon is further cleaved by the L cells to produce oxyntomodulin, which still retains the glucagon sequence; this peptide is secreted in smaller quantities than enteroglucagon, but is released into the circulation and inhibits secretion of gastric acid.

Glucagon-like Peptides

GLP-1 is highly conserved across species, suggesting that it is physiologically important. It is secreted in a cleaved form, GLP-1$_{7-36}$NH$_2$, which contains the thirty carboxy-terminal amino acids; this form inhibits secretion of gastric acid and is a more potent stimulus to insulin secretion than GIP. The physiological function of the thirty-five amino acid GLP-2 is unknown.

PANCREATIC POLYPEPTIDE AND PEPTIDE-TYROSINE-TYROSINE

Pancreatic polypeptide (PP) (Fig. 19.6) shares sequence homology with peptide-tyrosine-tyrosine (PYY), and neuropeptide Y (NPY), a neuropeptide found in adrenergic innervation (see Fig. 19.4).

Pancreatic Polypeptide

PP is a thirty-six amino-acid peptide produced by PP or F cells that are found mainly in the islets of Langerhans but are also scattered through the exocrine pancreas. It was first isolated as a contaminant

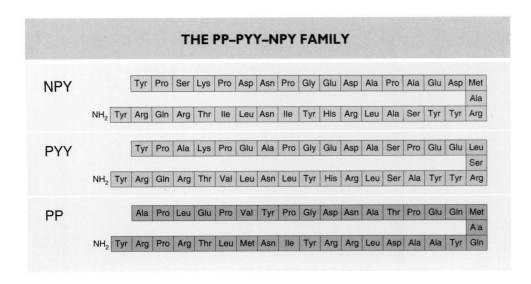

THE GASTRIN—CCK FAMILY

CCK33	Lys	Ala	Pro	Ser	Gly	Arg	Val	Ser	Met	Ile	Lys	Asn	Leu	Glu	Ser	Leu	Asp
																	Pro
	NH$_2$	Phe	Asp	Met	Trp	Gly	Met	Tyr(SO$_3$H)	Asp	Arg	Asp	Ser	Ile	Arg	His	Ser

G34	pGlu	Leu	Gly	Pro	Gln	Gly	Pro	Pro	His	Leu	Val	Ala	Asp	Pro	Ser	Lys	Lys
																	Glu
	NH$_2$	Phe	Asp	Met	Trp	Gly	Tyr	Ala	Glu	Glu	Glu	Glu	Glu	Leu	Trp	Pro	Gly

Fig. 19.5 The gastrin–cholecystokinin (CCK) family of peptides.

THE PP–PYY–NPY FAMILY

NPY			Tyr	Pro	Ser	Lys	Pro	Asp	Asn	Pro	Gly	Glu	Asp	Ala	Pro	Ala	Glu	Asp	Met
																			Ala
	NH$_2$	Tyr	Arg	Gln	Arg	Thr	Ile	Leu	Asn	Ile	Tyr	His	Arg	Leu	Ala	Ser	Tyr	Tyr	Arg

PYY			Tyr	Pro	Ala	Lys	Pro	Glu	Ala	Pro	Gly	Glu	Asp	Ala	Ser	Pro	Glu	Glu	Leu
																			Ser
	NH$_2$	Tyr	Arg	Gln	Arg	Thr	Val	Leu	Asn	Leu	Tyr	His	Arg	Leu	Ser	Ala	Tyr	Tyr	Arg

PP			Ala	Pro	Leu	Glu	Pro	Val	Tyr	Pro	Gly	Asp	Asn	Ala	Thr	Pro	Glu	Gln	Met
																			Ala
	NH$_2$	Tyr	Arg	Pro	Arg	Thr	Leu	Met	Asn	Ile	Tyr	Arg	Arg	Leu	Asp	Ala	Ala	Tyr	Gln

Fig. 19.6 The pancreatic polypeptide/peptide-tyrosine-tyrosine/neuropeptide Y (PP-PYY-NPY) family of peptides.

during the purification of insulin from the pancreas. It has no obvious physiological function. At pharmacological concentrations, PP is a weak inhibitor of gallbladder contraction, pancreatic secretion, and

gastric acid output. It is released into the circulation after meals, and in response to activation of cholinergic nerves from the vagus and to pancreatic exocrine stimulants such as CCK.

Peptide-tyrosine-tyrosine

PYY (the acronym PYY is derived from the IUPAC classification of amino acids, in which tyrosine is designated Y) is a thirty-six amino-acid peptide secreted by endocrine cells of the lower small intestinal and colonic mucosa, particularly of the rectum. Its distribution is similar to enteroglucagon, and in some areas, the two peptides are co-localised.

In mammals, PYY delays gastric emptying, decreases intestinal motility, and inhibits secretion of gastric acid. It also inhibits secretion of pancreatic exocrine juices and intestinal hormones, but probably at nonphysiological concentrations. There is a steep rise in PYY secretion after meals, particularly in response to carbohydrates and long-chain fatty acids, and PYY appears, by slowing intestinal transit, to allow more time for absorption. Its release occurs before nutrients have reached the ileum and so may result from a neuroendocrine reflex.

UNIQUE GUT PEPTIDES
Motilin

Motilin is a twenty-two amino-acid peptide secreted by M^0 cells of the duodenal and jejunal mucosa. It increases the contractility of gastrointestinal smooth muscle, accelerating gastric emptying and colonic transit. There is a high basal motilin output that sets the background muscle tone (with peaks in secretion coinciding with initiation of the myoelectric complex) and which causes interdigestive muscle contraction. Macrolide antibiotics such as erythromycin are motilin-receptor agonists, which explains the side effects of diarrhoea and abdominal cramps that are seen with use of such agents.

INHIBITORY ACTIONS OF SOMATOSTATIN

gastrointestinal tract

inhibition of
  secretion and action of gut hormones:
    secretin
    gastrin
    glucose-dependent insulinotrophic peptide
    motilin
    enteroglucagon
  gastric acid secretion
  gastric emptying and secretions
  nutrient absorption
  coeliac blood flow
  gallbladder contraction and secretions
  salivary excretions
  gastrointestinal motility

pancreas

inhibition of
  secretion and action of insulin and glucagon
  pancreatic enzyme and bicarbonate secretion

Fig. 19.7 Inhibitory actions of somatostatin in the gastrointestinal tract and pancreas.

Fig. 19.8 Nontumorous causes of elevated gut hormone levels.

NONTUMOROUS CAUSES OF ELEVATED GUT HORMONE LEVELS

gastrin	chronic renal failure hypercalcaemia H_2 blockers and proton pump inhibitors non-fasting sample
vasoactive intestinal polypeptide (VIP)	bowel ischaemia hepatic cirrhosis
glucagon	renal or hepatic failure stress prolonged fasting gonadotrophin-release inhibitors, e.g. danazol oral contraceptives familial hyperglucagonaemia
somatostatin	non-fasting sample
pancreatic polypeptide (PP)	non-fasting sample elderly pernicious anaemia
neurotensin	non-fasting sample

Neurotensin

Neurotensin is a thirteen amino-acid peptide that is produced by the N cells of the ileal mucosa and which is also present in enteric nerves. It inhibits secretion of gastric acid, gastric emptying, and gastric mucosal blood flow; stimulates release of pancreatic bicarbonate and intestinal secretions; and increases intestinal motor activity. It remains unclear, however, whether these are physiological functions. Neurotensin is released in response to mixed meals, particularly those with a high long-chain fatty acid content.

Somatostatin

Somatostatin is a peptide that is distributed widely in endocrine and neural tissues. It was initially discovered in the hypothalamus as the factor that inhibited GH release. At this site, it occurs predominantly as a fourteen amino-acid cyclic peptide that is linked by a disulphide bond. In the gastrointestinal tract, it occurs as fourteen and twenty-eight amino-acid peptides; both have an identical carboxy-terminal sequence, which is the biologically active region. Somatostatin is secreted by specific endocrine cells in the gastric and intestinal mucosa, and by the D cells on the inner rim of the pancreatic islets. It is also found in the enteric neural system.

Somatostatin is an inhibitor of hormone release and blocks the response to hormonal stimulation of the effector tissue. It inhibits a wide range of gastrointestinal functions (Fig. 19.7), the most clinically important being the inhibition of pancreatic secretions, gallbladder contraction, and insulin release. Somatostatin levels in plasma increase after food ingestion, with a more marked response seen with fat and protein than with carbohydrate, although the physiological importance of this response is unknown.

METHODS IN GASTROINTESTINAL ENDOCRINOLOGY

Understanding the pathophysiology of the gastrointestinal endocrine system relies upon hormone measurement by radioimmunoassay and visualisation of the endocrine cells by histochemical techniques.

Radioimmunoassay allows measurement of peptide levels, which are often as low as 10pmol/l in circulation and tissue. Although different antisera are used by different laboratories, thus preventing standardisation of results, there is consistency in the magnitude of hormone levels. Peptide assay is clinically most important in the diagnosis of gut hormone-secreting tumours. The elevation in circulating hormone levels is usually great, but a variety of gastrointestinal disorders (see below) and other conditions (Fig. 19.8) may be associated with more modest elevations.

In the normal gastrointestinal tract, immunocytochemistry is useful for determining the architecture of endocrine cells and the peptide hormone that is produced by individual cells, by using antibodies against specific peptides. Electron microscopy allows identification of secretory granules, which are often characteristic of a particular hormone (Fig. 19.9). *In situ* hybridisation, which detects hormone mRNA, is useful for demonstrating hormone synthesis in poorly granulated cells.

The histological features of gut hormone-secreting tumours are characteristic, with light microscopy showing a solid trabecular, glandular, or mixed pattern (Fig. 19.10). The techniques used to study normal cells can also be used to identify the particular peptides that are synthesised by tumours (Fig. 19.11). Furthermore, in tumours that are nonsecretory, nonspecific markers such as neuron-specific enolase and chromogranins can be used to demonstrate the endocrine nature of the tumour.

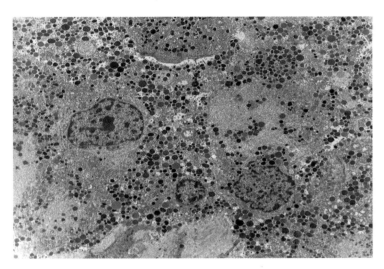

Fig. 19.9 An electron micrograph of a somatostatinoma with typical electron-dense granules.

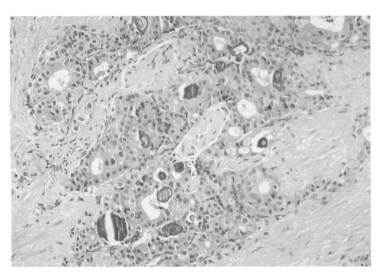

Fig. 19.10 Conventional histology of a duodenal somatostatinoma showing psammona bodies that are characteristic of these tumours.

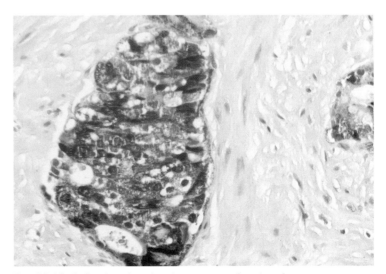

Fig. 19.11 A duodenal endocrine tumour showing dense immunoreactivity for somatostatin.

GUT HORMONES IN GASTROINTESTINAL DISEASE

The changes in gut hormones in gastrointestinal disease are usually the result of decreased hormone secretion from the affected region, and of compensatory elevation of other peptides that assist the adaptation of the gastrointestinal tract to loss of absorptive surface. Occasionally, the elevation in levels of gut peptide may contribute to the disease process.

GASTRIC PATHOLOGY

Gastrin levels are elevated in a variety of gastric disorders. Usually, gastrin is secreted in response to a diminished output of gastric acid as in atrophic gastritis (which is associated with achlorhydria) and following vagotomy. If the antrum is retained following surgery, gastrin-secreting cells are no longer exposed to gastric acid and so hypersecrete gastrin. G cell hyperplasia results in gastrin excess despite normal or elevated acid output.

In the postgastrectomy dumping syndrome, there is a gross exaggeration in the postprandial rise of VIP, PYY, enteroglucagon, and neurotensin levels, and a decrease in motilin levels. These changes may contribute to the impaired neural control of gastric emptying in this condition.

SURGERY

Following partial ileal resection, gastrin, enteroglucagon, PP, motilin, and PYY levels are all elevated (Fig. 19.12), leading to hypertrophy of the remaining small intestine and delayed intestinal transit and thus creating more area and time for nutrient absorption. Similar changes occur in association with colonic resection when the levels of gastrin and PP, but not of the principally colonic hormones, are elevated.

Jejuno-ileal bypass is an operation that at one time was performed for gross obesity. It resulted in almost complete loss of the postprandial rise in GIP, which is secreted by the bypassed segment, but the elevation of hormones from other segments (Fig. 19.12) led to compensatory hypertrophy of the remaining bowel so that the effect of the operation was ultimately negated.

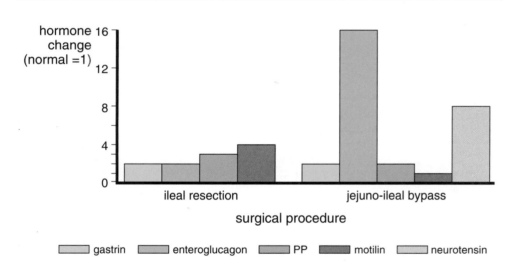

CHANGES IN GUT HORMONES AFTER SURGERY

Fig. 19.12 Changes in levels of gut hormones following bowel resection.

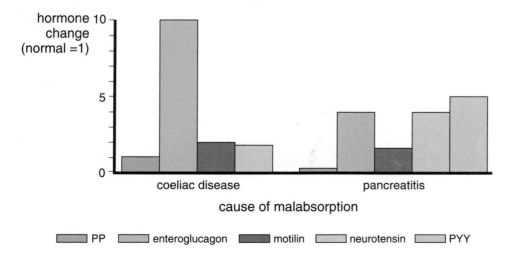

CHANGES IN GUT HORMONES IN MALABSORPTION

Fig. 19.13 Changes in levels of gut hormones associated with malabsorption.

MALABSORPTION

In chronic pancreatitis, the pancreatic endocrine cells are often affected to some extent, and this is reflected by decreased levels of PP. The excess of nutrients passing into the colon as a result of the steatorrhoea causes elevation of enteroglucagon and PYY levels, and neurotensin secretion also increases (Fig. 19.13). The gut adaptation resulting from these hormonal changes may explain the improvement in absorptive function seen with age in patients with cystic fibrosis.

Coeliac disease is associated with reduced secretion of hormones from the affected duodenum and jejunum, such as secretin, CCK, and GIP. This in turn leads to impaired pancreatic exocrine secretion, thus exacerbating the malabsorption. There is gross elevation of other hormones to compensate for the malabsorption, particularly neurotensin and enteroglucagon, the latter stimulating increased enterocyte turnover despite villous atrophy (Fig. 19.13). Similar changes occur in tropical sprue. Following successful treatment of these malabsorptive conditions, gut hormone levels return to normal.

ACUTE DIARRHOEA

There is a great elevation in motilin and enteroglucagon levels in acute infective diarrhoea (Fig. 19.14). These peptides may help in the repair process, or may contribute to the altered motility, particularly motilin. In Crohn's disease there is an elevation of PP levels, with a lesser increase in GIP, motilin and enteroglucagon levels; in ulcerative colitis there is a moderate elevation in PP, gastrin, GIP and motilin levels.

NEUROPATHIC DISEASE

In conditions in which local enteric nerves are destroyed, such as Hirschsprung's and Chagas' disease, there is a loss of local neuropeptides such as substance P, VIP, and somatostatin. These peptides are unaffected by diseases that affect distant neural gut innervation, such as the Shy–Drager syndrome.

GUT HORMONE TUMOURS

INTRODUCTION

Gut hormone tumours are rare, the most common being those associated with the carcinoid syndrome, with an annual incidence of one per five hundred thousand. Other functioning tumours occur with an annual incidence of one per million or less. The majority of gut hormone-secreting tumours originate in pancreatic islet cells, with the exception of carcinoid tumours, which usually occur in the midgut. Some fifty per cent of pancreatic islet cell tumours are nonfunctioning. The remainder are associated with a characteristic syndrome due to secretion of a particular hormone by the tumour (Fig. 19.15). The hormone secreted may be eutopic (from a tumour of the tissue from which the hormone is secreted normally – for example, insulin, glucagon, somatostatin or PP) or ectopic (for example, VIP or gastrin). The tumours may produce other hormones during the course of the

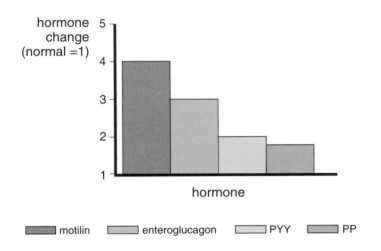

CHANGES IN GUT HORMONES IN ACUTE DIARRHOEA

Fig. 19.14 Gut hormone levels in acute diarrhoea.

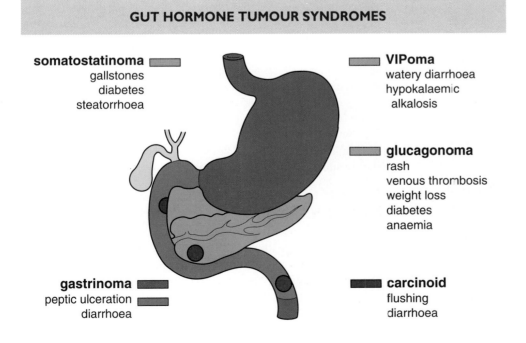

GUT HORMONE TUMOUR SYNDROMES

Fig. 19.15 Gut hormone tumour syndromes.

somatostatinoma
gallstones
diabetes
steatorrhoea

VIPoma
watery diarrhoea
hypokalaemic alkalosis

glucagonoma
rash
venous thrombosis
weight loss
diabetes
anaemia

gastrinoma
peptic ulceration
diarrhoea

carcinoid
flushing
diarrhoea

disease, giving rise to secondary hormone syndromes when secreted in sufficient amounts. Such secondary syndromes occur in some five per cent of cases, and so all patients should have their peptide levels assayed at least yearly to identify such cases. Approximately twenty-five per cent of pancreatic islet cell tumours, particularly gastrinomas and nonfunctioning tumours, occur in association with the autosomal dominant multiple endocrine neoplasia type 1 (MEN 1) syndrome, whose other characteristic features are parathyroid adenomas and, less commonly, pituitary adenomas.

Seventy per cent of sporadic islet cell tumours, and forty-five per cent of those associated with MEN 1, are malignant. The most common sites for metastases are the liver and regional lymph nodes, although they may occur in bone, the adrenals, the brain and the lungs, where they carry a much worse prognosis. Metastases are usually slow-growing so that prolonged survival is often possible, particularly if treatment can minimise the effects of hormone excess. Since these tumours and their associated syndromes are rare, there is often a delay in diagnosis following the onset of symptoms, averaging some three years. Following diagnosis, there is a fifty per cent chance of survival of around six years for those with sporadic tumours, and of fifteen years for those with MEN 1.

The aetiology of gut hormone-secreting tumours remains unclear. These tumours were originally classified as APUDomas. (The acronym APUD refers to the ability of these cells to perform amine precursor uptake and decarboxylation, and hence synthesise peptides.) It was proposed that these tumours arose from neural crest cells, and the APUD concept explained their ability to secrete a number of different hormones. The common origin of such cells from the neural crest has since been disproved, however, and it is now postulated that neuroendocrine and mucosal endocrine cells of the gastrointestinal tract and pancreas are derived from a common embryonic stem cell that divides and differentiates down a neuroendocrine or gastroenteropancreatic cell line. These tumours, therefore, are also referred to as gastroenteropancreatic or gut neuroendocrine tumours. The genetic basis for the majority of these

tumours is unknown, but in patients with MEN 1 there is a deletion on chromosome 11 in the q13 region, and this has been described in cases of sporadic insulinoma.

CARCINOID SYNDROME

Carcinoid tumours can occur throughout the gastrointestinal system, being derived from the embryonic foregut (bronchus, stomach and pancreas), midgut (small intestine and ascending colon) or hindgut (distal colon and rectum). The most common site of carcinoid tumours is the appendix, followed by the rectum and ileum (Fig. 19.16). The average age at presentation is around fifty years, and the annual incidence is one in one hundred and fifty thousand.

Carcinoid tumours account for up to thirty-five per cent of small bowel tumours. They are, however, usually slow-growing, and the malignant potential depends on the origin of the primary. Appendiceal and rectal carcinoids are usually incidental surgical findings and rarely metastasise, while small bowel carcinoids metastasise to the liver in some fifty per cent of cases.

The clinical manifestations of carcinoid tumours are varied and are often determined by the site of the tumour. The carcinoid syndrome occurs in around ten per cent of cases, usually in association with midgut tumours, and almost invariably in the presence of hepatic metastases. It results from the secretion of 5-hydroxytryptamine (5HT: serotonin) and a variety of other vasoactive substances such as histamine, bradykinins, prostaglandins and substance P. The cardinal features of the syndrome are diarrhoea and flushing. The diarrhoea is secretory and may be profuse, with passage of several litres per day, and there are occasionally associated electrolyte disturbances. It may also be associated with cramping abdominal pain. The flushing is paroxysmal and usually unprovoked, although it may occur in association with exertion or with ingestion of food or alcohol. It usually affects the face and upper thorax (Fig. 19.17), and may be associated with palpitations and postural hypotension, and rarely lacrimation and facial oedema. When flushing occurs over a prolonged period, patients often develop a permanent plethoric, cyanotic facial appearance (Fig. 19.18). This latter feature is more common in those with foregut tumours. Paroxysmal wheezing occurs in a small number of patients, attacks often occurring in association with flushing. Around twenty per cent of patients have cardiac valve abnormalities, usually affecting the right side of the heart. These lesions result from the formation of plaques on the valves, consisting of smooth muscle in a collagenous stroma. The most common findings are tricuspid incompetence and pulmonary stenosis, and these are often associated with severe right heart failure. Left-sided valve lesions in association with bronchial carcinoids are rarely found. Pellagra may occur, nicotinamide deficiency resulting from the increased conversion of 5-hydroxytryptophan into 5HT.

Diagnosis of the carcinoid syndrome is based on the finding of raised levels of 5-hydroxyindole acetic acid (5HIAA) in a twenty-four-hour urine collection. This is produced by the action of monoamine oxidase and aldehyde dehydrogenase enzymes on 5HT and accounts for over ninety-five per cent of the urinary excretion of 5HT.

GASTRINOMA SYNDROME

The gastrinoma syndrome has an annual incidence of one per million. Sixty per cent of gastrinomas are malignant, fifty per cent of patients having metastases at the time of diagnosis. Up to thirty per cent of patients with the gastrinoma syndrome will have MEN 1. The majority of tumours occur in the pancreas, but around twenty per cent of patients will have microadenomas (less than 1cm in diameter) in the duodenum, particularly those with MEN 1. Rarely, gastrinomas may be found in the stomach or ovary.

SITES OF CARCINOID TUMOURS

site	incidence (%)
appendix	40
small bowel	25
rectum	15
bronchus	10
colon	5
stomach	<5
duodenum	
pancreas	<1
ovary	
testis	

Fig. 19.16 Sites of carcinoid tumours.

The gastrinoma syndrome was first described in 1955 by Zollinger and Ellison, with the triad of fulminating ulcer diathesis, recurrent ulceration despite medical and surgical therapy, and a non-β-cell pancreatic islet tumour. Severe duodenal ulceration resulting from excess production of gastric acid is still the usual presenting feature, often associated with complications such as haemorrhage, perforation or pyloric stenosis. Ulceration may affect the oesophagus and upper small bowel with similar consequences, particularly stricture formation. The other increasingly recognised feature of the syndrome is diarrhoea or steatorrhoea. This results from acid inactivation of enzymes and mucosal damage in the upper small bowel, and may predate ulcer symptoms by up to twelve months.

Diagnosis of the gastrinoma syndrome depends on the demonstration of hypergastrinaemia in the presence of increased acid output. A basal acid output of greater than 10mmol/h (or 5mmol/h if the patient has previously undergone an acid-reducing operation), associated with a raised level of circulating gastrin, is diagnostic. Measuring the pentagastrin-stimulated acid output does not improve the diagnostic accuracy. If the acid output is equivocal and there is a strong clinical suspicion, the secretin test may be of value. In most normal individuals, secretin inhibits gastrin release and serum gastrin levels fall, but in patients with the gastrinoma syndrome, there is a paradoxical rise in levels of serum gastrin, usually greater than two-fold.

VIPOMA SYNDROME

The VIPoma syndrome results from the secretion of VIP and PHM by neuroendocrine tumours. Ten per cent of VIP-secreting tumours are extrapancreatic, usually occurring in children, and arise in neural crest tissue as ganglioneuromas, ganglioneuroblastomas, or neuroblastomas. The annual incidence of the VIPoma syndrome is one per ten million. Fifty per cent of VIPomas are malignant, and in such cases metastases are usually present at the time of diagnosis.

The characteristic feature of the syndrome is profuse secretory diarrhoea, with daily stool volumes usually exceeding 3 litres, and occasionally exceeding 20 litres. This results in profound dehydration and weakness, and there is usually a marked hypokalaemic alkalosis due to loss of potassium and bicarbonate ions in the stool. The diarrhoea may become severe enough to cause cardiovascular collapse. Other features of the syndrome are achlorhydria, glucose intolerance, hypercalcaemia and hypophosphataemia (probably due to secretion of parathyroid hormone-related protein: PTHrP), flushing, and rarely tetany due to hypomagnesaemia.

GLUCAGONOMA SYNDROME

The glucagonoma syndrome has an annual incidence of one per twenty million, and over ninety-nine per cent of cases result from pancreatic tumours that secrete glucagon. Over seventy-five per cent of glucagonomas are malignant, and fifty per cent of patients have metastases at the time of diagnosis.

The cardinal feature of the syndrome is a rash – necrolytic migratory erythema. This usually starts in the groins with the presence of erythematous blotches that become eroded and then heal leaving indurated pigmented areas. The rash migrates to the perineum, buttocks, and distal extremities (Fig. 19.19). All mucous membranes may be affected by the rash (Fig. 19.20). The aetiology of the rash remains unclear, but it may be the result of the action of glucagon on

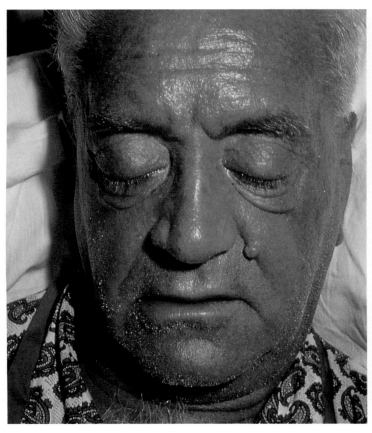

Fig. 19.17 Carcinoid syndrome. Acute flushing can be seen.

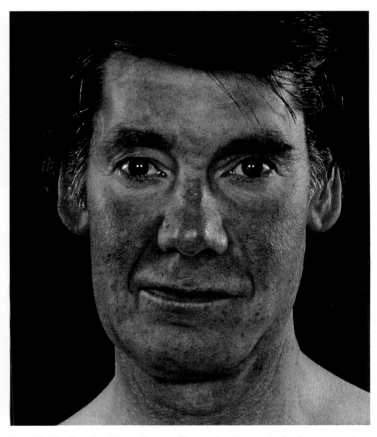

Fig. 19.18 Carcinoid syndrome. The patient has a plethoric, cyanosed facies.

the skin, prostaglandins in the epidermis, zinc deficiency, or hypoaminoacidaemia which occurs in the syndrome. Other features of the syndrome are impaired glucose tolerance and occasionally diabetes; weight loss, which may be extreme; normochromic normocytic anaemia; depression and mental slowing, which may be severe; and venous thrombosis, which can be extensive and life-threatening.

SOMATOSTATINOMA SYNDROME

Somatostatinomas are very rare tumours. Fifty per cent arise in the pancreas, with ninety per cent of these being malignant. The remaining fifty per cent arise from the duodenum, and over half of these occur in association with neurofibromatosis type 1. Duodenal tumours usually present early due to local effects such as intestinal obstruction, obstructive jaundice or gastrointestinal haemorrhage,

and so they are rarely associated with the somatostatinoma syndrome and rarely metastasise. The somatostatinoma syndrome reflects the inhibitory effects of somatostatin on biliary and pancreatic function, and is characterised by gallstones, steatorrhoea and diabetes. Occasionally, hypoglycaemia may occur due to greater inhibition of counterregulatory hormones rather than of insulin, and postprandial fullness, weight loss and anaemia are also described.

OTHER TUMOURS

Levels of PP are elevated in seventy-five per cent of pancreatic endocrine tumours, and neurotensin levels are elevated in ten per cent of VIPomas, but these hormones have not been associated with clinical syndromes. Tumours that secrete GHRH causing acromegaly

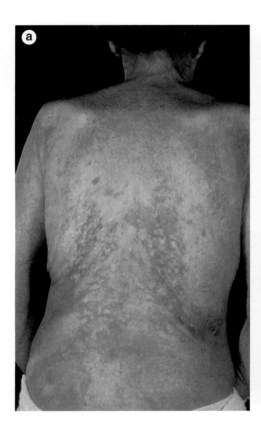
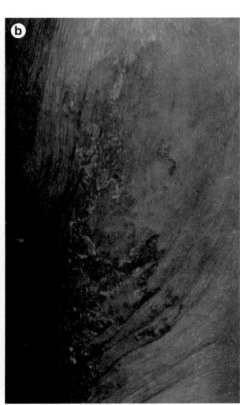

Fig. 19.19 *Glucagonoma syndrome: necrolytic migratory erythema.*

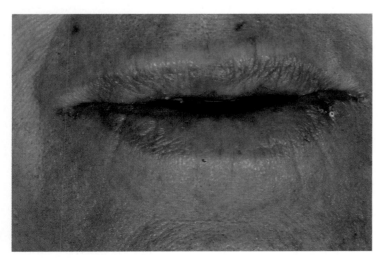

Fig. 19.20 *Glucagonoma syndrome: cheilitis.*

or gigantism, adrenocorticotrophic hormone causing Cushing's syndrome, and PTHrP resulting in hypercalcaemia, have all been reported. Up to fifty per cent of pancreatic tumours are nonfunctioning and these usually present late with metastases. The five-year survival chance of patients with nonfunctioning tumours is less than fifty per cent.

TUMOUR LOCALISATION

Tumours associated with the carcinoid syndrome, VIPomas, glucagonomas, somatostatinomas and nonfunctioning tumours are usually greater than 2cm in diameter, and over fifty per cent will have metastasised at the time of diagnosis. Localisation of these tumours and their metastases is easily accomplished with ultrasonography and computed tomography (CT) scanning (Figs. 19.21–19.23). Forty per

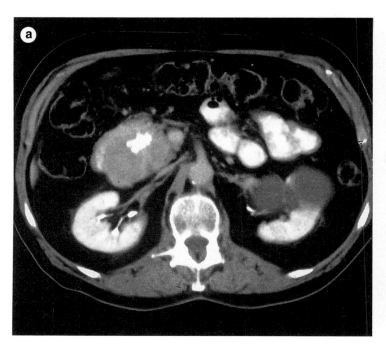

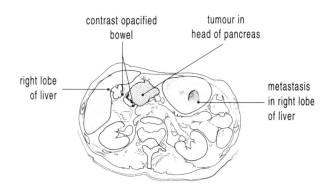

Fig. 19.21 *VIPoma syndrome showing a pancreatic tumour with liver metastasis.*

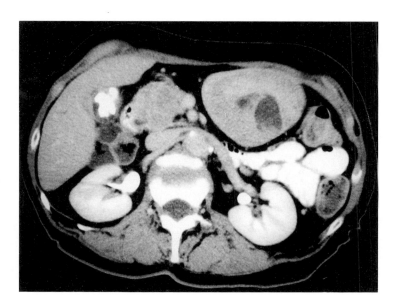

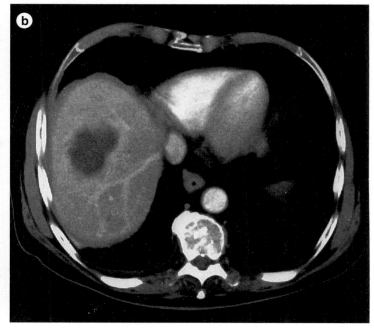

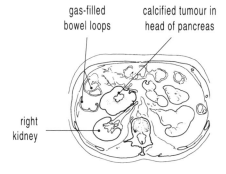

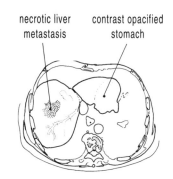

Fig. 19.22 *Glucagonoma syndrome.* (a) Calcified pancreatic tumour. (b) Necrotic liver metastasis following hepatic embolisation.

cent of gastrinomas, however, are less than 1cm in diameter, and localisation of these tumours and other microadenomas is best achieved with a combination of ultrasonography, rapid and dynamic CT scanning following a bolus injection of contrast, and highly selective visceral angiography (Fig. 19.24), which will identify some sev-

enty per cent of cases. Transhepatic portal venous sampling does not usually improve perioperative tumour localisation. Newer techniques such as endoscopic ultrasonography and radioisotope scanning with indium- or iodine-labelled somatostatin analogues (Fig. 19.25) may improve detection rates.

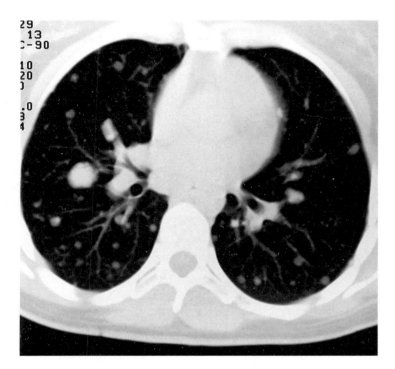

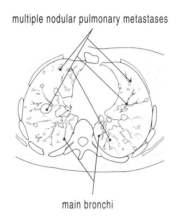

Fig. 19.23 A nonfunctioning pancreatic endocrine tumour with lung metastases.

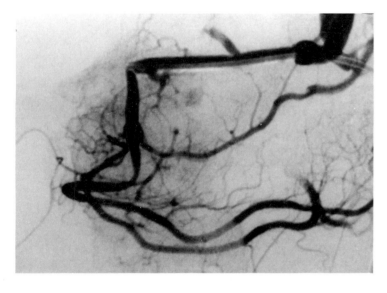

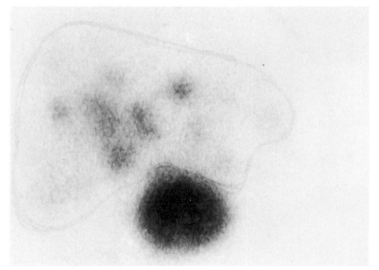

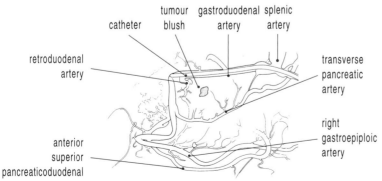

Fig. 19.24 A gastroduodenal arteriogram showing a gastrinoma blush in pancreatic head.

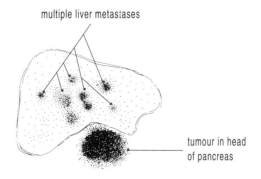

Fig. 19.25 An indium-labelled octreotide scan showing a pancreatic tumour and hepatic metastases (same patient as shown in Fig. 19.22).

TREATMENT
Surgery
Surgical excision offers the only chance of cure for patients with gut hormone-secreting tumours and should always be undertaken, if possible, when a primary tumour is identified and has not obviously metastasised. Such an approach is commonly of benefit only in gastrinomas or VIPomas, since other tumour types are usually malignant. Noncurative tumour debulking can provide excellent palliation, reducing hormone levels and morbidity from local effects. A few patients have successfully undergone hepatic transplantation for metastatic disease that is confined to the liver.

Cytotoxic Chemotherapy
A number of chemotherapeutic regimens have been used in the treatment of gut hormone tumours (Fig. 19.26). Most regimens have similar effects, VIPomas being particularly responsive to chemotherapy, while gastrinomas respond in only forty per cent of cases; carcinoids respond poorly, with as few as ten per cent of patients showing an objective improvement. The combination of streptozotocin and 5-fluorouracil is most commonly used. Interferon is not widely advocated because of the high incidence of severe side effects.

Hepatic Embolisation
The blood supply of the normal liver arises from the hepatic artery and the portal vein. Hepatic metastases, which are supplied only by the hepatic artery, can be devascularised by embolisation of the hepatic arterial tree (Figs. 19.27–19.29) without affecting normal liver parenchyma, providing that the portal vein is patent. Hepatic embolisation can provide good palliation in over fifty per cent of patients with symptomatic hepatic metastases, and the procedure can be repeated when symptoms recur. The somatostatin analogue octreotide should be administered to counter the effects of massive hormone release following embolisation, and broad-spectrum antibiotic prophylaxis is recommended.

CHEMOTHERAPY REGIMENS

regimen	response rate (%)	best response (%)	side effects
streptozotocin (500mg/m² on alternate days for ten days every three months)	40–60		anorexia, nausea and vomiting renal, hepatic and bone marrow toxicity
streptozotocin and 5-fluorouracil (400mg/m² schedule as above)	65	90 (VIPomas)	no additional side effects with 5-fluorouracil
interferon-α (3–6mU daily)	50–75	100 (VIPomas)	flu-like symptoms with high pyrexia hepatic and bone marrow toxicity
dacarbazine (250mg/m² for 5 days every 3–4 weeks)	50	100 (glucagonomas)	nausea

Fig. 19.26 Chemotherapy regimens for gut hormone tumours.

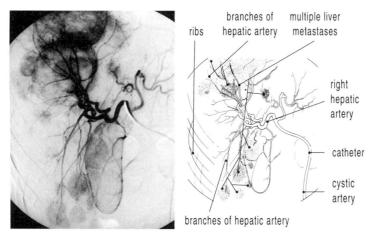

Fig. 19.27 An arteriogram of the right hepatic artery showing multiple liver metastases.

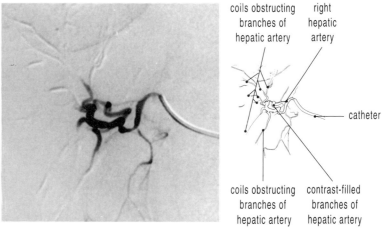

Fig. 19.28 An arteriogram showing branches of hepatic artery (as shown in Fig. 19.27) which are occluded by coils.

Octreotide

Octreotide, an octapeptide, is a long-acting analogue of somatostatin which contains the amino-acid sequence necessary for receptor binding (see Chapter 3). It inhibits the release of gut hormones from gastroenteropancreatic tumours and hence inhibits their peripheral actions. Up to ninety per cent of patients with hormonal syndromes respond to octreotide with a reduction in symptoms and hormone levels, and it can be life-saving in a VIPoma crisis. It is administered subcutaneously starting at doses as low as 50μg twice daily, increasing to a maximum of 500μg three times daily as effectiveness is progressively reduced.

Other Treatments

The diarrhoea and flushing of the carcinoid syndrome can often be controlled with the 5HT antagonists cyproheptidine and methysergide, although octreotide has proved to be more effective. Vitamin supplements containing nicotinamide are necessary when patients have pellagra, and may be used prophylactically.

Treatment of the gastrinoma syndrome has been much improved by use of the proton pump inhibitor omeprazole, which almost completely inhibits gastric acid production. It has greatly reduced morbidity in patients with unlocalised tumours or those with metastatic disease.

A variety of agents have been used in treating the diarrhoea of the VIPoma syndrome, the most effective being prednisolone. Octreotide has, however, again proved to be superior to these other drugs. VIPoma crises require intensive fluid and electrolyte support, and central venous pressure monitoring may be necessary.

Topical and oral zinc, a high-protein diet, amino-acid infusions, and blood transfusions may all lead to an improvement in the glucagonoma rash. The thrombotic tendency is unaffected by anticoagulants, but aspirin may be beneficial. Insulin may be needed to treat the diabetes of the glucagonoma and somatostatinoma syndromes.

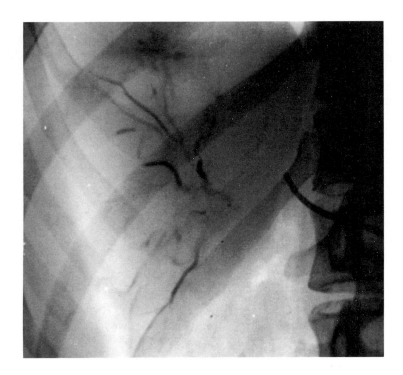

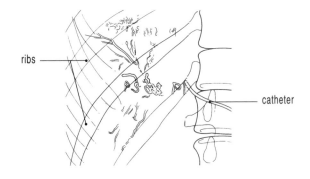

Fig. 19.29 A plain radiograph showing the position of the coils as shown in Fig. 19.28.

ribs

catheter

Hypoglycaemia and Insulinomas

Vincent Marks, MA, DM, FRCP, FRCPath

Hypoglycaemia is a biochemical description (Fig. 20.1). Although it has many causes, all are the result of an imbalance between the rate of entry of glucose into the glucose pool and the rate of removal of glucose.

THE GLUCOSE POOL IN HEALTH

The size of the glucose pool is normally tightly controlled by a number of quasi-independent homeostatic mechanisms that are co-ordinated by a hypothetical master centre (Fig. 20.2).

Although the exact size of the glucose pool is determined by both the volume of extracellular fluid and its glucose concentration, in practice it is only the latter that varies. The glucose pool rarely exceeds 27g (0.15mol) even after ingestion of a meal containing up to 360g (2mol) of glucose in the form of starch, and it does not shrink below 13g (0.075mol) even after prolonged fasting. The only route by which glucose normally enters the glucose pool is through the hepatic vein, which receives glucose either from hepatocytes during fasting or from the gut via the portal vein in the absorptive phase of a meal. During fasting, when the peripheral plasma insulin concentration falls below the level that is required to stimulate or permit free entry of glucose into insulin-dependent cells (such as muscle, fat, and connective tissues), outflow from the glucose pool is restricted to noninsulin-dependent tissues such as the brain and erythron. After feeding, and during the absorptive period, insulin is secreted by the B cells of the pancreas (Fig. 20.3) in response to nervous impulses that arise in the gut wall; to hormones that are liberated by endocrine cells in the intestinal mucosa; and to a rise in arterial glucose concentration. This has the effect of decreasing glucose output by the liver and increasing its uptake and conversion to glycogen, increasing outflow from the glucose pool into glucose-dependent tissues and producing a positive arteriovenous glucose difference across the forearm and other peripheral tissues.

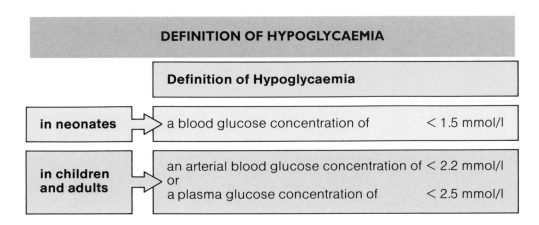

DEFINITION OF HYPOGLYCAEMIA

Definition of Hypoglycaemia	
in neonates	a blood glucose concentration of < 1.5 mmol/l
in children and adults	an arterial blood glucose concentration of < 2.2 mmol/l or a plasma glucose concentration of < 2.5 mmol/l

Fig. 20.1 The definition of hypoglycaemia. Hypoglycaemia is a biochemical description, which may or may not be accompanied by symptoms.

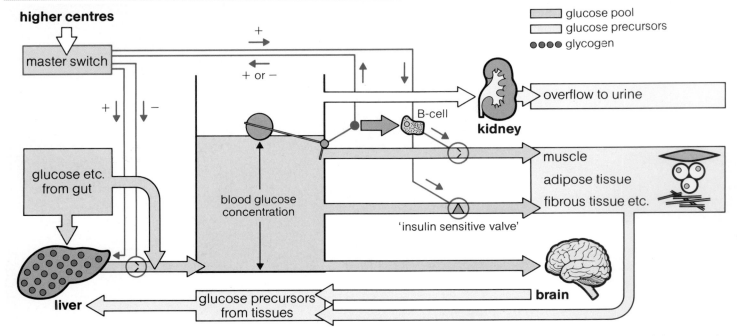

AUTOREGULATORY CONTROL OF THE BLOOD GLUCOSE POOL

glucose pool
glucose precursors
glycogen

higher centres
master switch
+
+ or −
+↓   ↓−
glucose etc. from gut
blood glucose concentration
B-cell
kidney
overflow to urine
muscle
adipose tissue
fibrous tissue etc.
'insulin sensitive valve'
liver
glucose precursors from tissues
brain

Fig. 20.2 A schematic representation of the autoregulatory control of the size of the blood glucose pool. Glucose homeostasis is presented as a self-regulating plumbing system. Blood glucose concentration rises as glucose enters the blood from the intestine. This in turn activates insulin secretion by direct action on the pancreas, and also through higher centres. Consequently, glucose inflow from the liver (from glycogen) is reduced, and outflow into the tissues is increased. During fasting, glucose inflow from the gut ceases; blood glucose concentration reaches basal levels; insulin secretion and outflow of glucose into the tissues almost cease; and glucose release from the liver (glycogen) is activated so that inflow exactly balances outflow into the brain and erythron. The 'insulin-sensitive valve' can be activated by both endogenous and exogenous insulin.

The small rise in arterial blood glucose concentration that follows the ingestion of a meal is not always reflected in venous blood; after a small early rise, there is often a postprandial fall in blood glucose to below fasting levels. In situations where the glucose homeostatic mechanisms become overwhelmed by excessively rapid absorption of glucose due to its precipitate entry into the duodenum, such as that which occurs after partial gastrectomy, or when insulin secretory capacity is reduced, the glucose pool may expand sufficiently to result in glycosuria.

In the postabsorptive state, the glucose needs of the body are confined almost exclusively to those of the brain and the erythron. These needs are met by hepatic release of glucose into the circulation, either by the breakdown of preformed glycogen (glycogenolysis) or by synthesis (gluconeogenesis) from glucose precursors. Gluconeogenesis occurs predominantly from lactate, pyruvate, alanine and glycerate, which are released into the circulation by somatic tissues, such as striatal muscle, during fasting.

HYPOGLYCAEMIA

Hypoglycaemia results when glucose outflow from the glucose pool is not balanced by glucose inflow from the liver (see Fig. 20.2). It most commonly arises from impaired hepatic glucose release under the influence of modest amounts of insulin. Most cases of hypoglycaemia are iatrogenic and result from pharmacologically large doses of exogenous insulin, or from drug-induced increased endogenous insulin secretion, reducing inflow of glucose from the liver to below its rate of outflow into the tissues. In a small number of cases, impaired release of glucose is secondary to some underlying, though not necessarily obvious, pathology elsewhere in the body and is referred to as 'spontaneous' hypoglycaemia.

NEUROGLYCOPENIA

Regardless of its immediate cause, most of the symptoms of hypoglycaemia arise as a result of alterations in cerebral metabolism (Fig. 20.4). The nature and severity of these neuroglycopenic symptoms depend largely upon the speed at which the blood glucose level falls, and whether habituation to hypoglycaemia has taken place. Acute neuroglycopenia is common in patients who have taken an insulin overdose, and warns them of the need to take sugar to prevent impairment of consciousness. Loss of these acute (sometimes referred to as adrenergic) symptoms is common in patients who have used insulin for many years to treat their diabetes, and gives rise to what is known as 'hypoglycaemia unawareness'. It then resembles subacute neuroglycopenia in its manifestations. The symptoms of subacute neuroglycopenia are relatively unobtrusive and generally more apparent to others than to the patients themselves.

Subacute neuroglycopenia is the symptom complex that is most commonly produced by overdosage with sulphonylureas and by diseases that cause spontaneous hypoglycaemia. Chronic neuroglycopenia and hyperinsulin neuropathy are both very uncommon and almost invariably result from persistent hypoglycaemia secondary to insulinoma or overenthusiastic treatment of diabetes. Normoglycaemic neuroglycopenia, which can be produced experimentally by 2-deoxyglucose and other substances that impair intraneuronal glucose metabolism, may be more common than was once thought. It occurs in children (and possibly in adults) during certain viral infections of the central nervous system which interfere with glucose transport into the brain, and also possibly as an inherited abnormality and in diabetes.

FUEL CONSUMPTION BY THE BRAIN

Under normal circumstances the human brain consumes approximately 120–130g glucose per day, which constitutes its main, if not sole, source of energy. During prolonged fasting or starvation the brain can metabolise ketones, such as aceto-acetate and β-hydroxybutyrate, as its main fuel (Fig. 20.5). In children, the switch from glucose to ketones as the main source of cerebral energy may occur as little as twenty-four hours after withdrawal of food. The supply of fuel to various parts of the brain is determined not only by its concentration in the plasma, but also by blood flow. Simultaneous reduction of both can lead to impairment of cerebral function, even when there is no discernible abnormality in either one alone. This probably accounts for the inability of many elderly subjects to withstand lowering of their blood glucose concentrations to levels that are well tolerated by young people. Similarly, it explains why elderly diabetic patients with unilateral cerebrovascular disease, who have been rendered hypoglycaemic by insulin, occasionally present with hemiplegia that is rapidly reversed by intravenous glucose.

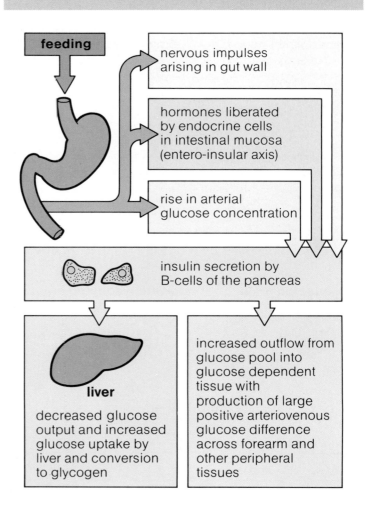

HYPOGLYCAEMIC EFFECT OF INSULIN

Fig. 20.3 The hypoglycaemic effect of insulin. Insulin secretion by the B-cells is stimulated during feeding and absorption of food by the nervous impulses that arise from the gut; by hormones that are secreted by endocrine cells in the intestinal mucosa; and by a rise in arterial blood glucose and/or amino-acid concentrations.

NEUROGLYCOPENIC SYNDROMES

acute neuroglycopenia
Sweating, malaise, anxiety, tachycardia, circumoral and/or carpal paraesthesia, unsteadiness, sleepiness progressing to stupor and coma; abnormal EEG present throughout: rapidly reversed by intravenous glucose but not by saline.

subacute neuroglycopenia
Lack of concentration, sleepiness, lassitude, inactivity progressing to stupor and coma; abnormal EEG throughout: rapidly reversed by intravenous glucose but not saline.

chronic neuroglycopenia (very rare)
Progressive mental deterioration simulating schizophrenia, depression or, most often, dementia; EEG may be normal. No immediate effect produced by glucose; partially reversible by permanent restoration of normoglycaemia.

normoglycaemic neuroglycopenia (very rare)
Caused by impaired intraneuronal glucose metabolism. Symptoms are a combination of those of acute and subacute neuroglycopenia and are partially or wholly relieved by sustained hyperglycaemia.

hyperinsulin neuropathy (extremely rare)
Paraesthesia in hands and feet, muscular weakness and wasting, fasciculation, reduced ankle jerks and high CSF protein concentration. Episodic, acute or subacute neuroglycopenia is common and chronic hypoglycaemia is invariably present.

Fig. 20.4 Features of the various neuroglycopenic syndromes. Acute neuroglycopenia is rare in patients with 'spontaneous' hypoglycaemia.

GLUCOSE HOMEOSTASIS

One popular, if simple, way of looking at glucose homeostasis is to consider it as the result of a balance between the actions of hormones and metabolic processes that increase blood glucose concentrations, and those that decrease it. The most important of the counterbalancing hormones are shown in Fig. 20.6. Although many more factors that can influence blood glucose levels are known, their physiological significance is not clear.

Insulin is normally the only blood glucose-lowering hormone to circulate in biologically significant amounts; however, in some very rare cases where patients have an inborn inability to form insulin from proinsulin, and in some patients with islet cell tumours, proinsulin and its partially split products are the dominant circulating hypoglycaemic hormones. Both insulin and proinsulin reduce hepatic glucose output and increase glucose uptake by insulin-dependent tissues after binding to specific insulin receptors. Insulin-like growth factors IGF1 and IGF2 are both able to produce hypoglycaemia when administered from an exogenous source, but only IGF2 is implicated in the pathogenesis of spontaneous hypoglycaemia. Like insulin and proinsulin, the IGFs suppress fatty acid release from adipocytes, and depress ketone production in the liver. They can therefore lower both plasma ketone levels and plasma glucose levels.

Pharmacologically, glucagon is the most potent of the hyperglycaemic hormones (Fig. 20.7). Its secretion is important, but not essential, in raising the concentration of blood glucose depressed by previous exogenous or endogenous insulin, providing that the sympathetic nervous system is intact. Glucagon exerts its hyperglycaemic effects exclusively through the liver by liberating glucose from preformed glycogen, by increasing glycogenolysis and, to a lesser extent, by increasing gluconeogenesis from glucose precursors (Fig. 20.8). Andidiuretic hormone (ADH; vasopressin) and adrenaline (epinephrine) are also potent glycogenolytic agents. It is doubtful, however, whether these exert a glycogenolytic effect at physiological concentrations except when they are grossly elevated in response to profound acute neuroglycopenia. Noradrenaline (norepinephrine),

FUEL UTILISATION BY THE HUMAN BRAIN

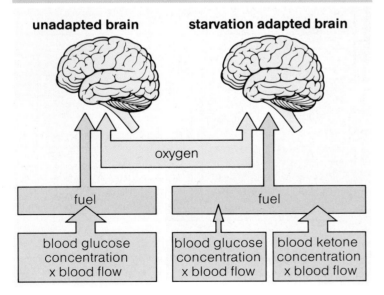

Fig. 20.5 Fuel utilisation by the human brain. Although the brain normally uses glucose as its sole fuel, it can adapt. It uses β-hydroxybutyrate and aceto-acetate in infants, and also in adults, during starvation.

HORMONES AND NEUROTRANSMITTERS INVOLVED IN GLUCOSE HOMEOSTASIS

hyperglycaemic

adrenaline	growth hormone
noradrenaline	prolactin
glucagon	placental lactogen
antidiuretic	cortisol
hormone (ADH)	thyroxine

— facilitative

hypoglycaemic

insulin

proinsulin

IGF1 and IGF2

Fig. 20.6 Hormones, neurotransmitters and growth factors which affect glucose homeostasis.

liberated at sympathetic nerve terminals in the liver, promotes glycogenolysis and liberation of glucose by hepatocytes through adrenoceptor activation, and probably represents one of the main physiological responses to hypoglycaemia. Growth hormone, prolactin, placental lactogen, cortisol and thyroxine indirectly impede glucose utilisation and promote its outflow from the liver.

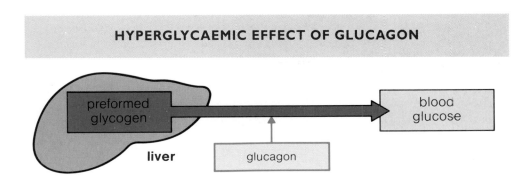

HYPERGLYCAEMIC EFFECT OF GLUCAGON

Fig. 20.7 The hyperglycaemic effect of glucagon. Glucagon works only on preformed glycogen to produce a rise in blood glucose. Thus, it does not cause hyperglycaemia if the liver is already depleted of glycogen, for example by prolonged fasting or alcohol intake.

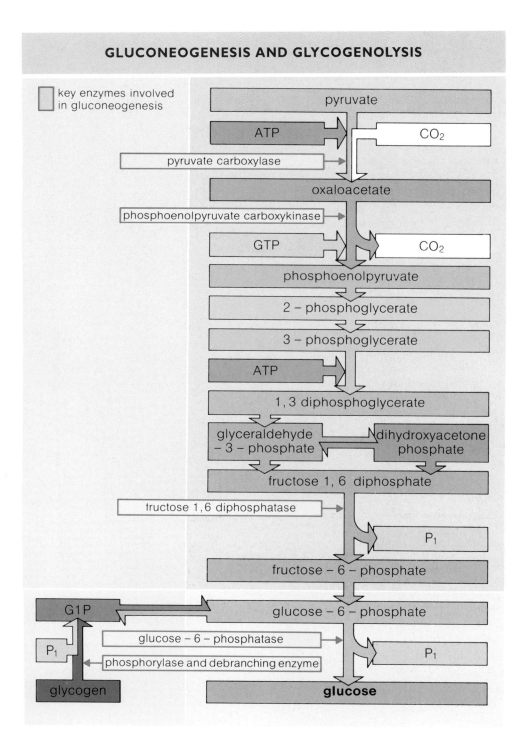

GLUCONEOGENESIS AND GLYCOGENOLYSIS

Fig. 20.8 Pathways of gluconeogenesis and glycogenolysis. Only those enzymes that are unique to these pathways and not shared by glycolysis and gluconeogenesis are shown.

CLINICAL CLASSIFICATIONS OF HYPOGLYCAEMIA

There are many ways of classifying hypoglycaemia clinically; the most useful is into fasting hypoglycaemia and stimulative hypoglycaemia. The former, as its name implies, occurs during fasting, but may also result in response to a specific stimulus. Stimulative hypoglycaemia occurs only in response to a stimulus such as a drug, or as a reaction to alimentary hyperglycaemia. In this context, starvation, but not simple fasting, is a 'stimulus' to hypoglycaemia.

Another useful classification of hypoglycaemic conditions is into those that are, and those that are not, associated with ketonaemia (plasma β-hydroxybutyrate levels greater than 600μmol/l). Most types of hypoglycaemia, apart from those due to endogenous or exogenous hyperinsulinism, autoimmune hypoglycaemia, or IGF2-secreting tumours, are accompanied by mild-to-moderate ketonaemia.

The main pathological causes of hypoglycaemia are shown in Fig. 20.9. Several conditions that may be confused clinically with hypoglycaemia and its associated symptomatology are listed in Fig. 20.10.

MAIN CAUSES OF CLINICAL HYPOGLYCAEMIA	
type	**example**
fasting hypoglycaemia inappropriate insulin secretion	insulinoma and nesidioblastosis
factitious hypoglycaemia	surreptitious insulin or sulphonylurea administration
drug and alcohol-induced hypoglycaemia	alcohol, aspirin, β-blockers
noninsulin-producing tumours	fibrosarcomas, carcinomas of stomach, adrenal, colon, prostate and breast
liver, heart or kidney failure	
endocrine disease	adrenocortical insufficiency, hypopituitarism
inborn errors of metabolism	glycogen storage disease types 1, 3 and 4; maple syrup urine disease; hereditary fructose intolerance
carbohydrate deprivation (especially in children)	'ketotic hypoglycaemia of children'
symptomatic neonatal hypoglycaemia of diverse aetiology	intrauterine malnutrition
infective	overwhelming septicaemia, malaria
autoimmune	anti-insulin receptor antibodies
stimulative rebound 'reactive' hypoglycaemia	post-gastrectomy, alcohol-induced, 'idiopathic' (rare), AIS
iatrogenic overtreatment with insulin	
overtreatment with sulphonylureas non-metabolised metabolised	chlorpropamide glibenclamide

Fig. 20.9 The main causes of clinical hypoglycaemia. These may be divided into three types: fasting, stimulative, and iatrogenic hypoglycaemia.

FASTING HYPOGLYCAEMIA: INSULINOMA

Insulinoma is a rare but important cause of hypoglycaemia and occurs with an incidence of approximately one case per million population per year. Hypoglycaemia and its associated neuroglycopenia are the presenting, and usually only the discernible, abnormalities. Characteristically there is a history, often going back several years, of episodic alterations in consciousness – these last from a few minutes to several hours and occur with increasing frequency and severity. Symptoms frequently occur in the morning before breakfast and commonly include difficulty in waking. Nevertheless, contrary to common belief, an episode of reactive hypoglycaemia in response to the ingestion of a meal is often the earliest sign of disease in patients with insulinoma. Measurement of the blood glucose concentration after an overnight fast almost always reveals hypoglycaemia, providing that it is performed on at least three occasions (Fig. 20.11). In suspected cases, glucose determinations of capillary blood (collected on filter paper during an attack and measured in a laboratory) are very informative. Sometimes episodes of hypoglycaemia occur only as a result of rigorous exercise or dieting. An association with fasting is seldom remarked upon spontaneously by patients, although paradoxically – because rebound hypoglycaemia is common – a relationship to eating and drinking may be mentioned. Weight gain and weight loss occur with almost equal frequency, although a few patients present with seemingly simple but intractable obesity as their sole complaint. Diagnosis depends upon the demonstration of symptomatic fasting hypoglycaemia in the presence of inappropriately high plasma insulin and C-peptide concentrations. This combination is almost pathognomonic of endogenous hyperinsulinism due to insulinoma, functional hyperinsulinism of infants (nesidioblastosis), or sulphonylurea poisoning.

Several factors determine the plasma insulin level in the blood, one of the most important being the arterial blood glucose concentration. Hypoglycaemia from any cause whatsoever (except endogenous hyperinsulinism) inhibits endogenous insulin and C-peptide secretion. This leads to a fall in peripheral venous plasma concentrations of insulin and C-peptide, to below 30pmol/l (5mu/l) and 300pmol/l (1ng/ml or 1μg/l), respectively. Values greater than these in the presence of proven hypoglycaemia indicate 'inappropriate' insulin secretion.

Patients who suffer from insulinoma demonstrate 'inappropriate' hyperinsulinaemia on some, but not necessarily all, occasions (Fig. 20.12). Factitious hypoglycaemia is associated with inappropriate hyperinsulinaemia during hypoglycaemic episodes, but is distinguished from endogenous hyperinsulinaemia by the associated appropriately low plasma C-peptide levels. All other types of spontaneous hypoglycaemia, apart from sulphonylurea poisoning and some forms of autoimmune hypoglycaemia, occur in conjunction with appropriately low plasma insulin and C-peptide concentrations.

CLINICAL CONDITIONS THAT MAY BE CONFUSED WITH HYPOGLYCAEMIA	
hysteria	vasovagal attacks or faint
anxiety neurosis	brain tumour
depression	angina pectoris
alcohol and drug intoxications	narcolepsy
epilepsy	syndrome of Klein and Levine

Fig. 20.10 Clinical conditions that may be confused with hypoglycaemia.

BLOOD GLUCOSE LEVELS IN INSULINOMA AND NESIDIOBLASTOSIS

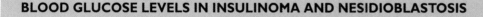
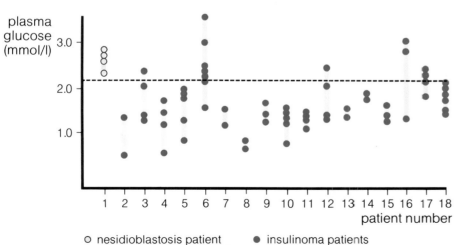

Fig. 20.11 Overnight fasting blood glucose levels in patients with insulinoma compared with those with nesidioblastosis. Seventeen patients with insulinoma and one with nesidioblastosis are shown. Each block represents one patient, and each dot represents the blood glucose concentration measured on one morning. Large differences in blood glucose concentration in the same individual on different occasions can be seen.

Large and spontaneous fluctuations in peripheral plasma insulin concentrations often occur in patients with insulinomas. Consequently, random plasma insulin measurements, except in the presence of chemically established hypoglycaemia, are of no diagnostic value.

Extensive hepatic extraction of insulin from portal venous blood can lead to the production of hypoglycaemia by inhibition of glucose release, without necessarily leading to abnormally high peripheral plasma insulin concentrations (Fig. 20.13). An appropriately low

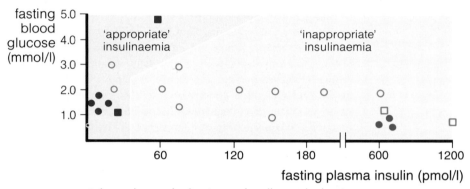

INSULIN AND GLUCOSE IN SPONTANEOUS HYPOGLYCAEMIA

- ● hypoglycaemia due to non insulin-producing tumour
- ○ benign insulinoma
- ◉ metastatic insulinoma
- □ factitious hypoglycaemia due to insulin
- ■ alcohol induced (fasting) hypoglycaemia

Fig. 20.12 The relationship of fasting plasma insulin with fasting blood glucose in several types of spontaneous hypoglycaemia. Plasma insulin and blood glucose concentrations that have been collected from patients with different types of hypoglycaemia are shown.

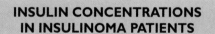

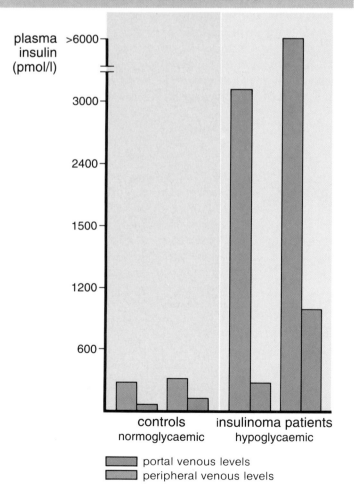

INSULIN CONCENTRATIONS IN INSULINOMA PATIENTS

- portal venous levels
- peripheral venous levels

Fig. 20.13 The fasting portal and peripheral venous plasma insulin concentrations during abdominal surgery in two insulinoma patients and two control subjects.

plasma insulin level in the presence of fasting hypoglycaemia does not, therefore, exclude the diagnosis of insulinoma, whereas a single inappropriately high one is highly suggestive of it and demands further investigation.

Approximately fifteen per cent of all insulinomas are metastatic; they are usually associated with the highest and most inappropriate plasma immunoreactive insulin levels.

Endogenous insulin is derived from proinsulin, which is synthesised exclusively on the rough endoplasmic reticulum of pancreatic B cells (Fig. 20.14). Proinsulin is cleaved enzymatically in the β-granules of the B cells to form two peptides, insulin and C-peptide, both of which are released into the circulation following an insulinotrophic stimulus. Intracellular cleavage of proinsulin into the two peptides is usually almost complete and, consequently, very little proinsulin enters the circulation, even in response to intensive B-cell stimulation. In most B-cell tumours, however, substantial amounts of intact proinsulin forms and partially split forms (Fig. 20.15) are released into the circulation where they are detected as immunoreactive insulin. In some cases proinsulin and partially split forms account for most, or even all, of the insulin immunoreactivity measurable in peripheral venous plasma. Proinsulin can now be measured specifically in peripheral venous plasma and may be very helpful in the differential diagnosis of obscure cases of fasting hypoglycaemia (Fig. 20.16).

Plasma C-peptide levels, like those of insulin, rise after B-cell stimulation but, because of its larger pool size and slower turnover rate, large fluctuations in plasma C-peptide are less common. Overnight fasting peripheral venous plasma C-peptide levels generally fall within the range 500–900pmol/l but, like plasma insulin levels, are suppressed by prolonged fasting, vigorous exercise, and hypoglycaemia. Except in the presence of endogenous hyperinsulinism, sulphonylurea poisoning and some forms of autoimmune hypoglycaemia, plasma C-peptide concentrations are invariably suppressed to below 300pmol/l by hypoglycaemia (Fig. 20.17). This is the basis of the insulin hypoglycaemia test for endogenous hyperinsulinism due to insulinoma. However, as ordinarily performed (Fig. 20.18) the test is neither very sensitive nor very specific; false-positive results can occur, especially in patients with factitious hypoglycaemia due to sulphonylurea abuse. False-negative responses can also occur because of suppression of C-peptide secretion in patients with insulinomas, possibly due to increases in circulating plasma adrenaline levels. Both the sensitivity and specificity of the insulin hypoglycaemic test can be improved by using an infusion of low doses of exogenous insulin under controlled conditions in order to maintain a constant and reduced blood sugar level (a hypoglycaemia clamp procedure), but this is expensive, tedious and has no advantage over simpler tests such as measurement of overnight or fasting insulin, C-peptide and proinsulin levels, and the vigorous exercise test.

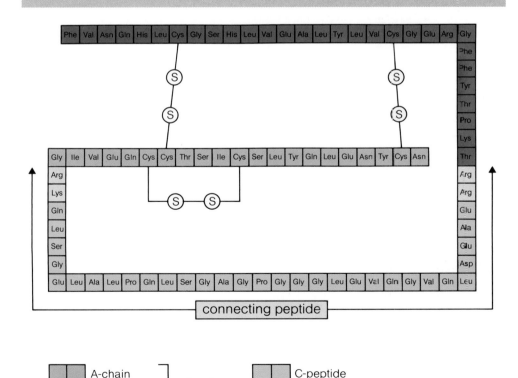

STRUCTURE OF HUMAN PROINSULIN

A-chain
B-chain
insulin
C-peptide
cleavage points

Fig. 20.14 The structure of human proinsulin. This molecule is enzymatically cleaved to yield two peptides, insulin and C-peptide, following an insulinotrophic stimulus.

The main clinical use of plasma C-peptide assay is in the differentiation of endogenous hyperinsulinism from exogenous (factitious) hyperinsulinism. In infants with functional hyperinsulinism, plasma C-peptide levels may reveal inappropriate insulin secretion when insulin assays themselves fail to do so because of insulin extraction by the liver.

MAIN HUMAN PROINSULIN-DERIVED PRODUCTS

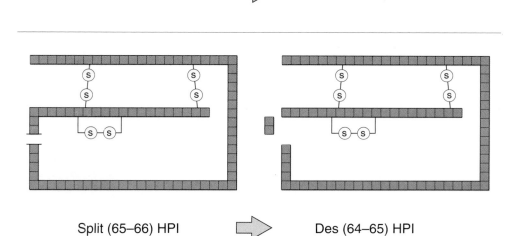

Split (32–33) HPI → Des (31,32) HPI

Split (65–66) HPI → Des (64–65) HPI

Fig. 20.15 The main human proinsulin (HPI)-derived products.

PROINSULIN LEVELS IN VARIOUS CLINICAL DISORDERS

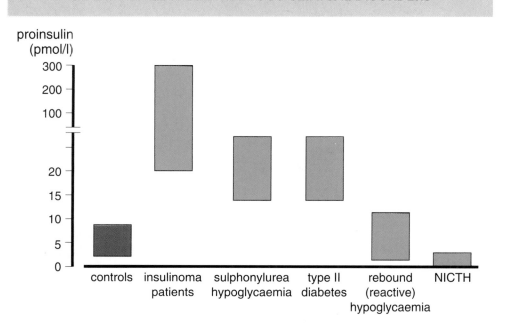

Fig. 20.16 Plasma proinsulin levels in diverse clinical disorders with and without hypoglycaemia. NICTH, non-islet cell tumoural hypoglycaemia.

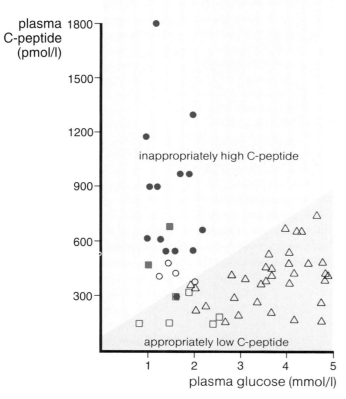

PLASMA GLUCOSE AND C-PEPTIDE CONCENTRATIONS IN CONTROLS AND HYPOGLYCAEMIC PATIENTS

Fig. 20.17 Comparison of fasting plasma glucose and C-peptide concentrations in healthy control subjects and in patients with various types of hypoglycaemia. Each symbol represents a single individual.

△ controls
○ nesidioblastosis
● insulinoma
□ factitious hypoglycaemia due to insulin
■ factitious hypoglycaemia due to sulphonylurea

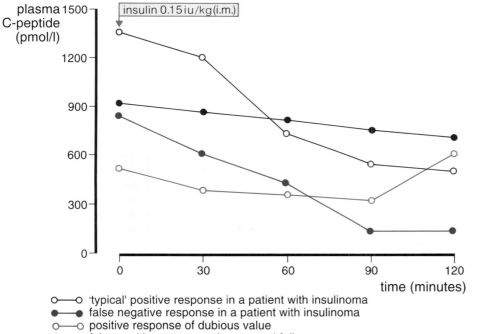

PLASMA C-PEPTIDE BEHAVIOUR IN INSULINOMA OR RENAL FAILURE

Fig. 20.18 Patterns of plasma C-peptide behaviour observed during insulin-induced hypoglycaemia in patients with insulinomas or renal failure.

○—○ 'typical' positive response in a patient with insulinoma
●—● false negative response in a patient with insulinoma
○—○ positive response of dubious value
●—● false positive response due to renal failure
▭ mean nadir +2s.d.in 15 healthy subjects
▭ limits of overnight fasting C-peptide levels in normoglycaemic subjects

CLASSIFICATION OF HYPOGLYCAEMIA IN THE NEONATAL PERIOD

type I early transitional adaptive hypoglycaemia
includes infants of diabetic mothers and those with erythroblastosis fetalis

type 2 secondary hypoglycaemia
secondary to asphyxia, infection, respiratory distress, pathology of the nervous system due to birth trauma, abrupt cessation of intravenous glucose infusions, etc.

type 3 'classical' neonatal hypoglycaemia
due to intra-uterine malnutrition, i.e. babies small for gestational age

type 4 recurrent functional hyperinsulinism
'nesidioblastosis'

type 5 self-limiting recurrent hypoglycaemia
e.g. Beckwith–Wiedemann syndrome

Fig. 20.19 Classification of hypoglycaemia that develops in the neonatal period.

FUNCTIONAL HYPERINSULINISM: NESIDIOBLASTOSIS

Functional hyperinsulinism (inappropriate hyperinsulinaemia in the presence of hypoglycaemia) is comparatively common in newborns but very rare in older children and in adults. It does not have a well-defined histopathological basis – the diffuse B-cell hyperplasia often referred to as nesidioblastosis is not necessarily confined to the well-demarcated islets of Langerhans, and occurs as an anatomical finding in many normal babies, and even in adults who never experience spontaneous hypoglycaemia. In its mildest form, functional hyper-insulinism of infants produces a transient lowering of blood glucose concentration and minimal inappropriate hyperinsulinaemia, often accompanied by slight and temporary neuroglycopenia during the first few days of life. In its most extreme form, gross interuterine hyperinsulinism is associated with obesity at birth and intractable symptomatic hypoglycaemia immediately thereafter. This can cause severe and permanent brain damage or death unless effective and continuous treatment is instituted at once. In the moderately severe case, however, the baby has a normal appearance at birth, and nothing untoward happens until the child is in its second or third month

Fig. 20.20 The sequence of events involved in the diagnosis and treatment of hyperinsulinism.

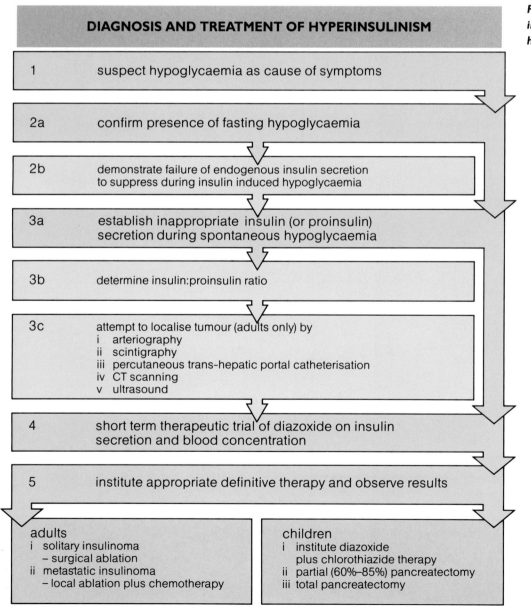

DIAGNOSIS AND TREATMENT OF HYPERINSULINISM

1 suspect hypoglycaemia as cause of symptoms

2a confirm presence of fasting hypoglycaemia

2b demonstrate failure of endogenous insulin secretion to suppress during insulin induced hypoglycaemia

3a establish inappropriate insulin (or proinsulin) secretion during spontaneous hypoglycaemia

3b determine insulin:proinsulin ratio

3c attempt to localise tumour (adults only) by
   i   arteriography
   ii scintigraphy
   iii percutaneous trans-hepatic portal catheterisation
   iv CT scanning
   v   ultrasound

4 short term therapeutic trial of diazoxide on insulin secretion and blood concentration

5 institute appropriate definitive therapy and observe results

adults
i   solitary insulinoma
    – surgical ablation
ii metastatic insulinoma
    – local ablation plus chemotherapy

children
i   institute diazoxide
    plus chlorothiazide therapy
ii partial (60%–85%) pancreatectomy
iii total pancreatectomy

of life, when failure of mental development or the onset of fits brings it to medical attention. Some of the cases are familial, especially those in which leucine sensitivity is a feature.

Recurrent functional hyperinsulinism (nesidioblastosis) must be distinguished from other types of neonatal hypoglycaemia (Fig. 20.19), many of which are epiphenomena of little clinical importance but which may, nevertheless, require temporary hyperglycaemic therapy.

DIAGNOSIS AND TREATMENT OF ENDOGENOUS HYPERINSULINISM

Diagnosis of endogenous hyperinsulinism takes place in four stages (Fig. 20.20), the first three of which are common to adults and infants: (i) suspicion that hypoglycaemia is the cause of the patient's symptoms; (ii) proof that hypoglycaemia is present during symptomatic episodes and can be provoked by fasting; (iii) proof that hypoglycaemia is accompanied by inappropriate hyperinsulinaemia and C-peptidaemia, and sulphonylurea abuse has been looked for and excluded; and (iv) localisation of the tumour, usually at surgery.

Preoperative localisation of an insulinoma rarely provides useful information and may be misleading. The most precise and specific localising procedure is percutaneous transhepatic portal vein catheterisation with venous sampling for insulin.

In infants below the age of two years, insulin-secreting tumours are so rare that either functional hyperinsulinism (nesidioblastosis) or malicious sulphonylurea administration must be considered the likely cause of endogenous hyperinsulinism.

Treatment of functional hyperinsulinism in infants varies from the introduction of frequent feeding, through the institution of combined diazoxide/chlorothiazide treatment, to total pancreatectomy in the most refractory cases. In children who respond to conservative

treatment, spontaneous recovery is almost invariable during the first ten to fifteen years of life.

In adults, surgical ablation of insulinomas is followed by complete and lasting remission, except in rare malignant insulinomas with hepatic metastases. In such cases palliative therapy, with diazoxide and chlorothiazide, or octreotide, may give prolonged symptomatic relief, as may chemotherapy with streptozotocin, 5-fluorouracil, CCNU, and other antineoplastic agents, with or without hepatic artery embolisation.

INSULIN-LIKE GROWTH FACTOR-II-SECRETING TUMOURS

Tumours of all histological varieties have long been recognised as being capable of inducing symptomatic hypoglycaemia (non-islet cell tumoral hypoglycaemia: NICTH) but, until recently, the mechanism by which they did so was unknown. The most common types of tumour involved are haemangiopericytomas, fibrosarcomas, and carcinomas of the gut, adrenal, breast or prostate although, in all but the first, hypoglycaemia is an extremely rare finding. In a minority, hypoglycaemia is the presenting symptom, and the symptomatology is indistinguishable from that of an insulinoma.

The immediate cause of the hypoglycaemia (Fig. 20.21) is overproduction by the tumour of either normal or a slightly altered form of IGF2, except in a tiny proportion of lymphomas in which autoantibodies to the insulin receptor appear to be involved. IGF2 that gains access to the plasma is normally avidly bound by the various specific IGF-binding proteins that are present in the circulation. Ordinarily, therefore, IGF2 in the circulation does not produce hypoglycaemia.

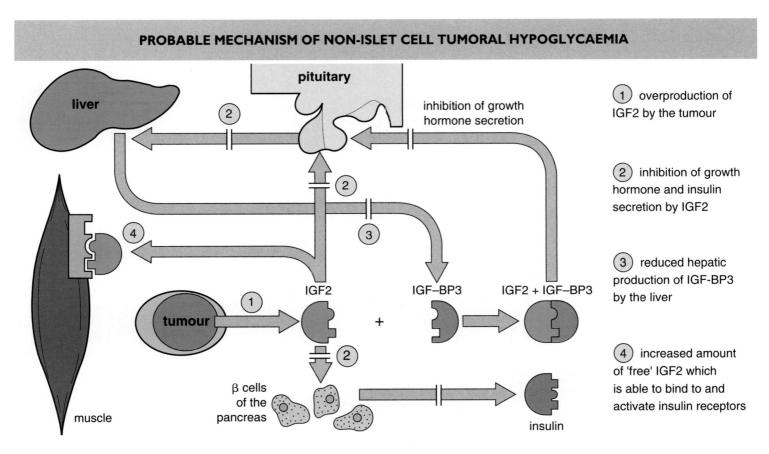

PROBABLE MECHANISM OF NON-ISLET CELL TUMORAL HYPOGLYCAEMIA

① overproduction of IGF2 by the tumour

② inhibition of growth hormone and insulin secretion by IGF2

③ reduced hepatic production of IGF-BP3 by the liver

④ increased amount of 'free' IGF2 which is able to bind to and activate insulin receptors

Fig. 20.21 The probable mechanism for production of hypoglycaemia by non-islet cell tumours.

The most important IGF-binding protein is IGF-BP3, which is produced in the liver under the influence of growth hormone. Hypoglycaemia caused by overproduction of IGF2 is the result of a sequence of events, rather than one single event. Initially, IGF2 released by the tumour is bound by IGF-binding proteins in the plasma and becomes unavailable for binding to the insulin receptors on cells, for which it has only a weak affinity. Eventually, however, the IGF2 suppresses production and secretion of pituitary growth hormone, possibly by a negative feedback mechanism, and this in turn reduces hepatic production of both IGF1 and IGF-BP3. This, it is postulated, leads to a further reduction in plasma IGF2 binding capacity and, consequently, the presence in the plasma of more free or nonprotein-bound IGF2 and/or IGF1 than normal. This can and does exert an insulin-like hypoglycaemic action. By reducing IGF2 production by removing the tumour (if this is surgically possible) or by temporarily increasing IGF-BP3 production by exogenous growth hormone administration (Fig. 20.22), the hypoglycaemia of NICTH may be relieved sufficiently to make surgery possible or to improve the quality of the remaining life of the patient.

The diagnosis of tumour-induced hypoglycaemia should be suspected whenever nonketotic fasting hypoglycaemia is found in association with suppressed levels of plasma insulin and C-peptide, and should be confirmed by the finding of an abnormally high IGF2 to IGF1 ratio due to normal or high plasma IGF2 levels and very low plasma IGF1 levels. Since tumours that cause hypoglycaemia are generally large or very large by the time they present with hypoglycaemia, localisation rarely presents a problem, though in some cases it is necessary to resort to the most modern imaging techniques.

REBOUND (REACTIVE) HYPOGLYCAEMIA

It has been known for more than sixty years, since the inception of widespread clinical blood glucose testing, that administration of a large glucose load is followed in most healthy subjects by an early rise in blood glucose concentration and that this is followed by a late rebound fall – often to hypoglycaemic levels (Fig. 20.23). The rise in blood glucose concentration is more marked in arterial blood than in venous blood. It is due to increased glucose uptake by peripheral tissues, under the influence of insulin released in response to the combined effects of arterial hyperglycaemia and alimentary stimuli.

Arterial glucose levels generally remain at or above fasting levels for much of the time, during which period glucose or food is still being absorbed. Sometimes, in response to oral glucose, but only very rarely in response to a solid meal, and towards the end of the absorptive phase, glucose is removed from the glucose pool faster than glucose enters it from the gut, and genuine arterial hypoglycaemia, capable of producing acute neuroglycopenia, may occur. Venous blood glucose concentrations commonly fall to well below fasting levels under these circumstances and are not necessarily pathological (Fig. 20.24). However, they have in the past been extensively misconstrued as being indicative of idiopathic rebound (reactive) hypoglycaemia, often abbreviated simply to hypoglycaemia and, as such, responsible for a number of vague disturbances experienced by patients in the course of their everyday life. The fluctuations in arterial blood glucose concentrations that occur after ingestion of solid meals are not usually as large as those that follow the ingestion of glucose solutions. Even so, large arteriovenous glucose differences may occur,

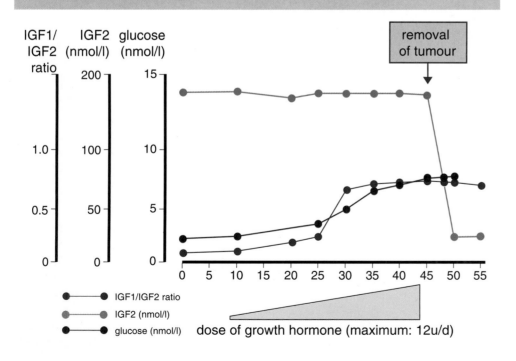

RESPONSE TO EXOGENOUS GROWTH HORMONE

Fig. 20.22 The responses of fasting blood glucose, plasma IGF2, and IGF1/IGF2 ratio to exogenous growth hormone administration.

giving an appearance of reactive hypoglycaemia if venous blood alone is analysed. Ordinarily, therefore, capillary or arterialised venous blood should be sampled whenever idiopathic reactive hypoglycaemia is suspected as the cause of a patient's symptoms. The best time to take a blood sample from a patient with suspected reactive hypoglycaemia is during the spontaneous symptomatic episodes that occur in the patient's natural environment. The patient, their spouse or another near relative can be taught how to collect capillary blood from a fingerprick onto specially prepared filter paper. If blood collected in this way shows a low glucose concentration on assay, the diagnosis of reactive hypoglycaemia can be seriously entertained.

Rebound reactive hypoglycaemia is often secondary to some underlying physical cause. It is common in patients with insulinomas and other varieties of fasting hypoglycaemia, and may be the only symptomatic feature of the autoimmune insulin syndrome (AIS). Contrary to former belief, reactive hypoglycaemia is not a common premonitory symptom of noninsulin-dependent diabetes. In practice, the most common cause is rapid gastric emptying, usually as a result of gastroduodenal surgery, but occasionally no pathoanatomical cause can be found.

Excessive secretion of insulin in response to hyperactivity of the enteroinsular axis has not been established as the cause of idiopathic reactive hypoglycaemia. However, evidence is accumulating that patients to whom this diagnosis has been given may experience symptoms which are attributable to neuroglycopenia at higher arterial blood glucose levels than in healthy subjects and which consequently do not meet the diagnostic criteria for hypoglycaemia.

ALCOHOL

Alcohol may produce hypoglycaemia in several different ways. The most important is by the inhibition of gluconeogenesis, which can result in a profound and particularly dangerous form of fasting hypoglycaemia, especially in children. Another is by increasing the amount of insulin that is secreted in response to an oral carbohydrate load. A special example of this occurs when a sugary drink mixed with alcohol (for example, a gin and tonic) is drunk on an empty stomach (Fig. 20.25). The ingestion of a small amount of predominantly starchy food with an alcoholic drink does not abolish, and may even enhance, this propensity to develop symptomatic reactive hypoglycaemia. Fig. 20.26 shows the occurrence of symptomatic hypoglycaemia in an otherwise healthy thirty-three-year-old woman. On two separate occasions she ingested a snack that provided 40g alcohol (as lager),

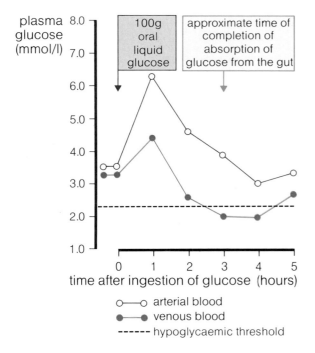

PRODUCTION OF SPONTANEOUS REACTIVE HYPOGLYCAEMIA

Fig. 20.23 The mechanism of apparent production of spontaneous reactive hypoglycaemia by oral glucose when venous blood is used for sampling. Plasma glucose values are taken from one patient. The disparity between arterial and venous plasma glucose levels can be seen.

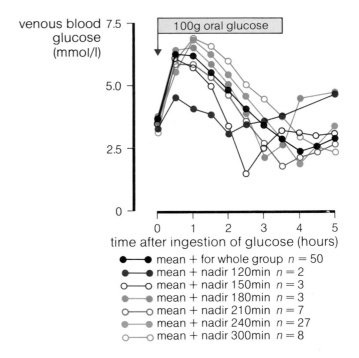

VENOUS BLOOD GLUCOSE LEVELS IN HEALTHY SUBJECTS

Fig. 20.24 Venous blood glucose levels in fifty healthy subjects. Each subject was given a 100g oral glucose load and grouped according to the time at which the nadir occurred. In two subjects, the lowest venous blood glucose level was observed at 120 minutes following glucose loading; however, in twenty-seven subjects it was at 240 minutes, and in eight it was at 300 minutes.

40g carbohydrate, and 20g protein. On each occasion, she experienced symptomatic reactive hypoglycaemia, which was relieved by the ingestion of food.

Treatment of uncomplicated rebound hypoglycaemia is mainly by avoidance of situations in which it is likely to arise, and by eschewing provocative stimulation.

AUTOIMMUNE HYPOGLYCAEMIA

Autoimmune disease is associated with spontaneous hypoglycaemia through three distinct mechanisms:
• Anti-insulin receptor antibody hypoglycaemia may be the presenting feature of a wide variety of autoimmune diseases, as well of lymphomas. In this condition, antibodies that are directed against insulin receptors may mimic insulin action and cause hypoglycaemia,

or block it and cause intractable hyperglycaemia. Plasma insulin and C-peptide levels may be high to very high when blood glucose levels are elevated due to excessive stimulation of the B cells, but are generally appropriately low during hypoglycaemia. The stimulatory antibodies may themselves be first-generation antibodies (Ab_1) against the insulin receptor (Fig. 20.27) or antibodies against insulin antibodies (that is, anti-idiotypes: Ab_2) (Fig. 20.28).
• AIS occurs mainly in Japan, where it is recognised as one of the most common causes of symptomatic spontaneous hypoglycaemia, especially in people with thyroid disease that has been treated with methimazole. It is characterised by the presence in plasma of autoantibodies to endogenous human insulin and high total plasma immunoreactive insulin. Plasma C-peptide levels may be normal, high, or very high, even during hypoglycaemic episodes that tend to be of the rebound variety more often than of the fasting variety. AIS is thought to be due to insulin that is secreted during the absorptive

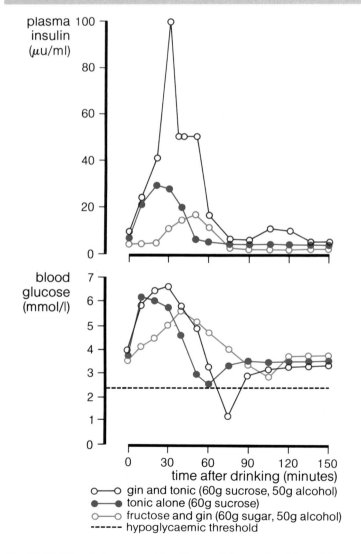

BLOOD GLUCOSE AND INSULIN LEVELS IN A HEALTHY SUBJECT FOLLOWING CONSUMPTION OF VARIOUS DRINKS

Fig. 20.25 Blood glucose and insulin levels in one healthy subject given drinks of different composition on three occasions. The drinks were consumed at 1300h on an empty stomach (from breakfast time).

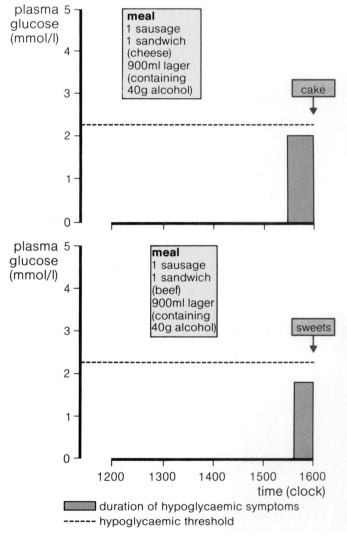

SYMPTOMATIC SPONTANEOUS ALCOHOL-INDUCED REACTIVE HYPOGLYCAEMIA

Fig. 20.26 Symptomatic spontaneous alcohol-induced reactive hypoglycaemia. A healthy 33-year-old woman was hypoglycaemic in the early afternoon on two separate occasions. This hypoglycaemia was overcome by eating cake or sweets.

phase of a meal being bound by anti-insulin antibodies and then being released from them during the postabsorptive phase when all the carbohydrate in the meal has been absorbed (Fig. 20.29).

• Graves' disease of the B cells has so far been described in very few patients, possibly because of the difficulty of demonstrating the presumed causal mechanism, namely the presence in the plasma of stim-

ulatory autoantibodies to pancreatic B cells. However, since antibodies of this type can be found in plasma from most patients with fasting hypoglycaemia, their pathogenetic importance must still be considered to be unproved.

The treatment for all three types of autoimmune hypoglycaemia is directed against the primary disease.

PRODUCTION OF HYPOGLYCAEMIA BY Ab₁

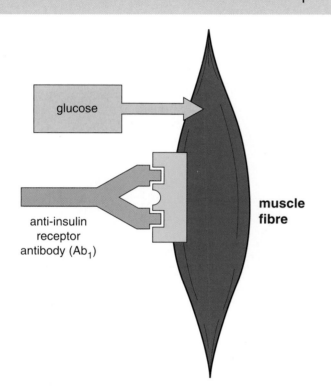

Fig. 20.27 The mechanism of production of hypoglycaemia by a (stimulatory) autoantibody (Ab₁) to the insulin receptor.

PRODUCTION OF HYPOGLYCAEMIA BY ANTI-IDIOTYPES

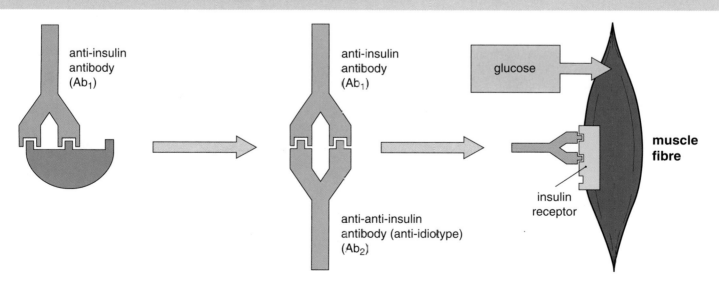

Fig. 20.28 The mechanism of production of hypoglycaemia by anti-idiotypes (Ab₂) to insulin antibodies (Ab₁), which are capable of binding to, and stimulating, insulin receptors.

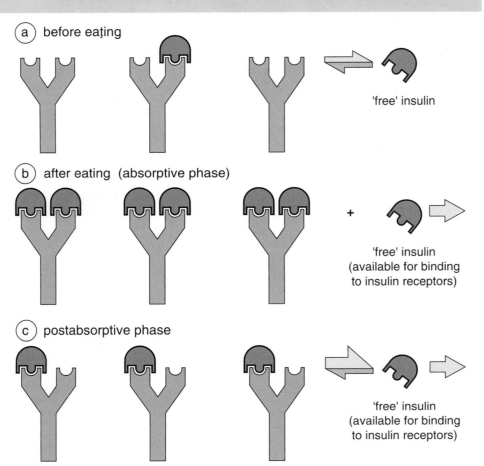

POSTULATED MECHANISM OF HYPOGLYCAEMIA BY AIS

(a) before eating

'free' insulin

(b) after eating (absorptive phase)

+

'free' insulin
(available for binding
to insulin receptors)

(c) postabsorptive phase

'free' insulin
(available for binding
to insulin receptors)

Fig. 20.29 The postulated mechanism of hypoglycaemia by the AIS. (a) Before eating, 'free' insulin is in equilibrium with antibody-bound insulin and the patient is normoglycaemic. (b) During the absorptive phase, hyperglycaemia stimulates insulin secretion, and insulin is taken up by circulating antibodies. (c) In the postabsorptive phase, insulin is released from circulating antibodies and becomes available to bind with insulin receptors.

21

Ectopic Humoral Syndromes

Ken Yamaguchi, MD,PhD

Patients with neoplasms develop various signs and symptoms, and the major clinical features are derived from the mass effect of the primary tumour, its invasion and distant metastases. In addition, neoplasms can produce a wide variety of clinical features at sites that are distant from the tumour mass; these are collectively referred to as paraneoplastic syndromes or remote effects of malignancy. Two major categories of paraneoplastic syndromes include humoral syndromes, described in this chapter, and neurogenic syndromes.

Ectopic humoral syndromes (Fig. 21.1) are clinical disorders in which the patient with neoplasms develops signs and symptoms explained by biologically active factors that are produced and secreted by the neoplasms. The term 'ectopic' indicates that the factors(s) causing the syndrome is not the physiological product of the tissue from which the neoplasm is derived. Conversely, humoral syndromes that are induced by the physiological product of the tissue are referred to as eutopic humoral syndromes.

Ectopic humoral syndromes induced by overproduction of peptide hormones, namely ectopic hormone syndromes, are best charac-

terised by their clinical features. The number of cancer patients who suffer from these syndromes is thought to be very small, and there is a tendency among physicians to pay little attention to such conditions. However, recent progress in endocrinology, cytokine research and oncology has provided new information regarding the mechanisms underlying the pathogenesis of these syndromes.

First, in some humoral syndromes, causative factors are now identifiable; the condition of humoral hypercalcaemia of malignancy (HHM) is a good example. Hypercalcaemia develops in approximately ten per cent of patients with advanced stages of cancer, and it is now established that a newly discovered calcium-regulating hormone, parathyroid hormone-related protein (PTHrP), is the causative factor in almost all patients with HHM. Second, an ectopic humoral syndrome that is induced by cytokine overproduction, or ectopic cytokine syndrome, is now known to occur. Moreover, evidence is accumulating to indicate the role of growth factors in the development of some humoral syndromes. Thus, it is reasonable to postulate that the clinical entities that are covered by the term ectopic humoral

ECTOPIC HUMORAL SYNDROMES

clinical syndromes	factors	common neoplasms
ectopic hormone syndromes		
syndromes frequently associated with endocrine tumours		
Cushing's syndrome	adrenocorticotrophic hormone (ACTH)	medullary thyroid cancer pancreatic endocrine tumour carcinoid tumour
WDHA (watery, diarrhoea, hypokalaemia, achlorhydria) syndrome	vasoactive intestinal polypeptide (VIP)	pancreatic endocrine tumour
Zollinger–Ellison syndrome	gastrin	pancreatic endocrine tumour
acromegaly	growth-hormone releasing hormone (GHRH)	pancreatic endocrine tumour carcinoid tumour
syndromes frequently associated with non-endocrine neoplasms with neuroendocrine nature		
hyperadrenocorticism (Cushing's syndrome)	ACTH	small-cell cancer (lung, oesophagus, uterus, etc.)
SIADH (syndrome of inappropiate ADH secretion)	andidiuretic hormone (ADH)	small-cell cancer (lung, uterus, etc.)
syndromes frequently associated with neoplasms without neuroendocrine nature		
hypercalcaemia	parathyroid-hormone related hormone (PTHrP)	various neoplasms
gynaecomastia	chorionic gonadotrophin (CG)	lung cancer
ectopic cytokine/growth factor syndromes		
leukocytosis	colony-stimulating facters (CSFs)	giant-cell lung cancer oesophageal cancer
erythrocytosis	erythropoietin	hepatocellular cancer renal-cell cancer

21.1 Classification of ectopic humoral syndromes.

syndrome will increase. Third, it is well established that neoplasms frequently produce hormones, cytokines, growth factors and other bioactive substances, although these neoplasms are rarely associated with clinical humoral syndromes. Increasing knowledge of the biological implications of bioactive substances produced by neoplastic cells indicates that these substances can act directly on neoplastic cells or tissues that surround the neoplastic cells, which in turn function to support neoplastic cell growth.

In this context, the concepts of ectopic humoral syndromes and ectopic production of bioactive substances by neoplasms are now attracting remarkable attention from clinical and scientific researchers in oncology as well as in endocrinology.

CLASSIFICATION

To understand ectopic humoral syndromes, it is necessary to differentiate between two separate conditions – ectopic humoral syndromes and ectopic production of bioactive substances – since these indicate different concepts (Fig. 21.2). In the case of peptide hormones, these two entities are referred to as ectopic hormone syndrome and ectopic hormone production, respectively. The former refers to clinically recognisable humoral syndromes caused by bioactive substances produced ectopically, while the latter indicates neoplasms that elaborate substances, irrespective of clinically obvious humoral manifestations.

This relation was clearly described when tissue concentrations of seventeen peptide hormones were examined in fifty tissue extracts of small-cell lung carcinomas, obtained at surgery or autopsy (Fig. 21.3). In this study, peptide hormones that were detected at a concentration of 10pmol or more per gram wet weight were considered to be producers; this criterion is very strict and probably underestimates the actual detection frequency. According to this criterion, the frequency of production of one of the seventeen peptides in small-cell lung carcinoma tissues was as high as eighty-four per cent, and that of two hormones or more was fifty per cent. This indicates that peptide hormone production is a very common phenomenon in small-cell lung carcinoma, as is multiple hormone production (Fig. 21.4).

It is important to clarify the conditions that determine the development of clinical syndromes. First, the neoplasm must produce large amounts of bioactive substances, and their plasma levels should be elevated enough to affect target tissues. The relationship between hormone production and the development of humoral syndromes in the fifty-case study already discussed is described in Fig. 21.3. In these cases, three patients developed ectopic adrenocorticotrophic hormone (ACTH) syndrome, and two developed ectopic antidiuretic hormone (ADH: vasopressin) syndrome. Ectopic ACTH and ADH syndromes developed in patients with tumours that produced large amounts of ACTH and ADH, respectively; greater numbers of cases were found to produce the respective peptides in smaller amounts, but these were not associated with the clinical syndrome.

ECTOPIC HUMORAL SYNDROME AND ECTOPIC PRODUCTION OF BIOACTIVE SUBSTANCES

Fig. 21.2 The ectopic humoral syndrome and the ectopic production of bioactive substances.

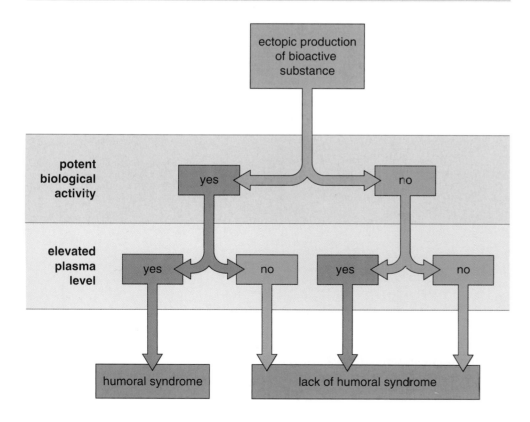

Second, the factor produced by the neoplasm must possess sufficiently potent biological activity to develop humoral syndromes. As shown in Fig. 21.3, detection frequencies and tissue concentrations of peptides such as gastrin-releasing peptide (GRP), calcitonin and growth hormone-releasing hormone (GHRH) have a tendency to be higher than those of ACTH and ADH in tumours although clinical syndromes associated with these peptide hormones were not observed. It is well established that overproduction of calcitonin is not associated

PEPTIDES IN SMALL-CELL LUNG CANCER

peptide	IR-peptide (pmol/g)	positive cases (%)
GRP		62
calcitonin		26
GHRH		20
ACTH		18
somatostatin		18
neurotensin		12
calcitonin-gene-related peptide (CGRP)		12
ME–AGL		8
ADH		8
VIP		6
neuropeptide Y (NPY)		6

• tumours inducing ectopic humoral syndrome

Fig. 21.3 Tumour concentrations of peptides in the extracts prepared from fifty small-cell lung cancer tissues. Leucomorphin, pancreatic polypeptide, peptide tyrosine tyrosine (PPY), secretin, big gastrin (1–15) , and motilin were not detected in any of the tumour extracts and thus are excluded from the results. Modified from Yamaguchi (1986), by courtesy of the *Japanese Journal of C'inical Oncology.*

HORMONE PRODUCTION BY SMALL-CELL LUNG CANCERS

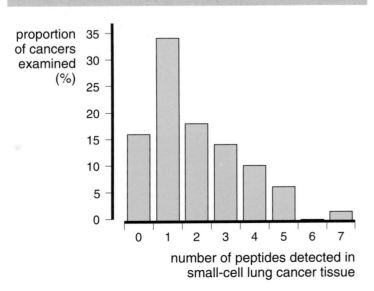

Fig. 21.4 The frequency of hormone production by small-cell lung cancers. Modified from Yamaguchi (1986), by courtesy of the *Japanese Journal of Clinical Oncology.*

with any humoral syndrome, because calcitonin has no clinically detectable biological activity. However, overproduction of GRP or GHRH from neuroendocrine tumours has been reported to induce Cushing's syndrome or acromegaly, respectively. These syndromes were not observed in the patients with small-cell lung carcinoma; therefore it is reasonable to speculate that the biological activities of these peptide hormones are rather weak, and that the amount of peptide hormone that was produced by each small-cell lung neoplasm was not great enough to develop humoral syndromes. These features are not limited to small-cell lung carcinoma or to ectopic hormone production, but are common to a variety of carcinoma that produce bioactive substances (Fig. 21.5).

CHARACTERISTICS OF NEOPLASMS ASSOCIATED WITH ECTOPIC HUMORAL SYNDROMES

Ectopic humoral syndromes can be classified by clinical features, by the factors responsible for the humoral syndrome, or by the type of neoplasms frequently associated with the syndromes; representative syndromes are summarised in Fig. 21.1.

Three categories of neoplasm are associated with ectopic humoral syndromes. First, these syndromes develop frequently in patients with a neuroendocrine tumour, although the hormone responsible for the syndromes is not the normal product of the original endocrine organ: for instance, when a patient with a typical endocrine tumour such as a medullary thyroid carcinoma, carcinoid tumour or pancreatic endocrine tumour develops Cushing's syndrome due to the production of ACTH, this entity is categorised as the ectopic ACTH syndrome, since ACTH is not the physiological product of these endocrine organs.

Second, an ectopic hormone syndrome may develop in a patient with a neoplasm derived from a tissue that does not normally produce hormones at all. The lung does not normally produce ACTH; when lung cancer cells produce ACTH, which in turn results in

Cushing's syndrome, then this clinical entity is referred to as ectopic ACTH syndrome. It is worth noting that lung cancers associated with the ectopic ACTH syndrome are always small-cell cancers, which possess neuroendocrine characteristics.

Third, some ectopic hormone syndromes develop in patients with nonendocrine neoplasms without neuroendocrine characteristics. HHM is now regarded as ectopic PTHrP syndrome; the neoplasms associated with this syndrome do not always possess neuroendocrine characteristics.

As described later, each of these categories requires a different explanation from the standpoint of its pathogenesis.

BIOLOGICAL EFFECTS OF ECTOPIC PRODUCTION OF BIOACTIVE SUBSTANCES

Ectopic humoral syndromes are caused by the bioactive substances produced by the neoplasm (Fig. 21.5) and secreted into the systemic circulation. The substances reach the target organs where they induce responses, which in turn cause the clinical syndrome(s). This outcome would be classified as an endocrine mechanism. The products of cancer cells can also act in a paracrine fashion locally on normal tissues or can infiltrate immune cells surrounding the cancer cells. It is reasonable to speculate that some of these cancer cell products play a role in stimulating cellular growth of mesenchymal cells, resulting in modulation of stromal tissues, tumour angiogenesis or cellular immune responses. Bioactive substances may be produced by neoplastic cells to act on the same neoplastic cells (autocrine effects). The hypothesis has been proposed that cancer cells have the ability to produce growth factors and to stimulate tumorigenesis by responding to these factors. This mechanism is now known as the autocrine growth mechanism of cancer cells: factors responsible for it are referred to as autocrine growth factors. Growth factors such as platelet-derived growth factor, transforming growth factor α (TGF-α) and insulin-like growth factor 1 (IGF-I), cytokines such as interleukin-2 (IL-2) and

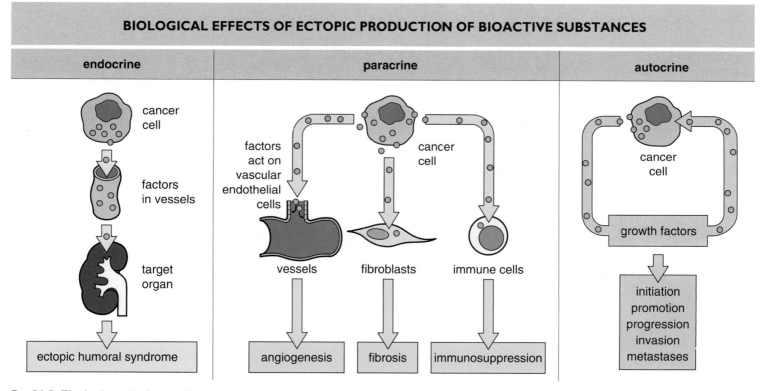

Fig. 21.5 *The biological effects of ectopic production of bioactive substances by neoplasms.*

interleukin-6 (IL-6), and peptide hormones with activity to stimulate cellular growth, such as GRP, are now regarded as autocrine growth factors in a variety of cancer cell lines.

Although bioactive substances produced and functioning in a paracrine or autocrine fashion are not associated with ectopic humoral syndromes, the biological implications of these substances are now recognised to be important in understanding the biological characteristics of neoplastic cells and in developing new modalities of cancer therapies.

MECHANISMS OF ECTOPIC HORMONE PRODUCTION IN MULTISTAGE CARCINOGENESIS

transformation of neuroendocrine cells and subsequent expression of ectopic hormone gene

neuroendocrine differentiation of transformed totipotential stem cells and subsequent expression of ectopic hormone gene

expression of ectopic hormone gene by transformed non-endocrine cells

Fig. 21.6 Proposed mechanisms of ectopic hormone production by neoplasms in the process of multistage carcinogenesis.

PATHOGENESIS

The development of neoplastic cells is associated with several carcinogenic steps; some clones of neoplastic cells acquire an ability to invade and metastasise, which may finally characterise the prognosis. Although these carcinogenic steps, or multistage carcinogenesis, were rather hypothetical, recent progress in molecular oncology has revealed that the carcinogenic steps result from cumulative somatic mutations in oncogenes and tumour-suppressor genes, and from phenotypical abnormalities in growth-factor signal transduction pathways. The basic abnormality in the ectopic humoral syndrome or in ectopic production of bioactive substances indicates that neoplastic cells acquire the ability to express a gene that codes for bioactive substances; the gene would not otherwise have been expressed by the mature cells of that organ. Although the information available at present is insufficient to explain this phenomenon fully, it appears to be associated with sequences of events that occur in the carcinogenic process for neoplastic cells.

The hypotheses for explaining ectopic production of biologically active substances focus mainly on peptide hormones. The proposed mechanisms to explain ectopic elaboration of hormones fall into three categories (Fig. 21.6). The first is that the normal cell to be transformed possesses neuroendocrine characteristics. Although the cell does not initially express a gene encoding the hormone concerned, neoplastic cells possess the ability to express the gene during one or more of the carcinogenic steps. Ectopic hormone production by neuroendocrine tumours is the representative case; medullary thyroid carcinoma and pancreatic endocrine tumours can express the ACTH gene, which is normally suppressed in adult thyroid C-cells and pancreatic islet cells. Another example in this category is the development of carcinogenic steps in cells that possess neuroendocrine potential, but in which this potential remains dormant in

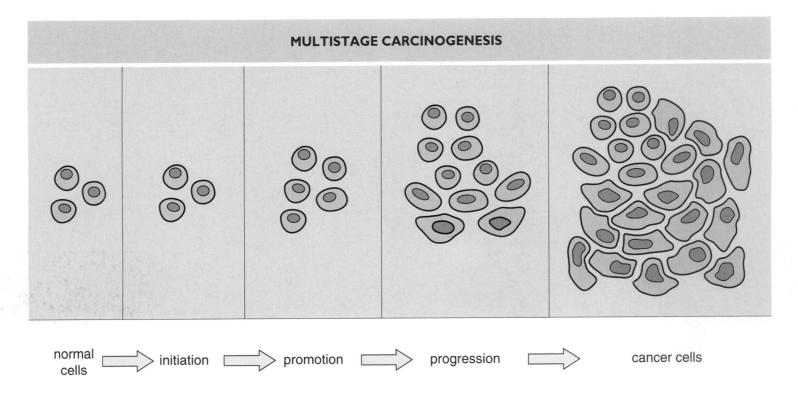

MULTISTAGE CARCINOGENESIS

normal cells ⟹ initiation ⟹ promotion ⟹ progression ⟹ cancer cells

Fig. 21.7 Multistage carcinogenesis. Genetic and phenotypic alterations responsible for multistage carcinogenesis in small-cell lung carcinoma include inactivation of tumour-suppressor genes (p53, Rb, chromosome 3p locus), activation of oncogenes (c-*myc*, L-*myc*, and N-*myc*), and autocrine growth mechanisms (GRP and IGF-I).

the adult nonendocrine tissues. It is possible to speculate that this hypothesis could explain ectopic GRP production by small-cell lung carcinoma. It is well known that fetal lung possesses a large number of neuroendocrine cells, and that many of these express the GRP gene. In adult lung, neuroendocrine cells are very rarely detected. If neoplastic transformation of these dormant cells can explain the development of small-cell lung carcinoma, the very high detection frequency of GRP in small-cell lung carcinoma could be explained.

According to the second hypothesis, neoplastic transformation develops in totipotential dormant stem cells; at the start of multistage carcinogenesis, the neoplastic stem cell differentiates in various directions; if a clone of neoplastic cells differentiates into a neuroendocrine cell lineage and acquires potent growth-promoting carcinogenic activity, a clinically detectable neoplasm composed of neuroendocrine cells may arise, which in turn would lead to the development of humoral syndromes.

The third hypothesis is based on the case of ectopic hormone production in which neuroendocrine differentiation is not always observed in neoplastic cells. The ectopic PTHrP syndrome, namely HHM, is the illustrative case. The list of the neoplasms that elaborate this protein and then develop HHM includes squamous cell carcinomas of the lung and oesophagus, breast carcinoma, ovarian adenocarcinomas, endocrine tumours, fibrosarcomas, and haematological malignancies, especially adult T-cell leukaemia. It is possible that a fundamental change has occurred in a gene encoding the hormone; deletion of, or point mutation at, the regulatory unit of the hormone gene may increase the expression of the gene. However, this mechanism may not explain most of the cases of HHM, because the frequency of development of such an abnormality is likely to be rather low. As described in Fig. 21.7, several somatic changes may occur in the development of neoplastic cells. Some of these changes, or as yet unidentified somatic changes, in genes that regulate hormone gene expression, might play a role in this type of ectopic hormone production. With regard to these molecules, transcriptional factors with activity to bind to DNA and regulate gene expression might be candidates.

It is likely that the phenomenon of ectopic hormone production is multifactorial, and that all of the possibilities described above may work in various situations of ectopic hormone production. The major reason why it is difficult to determine which mechanism occurs in a given case is the lack of methodology to detect, at a very early stage, the neoplastic cells that will develop into neoplasms that are associated with ectopic hormone production.

CLINICAL FEATURES OF ECTOPIC HUMORAL SYNDROMES

There are common clinical characteristics in ectopic humoral syndromes which undoubtedly play key roles in the diagnosis of these clinical entities, but careful observation during routine laboratory tests of cancer patients will make it possible to detect the early stages of the diseases before clinical symptoms become evident (Fig. 21.8). Electrolyte imbalances such as hypokalaemia, hyponatraemia and hypercalcaemia suggest the presence of ectopic ACTH, ADH and PTHrP syndromes, respectively, and metabolic abnormalities such as diabetes mellitus are associated with the ectopic ACTH syndrome. These electrolyte and metabolic imbalances are frequently encountered as the only detectable signs of ectopic humoral syndromes. Patients with an ectopic humoral syndrome frequently have neoplasms at the advanced stage, for which curable surgery is impossible, with the exception of cases of classical neuroendocrine tumours.

Demonstration of the neuroendocrine characteristics of neoplastic cells is useful for the definite diagnosis in many cases of ectopic hormone syndromes. Several neuroendocrine features of neoplastic cells are described in Fig. 21.9.

TESTS FOR ECTOPIC HUMORAL SYNDROMES	
syndromes	abnormal in routine tests
ectopic ACTH syndrome	hypertension, hypokalaemia, diabetes mellitus
ectopic ADH syndrome	hyponatraemia
humoral hypercalcaemia of malignancy	hypercalcaemia
ectopic cytokine syndrome	leukocytosis, erythocytosis

Fig. 21.8 Routine laboratory tests indicating the presence of ectopic humoral syndromes.

NEUROENDOCRINE CHARACTERISTICS OF NEOPLASTIC CELLS	
histology	cellular morphology specific staining
electron microscopy	neuroendocrine granules
immunohistochemistry and/or biochemical assays for substances expressed in neuroendocrine cells	peptide hormones: enzymes (neurone-specific enolase, creatine kinase BB, l-amino acid decarboxylase, ADCC) adhesion molecules: N-CAM (cluster-1 antigen)

Fig. 21.9 Neuroendocrine characteristics of neoplastic cells.

The clinical features of ectopic humoral syndromes are in many ways similar to those of eutopic humoral syndromes. Therefore, the features that differentiate between these syndromes will be emphasised.

ECTOPIC ADRENOCORTICOTROPHIC SYNDROME

The ectopic ACTH syndrome (Fig. 21.10) is one of the most extensively studied ectopic humoral syndromes. The production of large amounts of ACTH by the neoplasms results in the elevation of plasma ACTH levels, which in turn stimulates cortisol secretion from the adrenal cortex.

Hypercortisolism accounts for most signs and symptoms of ectopic ACTH syndrome. The hyperpigmentation of the ectopic ACTH syndrome is due to the pigmentary action of the very high levels of ACTH, although occasionally an additional melanocyte-stimulating hormone (MSH) derived from its ACTH precursor molecule (pro-opiocortin) is produced. Patients with the ectopic ACTH syndrome due to low-grade malignancies, such as a medullary thyroid carcinoma, carcinoid tumours or pancreatic endocrine tumours, develop typical features of Cushing's syndrome, because such patients survive for a sufficient period to develop the full-blown syndrome. However, in the case of high-grade malignancies, such as small-cell carcinomas of the lung and uterus, the patient's condition becomes rapidly worse, which in turn makes it impossible to develop typical physical changes; such patients frequently present only an electrolyte imbalance, metabolic derangement and hyperpigmentation. Since a medical history indicating that the patient had suffered from a neoplasm often precedes the development of ectopic ACTH syndrome, diagnosis of the latter condition is not very difficult. If, however, the ectopic ACTH syndrome is due to an endocrine tumour, especially in the case of a carcinoid tumour, it sometimes precedes the discovery of the neoplasm. The diagnosis of this syndrome is confirmed by the following observations: elevation of plasma ACTH and cortisol levels and urinary free cortisol excretion; and failure to suppress plasma cortisol and urinary free cortisol after high-dose dexamethasone administration (8mg/d for two days).

Treatment of the ectopic ACTH syndrome is difficult. Surgical removal of the ACTH-producing tumour is desirable but difficult in most cases. Effective chemotherapy and/or radiotherapy of the neoplasms may produce relief from the syndrome. The metabolic abnormalities that are induced by hypercortisolism can be controlled by either surgical bilateral adrenalectomy or medical treatment with metyrapone, o,p-DDD, ketoconazole, or aminoglutethimide (see Chapter 8).

ECTOPIC ANTIDIURETIC HORMONE SYNDROME

The ectopic ADH syndrome (Fig. 21.11) is caused by the production of ADH by neoplasms with endocrine characteristics. This syndrome is also referred to as the Schwarz–Bartter syndrome or the syndrome of inappropriate ADH secretion (SIADH). Although ectopic ACTH syndrome is observed in patients with various types of neoplasms, almost all cases of the disorder develop in patients with small-cell lung carcinoma (see Chapter 2).

Physiologically, ADH is produced at the hypothalamus and stored in the posterior pituitary gland. When water loss develops, secretion of ADH is stimulated. ADH acts on the renal distal tubules and enhances the reabsorption of water, so serum osmolality is maintained at the normal level. In ectopic ADH syndrome, secretion of ADH by neoplasms continues even though the body water has increased, and serum osmolality is lowered. This 'inappropriate ADH secretion' brings about severe water excess, and serum osmolality and sodium concentration are decreased. This abnormality results in movement of water from the extracellular space to the intracellular space, which in turn induces water intoxication.

The signs and symptoms that develop in patients with ectopic ADH syndrome are due to the effect of water intoxication on the nervous system. If the serum sodium concentration does not fall below 120mmol/l, the patient may have no complaints. If the level falls lower than this value, a variety of signs and symptoms, as described in Fig. 21.11, usually appear.

Diagnosis of ectopic ADH syndrome is made on the basis of the criteria described in Fig. 21.11. Under physiological conditions, hyponatraemia and low osmolality inhibit the excretion of urinary sodium. Therefore, urinary sodium concentration and osmolality

ECTOPIC ACTH SYNDROME

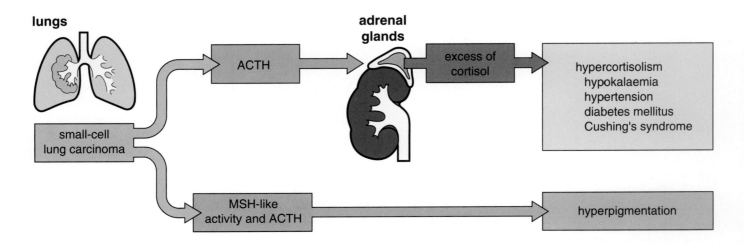

Fig. 21.10 Mechanisms and clinical features of ectopic ACTH syndrome.

decrease (urinary sodium concentration below 10mmol/l). In the case of ectopic ADH syndrome, urinary sodium excretion continues, which further aggravates hyponatraemia and low serum osmolality. The mechanism responsible for the continuation of urinary sodium excretion has not yet been elucidated, and a 'third factor' has been proposed. Recently discovered natriuretic peptides – atrial natriuretic peptide and brain natriuretic peptide – may play a role in the development of ectopic ADH syndrome.

Under rare conditions, inappropriate ADH secretion from the posterior pituitary gland in cancer patients is observed. Certain drugs, including vinca alkaloids, cyclophosphamide, barbiturates and morphine, may cause SIADH by stimulating ADH secretion from the posterior pituitary. Metastatic tumours in the hypothalamus and inflammatory changes, as well as the tumour mass present in the intrathoracic cavity, may stimulate the secretion of ADH from the posterior pituitary gland. Since these disorders are sometimes difficult to differentiate from ectopic ADH syndrome, the final diagnosis of this syndrome is made by demonstration that the neoplasm produces a large amount of ADH.

HUMORAL HYPERCALCAEMIA OF MALIGNANCY

Hypercalcaemia is the most frequent paraneoplastic syndrome observed in cancer patients; it is also known as malignancy-associated hypercalcaemia. Analysis of data on all inpatients from 1983 to 1985 at the National Cancer Center Hospital, Tokyo, showed the frequency of hypercalcaemia (>2.65mmol/l; 10.6mg/dl) to be over three per cent among all inpatients and ten per cent among inpatients with advanced cancers.

Malignancy-associated hypercalcaemia can be divided into two categories: hypercalcaemia induced by severe bone metastases; and the elaboration of hypercalcaemic factors by neoplastic cells, termed HHM. It is roughly estimated that more than seventy per cent of malignancy-associated hypercalcaemia belongs to the latter cause – HHM.

Humoral factors responsible for HHM have long been sought, and the factors with bone-resorbing activity, including PTH, prostaglandins, TGF-α, TGF-β, epidermal growth factor, IL-1α and IL-Iβ, were claimed to be candidates but were shown not to be the major factors responsible for this morbidity. Recently, a protein with PTH-like activity, referred to as PTHrP, was isolated from a cancer cell line that was established from lung cancer tissue from a hypercalcaemic patient, and the structure of PTHrP mRNA was identified. Since biological activities of PTHrP explain most of the clinical and laboratory findings of HHM patients, and several clinical studies on a large number of HHM patients have clarified that PTHrP substantially contributes to the development of HHM, PTHrP is now the primary candidate for the factor responsible for HHM.

HHM develops in patients with a variety of neoplasms described in Fig. 21.12. Although there is a tendency for patients with squamous cell carcinoma to develop HHM most frequently, patients with adenocarcinoma also develop this condition. Moreover, recent observations have shown that more than sixty per cent of patients with adult T-cell leukaemia develop severe hypercalcaemia of the HHM type. PTHrP is the primary candidate as the causative factor in these patients. Thus, HHM in patients with solid tumours as well as haematological malignancies have the common aetiology of PTHrP production by neoplastic cells. In solid neoplasms, the development

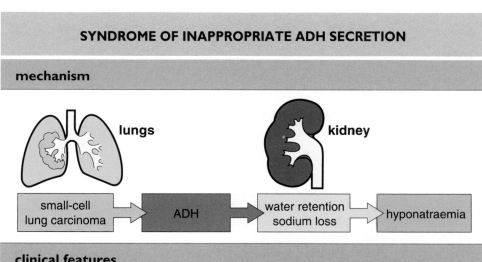

Fig. 21.11 The syndrome of inappropriate ADH secretion.

SYNDROME OF INAPPROPRIATE ADH SECRETION

mechanism

lungs → small-cell lung carcinoma → ADH → water retention sodium loss → hyponatraemia ← kidney

clinical features

serum sodium level	signs and symptoms
120–130mmol/l	often asymptomatic
lower than 120mmol/l	anorexia, nausea, vomiting anxiety, lethargy, weakness headache, convulsion, coma

laboratory data of a representative case

	blood	urine
sodium	108mmol/l	94mmol/l/day
osmolarity	200mosmol/l	532mosmol/l

of HHM has been shown to be closely associated with the stage of the disease: a study of three hundred and seventy-six consecutive patients with primary oesophageal carcinoma treated at the National Cancer Center Hospital, Tokyo, from 1983 to 1988, demonstrated that only five patients (1.3%) with operable cancer presented with hypercalcaemia. Following surgery, serum calcium levels were normal in all five patients. In contrast, among one hundred and twenty

patients whose serum calcium levels were evaluated within two months of death from advanced oesophageal carcinoma, forty-five (thirty-eight per cent) developed hypercalcaemia. In other types of neoplasm the same relationship was observed, indicating that this electrolyte imbalance develops mainly in patients with advanced cancers.

The mechanisms that are responsible for the development of HHM, and its clinical features, are summarised in Fig. 21.13. The signs and symptoms that develop in patients with HHM are due to hypercalcaemic nephropathy and neurological complications. If the total serum calcium level rises to >3mmol/l (12mg/dl), a variety of signs and symptoms, described in Fig. 21.13, usually appear. In contrast to hypercalcaemia of primary hyperparathyroidism, serum calcium levels in HHM patients increase rapidly, and the symptoms and signs are therefore always more severe than those in patients with primary hyperparathyroidism; often, a patient with advanced cancer has a normal calcium level, but a week later the patient develops severe hypercalcaemia. In the case of primary hyperparathyroidism, the serum calcium levels are stable, except in patients with parathyroid carcinoma.

The diagnosis of HHM is currently based on differential diagnosis from other diseases that have the capacity to develop hypercalcaemia (Fig. 21.14). Ongoing clinical trials to measure serum PTHrP levels by immunoassay systems that recognise the amino-terminal and/or carboxyl-terminal portion of PTHrP show promising results. These assays may play a definitive role in diagnosing HHM due to PTHrP-producing tumours.

ECTOPIC CHORIONIC GONADOTROPHIN SYNDROME

Neoplasms that arise from trophoblastic cells, notably choriocarcinomas of the placenta and testes, secrete excessive amounts of chorionic gonadotrophin (CG); this entity falls into the category of eutopic hormone production. Alternatively, ectopic CG production is associated with hepatocellular carcinomas, gastrointestinal cancers, brain germinomas, or pineal tumours and lung cancers. Clinical syndromes caused by ectopic CG production include precocious puberty in children, gynaecomastia in adult males, and menstrual irregularities in women. From the standpoint of clinical oncology, the second clinical

MALIGNANCIES ASSOCIATED WITH HHM

squamous cell carcinoma	oesophageal carcinoma laryngeal carcinoma tongue carcinoma lung carcinoma uterus carcinoma
adenocarcinoma	renal cell carcinoma ovarian carcinoma
transitional cell carcinoma	bladder carcinoma
haematological malignancies	multiple myeloma malignant lymphoma adult T-cell leukaemia

Fig. 21.12 Malignancies frequently associated with HHM.

MECHANISMS AND FEATURES OF HHM

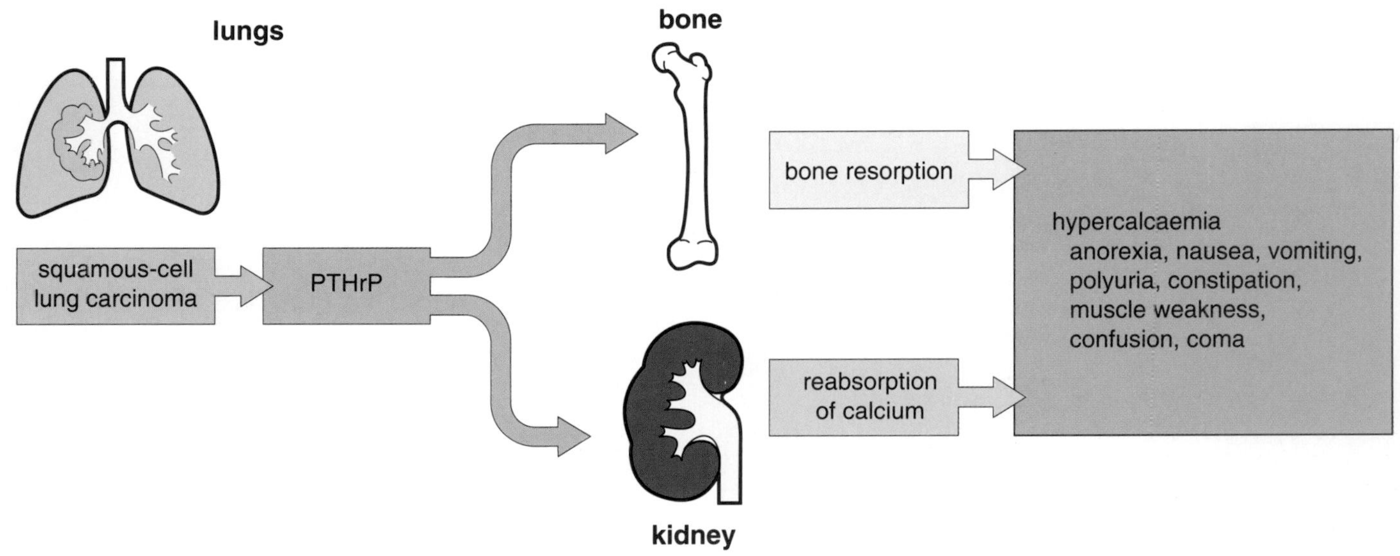

Fig. 21.13 Mechanisms and clinical features of HHM.

syndrome is important, since a greater number of adult patients than children have ectopic CG syndrome.

The diagnosis of ectopic CG syndrome could be achieved by the measurement of plasma CG or the β-subunit of CG by immunoassays; routine urinary pregnancy tests should be avoided since they are not always sensitive. It is worth noting that in the male patient with bilateral gynaecomastia and plasma CG elevation, the presence of lung cancer or germ cell tumours of the testis or extragonadal sites should be sought vigorously.

The presence of gynaecomastia may be unpleasant since it is sometimes painful and may be emotionally distressing. This abnormality can be treated by surgical reduction.

ECTOPIC HORMONE SYNDROMES ASSOCIATED WITH NEUROENDOCRINE TUMOURS

Neoplasms derived from endocrine organs develop syndromes induced by hormonal excess – eutopic humoral syndromes – as described in other chapters. The major ectopic hormone syndromes that develop in patients with endocrine tumours are those induced by overproduction of ACTH, gastrin, vasoactive intestinal polypeptide (VIP) and GHRH.

Ectopic Adrenocorticotrophic Hormone Syndrome Associated with Neuroendocrine Tumours

Endocrine tumours frequently associated with ectopic ACTH syndrome are carcinoid tumours, medullary thyroid carcinomas and pancreatic endocrine tumours. It is worth noting that a full-blown Cushing's syndrome always develops in these cases, because these endocrine tumours characteristically grow slowly and hence there is enough time for the patient to develop the syndrome. This is quite different from the clinical features observed with ectopic ACTH syndrome in patients with small-cell lung carcinoma.

Zollinger–Ellison Syndrome

The production of gastrin, a product of gastric G-cells, by pancreatic endocrine tumours results in gastric acid hypersecretion and subsequently induces peptic ulcer disease; this entity is referred to as the Zollinger–Ellison syndrome (gastrinoma). Since gastrin is a physiological product of gastric G-cells regulating gastric acid secretion, and this hormone is not produced physiologically by islet cells of the pancreas, the Zollinger–Ellison syndrome is categorised as an ectopic hormone syndrome.

Watery Diarrhoea, Hypokalaemia, and Achlorhydria Syndrome

The watery diarrhoea, hypokalaemia, and achlorhydria (WDHA) syndrome is a clinical entity in which profuse watery diarrhoea, hypokalaemia, and achlorhydria or hypochlorhydria are induced by the overproduction of a VIP – a brain and gut peptide with potent biological activity for stimulating vasodilatation and intestinal secretion. The syndrome is also known as VIPoma, pancreatic cholera and the Verner–Morrison syndrome. The tumours responsible for this morbidity are, in adults, pancreatic neuroendocrine tumours and, in children, neuroblastic tumours, including ganglioneuroblastoma, ganglioneuroma and neuroblastoma. Based on the normal distribution of this peptide, the syndrome induced by the VIP-producing pancreatic endocrine tumour fits the criteria of the ectopic humoral syndrome. The most serious clinical problem in WDHA patients is watery diarrhoea and the resultant imbalances of water and electrolytes, which in turn threaten the patient's life. Complete surgical resection of the tumour is the optimal goal of treatment.

Recently, a long-acting and potent somatostatin analogue, octreotide, has been developed (see Chapter 3). Short-term adminis-tration of this agent is useful for improving the condition of WDHA patients at the preoperative stage, and this agent is also effective in reducing watery diarrhoea in inoperable WDHA patients. The somatostatin analogue acts on tumour cells to inhibit VIP secretion, as well as directly on the small intestine and exocrine pancreas, thus inhibiting the exocrine intestinal and pancreatic secretion stimulated by VIP.

Ectopic Growth Hormone-releasing Hormone Syndrome

GHRH is a hypothalamic hormone that stimulates growth hormone secretion from the anterior pituitary gland. Since the discovery of ectopic GHRH syndrome, an appreciable number of patients who suffer from acromegaly caused by GHRH production have been reported; neoplasms associated with ectopic GHRH syndrome are thus far limited to bronchial carcinoid and pancreatic endocrine tumour, although ectopic GHRH production is frequent in a variety of neoplasms with neuroendocrine characteristics, including small-cell lung carcinoma. It appears that this is not a frequent cause of acromegaly (much less than one per cent), but this entity is very important for the differential diagnosis of multiple endocrine neoplasia (MEN) type I. When a patient suffering from acromegaly is found to have a pancreatic endocrine tumour and the latter does not show any humoral syndrome, then two possibilities will be considered: one is that the patient has MEN type I, possessing both a pituitary tumour and an asymptomatic pancreatic endocrine tumour; the other is that the patient's pancreatic endocrine tumour produces GHRH, which in turn stimulates growth hormone secretion from the pituitary, resulting in acromegaly. In the latter case, the plasma GHRH level is one hundred- to one thousand-fold higher than the normal value (upper limit of normal is approximately 100pg/ml) and is useful for the differential diagnosis.

DIFFERENTIAL DIAGNOSIS OF HYPERCALCAEMIA

malignancy-associated hypercalcaemia	humoral hypercalcaemia of malignancy extensive bone metastasis
coexistence of other diseases	primary hyperparathyroidism Cushing's syndrome hyperparathyroidism adrenocortical insufficiency sarcoidosis Paget's disease
drug-induced hypercalcaemia	calcium vitamin D analogues anti-tumour hormonal agents (tamoxifen) thiazide

Fig. 21.14 Differential diagnosis of hypercalcaemia in patients with malignancy.

ECTOPIC CYTOKINE SYNDROMES

Recent development in cytokine and growth factor research has demonstrated that the production of cytokines or growth factors by cancer cells induces typical humoral syndromes in patients with various types of neoplasms. Thus, ectopic cytokine syndrome is now an important component of ectopic humoral syndromes. Two conditions – granulocytosis syndrome and polycythaemia syndrome – are now well characterised. Two other possible entities, tumour hypoglycaemia syndrome and cancer cachexia syndrome, are clinically well recognised, but which factor (or factors) is responsible for these syndromes is not established; candidates are cytokines or growth factors.

Granulocytosis Syndrome

Granulocytosis syndrome is a rare but well-recognised haematological abnormality that develops in cancer patients. Although several mechanisms responsible for this morbidity have been proposed in patients with neoplasms, recent studies have revealed that the production of granulocytosis-stimulating factors is the major cause of this paraneoplastic syndrome. Recent developments in haematology have revealed that there are at least four types of cytokines responsible for this condition: granulocyte (G)-colony-stimulating factor (CSF), granulocyte macrophage (GM) CSF macrophage (M) CSF, and multi-CSF (IL-3). In a small number of cancer patients with granulocytosis syndrome, G-CSF, GM-CSF and M-CSF have been shown to be the cause. Neoplasms that are associated with the granulocytosis syndrome are found in the lung, oesophagus, stomach and pancreas. These patients always present with remarkable granulocytosis (greater than 20,000/μl), fever refractory to antibiotics (greater than 38°C) and hepatomegaly. In most cases this syndrome, associated with lung cancer, develops at a rather early stage of the disease compared with other ectopic humoral syndromes. Postoperatively, following successful tumour resection, fever and hepatomegaly disappear acutely, and granulocytosis disappears more gradually. The differential diagnosis in these patients includes the possibility of a leukaemoid reaction that is induced by overt infection, or of coexistent chronic myelogenous leukaemia.

Erythrocytosis

Polycythaemia caused by increased erythropoietin secretion occurs in association with renal cell carcinoma, cerebellar haemangioblastomas and, less commonly, with adrenal, ovarian and hepatic neoplasms. Since erythropoietin is normally produced by the kidney, the syndrome that develops in patients with renal cell carcinoma does not fit into the category of the ectopic humoral syndrome. At present, the assay for plasma erythropoietin levels is not sufficiently reliable, making the differential diagnosis between ectopic erythropoietin syndrome and other mechanisms that generate erythrocytosis in cancer patients sometimes difficult; the latter mechanisms include the production of substances with erythropoietic activities or activities to stimulate erythropoietin production, such as androgenic hormones, prostaglandins, and β-adrenergic antagonists. Erythrocytosis usually does not require treatment.

Tumour Hypoglycaemia Syndrome

It is well established that severe fasting hypoglycaemia occurs in association with nonpancreatic neoplasms. Three types of neoplasms, including mesenchymal, hepatocellular and adrenal tumours, account for ninety-five per cent of the cases. Mesenchymal tumours include fibrosarcomas, mesotheliomas, neurofibromas, neurofibrosarcomas, spindle cell carcinomas, rhabdomyosarcomas and leiomyosarcomas (see Chapter 20).

Cancer Cachexia Syndrome

Progressive weight loss is a common clinical feature in cancer patients. In most cases, weight loss can be explained partly by anorexia or decreased oral intake as a result of therapeutic toxicity, chronic pain, a depressive state, obstruction of the gastrointestinal tract, hypercalcaemia, uraemia, and so on. It is also well recognised that weight loss appears at an early stage of malignancy and disappears with the resection of the tumour. This clinical observation fits into the category of humoral syndrome. The best evidence that the cancer cachexia syndrome is induced by humoral factor(s) produced by cancer cells is obtained by analyses of human tumour xenografts in mice, which develop severe cachexia; tumour resection in these mice brings about rapid regain of the lost weight. The hypothetical factor responsible for this syndrome, originally referred to as 'toxohormone', has long been sought. Recent experimental studies demonstrate that two cytokines, leukaemia and IL-6 inhibitory factor, are the most likely candidates for this syndrome. Since the mechanisms responsible for cachexia in cancer patients are multifactorial, evaluation of the role of these cytokines in the development of the syndrome is difficult.

ECTOPIC SUBSTANCES AS MARKERS FOR NEOPLASIA

With the initial recognition of ectopic humoral syndrome, namely ectopic hormone syndrome, it was hoped that by measuring the amounts of hormones in the plasma, a screening process for clinically silent tumours would become available. To ascertain whether this would prove to be correct, several ectopically produced hormones such as ACTH, calcitonin and CG have been extensively studied. Although initial studies were optimistic, further clinical investigation demonstrated that these markers were not reliable. Further study is required to identify reliable markers of cancer.

Hormone Assay Techniques

Tony E Torresani, PhD

In the clinical laboratory, the need for sensitive and specific *in vitro* tests for the determination of endocrinological compounds has been dictated by the low concentration of hormones present in blood. The enzymatic methods that are usually employed in clinical chemistry are capable of detecting substances in the range of 5–10µg/ml, but this sensitivity is not well suited for the quantitative determination of hormone concentrations. The use of specific binding reagents, however, has made the measurement of hormones possible: protein-binding assays, receptor assays and immunoassays are all binding assay methodologies that can be used for this purpose (Fig. 22.1).

Protein-binding assays use proteins, extracted from plasma or tissues, which are capable of binding an endocrinological substance. An example of such a technique is the thyroxine (T_4) test which uses the specific thyroxine-binding globulin for the determination of T_4. Protein-binding assays, however, have limited usage, due to their low binding affinity and specificity.

Receptor assays use the receptor that is specific for the hormone to be measured as a ligand. Such ligands are either soluble receptor proteins or suspensions of membrane-bound receptors. The binding mechanism in the receptor assay involves the biologically active part of the hormone that is to be measured. A receptor assay can therefore give information on whether the structure of a circulating hormone might be pathologically altered. Furthermore, the assay allows the detection of autoimmune antibodies that are directed against the receptor itself. An example of this type of receptor assay is the detection of antibodies to the thyroid receptor for thyroid-stimulating hormone (TSH). The use of receptor assays is restricted by the difficulty in finding and isolating the appropriate receptor for every hormone to be measured.

Immunoassays use antibodies that are raised against the hormones to be measured. The binding mechanism in the immunoassay involves the immunologically active epitopes on the hormone molecule. These binding sites, however, are not necessarily related to the biological activity of the hormone. Immunoassays, nevertheless, have become the method of choice since, on practical grounds, they are much easier to perform than receptor assays.

Since the first description of a radioimmunoassay (RIA) by Yalow and Berson in 1959, the immunological tests for the determination of hormones have seen a continuous development and improvement. Today's endocrinological investigations rely heavily on the use of such tests for the determination of peptide and steroid hormones.

The basic mechanism of a hormone immunoassay is the reaction between an antigen, the hormone to be measured, and an antibody capable of binding to that antigen (Fig. 22.2). Since the complex that is formed cannot be directly detected, due to its low concentration, an additional reagent needs to be introduced into the reaction, namely the label. The label shown in Fig. 22.2 is coupled to the antigen and produces a signal that can easily be measured. The hormone that is bound in the antigen–antibody complex can thus be detected and quantified.

THE ANTIBODY

BASICS

The keystone of an immunoassay is the reaction between the antigen and the antibody. The easiest way to describe this process is to imagine the antigen as a key and the antibody as a lock. Only one key will properly fit and operate the lock (Fig. 22.3). Thus, the antibody will selectively recognise the antigen among the myriad of structurally related substances that are present in the sample. The selectivity of an immunoassay is, in consequence, predominantly dependent on the specificity of the reaction between the antigen and antibody.

Antibodies that are used in immunoassays belong to the IgG class of immunoglobulins and have a molecular weight of some one hundred and fifty thousand. Structurally, the antibodies are composed of two 'heavy' and two 'light' peptide chains, which are linked together

BINDING ASSAYS

method	binding reagent
protein-binding assay	binding protein extracted from plasma or tissue
receptor assay	hormone-specific receptor
immunoassay	antibody

Fig. 22.1 *Different types of binding assays.* Endocrinological substances can be measured with different assay techniques, all based on a binding reaction between an analyte and a binding agent.

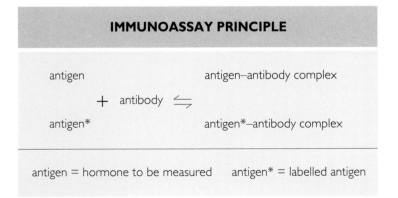

IMMUNOASSAY PRINCIPLE

antigen   antigen–antibody complex

$+$ antibody $\rightleftharpoons$

antigen*   antigen*–antibody complex

antigen = hormone to be measured   antigen* = labelled antigen

Fig. 22.2 *The principle of the immunological reaction.* An antigen reacts, in competition with a labelled antigen, with the binding sites of a specific antibody. Two complexes are formed, their concentration being dependent on the initial concentration of the antigen to be measured.

by disulphide bonds; their structure resembles a large 'Y' (Fig. 22.4). The amino-terminal part of the heavy and the light chains is involved in the binding with the antigen. The three-dimensional structure of the binding domain recognises the antigen with the correct corresponding structure and reacts only with such antigen, forming the antigen–antibody complex (Fig. 22.5), while antigens with another structure cannot bind to the antibody.

SPECIFICITY AND CROSSREACTIVITY

The specificity of an antibody for a given antigen is characterised by the crossreactivity. Crossreactivity describes the structural relationship between the antigen and the binding domain on the antibody. An antibody is classified as highly specific when it binds exclusively with one defined antigen. In practice, the ideal antibody with one hundred per cent specificity does not exist. Every antibody, to a certain

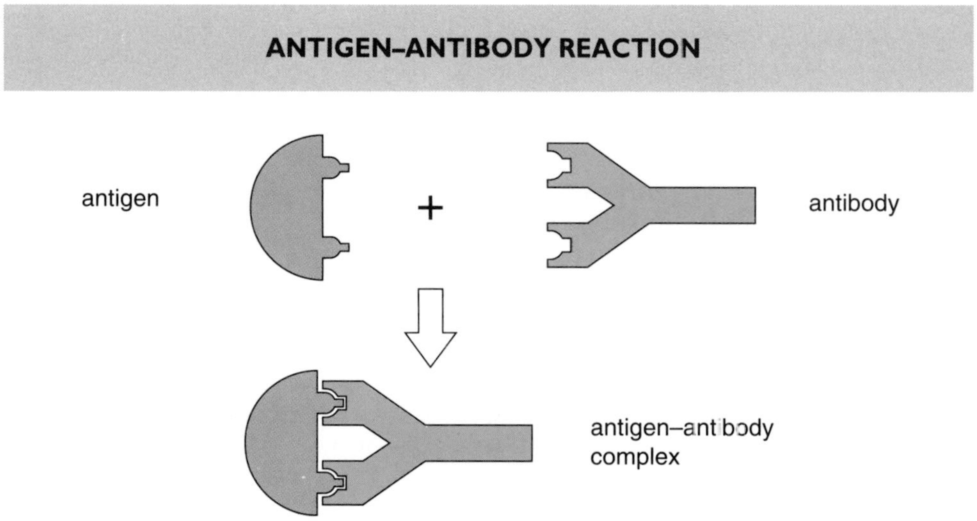

ANTIGEN–ANTIBODY REACTION

antigen + antibody

antigen–antibody complex

Fig. 22.3 The mechanism of the antigen–antibody reaction.
In order to bind with an antibody, the structure of the antigen must fit the corresponding structure of the antibody.

STRUCTURE OF IgG

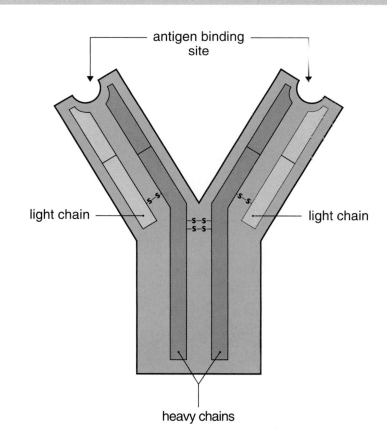

antigen binding site

light chain — — light chain

heavy chains

Fig. 22.4 A simplified structure of an antibody molecule (IgG). The antigen binding site is at the amino-terminal part.

22

degree, also recognises antigens with structural homology (Fig. 22.6). The glycoprotein hormones, luteinising hormone, follicle-stimulating hormone and TSH, for example, are each composed of two subunits, and the α-subunit is identical in all three hormones. Polyclonal antibodies prepared against one of these glycoprotein hormones will also partially recognise the others; this partial recognition can be measured and expressed as a percentage. A high degree of crossreactivity of the antibody will inevitably result in interference in the immunoassay.

The choice of an antibody is therefore of paramount importance in the design of an immunoassay; monoclonal and polyclonal antibodies can be used for such assays. Polyclonal antibodies are characterised by having a high binding affinity and are somewhat easier to prepare than monoclonal antibodies; by definition, they are not homogenous with respect to binding and therefore are less specific than monoclonal antibodies. Monoclonal antibodies are characterised by the homogeneity of their binding affinity and specificity. They are currently used in most commercial immunoassays since they can be produced in large quantities.

THE LABEL

As previously mentioned, the immunological reaction involved in the measurement of hormones cannot be directly detected with the conventional means of clinical chemistry. The endpoint signal therefore needs to be amplified by the introduction of a further compound, a label, which is capable of generating a signal of high specific activity. This label should be coupled to one of the components of the immunological reaction, without interfering with it. Among the substances used as labels, the following are more common: radioactive isotopes, enzymes, fluorescent substances, and bioluminescent and chemiluminescent compounds.

RADIOACTIVE LABELS

Radioactive substances were the first types of labels to be used in immunoassays. The iodine isotopes ^{125}I or ^{131}I are ideal for the labelling of proteins and peptides that contain the amino acid tyrosine. During the labelling reaction, one hydrogen in the tyrosine is substituted by one iodine. Although iodine is larger than hydrogen, there is usually no disturbance of the immunological characteristics of the labelled compound. For the labelling of steroid hormones, the isotopes ^{3}H and ^{14}C are more commonly used because they can be directly incorporated into the structure of the steroid molecule.

The activity of the label that is bound in the antigen–antibody complex is measured in γ- or β-counters, according to the type of radiation specific for the isotope. The low detection limit of RIAs is determined by the high specific activity of the label and by the fact that radioactivity is usually absent from the samples in which the assays are performed.

The use of radioactive labels has paved the way for the introduction of RIAs, and has for the first time made the direct *in vitro* measurement of hormones possible. Unfortunately the RIA technique has some major drawbacks, and the laboratories that perform RIAs are subject to more and more stringent regulations concerning radiation protection, storage of isotopic materials, and disposal of radioactive waste, although the isotopic activities that they use are very small.

SPECIFICITY OF AN ANTIBODY

correct antigen

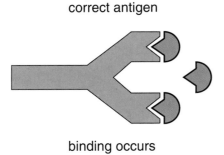

binding occurs

wrong antigen

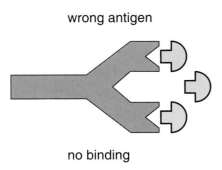

no binding

CROSS REACTIVITY

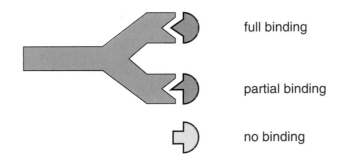

full binding

partial binding

no binding

Fig. 22.5 Specificity of an antibody. Only the antigen with the correct structure will bind to the antibody. Other antigens in the sample will not bind to the antibody.

Fig. 22.6 Crossreactivity. Antigens with a related structure may bind partially with the antibody. Such crossreactivity can negatively affect the assay.

The labelled compounds that are used are relatively unstable, due to the short natural half-life of the isotopes, and to radiolysis of the labelled compounds during storage. These problems thus prompted a search for alternative methods of labelling which, by preserving the high specificity and sensitivity of the RIA, would allow a simpler handling of the immunoassays. The first such alternative labelling method involved the coupling of enzymes, instead of radioactive substances, to antigens or antibodies.

ENZYMATIC LABELS

It soon became quite clear that the coupling of enzymes (which have much larger molecular weights than, for instance, ^{125}I) had no adverse effects either on the immunological reaction or on the activity of the enzyme itself. The prerequisite of the immunoassay, the antigen–antibody reaction, is thus preserved, but instead of a radioactive tracer, an enzyme is used, thereby allowing immunoassays to be handled in ordinary laboratories. The main difference between RIAs and enzyme immunoassays (EIAs) is in the colour-development reaction that follows the immunological reaction in order to measure the activity of the enzyme in the antigen–antibody complex. Colour development can be measured in ordinary photometers, which are found in most laboratories. The sensitivity that is necessary for the low detection limit is determined by the velocity of the enzymatic reaction. The characteristics of an enzyme that is suitable to be used in an immunoassay are therefore high specific activity, absence from the sample used in the assay, freedom from interference with other substances that are present in the sample, and no loss of activity during the coupling procedure. Commonly used enzymes that fulfil these criteria include, among others, glucose-6-phosphate dehydrogenase, horse-radish peroxidase, alkaline phosphatase, and β-galactosidase.

FLUORESCENT LABELS

Other nonisotopic immunoassays use fluorescent labels. Apart from use in the more conventional fluoroimmunoassays (FIAs, IFMAs), fluorescent labels are also used in fluorescence polarisation assays and time-resolved FIAs. These latter two assays require special measuring equipment: ordinary fluorimeters and fluorimeters that are capable of time-resolved counting for manual and semiautomatic operation, or fluorescence polarisation equipment that is usually used for fully automated immunoassays.

Fluorescent dye labels such as fluorescein isothiocyanate (FITC) have been used for quite some time now. Although it is theoretically possible to achieve great sensitivity in assays using fluorescent labels, there are some disadvantages. First, there is the problem of the natural fluorescence of substances that are contained in the samples to be measured. This results in high nonspecific fluorescence, which reduces the assay sensitivity. Fluorescent labels have the closest resemblance to radioactive labels since their activity can be measured directly, as in γ-counting, or after placing them in a special signal-amplifying solution, as in β-counting.

In recent years, a very promising alternative to organic fluorescent labels has been found, namely in the rare earth chelates. These compounds, when used with the time-resolved counting technique, can be used for very sensitive immunoassays. Typical representatives of these labels are the chelates of europium, terbium and samarium. Intrinsic to the rare earth chelates are a series of characteristics that are ideally suited to a fluorescent label: large Stokes shifts (Fig. 22.7) and narrow emission spectra; long-lasting fluorescence, which is ideal for the time-resolved technique (Fig. 22.8); and high specific activity. The sum of such characteristics results in minimal background fluorescence and in low limits of detection.

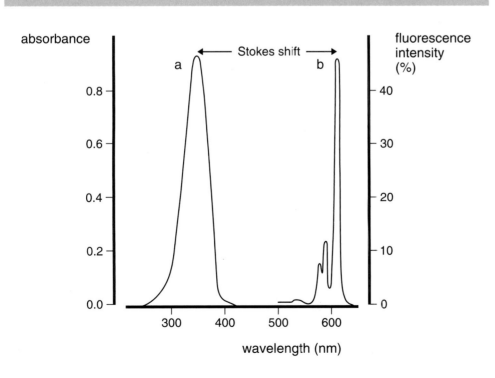

EXCITATION AND EMISSION SPECTRA

absorbance

fluorescence intensity (%)

Fig. 22.7 Excitation and emission spectra of europium chelates. The difference between the peak of the excitation wavelength (a) and the peak of the wavelength of the fluorescent emission (b) is known as Stokes shift. The large shift permits, in the measuring equipment, a clear-cut separation of the two wavelengths, leading to very low background, which is further reduced by the narrow emission peak.

CHEMOLUMINESCENT AND BIOLUMINESCENT LABELS

Another type of nonisotopic immunoassay involves the use of chemoluminescent and bioluminescent labels. By analogy to the EIAs, the activity of these labels can only be measured with a light-developing reaction, which follows the immunological reaction. The emission of photons in the chemoluminescent step is a very rapid process and involves the light-developing reaction taking place in the measuring equipment.

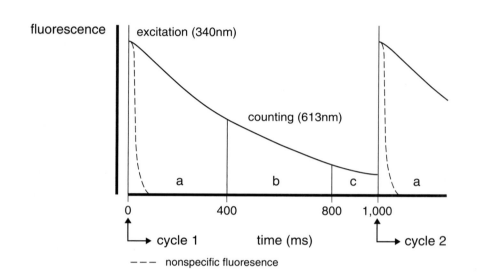

TIME-RESOLVED COUNTING

Fig. 22.8 The principle of time-resolved counting. Each counting cycle in the time-resolved fluorimeter has the duration of 1ms. After excitation of the sample, nonspecific fluorescence of short duration, originating from the assay tube material, is emitted. During this period of time (a), the fluorescence detector is not measuring. The detector is then activated for a short period of time and the specific fluorescence is measured (b). The detector is again deactivated and the system prepared for a new counting cycle (c). One sample measurement has the duration of 1s, or 1,000 cycles.

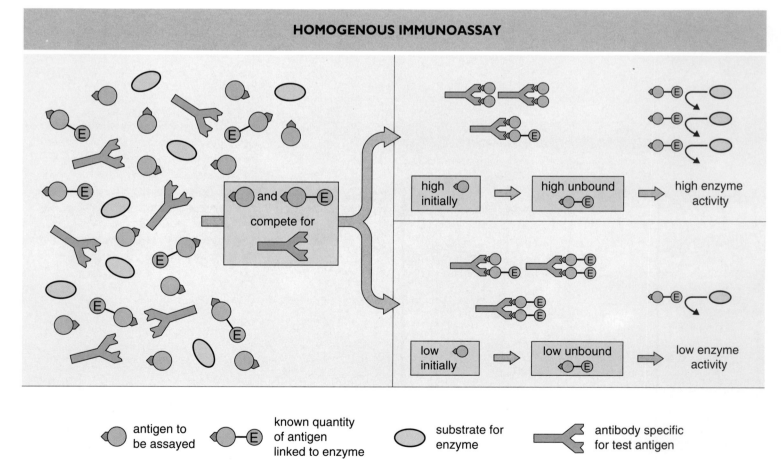

HOMOGENOUS IMMUNOASSAY

Fig. 22.9 A homogenous immunoassay. The reaction mixture contains the antigen to be measured, the specific antibody, the enzyme–antigen conjugate, and the substrate for the enzyme. When the antibody binds to the enzyme–antigen conjugate, the substrate cannot react with the enzyme. The enzymatic activity is directly proportional to the concentration of the antigen.

Several compounds have been used as luminescent labels, the most common being luminol and its derivatives, enzymes such as firefly luciferase and alkaline phosphatase, and a variety of acridinium esters. The acridinium esters characteristically have good stability and specific activity, giving them low detection limits. The light that is produced by acridinium esters is easily measured and generated by a simple chemical reaction. Future development of immunoassays using luminescent labels will concentrate on the preparation of new substrates that are capable of generating more and longer-lasting light.

THE ASSAY

SEPARATION OF BOUND AND FREE

Assays are referred to as homogenous or heterogenous, according to whether the measurement of the endpoint of the assay can be carried out directly or after separation of the antigen–antibody complex from the nonreacted assay components; however, the vast majority of immunoassays are of the heterogenous type.

Homogenous Assays

The homogenous assays are usually EIAs of the enzyme-multiplied immunoassay technique (EMIT) type. Their principle consists in either the blocking or enhancing of the activity of the enzyme that is used as a label (Fig. 22.9). The formation of the antigen–antibody complex can result in hindrance of the substrate–enzyme reaction. Homogenous assays are somewhat easier to perform and can easily be automated. They are, however, less sensitive than conventional immunoassays that require separation and can therefore be used for measuring substances of low molecular weight and which are present in the sample in relatively high concentrations, such as T_4.

Heterogenous Assays

The heterogenous assay technique involves separation of bound and free reactants after the immunological reaction has taken place. The separation can be in liquid or solid phase.

In the liquid-phase separation procedure, a precipitating agent, usually a second antibody that is directed against the hormone-binding antibody, is used. The precipitate thus formed is separated by centrifugation.

Less time-consuming and easier to perform is the solid-phase separation. With this technique, either the antibody or the antigen is fixed on a solid support; this support can be the wall of the reaction vessel or a solid particle. The solid-phase separation technique is the most widely used.

REACTION TYPES

According to the reaction type and whether the antigen or the antibody is coupled to the label, immunoassays can be classed as two main types: competitive assays and immunometric assays (Fig. 22.10).

Competitive Assays

Competitive immunoassays are based on the competition between the antigen in the sample and the labelled antigen for the antibody binding sites (Fig. 22.11).

During the immunological reaction, the antigen to be measured and the labelled antigen are incubated with a specific antibody that can be either in liquid form or coupled to a solid phase. The antibody is present in limited amount so that only a part of the antigen, both labelled and unlabelled, can be bound. The distribution of the bound antigens reflects their relative concentrations in the assay. The separation step eliminates all nonreacted components. According to the label used, the activity of the bound fraction is directly measured

Fig. 22.10 Characteristics of immunoassay methods. Sensitivity and specificity of an immunoassay are dependent on the methodology and the type of antibody used.

CHARACTERISTICS OF IMMUNOASSAY METHODS

method	sensitivity (g)	specificity
competitive RIA/EIA/FIA	10^{-9}–10^{-12}	average polyclonal antibodies
immunoradiometric assay enzyme-linked immunospecific assay	10^{-12}	good monoclonal antibodies
immunometric LIA immunometric time-resolved FIA	10^{-12}–10^{-15}	good monoclonal antibodies

(RIA, FIA) or a further reagent is added for development of colour or light (EIA, chemoluminescent assay). By plotting the concentration of the standards against their measured response, a standard curve can be constructed. In the competitive assay, the response is inversely related to the concentration of the antigen in the sample (Fig. 22.12).

COMPETITIVE IMMUNOASSAY

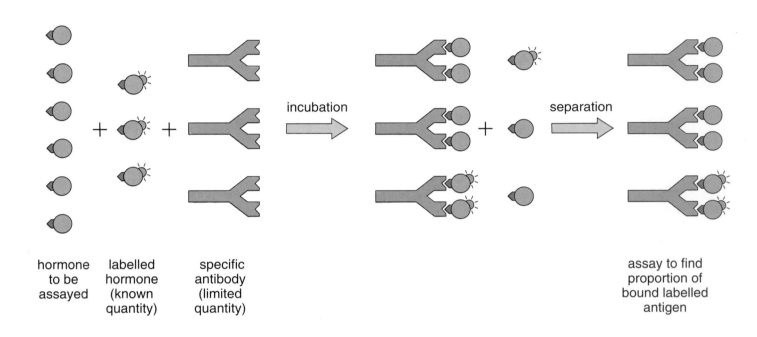

| hormone to be assayed | labelled hormone (known quantity) | specific antibody (limited quantity) | | | assay to find proportion of bound labelled antigen |

Fig. 22.11 The principle of the competitive immunoassay. The hormone to be measured and the labelled hormone compete for the antibody that is present in limited amount.

Fig. 22.12 A dose–response curve for a RIA. The measured radioactivity of the antibody-bound label is plotted against the concentration of the standard samples.

DOSE–RESPONSE CURVE FOR A RIA

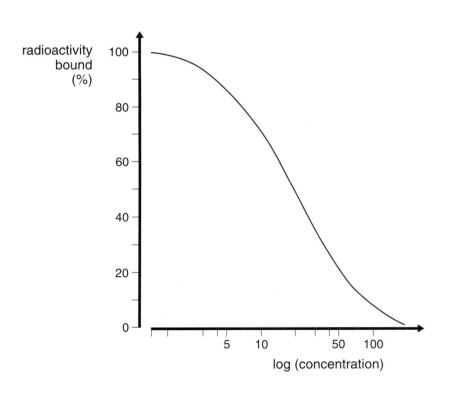

Polyclonal antibodies and labelled antigens are normally used for competitive assays. Furthermore, antigens with low molecular weight or low antigenicity are easier to measure with competitive assays.

Immunometric Assays

For the measurement of larger antigens with several different antibody binding sites, the immunometric or sandwich assay technique is more often used. In the former technique, the label is coupled to one of the antibodies (Fig. 22.13). This assay is a reagent excess assay and requires shorter incubation times than competitive assays. Two different monoclonal antibodies are used for this type of assay: one is fixed to a solid phase, usually the wall of the reaction vessel, while the other is coupled to the label. During the immunological reaction, the antigen binds the solid-phase antibody on one epitope and the labelled antibody on another. The so-formed 'sandwich' complex is then separated from nonreacted components. Measurement of the label activity is carried out in the same manner as in the competitive technique. In this instance, however, the concentration of the measured signal is directly proportional to the concentration of the antigen in the sample (Fig. 22.14).

STANDARD MATERIAL

The preparation of standard material that is suitable for use in immunoassays represents a complex problem, with many open questions still remaining. Since commercial immunoassay suppliers use secondary standard material from various sources, the direct comparison of results obtained in different laboratories remains difficult. The problem is particularly true for protein hormones, where the structure and sequence are not always completely known. The standard preparations that are obtained by extraction from biological material

are quite heterogenous and of different purity. A certain degree of uniformity in results can be achieved by using, whenever possible, standard material supplied by agencies such as the National Institute for Biological Standards and Control (in the UK) and the National Institutes of Health (in the USA).

Fortunately, recent progress in the field of molecular biology has made the preparation of recombinant material for some hormones (for example insulin and growth hormone) possible. It can be foreseen that such recombinant material, available in sufficient quantities, will also be used as standards in immunoassays.

Another point of concern is the medium in which standards are prepared. The ideal diluent is hormone-free serum, but this is almost impossible to obtain in satisfactory quality. The extraction procedures that are used to prepare such materials also invariably modify the natural characteristics of the serum.

THE SAMPLE

Another important component of an immunoassay is the sample. The versatility of immunoassays permits the measurement of hormones in almost every biological fluid. Serum, plasma, urine, saliva, spinal or amniotic fluid, or even whole blood that has been dried on filter paper, are all sample materials that can be used in immunoassays.

The conditions under which a sample is drawn, however, can influence the results of the immunoassay to a great extent. Many hormones are secreted in pulsatile manner and/or with a circadian rhythm; others are influenced by factors such as stress or food intake. Thus, correct interpretation of laboratory results is highly dependent on sampling time and conditions: for example, blood sampling for the measurement of cortisol should always be carried out at a certain time of day and under rested conditions.

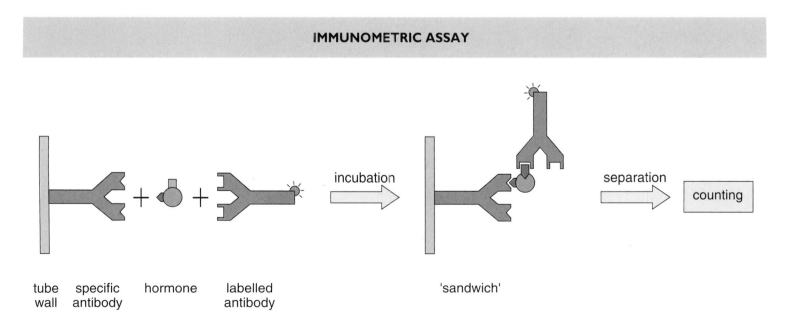

IMMUNOMETRIC ASSAY

tube wall | specific antibody | hormone | labelled antibody | incubation | 'sandwich' | separation | counting

Fig. 22.13 The principle of immunometric assay. The hormone to be measured reacts with two different antibodies, one of them labelled.

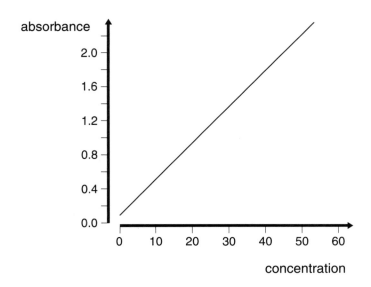

DOSE–RESPONSE CURVE FOR AN ENZYME-LINKED IMMUNOSPECIFIC ASSAY

Fig. 22.14 A dose–response curve for an enzyme-linked immunospecific assay. The colour absorption is plotted against the concentration of the standard samples.

When collecting plasma samples, the choice of anticoagulants can also affect the results by interfering with the immunological or the enzymatic reaction.

When assaying certain parameters, the temperature at which the sample is drawn and maintained is critical. For the measurement of adrenocorticotrophic hormone or antidiuretic hormone (arginine vasopressin), for example, the samples must be drawn in chilled tubes that are kept on ice, and the serum should be immediately separated at 4°C from the red blood cells and frozen. Furthermore, the addition of protease inhibitors is necessary in order to prevent degradation of the analyte.

Samples for immunoassay are usually stored at −20°C. These conditions are adequate for most analytes, provided it is not necessary to store the samples for more than six months – when a storage temperature of −70°C is advisable.

Similar care has to be taken when transporting or shipping samples to a laboratory. Although many analytes are fairly stable for up to forty-eight hours at room temperature, the transfer time between the place of sampling and the laboratory should be kept as short as possible. If it becomes necessary to transport a sample over a long distance, packaging of serum or plasma in insulated containers with dry ice is desirable.

23

Radiology of Endocrine Disease

Janet E Dacie, FRCP, DMRD, FRCR

F Elizabeth White, MRCP, DMRD, FRCR

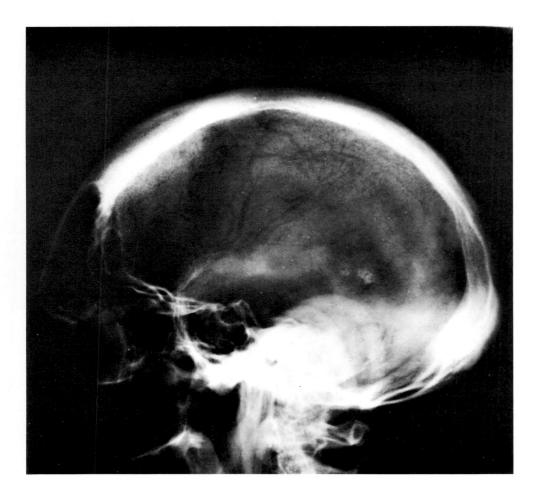

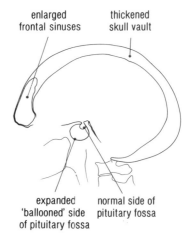

Fig. 23.1 Acromegaly: lateral skull film showing vault changes and a 'ballooned' pituitary fossa. The main role of radiology in the assessment of acromegaly is to confirm the presence of a pituitary tumour and to provide information necessary for treatment and follow-up. (See Chapter 24 for a discussion of pituitary tumours.) Certain characteristic systemic changes do, however, occur in acromegaly and this lateral skull film demonstrates typical diffuse hyperostosis of the calvarium and abnormally large frontal sinuses. A double floor to the pituitary fossa can be seen. One side is of normal calibre and the other is grossly expanded i.e. 'ballooned'. (See Fig. 23.3 for details.)

enlarged frontal sinuses

thickened skull vault

expanded 'ballooned' side of pituitary fossa

normal side of pituitary fossa

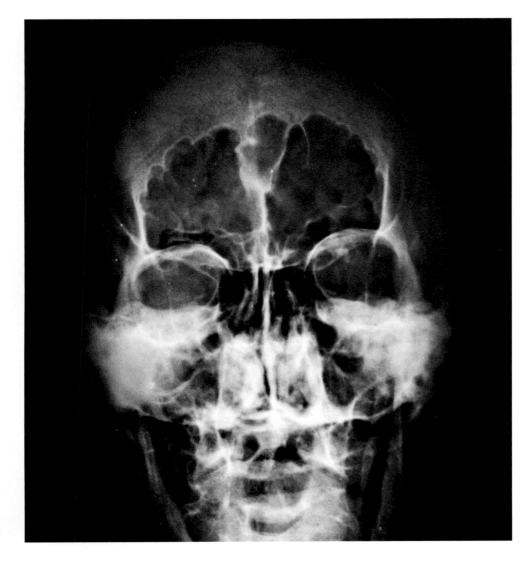

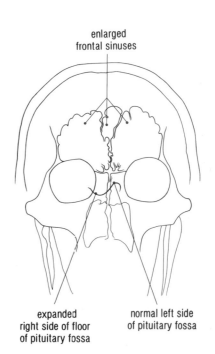

Fig. 23.2 Acromegaly: postero-anterior (PA) skull film showing enlarged frontal sinuses. This PA skull film of the same patient as in Fig. 23.1 demonstrates the marked enlargement of the frontal sinuses. The floor of the pituitary fossa is seen to be grossly enlarged on the right side by a large but asymmetric pituitary tumour.

enlarged frontal sinuses

expanded right side of floor of pituitary fossa

normal left side of pituitary fossa

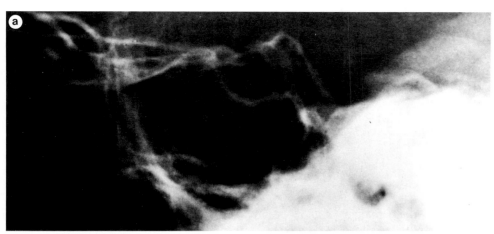

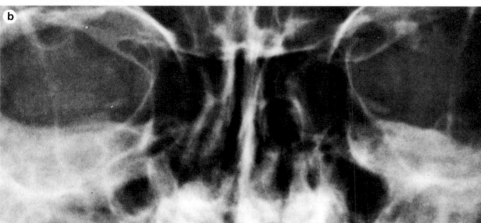

Fig. 23.3 Acromegaly: coned views of 'ballooned' pituitary fossa. These coned lateral (a) and PA (b) views of the pituitary fossa are of the same patient as in Figs. 23.1 and 23.2. They demonstrate more clearly the gross asymmetric expansion of the right side of the floor of the pituitary fossa.

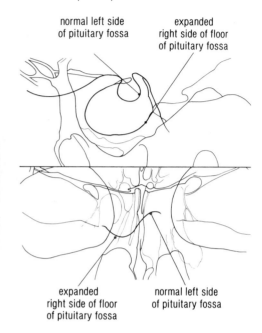

Fig. 23.4 Acromegaly: prognathic jaw. The lateral skull film of another patient shows characteristic prognathism with increase in the normal angle of the mandible. The pituitary fossa is grossly enlarged and the skull vault is markedly thickened, particularly anteriorly, although in this patient the frontal sinuses are not enlarged.

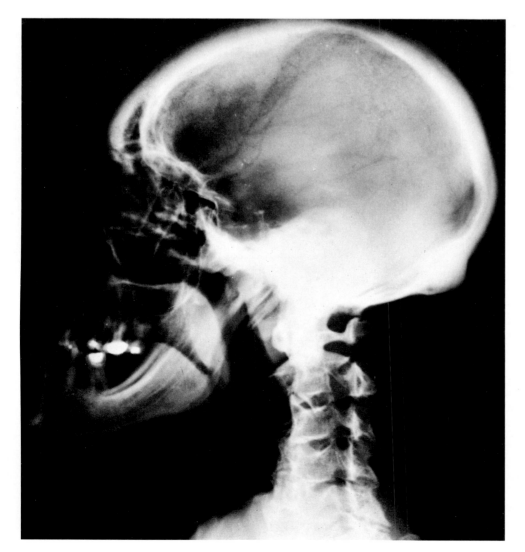

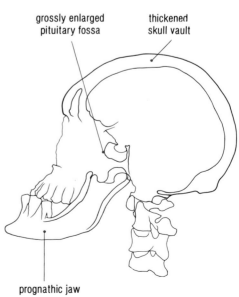

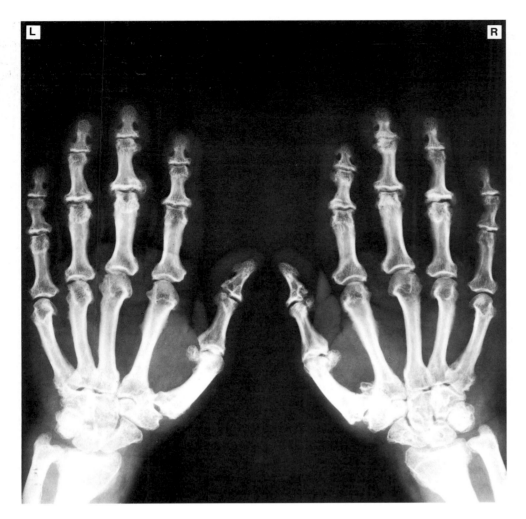

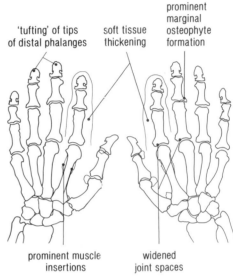

Fig. 23.5 Acromegaly: hands. In acromegaly the hands are large and the classical radiological features include generalised soft tissue thickening, widening of the joint spaces due to hypertrophy of the articular cartilages, prominent muscle insertions particularly along the metacarpal shafts, tufting of the tips of the terminal phalanges and prominent osteophyte formation. In addition, in this patient, degenerative cysts are present in some of the carpal bones, particularly in the right carpus.

'tufting' of tips of distal phalanges   soft tissue thickening   prominent marginal osteophyte formation

prominent muscle insertions   widened joint spaces

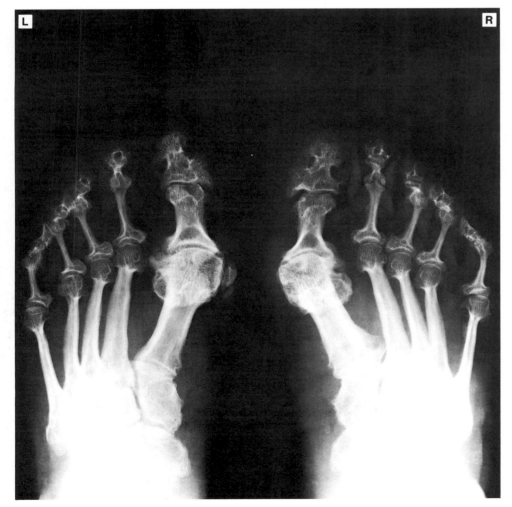

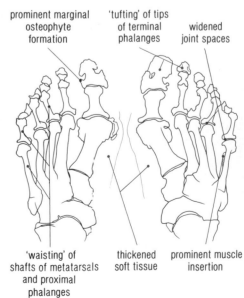

Fig. 23.6 Acromegaly: feet. The radiological changes in the hands in acromegaly are also seen in the feet but, in addition to new bone formation, bone resorption occurs giving rise to typically thinned metatarsals. Thinning of the shafts of the phalanges may also occur, as in this patient.

prominent marginal osteophyte formation   'tufting' of tips of terminal phalanges   widened joint spaces

'waisting' of shafts of metatarsals and proximal phalanges   thickened soft tissue   prominent muscle insertion

Fig. 23.7 Acromegaly: lateral dorsal spine. In acromegaly new bone formation may occur around the vertebral bodies. This lateral view of the dorsal spine shows such changes at the anterior margins of the vertebrae. The anterior edge of the intervertebral discs can be clearly identified and the vertebral bodies are increased in their anteroposterior diameter. The new bone formation is usually more marked in the dorsal than in the lumbar spine.

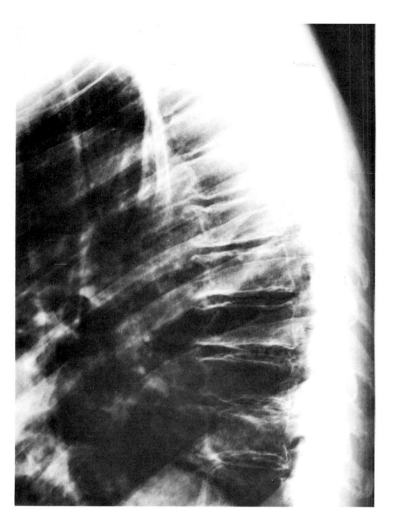

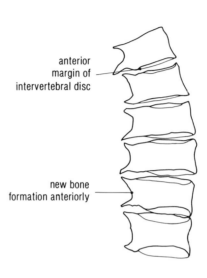

Fig. 23.8 Acromegaly: lateral lumbar spine. In addition to new bone formation anteriorly this lateral view of the lumbar spine shows prominent marginal osteophyte formation and characteristic scalloping of the posterior margins of the vertebral bodies. Although such scalloping may be seen in the dorsal spine, the lumbar spine is most commonly affected.

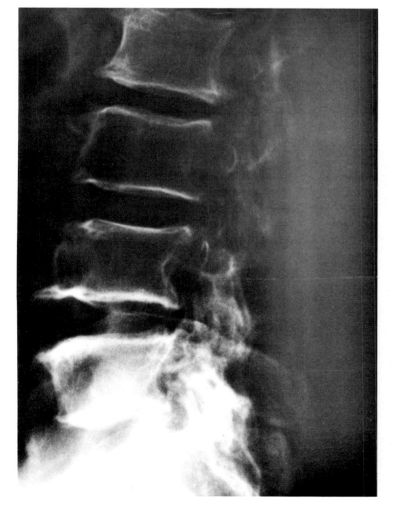

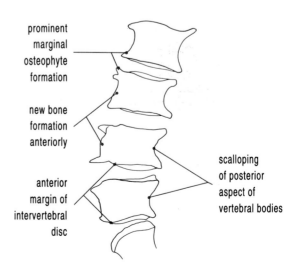

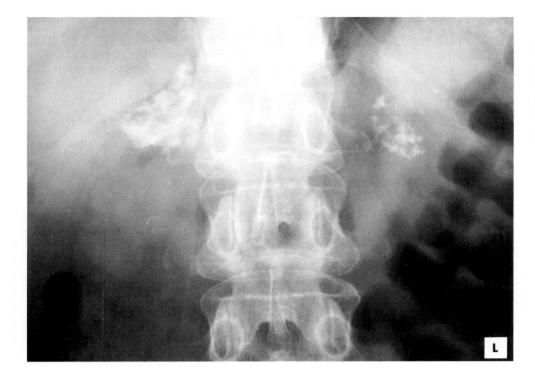

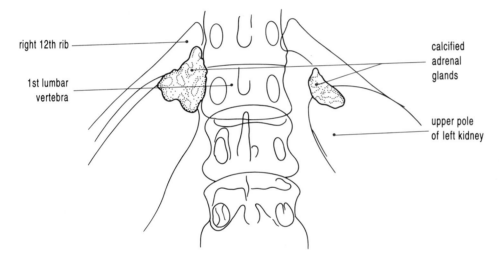

Fig. 23.9 Addison's disease: calcified adrenal glands. This coned anteroposterior (AP) film of the upper abdomen demonstrates calcified adrenal glands, seen in some patients with Addison's disease. An identical appearance, however, may be found incidentally in patients without evidence of adrenal disease (the so-called 'idiopathic' calcification of the adrenals).

right 12th rib

1st lumbar vertebra

calcified adrenal glands

upper pole of left kidney

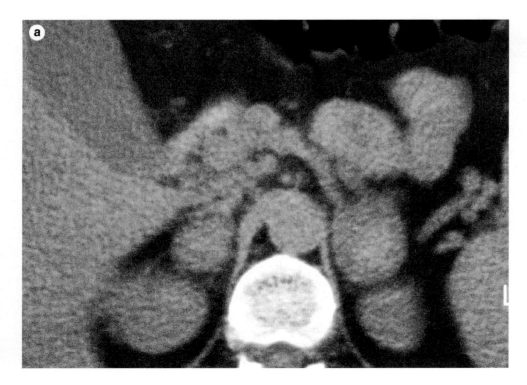

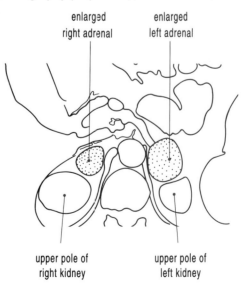

Fig. 23.10a Addison's disease: enlarged adrenal glands demonstrated by computed tomography (CT). See opposite for description.

enlarged right adrenal

enlarged left adrenal

upper pole of right kidney

upper pole of left kidney

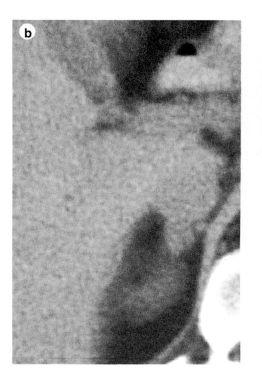

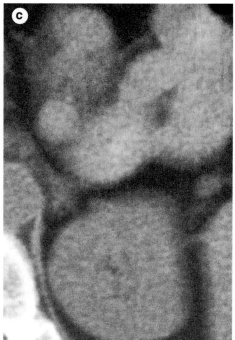

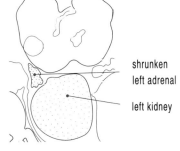

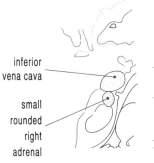
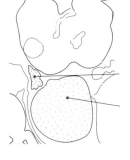

inferior
vena cava

small
rounded
right
adrenal

shrunken
left adrenal

left kidney

*Fig. 23.10 (cont) **Addison's disease: enlarged adrenal glands demonstrated by computed tomography (CT).*** The CT scan (a) shows bilateral adrenal enlargement in a patient taking anticoagulant therapy who presented with the features of acute adrenal insufficiency. The adrenals show increased density compared with the soft tissues indicating recent haemorrhage. The follow-up scan seven months later, shows shrinkage of both the right (b) and left (c) adrenal glands, which have lost their normal contour.

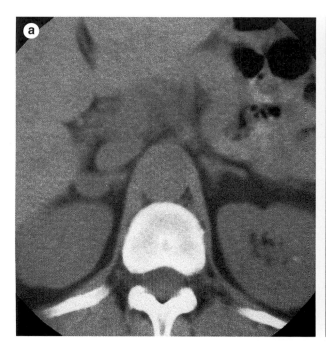

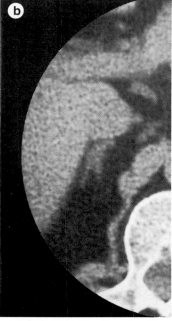

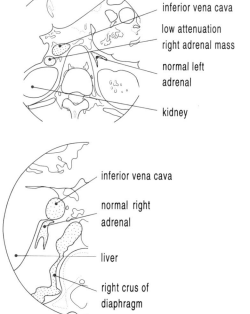

inferior vena cava

low attenuation
right adrenal mass

normal left
adrenal

kidney

inferior vena cava

normal right
adrenal

liver

right crus of
diaphragm

*Fig. 23.11 **Conn's syndrome: right adrenal adenoma demonstrated by CT (with normal adrenal glands for comparison).*** Conn's syndrome is caused by either adrenal hyperplasia or an adrenal tumour, the majority of which are small adenomas. Scan (a) shows a 1cm tumour in the right adrenal gland, lying between the inferior vena cava (IVC) and the right kidney, and a normal left adrenal gland. The tumour is of low attenuation when compared with the soft tissues. This feature is often seen in Conn's

tumours. Venous sampling to measure aldosterone levels may be required to confirm the CT findings and may detect tumours too small to be visualised on CT. Significantly elevated aldosterone levels from both adrenal glands usually indicates bilateral hyperplasia. Scan (b) shows a normal right adrenal gland for comparison. The short adrenal body is situated immediately posterior to the IVC. It divides into two parallel limbs which lie between the liver and the right crus of the diaphragm.

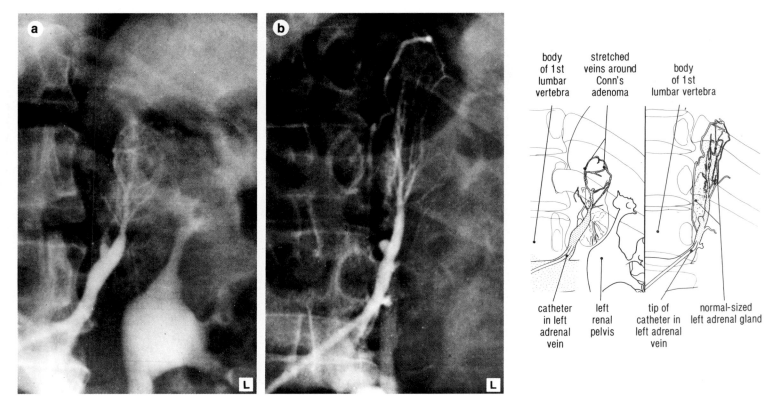

Fig. 23.12 Conn's adenoma in the left adrenal gland: demonstrated by venography (with normal venogram for comparison). Film (a) shows the typical venographic appearance of a Conn's adenoma. The catheter tip is in the left adrenal vein and contrast medium has filled veins stretched around a 1cm tumour in the superior pole of the adrenal gland. This appearance should be compared with that of a normal left adrenal venogram (b). Blood for aldosterone estimation should be taken from the adrenal vein prior to venography because of the risk of extravasation of contrast medium during that procedure. Even careful venography carries a small risk of adrenal infarction which could result in adrenal insufficiency if both adrenal glands are compromised. Adrenal venography alone is rarely carried out today, except to identify the catheter position during venous sampling.

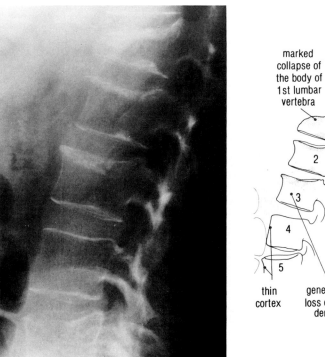

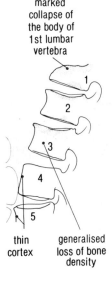

Fig. 23.13 Cushing's syndrome: osteoporosis and vertebral fractures. Cushing's syndrome, when severe, results in generalised osteoporosis and this lateral film of the lumbar spine shows the typical appearance. The bone density is reduced and the cortical margins of the bones are thin. There is marked collapse of the body of the first lumbar vertebra, with marginal condensation of the superior borders of the bodies of the second and third. In the dorsal spine multiple vertebral fractures may lead to a pronounced kyphosis. It should be noted that the radiological appearances of osteoporosis affecting the spine are similar whatever the cause.

Fig. 23.14 Cushing's syndrome: rib fracture. Spontaneous asymptomatic rib fractures are characteristic of Cushing's syndrome and this coned view shows the typical appearance. Multiple rib fractures are surrounded by excessive callus formation. In some patients, in addition to obvious rib fractures, characteristic widening of the anterior ends of the ribs resulting from numerous stress infractions may be seen.

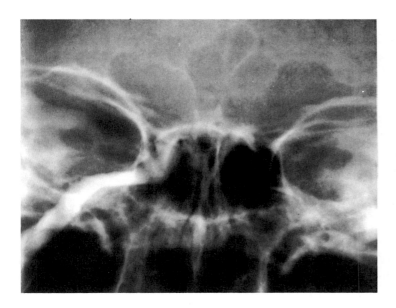

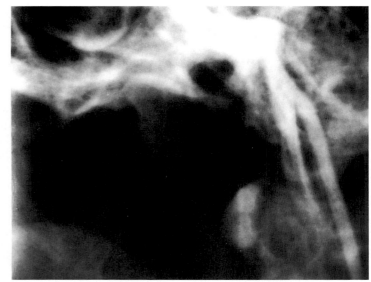

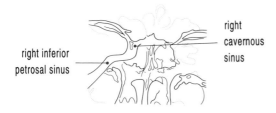

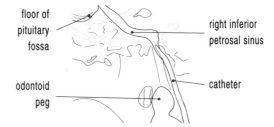

Fig. 23.15 Cushing's syndrome: inferior petrosal sinus venography (PA and lateral) to confirm catheter position prior to venous sampling. Percutaneous catheterisation of one inferior petrosal sinus, or if possible both simultaneously, is useful in the investigation of ACTH-dependent Cushing's syndrome. The finding of a 2:1 gradient in ACTH levels in venous samples from the inferior petrosal sinus(es) compared with peripheral blood suggests that the syndrome is likely to be of pituitary origin

but is only seen in 50 per cent of cases. However, if 100μg corticotrophin releasing hormone, CRH₄₁, is given intravenously, a rise in ACTH levels in the petrosal sinuses of over twice the basal value establishes a diagnosis of pituitary dependent Cushing's disease in 80 per cent of cases and may lateralise a microadenoma to one side of the fossa. Venous sampling from other sites may help to locate an ectopic source of ACTH production (see chapter 8).

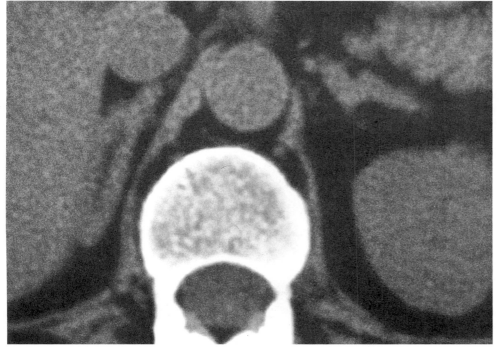

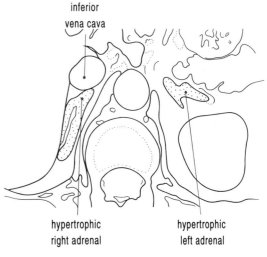

Fig. 23.16 Cushing's syndrome: hypertrophy of the adrenal glands demonstrated by CT. Most cases of Cushing's syndrome are caused by increased ACTH production by the pituitary gland. The remainder are due either to an ectopic ACTH-producing tumour or to a primary adrenal tumour (adenoma or carcinoma). Increasing ACTH levels result in adrenal

hyperplasia with accompanying hypertrophy. Small changes in size cannot be detected by CT and the adrenals may therefore appear normal. More marked hypertrophy can be shown as thickening of the limbs of the gland with convexity of the margins. The normal configuration is, however, retained. (Compare with the CT appearance of normal adrenals Fig. 23.11.)

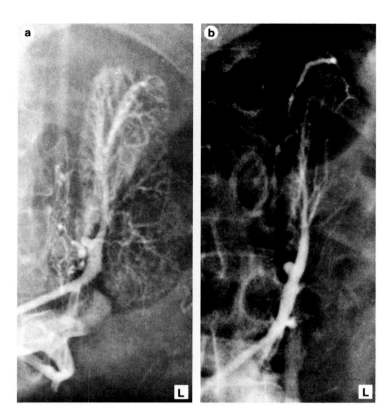

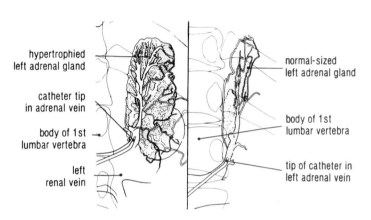

Fig. 23.17 Cushing's syndrome: hypertrophied left adrenal gland demonstrated by venography (with normal venogram for comparison). Film (a) was obtained prior to venous sampling and shows the venographic appearances of one of a pair of hypertrophied adrenal glands. The tip of the catheter is in the left adrenal vein and contrast medium has filled small veins within the enlarged gland. A segment of the left renal vein has been partially outlined. The appearances should be compared with those of a normal-sized left adrenal gland (b).

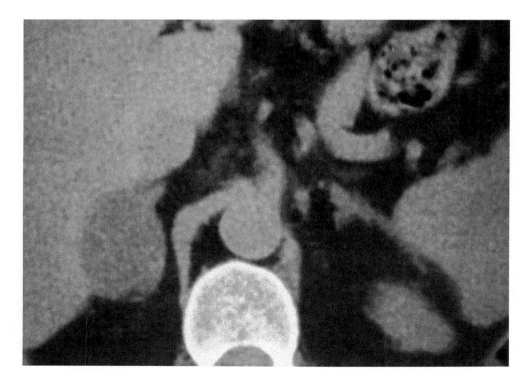

Fig. 23.18 Cushing's syndrome: right adrenal adenoma demonstrated by CT. Adrenal adenomas causing Cushing's syndrome are usually 2–5cm in size. They are readily detected by CT because of the contrast provided by the abundant retroperitoneal fat which is present in most patients. This scan shows a 3.5cm rounded mass in the right adrenal gland. It lies immediately behind the IVC and between the liver and the right crus of the diaphragm.

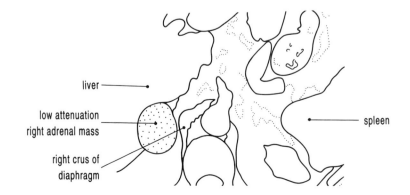

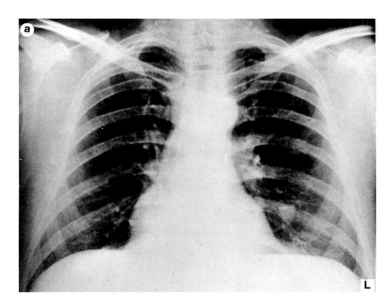

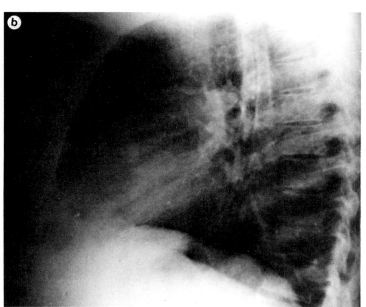

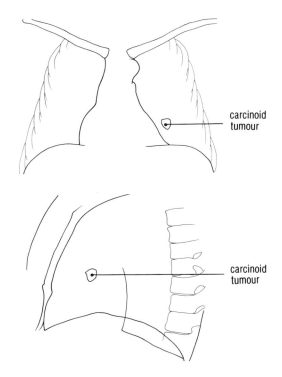

Fig. 23.19 Cushing's syndrome: ectopic ACTH production by a carcinoid tumour of the lung. Cushing's syndrome sometimes results from ectopic ACTH production by tumours, particularly of the lung, thymus or pancreas. Such tumours may be very difficult to locate. Although a few may be detected by conventional radiographic techniques, others require CT scanning or venous sampling for their identification, and some are never found. The PA chest film (a) shows a small mass in the left lower zone. There is some generalised loss of bone density and the patient appears fat. On the lateral view (b) the mass is shown to lie in the lingular segment of the left upper lobe. The patient had Cushing's syndrome secondary to ectopic ACTH production by a benign bronchial carcinoid tumour of the lung.

carcinoid tumour

carcinoid tumour

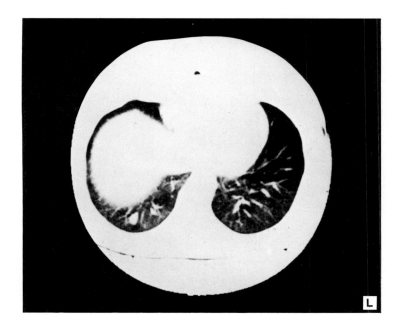

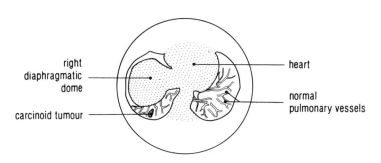

Fig. 23.20 Cushing's syndrome: ACTH-secreting carcinoid tumour of the lung demonstrated by CT. The 7mm nodule in the right costophrenic recess represents a small malignant carcinoid tumour secreting ACTH. It could not be seen on either chest radiography or conventional tomography. Removal of the tumour cured the patient. Reproduced by courtesy of the British Medical Journal.

right diaphragmatic dome

heart

carcinoid tumour

normal pulmonary vessels

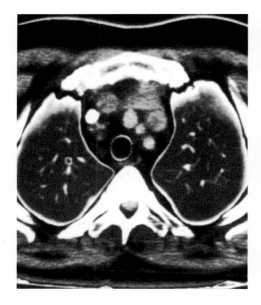
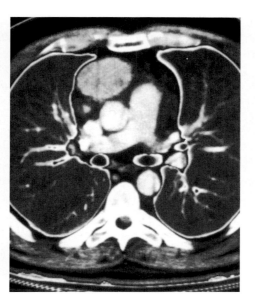

Fig. 23.21 Cushing's syndrome: malignant thymic ACTH-secreting carcinoid tumour demonstrated by CT. Ectopic ACTH can be produced by carcinoid tumours of the thymus. These enhanced CT scans show in the right picture a 4cm ACTH-producing tumour lying just in front of the ascending aorta. The tumour has enhanced slightly with contrast medium but not as markedly as the vascular structures. The left scan shows enlarged anterior mediastinal lymph nodes at a higher level.

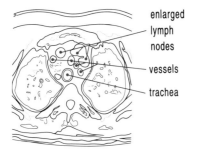

enlarged
lymph
nodes

vessels

trachea

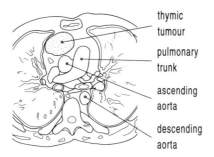

thymic
tumour

pulmonary
trunk

ascending
aorta

descending
aorta

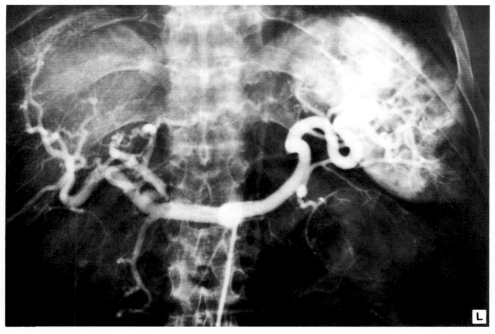

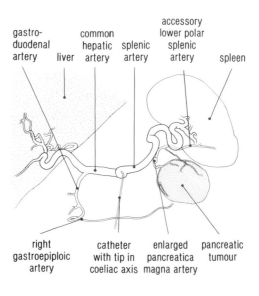

gastro-
duodenal
artery

liver

common
hepatic
artery

splenic
artery

accessory
lower polar
splenic
artery

spleen

right
gastroepiploic
artery

catheter
with tip in
coeliac axis

enlarged
pancreatica
magna artery

pancreatic
tumour

Fig. 23.22 Cushing's syndrome: ectopic ACTH production by an islet cell tumour of the pancreas demonstrated by angiography. This picture shows the arterial phase of a coeliac axis arteriogram. The procedure was carried out to define the blood supply of a pancreatic tumour which had been previously demonstrated by CT. The pancreatica magna artery is enlarged and its branches are stretched over the surface of a large pancreatic tumour. The splenic vein was shown to be patent on later films. At operation a large tumour of the pancreas was removed. Histological examination showed an islet cell tumour which was thought to be malignant. The tumour contained ACTH and the patient was cured of his Cushing's syndrome upon its removal.

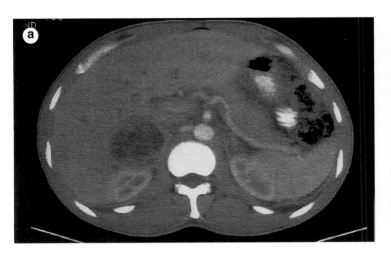

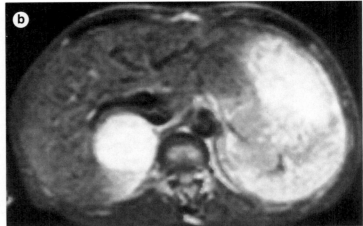

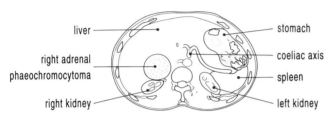

liver — stomach
right adrenal phaeochromocytoma — coeliac axis
right kidney — spleen
— left kidney

liver — stomach
right adrenal phaeochromocytoma —
— spleen

Fig. 23.23 Adrenal phaeochromocytoma: right adrenal tumour demonstrated by CT and MRI. Most adrenal phaeochromocytomas can be detected by CT because they are usually 3cm or more in size. The enhanced CT scan (a) shows an inhomogeneous, predominantly low density 5cm mass replacing the right adrenal gland. Small tumours may show uniform contrast enhancement. Larger tumours often show areas of low density due to tumour necrosis, as in this case. Magnetic resonance imaging (MRI) can also demonstrate adrenal masses well. Phaeochromocytomas show most clearly on MRI in the T2-weighted images as a mass with high signal, as in scan (b).

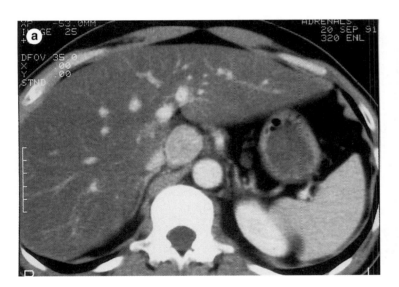

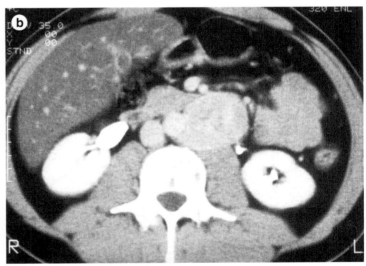

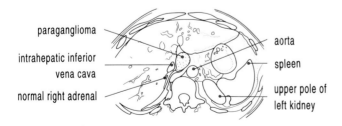

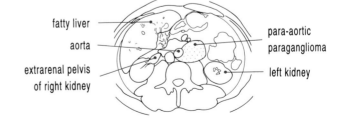

paraganglioma — aorta
intrahepatic inferior vena cava — spleen
normal right adrenal — upper pole of left kidney

fatty liver — para-aortic paraganglioma
aorta —
extrarenal pelvis of right kidney — left kidney

Fig. 23.24 Para-aortic paragangliomas demonstrated by CT. If an adrenal tumour is not shown on CT in a patient with strong clinical evidence of a phaeochromocytoma, it is likely that the tumour lies at an ectopic site along the sympathetic chain. The majority of such paragangliomas occur in the para-aortic region or around the renal hilum, and may be visible on CT. Scan (a) shows a small tumour lying anterior to and separate from the right adrenal. A second larger tumour is present to the left of the aorta at the level of the kidneys (b). Both were confimed as benign paragangliomas at surgery. To detect tumours at other ectopic sites or those too small to be seen on CT, ^{123}I meta-iodobenzylguanidine (MIBG) radionuclide scanning (see Chapter 25 Figs. 25.16 & 25.19) or venous sampling for catecholamine levels is required.

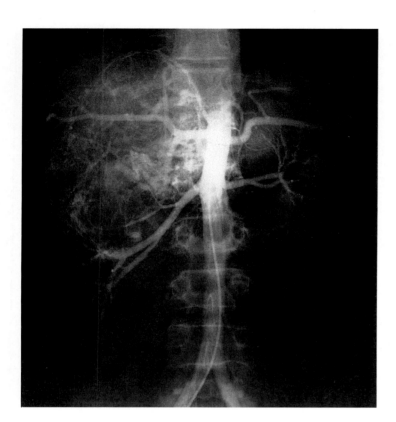

Fig. 23.25 Adrenal phaeochromocytoma: large vascular tumour demonstrated by arteriography. Arteriography has now been largely superseded by CT, MIBG scanning and venous sampling for the detection of phaeochromocytomas. The procedure is hazardous unless adequate medical α- and β-adrenergic blockade has been given and should be undertaken only if really essential. In this patient angiography was carried out to determine the arterial supply and venous drainage of the known tumour prior to surgery. Arteriography still has a place in identifying an ectopic phaeochromocytoma when its approximate location has been shown by venous sampling or MIBG scanning, and CT examination is negative.

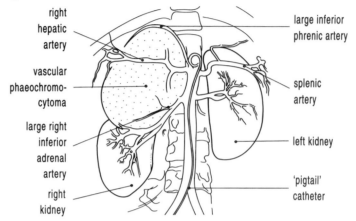

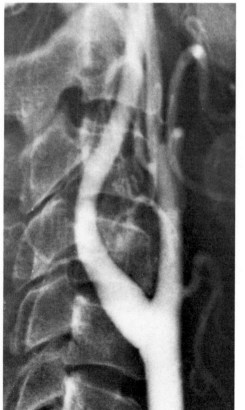

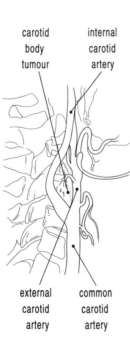

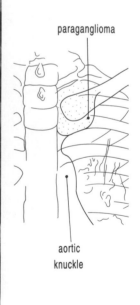

Fig. 23.26 Carotid body tumour: demonstration by angiography.
This patient with persistent hypertension after the removal of a left adrenal phaeochromocytoma had elevated levels of catecholamines in the right side of the neck on venous sampling. Subsequent carotid arteriography demonstrated a typical carotid body tumour. On this lateral film the carotid bifurcation is seen to be splayed by the tumour which lies between the origins of the internal and external carotid arteries. The blood supply of the tumour arises from the proximal external carotid artery and a tumour blush is present.

Fig. 23.27 Malignant paraganglioma in the left upper chest.
This coned view shows a mass with a well-defined margin lying in the left upper paravertebral region. The patient complained of occaisional headaches and sweating but was normotensive. At operation, however, the blood pressure rose steeply while the tumour was being handled. Histological examination showed a paraganglioma which was originally thought to be benign. Seven years later, however, the tumour recurred in the chest and metastatic paraganglioma was found on biopsy of a skull lesion. The patient is still alive, seventeen years after initial presentation, after treatment with 131IMIBG (see Chapter 25).

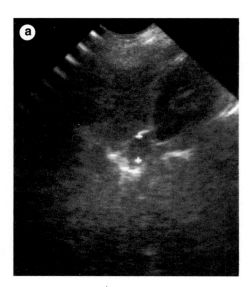
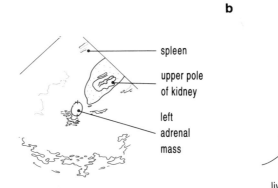
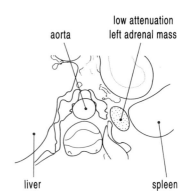

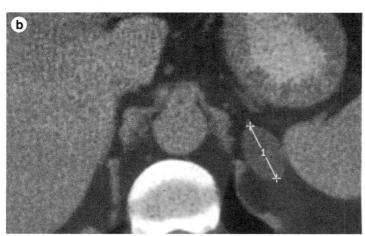

Fig. 23.28 Nonfunctional left adrenal tumour: ultrasound and CT scans. This 2cm mass was an incidental finding on ultrasonography (a). CT (b) confirmed that the mass was of adrenal origin and also showed that it had a relatively low attenuation suggestive of adrenocortical origin. In this situation, a biochemical screen is indicated to determine whether or not there is evidence of endocrine disease. If this is normal a follow-up scan should be done to exclude an increase in size, indicative of malignancy. Nonfunctional adrenal masses are quite frequently found on CT and surgery is unwarranted in most cases.

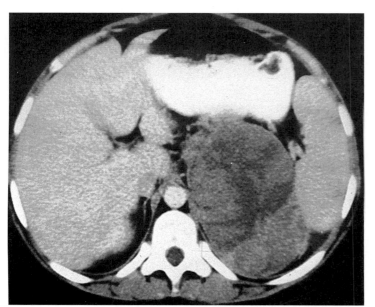
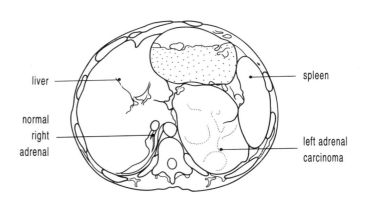

Fig. 23.29 Adrenal carcinoma: CT scan. This 10cm left adrenal mass shows the characteristic CT appearances of an adrenal carcinoma. Adrenal carcinomas usually measure 6cm or more at the time of presentation and show inhomogeneous enhancement following the injection of intravenous contrast medium. Enlarged lymph nodes or metastatic spread elsewhere may also be shown. This patient had a pulmonary metastasis on chest X-ray.

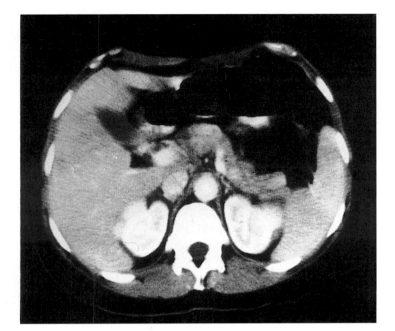

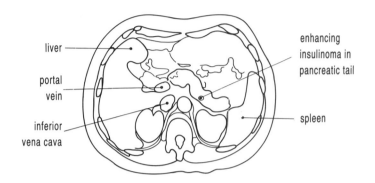

Fig. 23.30 Insulinoma: demonstrated by contrast-enhanced CT.
These islet cell tumours of the pancreas are often less than 1.5cm in diameter, are multiple in 10 per cent of cases and are occasionally malignant. Their demonstration by CT requires a meticulous technique, using thin contiguous sections and rapid sequence scanning after a bolus of contrast medium. Even small insulinomas can be detected by CT because of their intense enhancement, as seen in this scar.

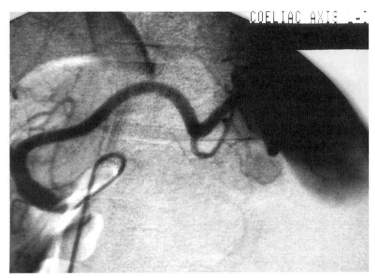

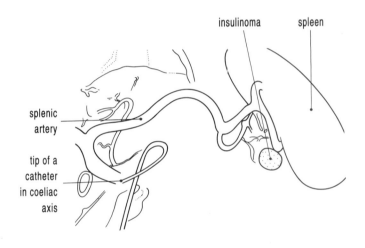

Fig. 23.31 Insulinoma: demonstrated by intra-arterial digital subtraction angiography (DSA). Selective or superselective arterial catheterisation is required together with gas distension of the stomach and paralysis of the bowel. Multiple projections may be necessary, as in this patient where the small insulinoma in the tail of the pancreas (confirmed

surgically) was only clearly shown on DSA films obtained in the 45° left anterior oblique projection. Angiography may produce a false positive 'blush' from the gut or splenunculus and this problem can be resolved by combining angiography with CT, which will show whether the 'blush' is truly pancreatic (see Fig. 23.32).

Fig. 23.32 Insulinoma: demonstrated by CT angiography.
CT angiography is probably the most sensitive means of detecting small islet cell tumours pre-operatively. This CT scan was obtained immediately after the injection of contrast medium into the coeliac axis. It shows a small insulinoma in the tail of the pancreas, lying at the splenic hilum, which was not detected on the initial angiogram. Transhepatic venous sampling may be helpful in locating an insulinoma not detected by CT and/or angiography.

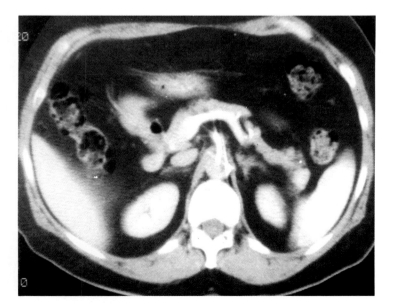

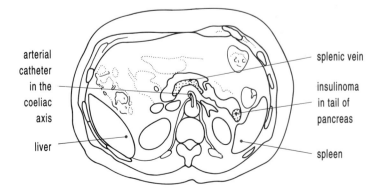

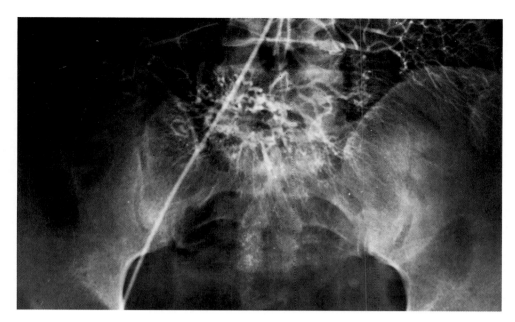

Fig. 23.33 Carcinoid tumour: characteristic angiographic appearance of mesenteric involvement. This film from the arterial phase of a superior mesenteric arteriogram demonstrates the typical angiographic appearance of a carcinoid tumour which has invaded the mesentery. Invasion results in thickening and foreshortening of the mesentery. The arteries become very tortuous and are drawn into a characteristic stellate pattern. Arterial narrowing distal to the tumour frequently occurs.

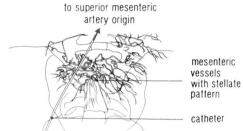

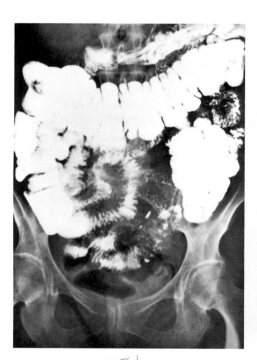

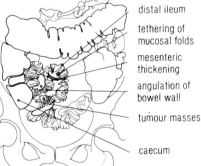

Fig. 23.34 Carcinoid tumour: distal ileal involvement. This 80 minute follow-through film shows an abnormal distal ileum with mesenteric thickening, nodular masses invading the bowel wall and angulation and tethering of mucosal folds. These appearances are characteristic of carcinoid tumour and reflect invasion by the tumour with an extensive fibroblastic response. Metastatic carcinoma to the mesentery can cause a similar appearance.

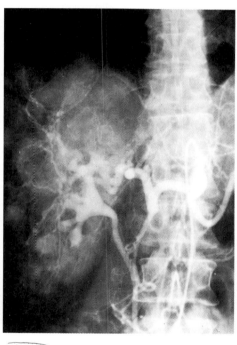

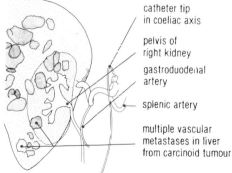

Fig. 23.35 Carcinoid tumour: hypervascular hepatic metastases.
Hepatic metastases from a carcinoid tumour are characteristically hypervascular and this film of the arterial phase of a coeliac axis arteriogram shows multiple tumour blushes throughout the liver. A similar appearance is produced by other hypervascular hepatic metastases such as those from a renal cell carcinoma.

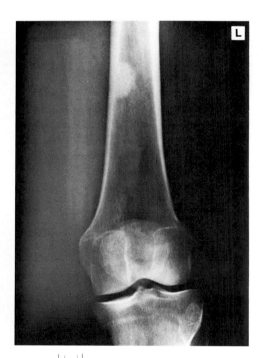

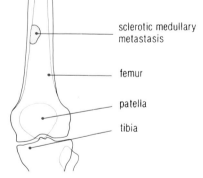

Fig. 23.36 Carcinoid tumour: sclerotic bony metastasis. Bony metastases from malignant carcinoid tumours are characteristically densely sclerotic. This AP film of the distal femur and knee shows the typical appearance of such an intramedullary lesion. The primary tumour was in the rectum. (Carcinoid tumour: ectopic ACTH production. See under Cushing's syndrome Figs. 23.19–23.21.)

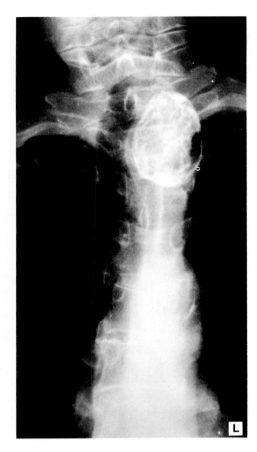
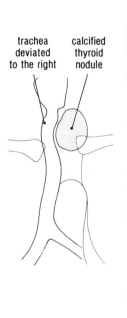

Fig. 23.37 Goitre: calcified thyroid nodule. This AP film of the thoracic inlet shows the typical appearance of a large calcified thyroid nodule which is slightly displacing the trachea to the right side. Most goitres, however, do not show calcification. Calcified goitres are usually benign but may be malignant.

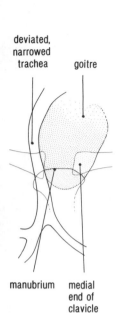

Fig. 23.38 Goitre: deviation and narrowing of the trachea. This AP view of the thoracic inlet shows marked displacement of the trachea to the right by a large left-sided goitre which extends inferiorly to just below the sternal notch. The trachea is slightly narrowed in its transverse diameter just above the level of the thoracic inlet. No calcification can be seen within the goitre. Although any displacement or narrowing of the trachea in the AP plane can be readily assessed on a lateral view of the thoracic inlet, it may be difficult to determine whether or not there is any significant extension of a cervical goitre into the mediastinum.

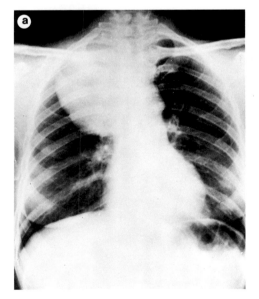
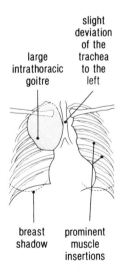

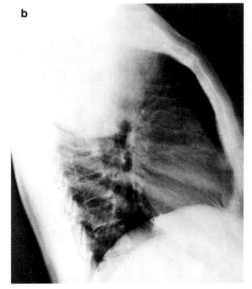
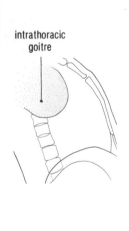

Fig. 23.39 Intrathoracic goitre in acromegaly. The PA chest film (a) shows a large mass in the right upper chest which is confluent with the mediastinum medially and has a well-defined lateral margin. The mass does not contain any obvious calcification and is only slightly displacing the trachea to the left. The right lateral view (b) shows a clearly defined mass lying posteriorly. The patient had presented with a goitre and had noticed some enlargement of the hands and feet. There were no symptoms of dysphagia or of thyrotoxicosis. The mass in the chest was subsequently shown on radionuclide and CT scans to be in continuity with the cervical goitre. The patient was also found to have a pituitary tumour and acromegaly. Prominent muscle insertions can be seen on the PA chest film at the lower borders of the ribs but no bony changes of acromegaly are present in the dorsal spine (see Fig. 23.7). At the combined surgical approach of cervical incision and a right posterolateral thoractomy, the large mass in the right side of the mediastinum was confirmed to be continuous with an enlarged right lobe of the thyroid gland and was removed. Histological examination showed that the mass was a large colloid goitre.

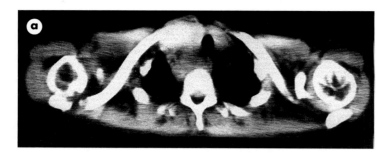

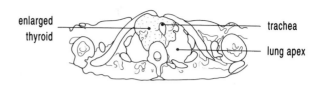

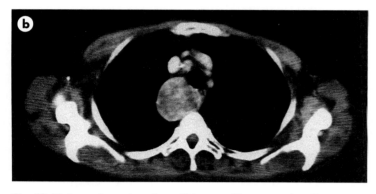

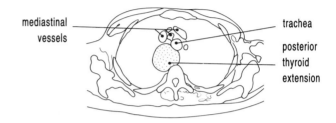

Fig. 23.40 Intrathoracic goitre: CT scans. These are of a different patient to Fig. 23.39. The higher scan (a) shows bilateral thyroid enlargement with narrowing and displacement of the trachea. The density of thyroid tissue on unenhanced CT is usually higher than that of other soft tissues because of the iodine content of the gland. This is not particularly obvious in this patient. The lower scan (b) shows extension of the right lobe into the posterior mediastinum with patchy enhancement following intravenous contrast.

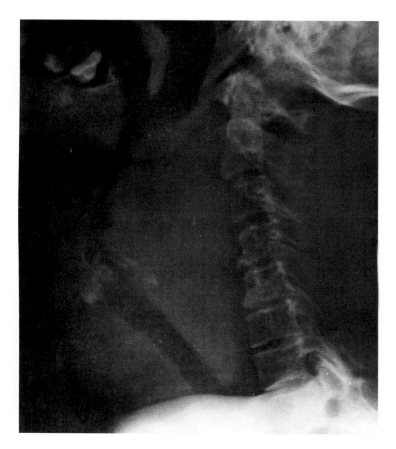

Fig. 23.41 Carcinoma of the thyroid: retrotracheal extension of tumour. This lateral view of the neck shows massive soft tissue swelling with marked anterior displacement of the trachea which is compressed in its anteroposterior diameter. The displacement is due to gross retrotracheal extension of the thyroid and is indicative of malignancy. This patient had an anaplastic carcinoma of the thyroid.

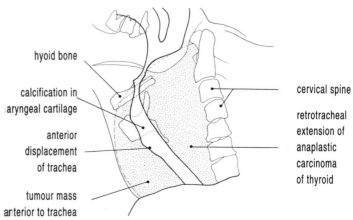

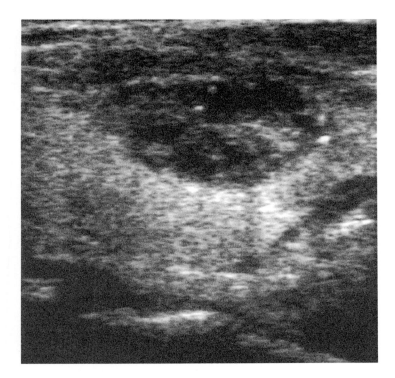

Fig. 23.42 Multinodular goitre: ultrasound scan. This longitudinal scan shows a large nodule containing specks of calcium which was 'cold' on radionuclide scanning (see Chapter 25, Fig. 25.6). Ultrasound revealed further nodules, consistent with a multinodular goitre. Fine needle aspiration confirmed the benign nature of the 'cold' nodule. In patients who appear to have a solitary thyroid nodule clinically, which is 'cold' on radionuclide scanning, neck ultrasound can be of value. It will show if the nodule is cystic or solid. Solitary solid thyroid lesions need further investigation because they may be malignant. The presence of unsuspected further nodules, however, usually indicates a multinodular goitre.

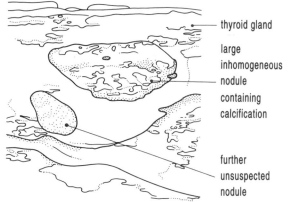

thyroid gland

large inhomogeneous nodule containing calcification

further unsuspected nodule

Fig. 23.43 Thyroid carcinoma: ultrasound scan. This transverse scan shows an irregular, hypoechoic mass in the left lobe of the thyroid in a patient with metastatic disease but no known primary. Ultrasound-guided fine needle aspiration yielded abnormal cells consistent with an anaplastic carcinoma.

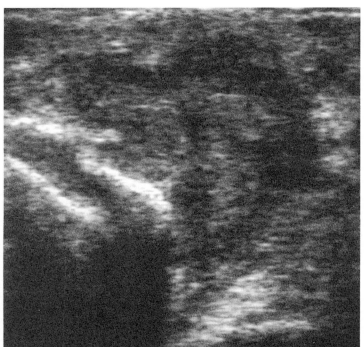

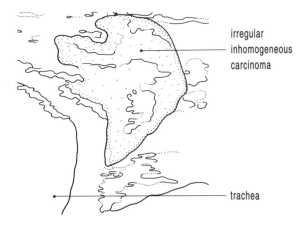

irregular inhomogeneous carcinoma

trachea

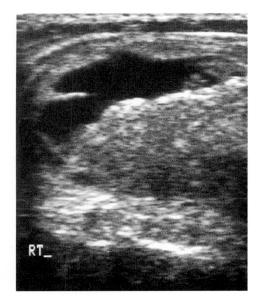

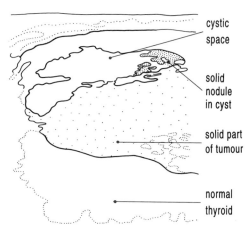

cystic space

solid nodule in cyst

solid part of tumour

normal thyroid

Fig. 23.44 Hürthle cell tumour: ultrasound scan. This transverse scan shows an unusual partly cystic mass in the right lobe of the thyroid in a patient with gradual thyroid enlargement over two years. Fine needle aspiration showed large numbers of Hürthle cells and surgery confirmed a Hürthle cell tumour.

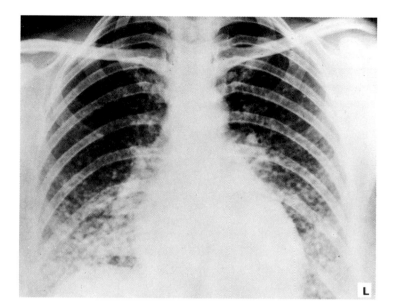

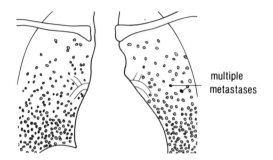

Fig. 23.45 Carcinoma of the thyroid: 'snow storm' appearance of pulmonary metastases. This PA chest film shows multiple small nodular opacities throughout both lungs, most marked at the bases, the characteristic 'snow storm' appearance of pulmonary metastases from carcinoma of the thyroid. Such metastatic deposits may remain unchanged over a long period of time due to a very low grade of malignancy and may take up and be treated with ^{131}I.

multiple metastases

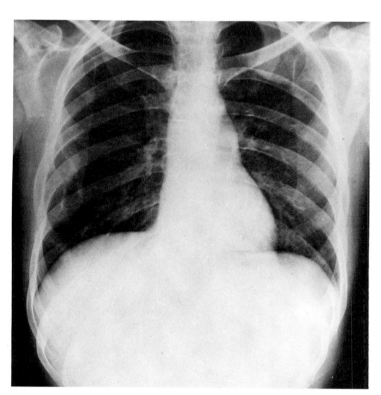

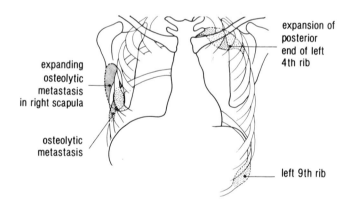

Fig. 23.46 Carcinoma of the thyroid: chest radiograph showing expanded bony metastases. This PA chest film shows multiple osteolytic bony metastases. Those involving the right scapula and the left fourth and ninth ribs show marked expansion of bone. Carcinoma of the thyroid characteristically gives rise to osteolytic metastases, sometimes accompanied by marked expansion of bone, as in this patient. The appearance is, however, not diagnostic because metastatic renal cell carcinoma, multiple myeloma, and occasionally metastatic carcinoma of the breast may also cause similar bone expansion. Such thyroid carcinoma metastases may, but do not necessarily, show up on routine radionuclide bone scanning.

expanding osteolytic metastasis in right scapula

osteolytic metastasis

expansion of posterior end of left 4th rib

left 9th rib

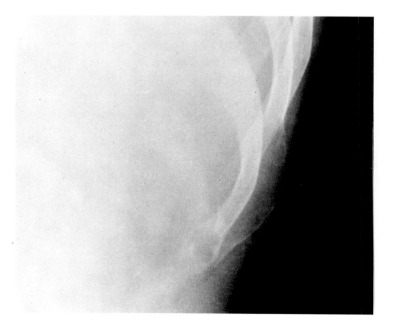

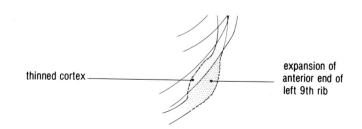

Fig. 23.47 Carcinoma of the thyroid: close-up view of an expanded rib metastasis. This coned view of the left ninth rib of the same patient as in Fig. 23.46 clearly shows the medullary destruction and expansion with thinning of the overlying cortex.

thinned cortex

expansion of anterior end of left 9th rib

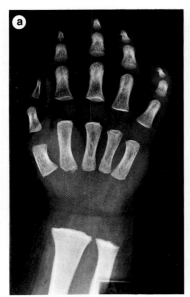
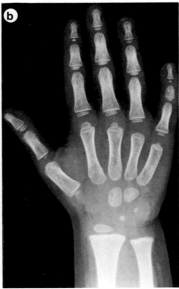

Fig. 23.48 Hypothyroidism in childhood: delay in skeletal maturation (with normal hand for comparison). This PA film (a) of the hand of a three-year-old hypothyroid boy demonstrates the characteristic retardation of skeletal growth. The bones of the hand are smaller than normal reflecting the generalised delay in growth that occurs and ossification has not yet started in any of the carpal bones or secondary epiphyses. Irregularity and increased density of the metaphyses occurs and, in this view, these changes are best seen in the distal radius and ulna. The appearances should be compared with those of the hand of a normal boy of similar age (b).

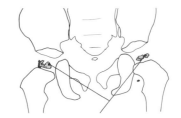

Fig. 23.49 Hypothyroidism in childhood: fragmentation of the femoral capital epiphyses. This AP view of the pelvis shows delay in ossification, with fragmentation and hypoplasia of the femoral capital epiphyses. Fragmentation of the ossification centres of the femoral heads might suggest the diagnosis of bilateral Perthes' disease; however, symmetrical involvement would be excessively rare in that condition.

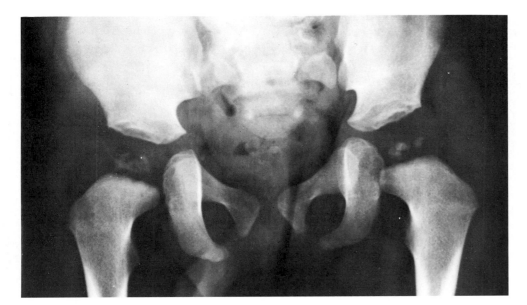

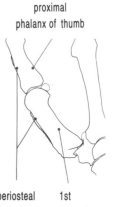

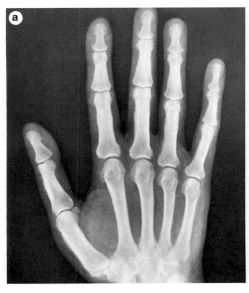
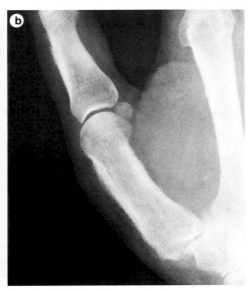

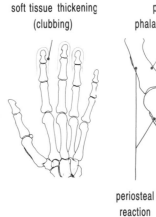

Fig. 23.50 Thyroid acropachy: hand radiograph showing periosteal reaction and clubbing. Thyroid acropachy occurs as part of Graves' disease and consists of clubbing of the fingers and toes, usually associated with exophthalmos and pretibial myxoedema. Bone changes are not necessarily part of the syndrome although they are frequently present. The PA film (a) of a hand shows the characteristic periosteal reaction of thyroid acropachy along the radial aspect of the shaft of the first metacarpal, the typical site. Soft tissue thickening is evident around some of the distal phalanges. The coned view (b) of the thumb and first metacarpal better demonstrates the characteristic lace-like appearance of the periosteal reaction. Besides the typical involvement of the first metacarpal, periosteal new bone formation may also occur along the shafts of other metacarpals and the proximal phalanges. In this patient a slight periosteal reaction is also present along the shaft of the proximal phalanx of the thumb.

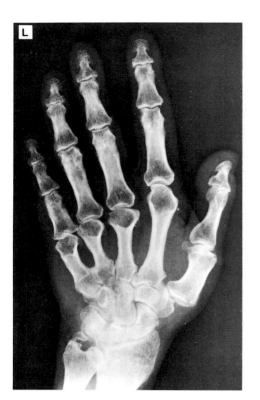
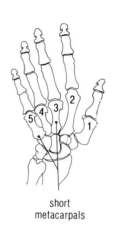

Fig. 23.51 *Pseudohypoparathyroidism: short metacarpals.*
This PA view of the hand shows short, rather broad metacarpals, an appearance seen in pseudohypoparathyroidism. In this patient, all the metacarpals except the second are rather short but the number involved may be variable.

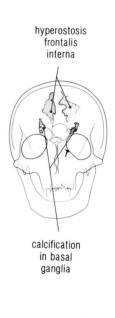

Fig. 23.52 *Pseudohypoparathyroidism: short metatarsals.*
This AP view of the foot shows a similar appearance to that of the hand, with shortening of the third and fourth metatarsals.

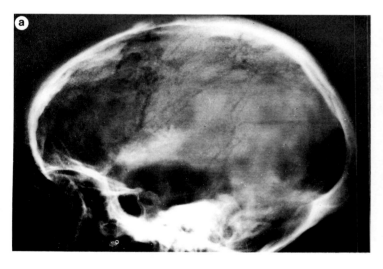
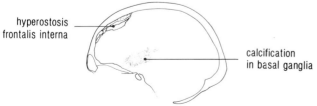
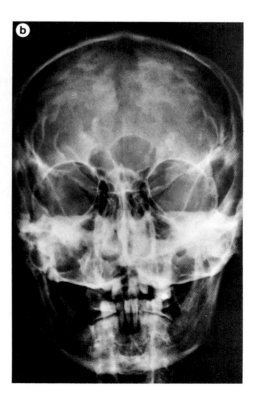

Fig. 23.53 *Pseudohypoparathyroidism: calcification in the basal ganglia.* In pseudohypoparathyroidism, heterotopic deposits of calcium phosphate occur in the soft tissues and most commonly affect the basal ganglia. The lateral (a) and PA (b) skull films show characteristic symmetrical punctate calcification in the basal ganglia. Similar calcification, however, also occurs in hypoparathyroidism. In this patient, slight hyperostosis frontalis interna is also present.

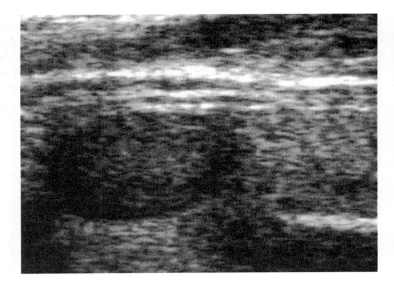

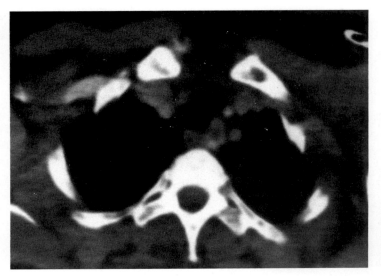

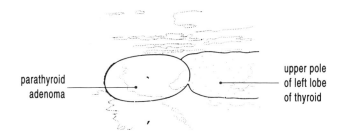

parathyroid
adenoma

upper pole
of left lobe
of thyroid

air in trachea

ectopic
parathyroid
adenoma

oesophagus

Fig. 23.54 Parathyroid adenoma: ultrasound scan. The vast majority of parathyroid adenomas are found on exploration of the neck, providing that the surgeon is experienced. Pre-operative ultrasonography can, however, be helpful, as in this patient where an enlarged parathyroid was demonstrated adjacent to the upper pole of the left lobe of the thyroid. The finding of a solitary enlarged parathyroid gland is likely to indicate an adenoma rather than parathyroid hyperplasia and is an aid to planning surgery. Intrathyroid parathyroid glands cannot be distinguished on ultrasonography from other thyroid nodules. (See also Chapter 25, Fig. 25.11.)

Fig. 23.55 Mediastinal parathyroid adenoma: CT scan. CT can be used to try to locate a parathyroid adenoma when neck exploration has failed to identify either a tumour or hyperplasia, or if hypercalcaemia recurs after surgery. This CT scan shows an ectopic parathyroid adenoma lying immediately to the left of the oesophagus. There is rim enhancement following the injection of intravenous contrast medium.

Fig. 23.56 Venous sampling for parathyroid hormone: inferior thyroid venogram. Venous sampling can be undertaken if CT has failed to locate an ectopic tumour. Samples should be taken from mediastinal as well as from thyroid veins. The right and left inferior thyroid veins may join to form a common trunk, as in this patient. The venous anatomy and pattern of drainage may have been altered by previous surgery and not all ectopic tumours will be located by this technique.

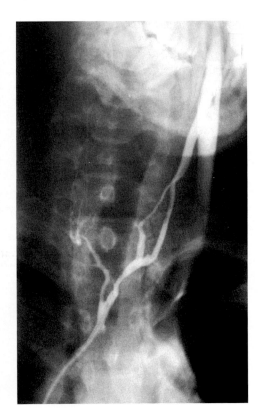

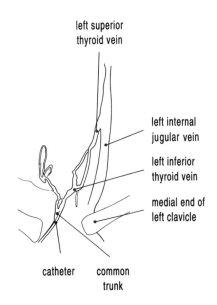

left superior
thyroid vein

left internal
jugular vein

left inferior
thyroid vein

medial end of
left clavicle

catheter   common
trunk

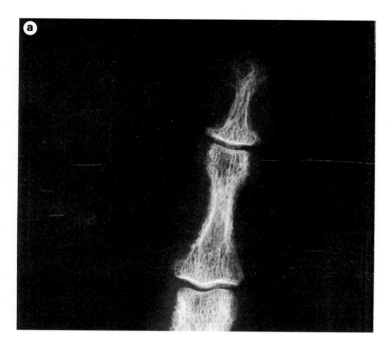

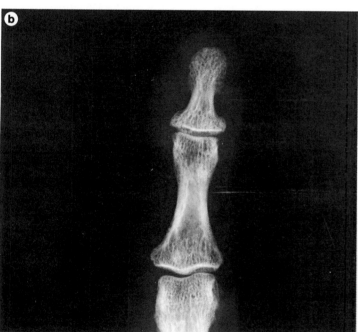

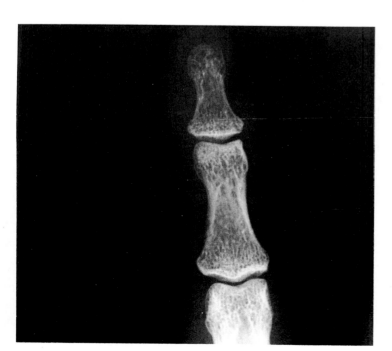

Fig. 23.57 Primary hyperparathyroidism: phalanges showing gross subperiosteal bone resorption (with appearance after healing for comparison). Bony changes are now evident radiologically in a minority of patients with primary hyperparathyroidism. Subperiosteal bone resorption is the earliest radiological sign and is specific for hyperparathyroidism. Generalised skeletal demineralisation is a late finding. The film (a) of the middle and distal phalanges of the index finger shows gross subperiosteal bone resorption of the shafts of the phalanges and also of the tip of the distal phalanx. The bone density is decreased and the texture of the cortex shows a 'basket-work' pattern with loss of definition of the normal corticomedullary junction. These appearances of gross hyperparathyroidism should be compared with those in (b) where healing had occurred following removal of a parathyroid adenoma. Although subperiosteal bone resorption classically involves the phalanges, it may also occur at many other sites. These include the outer ends and under-surface of the clavicles, the metaphyseal regions of the growing ends of the long bones, the ischial tuberosities, the pubic bones at the symphysis, the sacroiliac joints and the inner wall of the dorsum sellae.

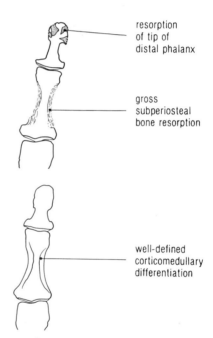

resorption
of tip of
distal phalanx

gross
subperiosteal
bone resorption

well-defined
corticomedullary
differentiation

Fig. 23.58 Primary hyperparathyroidism: magnification film of the index finger showing early subperiosteal bone resorption. This magnified film of the middle and distal phalanges of the index finger shows the early bony changes of hyperparathyroidism. Slight subperiosteal bone resorption is present along the radial aspect of the middle phalanx, the characteristic site for early change. There is also poor definition of the cortical outline of the tip of the distal phalanx, The technique of magnification radiography using a fine-focus X-ray tube is helpful in identifying these subtle appearances.

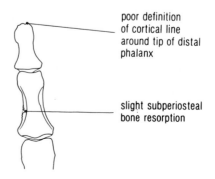

poor definition
of cortical line
around tip of distal
phalanx

slight subperiosteal
bone resorption

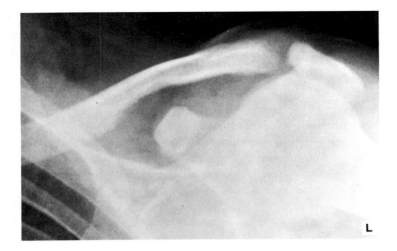

Fig. 23.59   Primary hyperparathyroidism: erosion of the outer end of the clavicle. This coned AP view of the lateral half of the left clavicle shows subperiosteal bone resorption of the outer end of the clavicle with slight widening of the acromioclavicular joint. There is also erosion of the under surface of the clavicle above the coracoid process of the scapula.

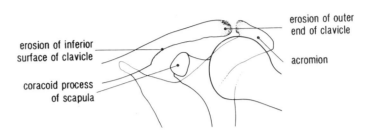

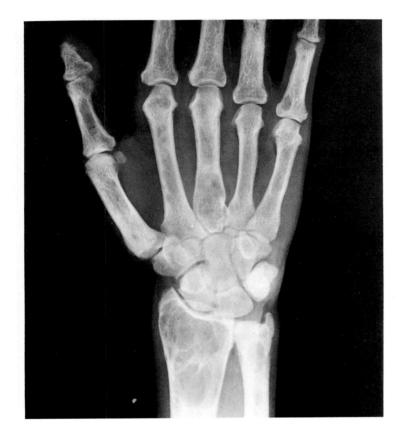

Fig. 23.60   Primary hyperparathyroidism: brown tumours. Brown tumours sometimes occur in primary hyperparathyroidism but are relatively uncommon in secondary hyperparathyroidism. This PA film of the wrist shows the typical appearance of brown tumours. Osteolucent bony defects are present in the distal radius and ulna, the base of the third metacarpal and the proximal phalanx of the little finger. The bone density is generally decreased. After parathyroidectomy brown tumours fill slowly with new bone from the periphery. Incomplete healing results in an appearance which may closely resemble that of fibrous dysplasia.

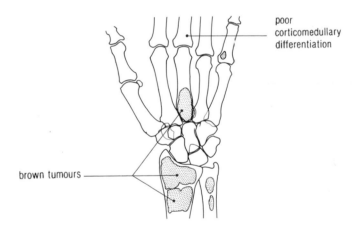

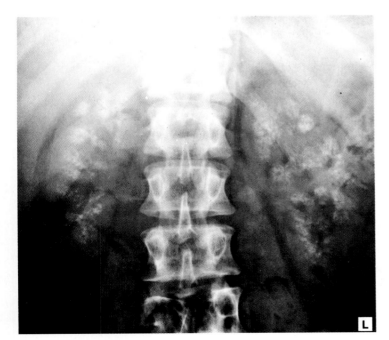

Fig. 23.61   Primary hyperparathyroidism: nephrocalcinosis and a brown tumour. Although pathologically about 60 per cent of patients with primary hyperparathyroidism have renal calculi or nephrocalcinosis, the radiological demonstration of such abnormalities is far less common. This coned abdominal film shows extensive nephrocalcinosis of the fine type seen in primary hyperparathyroidism. Generalised loss of bone density is present and a brown tumour has resulted in the partial collapse of the body of the fourth lumbar vertebra.

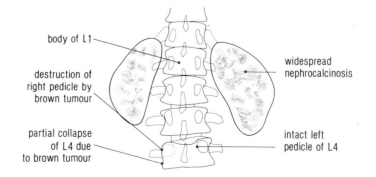

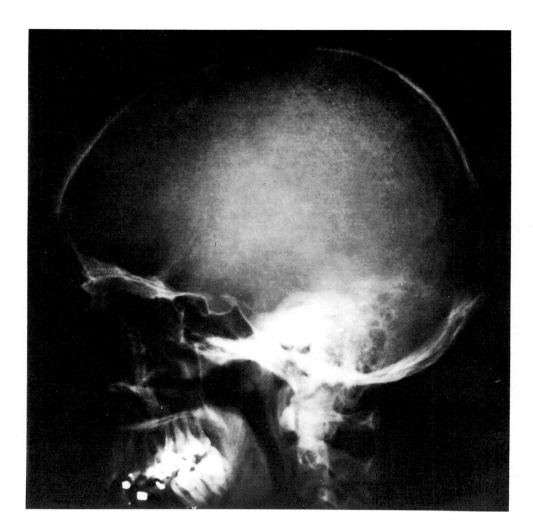

Fig. 23.62 Primary hyperparathyroidism: 'pepper pot' skull. This lateral film shows the classical changes in the skull vault of primary hyperparathyroidism. Generalised skeletal demineralisation is reflected by diffuse porotic mottling of the calvarium giving a granular or 'pepper pot' appearance. The vascular grooves are poorly defined and there is absence of the lamina dura of the teeth. The latter appearance is, however, not specific because it may occur in other dimineralising disorders such as osteoporosis and osteomalacia. In some patients with primary hyperparathyroidism the dorsum sellae may be eroded and in those with polyglandular adenomatosis and an associated pituitary tumour there may be enlargement of the pituitary fossa.

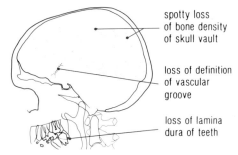

spotty loss of bone density of skull vault

loss of definition of vascular groove

loss of lamina dura of teeth

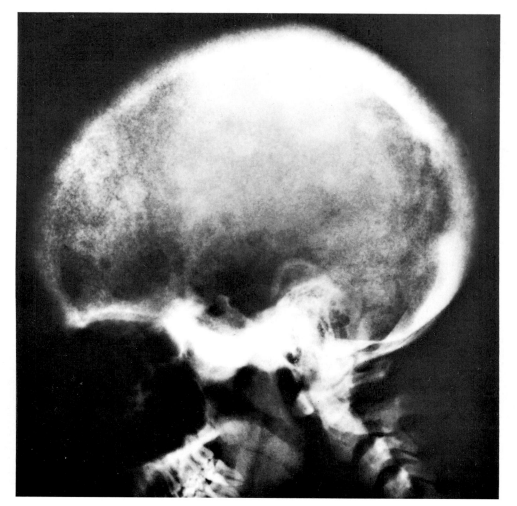

Fig. 23.63 Renal osteodystrophy: skull changes. The radiological appearances of renal osteodystrophy consist of areas of both demineralisation and sclerosis. These changes are thought to be due to a combination of osteomalacia, secondary hyperparathyroidsm and a calcitonin effect. This lateral film of the skull of a 17-year-old girl with chronic renal failure shows marked calvarial thickening with considerable mottling. Sometimes such change may resemble Paget's disease. The skull base and the cervical spine are dense and there is loss of the lamina dura of the teeth.

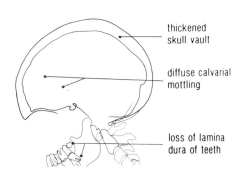

thickened skull vault

diffuse calvarial mottling

loss of lamina dura of teeth

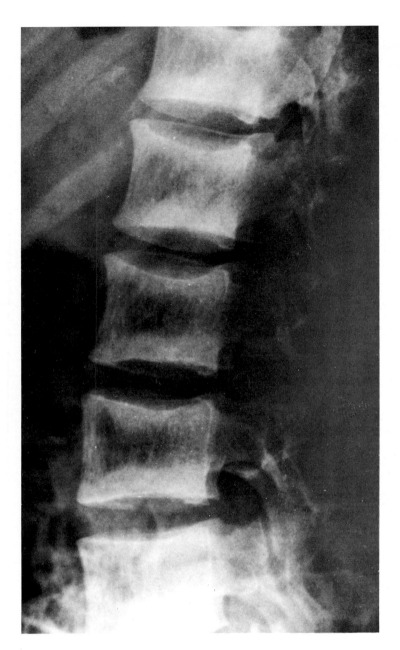

Fig. 23.64 Renal osteodystrophy: 'rugger jersey' spine. This lateral film of the lumbar spine shows central demineralisation and linear bands of subarticular density at the superior and inferior margins of the vertebral bodies – the classical appearance of a 'rugger jersey' spine.

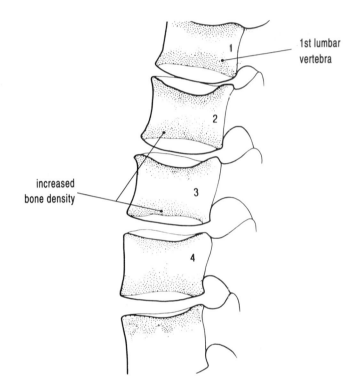

Fig. 23.65 Renal rickets: characteristic radiological appearance of the shoulder. This AP view of the right shoulder of a 16-year-old boy with chronic renal failure shows marked widening of the epiphyseal plate of the humerus with irregularity and splaying of the metaphysis, characteristic features of rickets. Subperiosteal erosion of the outer end of the clavicle and of the acromion with widening of the acromioclavicular joint indicate secondary hyperparathyroidism. The bone density is generally decreased and the humeral shaft in particular demonstrates thinning of the cortex and poor definition of the corticomedullary junction. The bone age is delayed.

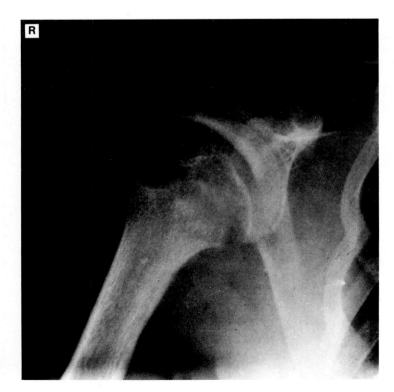

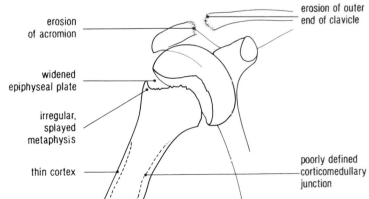

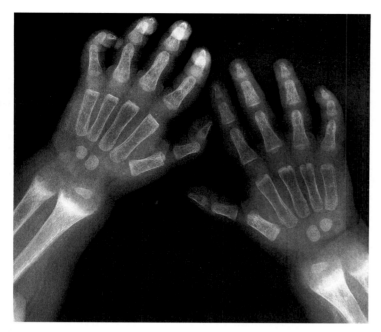

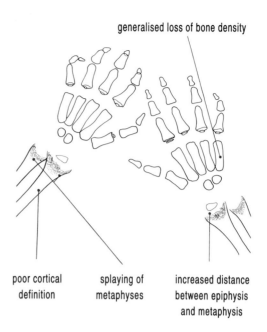

generalised loss of bone density

poor cortical definition   splaying of metaphyses   increased distance between epiphysis and metaphysis

Fig. 23.66 Nutritional rickets: characteristic radiological appearance of the hands. Rickets is the term used when inadequate osteoid mineralisation affects the growing skeleton. This PA film of the hands of a two-year-old boy illustrates the characteristic appearance of nutritional rickets. Gross demineralisation of the bones is present and ossification of the secondary epiphyseal centres is delayed. Wide bands of translucency in the metaphyses and irregularity of the metaphyseal margins are characteristic. The distal radial metaphyses are cupped or splayed due to the effects of weight bearing (i.e. crawling) on the weakened bones.

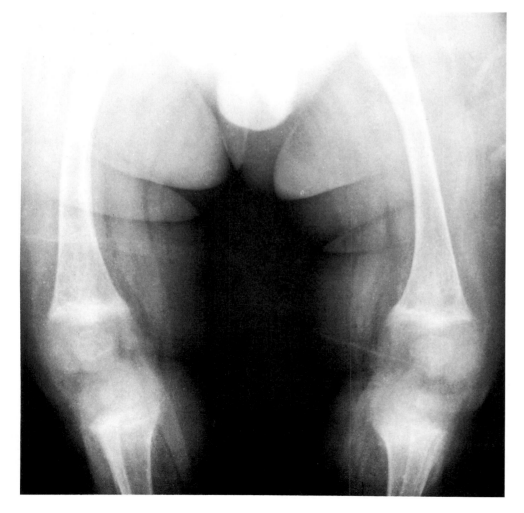

Fig. 23.67 Nutritional rickets: bowing of the femora and genu vara. Gross demineralisation of the bones is seen in this AP film of the femora and knees of the same child as in Fig. 23.66. Bowing of the femora and genu vara result from the effects of weight bearing on the weakened bones. The film also shows typical splaying and irregularity of the metaphyses and poorly ossified epiphyseal centres.

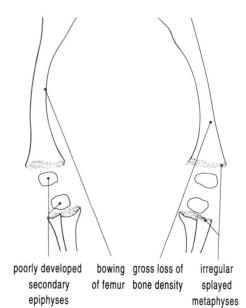

poorly developed secondary epiphyses   bowing of femur   gross loss of bone density   irregular splayed metaphyses

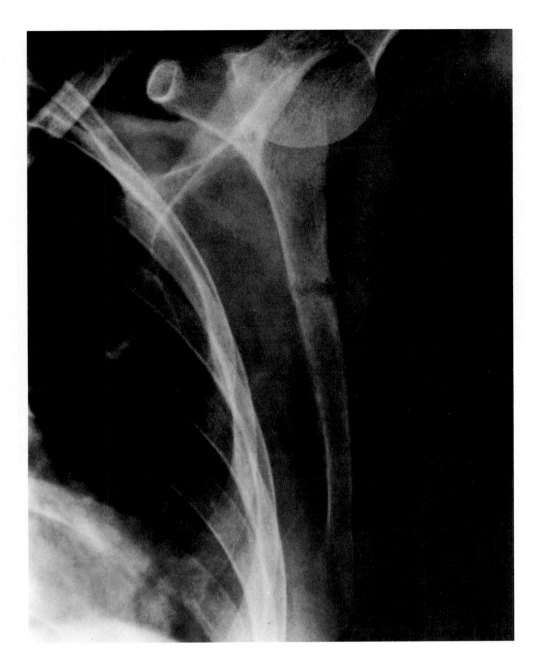

Fig. 23.68 Osteomalacia: Looser zone in the scapula. Osteomalacia is the term used to describe inadequate osteoid mineralisation in the adult. Stress fractures of the weakened bones are common and the resultant seams of osteoid are known as Looser's zones. This film of the left scapula of a woman with vitamin D deficiency illustrates the typical appearance of a Looser zone. There is little or no evidence of healing. Because Looser's zones are due to stress induced by normal activity they tend to occur at constant symmetrical sites: these include the ribs, the scapulae, the obturator rings of the pelvis, the metatarsal shafts, and the femoral necks (see Fig. 23.69). Osteomalacia results in generalised demineralisation of the bones but this may be evident radiologically only when the disease is severe. When gross osteomalacia is present deformities of the weakened bones may occur: these include triradiate pelvis, kyphosis, bowing of the limbs, 'hour-glass' shaped thoracic cage and basilar invagination of the skull.

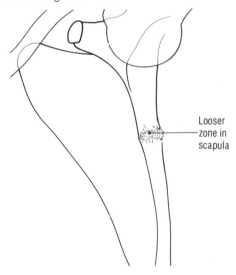

Looser zone in scapula

Fig. 23.69 Osteomalacia: Looser zone in the femoral neck. This coned AP view of the upper part of the right femur shows a linear lucency in the medial aspect of the femoral neck, a typical site for a Looser zone.

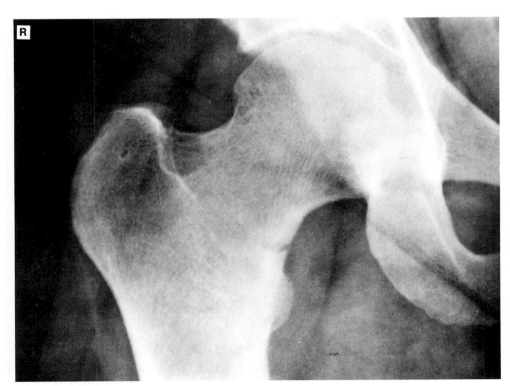

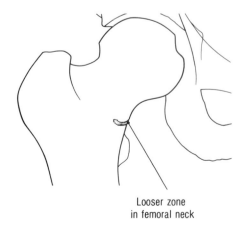

Looser zone in femoral neck

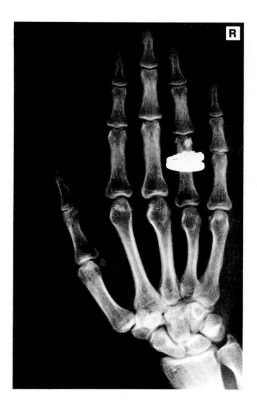
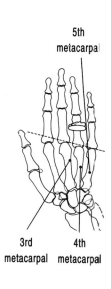

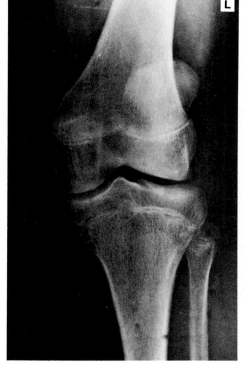
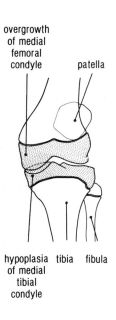

Fig. 23.70 Gonadal dysgenesis (Turner's syndrome): short fourth metacarpal. The fourth metacarpal is often short in gonadal dysgenesis, as in this patient. Normally, a line tangential to the distal ends of the third and fifth metacarpals will transect the head of the fourth. If the fourth metacarpal is short, it will touch or lie below such a line. In gonadal dysgenesis the fifth metacarpal is often also short and occasionally the third metacarpal may be similarly affected. Premature fusion of the ossification centres of the involved metacarpals may be seen in young patients.

Fig. 23.71 Gonadal dysgenesis (Turner's syndrome): impaired development of the medial tibial condyle. This AP film of the knee shows hypoplasia of the medial tibial condyle which is often a feature of gonadal dysgenesis. The medial tibial condyle appears depressed and there is corresponding overgrowth of the medial femoral condyle.

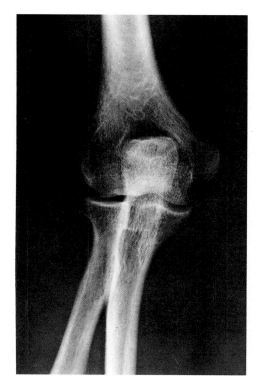
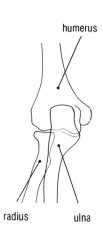

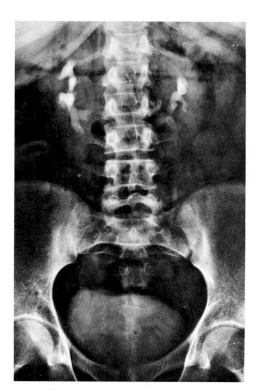
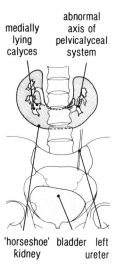

Fig. 23.72 Gonadal dysgenesis (Turner's syndrome): cubitus valgus. Bilateral cubitus valgus is frequently present in gonadal dysgenesis and this AP film of the elbow demonstrates the increase in the carrying angle, as shown by lateral deviation of the radius and ulna.

Fig. 23.73 Gonadal dysgenesis (Turner's syndrome): fused or 'horseshoe' kidney. This full length film of an intravenous urogram shows a fused or 'horseshoe' kidney, one of the commonest associated anomalies in gonadal dysgenesis. The lower poles of the kidneys are joined in the midline and this results in abnormal orientation of the pelvicalyceal systems and medially lying calyces. Other renal anomalies, in particular those involving rotation and ectopia, are also common in gonadal dysgenesis.

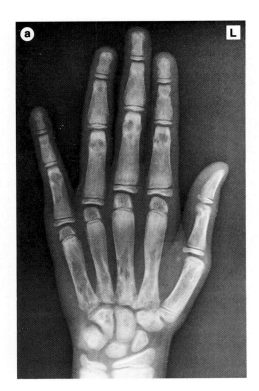 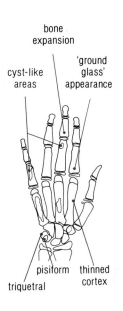

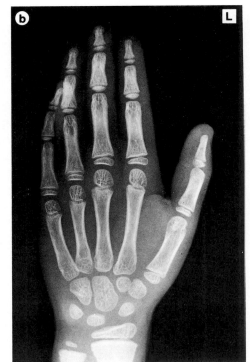 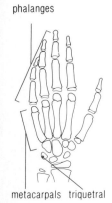

Fig. 23.74 McCune-Albright's syndrome: hand with normal for comparison. This PA film (a) of the hand of a six-year-old girl with skin pigmentation and precocious puberty shows the characteristic appearances of polyostotic fibrous dysplasia. Both bone replacement and new bone formation are evident. The affected spongiosa has an amorphous appearance resembling that of 'ground glass' and the bones show areas of expansion with thinning of the overlying cortex. Small cyst-like lesions are also present with reactive sclerosis around some of their margins. The carpal bones and secondary epiphyses are well developed and the pisiform bone, which normally starts to ossify at about nine years in the female, is seen superimposed on the triquetral. The bone age is advanced to ten years and this film should be compared with (b), that of a normal six-year-old girl, which shows the degree of bony development which usually occurs by that age.

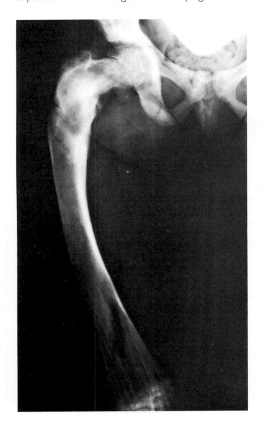 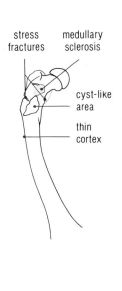

Fig. 23.75 McCune-Albright's syndrome: deformity of the femur. This AP film shows marked coxa vara and bowing of the shaft. The cyst-like lesions and areas of medullary sclerosis are typical of fibrous dysplasia. The cortex is thin, particularly at the lateral margin and stress fractures are present in the proximal femoral shaft. Such changes often progress and may result in a 'shepherd's crook' deformity of the upper femur.

Fig. 23.76 McCune-Albright's syndrome: skull showing leontiasis ossea. Involvement of the skull by fibrous dysplasia is usually manifest by extensive new bone formation and this lateral film of the same girl as in Fig. 23.74 shows the characteristic appearance of leontiasis ossea. The convexity of the calvarium is thickened and there is considerable sclerosis of the floor of the anterior fossae, the base of the skull, the maxillae and the frontal bones, making the radiograph features indistinct.

Imaging of the Pituitary and Hypothalamus

Robert J Witte, MD

Leighton P Mark, MD

Victor M Haughton, MD

Imaging of the pituitary and hypothalamus has evolved with the development of new imaging modalities such that positive contrast cisternography and pneumoencephalography are now only of historical interest. Although skull radiography is rarely used as a primary means of investigation of the sella it should always be evaluated when the study is obtained for other purposes (Fig. 24.1).

MAGNETIC RESONANCE IMAGING (MR)

Since its introduction, magnetic resonance imaging (MR) has taken on a major role in imaging the sella and hypothalamus. Few would argue that with its multiplanar capability and superior tissue contrast differentiation, MR imaging is the preferred initial modality, surpassing computed tomography, for patients with pituitary dysfunction or visual field defects.

MR imaging allows multiplanar images of the pituitary to be obtained with the patient's head in the neutral position. The strength of the signal depends on proton density and on two relaxation times, T1 and T2. T1 depends on the time the protons take to return to the axis of the magnetic field and T2 depends on the time the protons take to dephase. A T1-weighted image is one in which the contrast between tissues is mainly due to their T1 relaxation properties while in a T2-weighted image the contrast is due to the T2 relaxation properties. Routinely, T1-weighted images are obtained before and after intravenous contrast administration of a gadolinium chelate (i.e. gadopentatate dimeglumine). T2-weighted images are obtained when further tumour delineation or characterisation is felt necessary: images are acquired in the coronal and sagittal planes.

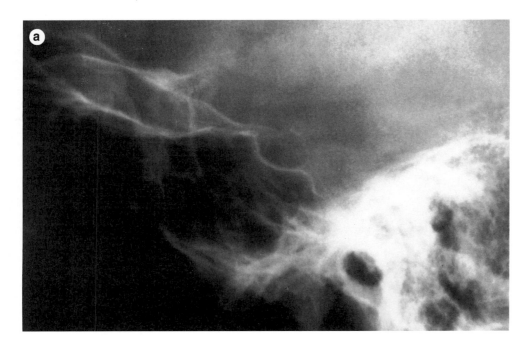

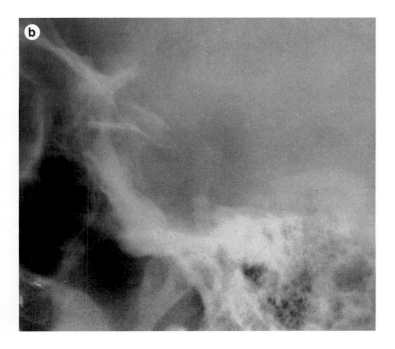

Fig. 24.1 Plain skull radiographs. Normal sella (a) and enlarged sella from pituitary macroadenoma (b).

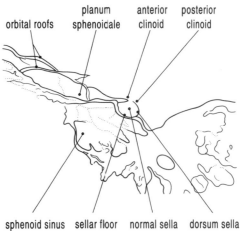

orbital roofs · planum sphenoidale · anterior clinoid · posterior clinoid

sphenoid sinus · sellar floor · normal sella · dorsum sella

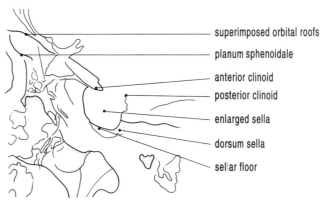

- superimposed orbital roofs
- planum sphenoidale
- anterior clinoid
- posterior clinoid
- enlarged sella
- dorsum sella
- sellar floor

COMPUTED TOMOGRAPHY (CT)

Computed tomography was considered for many years to be the gold standard for imaging the pituitary and hypothalamus with its high resolution and reformatting capabilities providing excellent anatomic detail of this area. Even though today MR is the preferred initial imaging modality, CT still provides a quick means to visualise thin sections of this area.

Certain patients are unable to undergo an MR examination for various reasons (e.g. a pacemaker or claustrophobia). Aneurysm clips may also be deflected in the magnetic field or may degrade MR image quality. In these patients CT still provides excellent evaluation of the sellar region. CT also provides valuable additional information to MR imaging when evaluating sellar masses with respect to bone involvement, tumour calcification and acute haemorrhage. Direct coronal images are obtained with the patient positioned in a head-holder and the neck extended comfortably to a maximal point. Gantry tilt is utilised to obtain an optimal coronal positioning, perpendicular to the sellar floor, while avoiding dental amalgam artefacts. A lateral localiser image is used to select contiguous coronal images, with a slice thickness of about 1.5mm. If the patient cannot be positioned for direct coronal imaging, reformatted coronal images can be obtained from axial images. Intravenous contrast medium (containing 30–40g of iodine) is administered immediately prior to the scan. Patients with a contrast allergy need to be premedicated with corticosteroids given twenty-four hours, twelve hours, and two hours prior to the study.

ANATOMY

The pituitary rests in the sella turcica, a shallow impression in the posterior sphenoid when viewed in the sagittal plane (Fig. 24.2). The anterior pituitary (adenohypophysis) accounts for about seventy-five per cent of the gland, and is the same intensity as grey matter on T1-weighted images. The contents of the posterior part of the fossa usually appear as a 'bright spot' on T1-weighted images. Proposed sources of this bright signal include phospholipids and/or hormones in the posterior gland (neurohypophysis) or tissue adjacent to the gland. The infundibulum can be seen extending from the tuber cinereum of the hypothalamus through the diaphragma sellae to the superior surface of the gland. The optic chiasm is anterior to, and the mammillary bodies posterior to the, tuber cinereum. The midline third ventricle lies immediately above the optic chiasm and the tuber cinereum.

In the coronal plane (Figs. 24.3 & 24.4), the sella is bordered laterally by the dural reflection of the cavernous sinuses. Cranial nerves III (oculomotor), IV (trochlear), V1 (ophthalmic), and V2 (maxillary) course along the lateral wall of the cavernous sinus. Cranial nerve VI

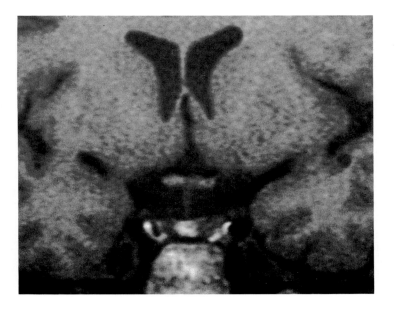

Fig. 24.2 Normal pituitary. Unenhanced sagittal T1-weighted MR image showing normal anatomic structures; anterior pituitary, posterior sella 'bright spot', infundibulum, optic chiasm and mammillary bodies.

Fig. 24.3 Normal sella: magnetic resonance imaging. Coronal T1-weighted MR image following contrast administration. Normal anatomic structures include the anterior pituitary, cavernous sinus, cavernous carotid artery, infundibulum, optic chiasm and lateral ventricles.

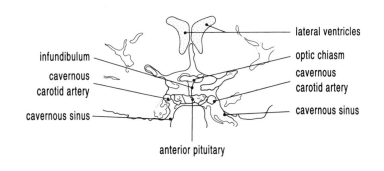

(abducens) courses more medially along the sinus trabeculae. The pituitary stalk usually reaches the pituitary gland in the midline. However, up to forty per cent of the normal population may have an eccentric insertion. The gland usually measures 4–8mm in vertical dimension with a flat or concave superior border. The optic chiasm and third ventricle are identified superiorly, as well as the hypothalamus forming the floor of the third ventricle. Since the infundibulum and pituitary lack a blood-brain barrier, intense enhancement is seen in these structures and the cavernous sinuses following contrast administration. Mild superior glandular convexity may be seen at puberty or in lactating females (Fig. 24.5).

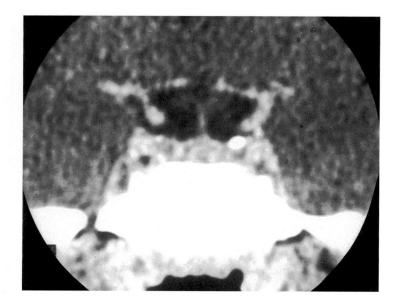

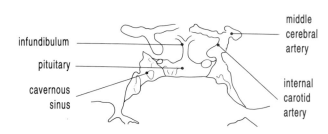

Fig. 24.4 Normal sella: computed tomography. Normal anatomic structures include the pituitary, infundibulum, optic chiasm, cavernous sinus, internal carotid artery and middle cerebral artery.

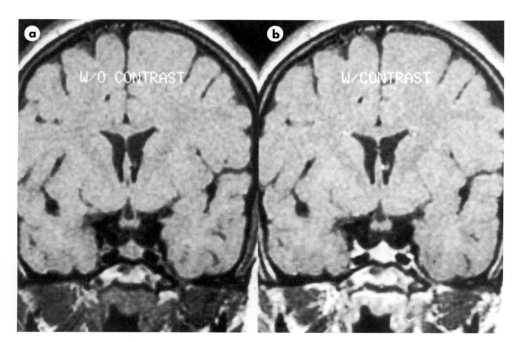

Fig. 24.5 Normal anatomic variant: magnetic resonance imaging. T1-weighted coronal images of the sella pre-contrast administration (a) and post-contrast administration (b), show a convex superior margin of the pituitary, a normal variant in adolescent and lactating females.

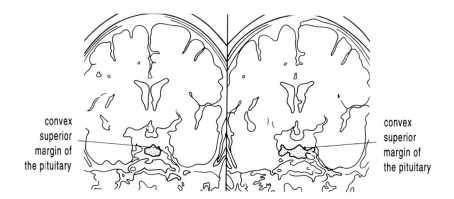

EMPTY SELLA

Defects in the diaphragma sella may allow passage of cerebrospinal fluid (CSF) from the suprasellar cistern into the sella turcica, although it may also result from infarction or irradiation of a pituitary tumour. The condition is termed 'empty sella' and is usually an incidental finding. Differentiation from an intra- or suprasellar cyst is based on the normal location of the infundibulum, extending from the tuber cinereum to a small posteriorly displaced pituitary gland (Fig. 24.6). The clinical condition of 'empty sella syndrome' has been applied to the combination of an 'empty sella' with the constellation of symptoms: headache, endocrine dysfunction, and visual disturbances.

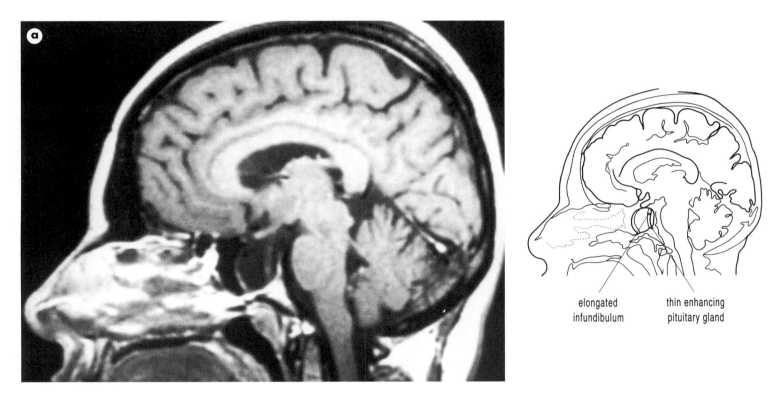

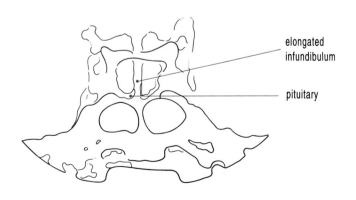

Fig. 24.6 *Empty sella.* Sagittal T1-weighted post-contrast MR image (a) showing a large 'empty sella', with an elongated infundibulum inserting into a thin enhancing pituitary gland. Coronal CT (b) in a different patient showing insertion of the infundibulum into a thin pituitary.

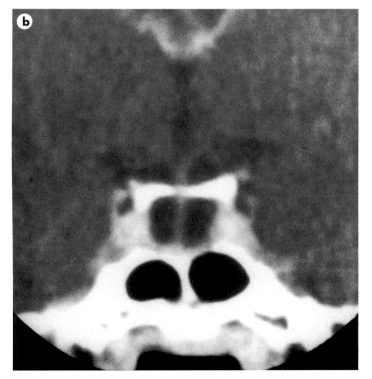

ADENOMAS

Adenomas are classified radiographically by size. Microadenomas are considered to be less than 1cm, and macroadenomas, greater than 1cm. Microadenomas are often functional and come to clinical attention due to signs and symptoms of excess hormone secretion (i.e. prolactin, ACTH, or growth hormone). Microadenomas are usually hypointense compared with the normal pituitary on T1-weighted images. Small incidental pars intermedia cysts located between the anterior and posterior lobes may have a similar appearance or a high intensity signal. On intravenous contrast administration the microadenoma frequently enhances to a lesser degree than the surrounding gland, accentuating its hypointense appearance. Microadenomas are often asymmetrically located in the gland.

Secondary signs caused by the mass effect of the microadenoma include deviation of the infundibulum away from the mass and upward convexity of the superior margin of the gland (Fig. 24.7). However, as stated above, the secondary signs are nonspecific and may be seen in the normal population. These signs are less reliable than the identification of a hypointense lesion in a symptomatic patient. A small percentage of microadenomas may show greater enhancement than the remainder of the gland following contrast administration (Fig. 24.8).

Macroadenomas usually present clinically with signs and symptoms associated with the displacement of the optic chiasm, cavernous sinus, and hypothalamus. These tumours are often homogeneous in appearance, isointense with grey matter on T1-weighted images and enhance homogeneously after contrast administration (Fig. 24.9).

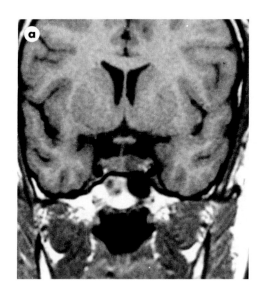
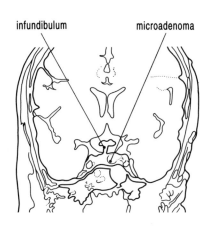
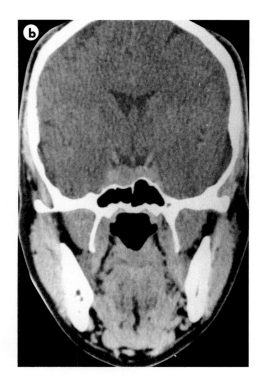
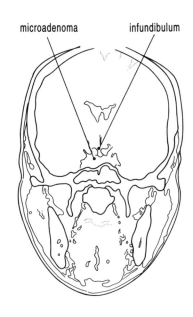

Fig. 24.7 Microadenoma. T1-weighted coronal MR image (a) showing hypointense microadenoma in the left side of the pituitary. The mass causes a convex superior margin of the gland and displacement of the infundibulum to the right. Coronal CT (b) in a different patient with a microadenoma in the right side of the pituitary displacing the infundibulum to the left.

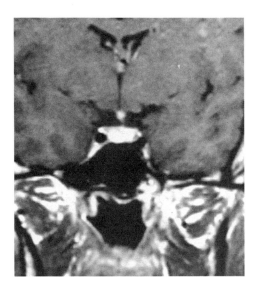

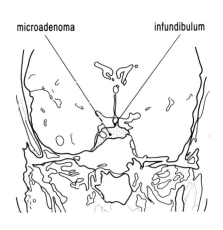

microadenoma   infundibulum

Fig. 24.8 Enhancing microadenoma: magnetic resonance imaging. Contrast enhanced T1-weighted coronal MR image showing an enhancing microadenoma in the right side of the pituitary. The infundibulum is displaced to the left.

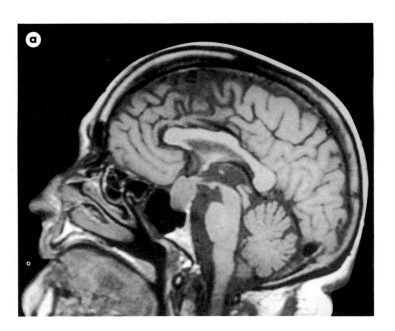

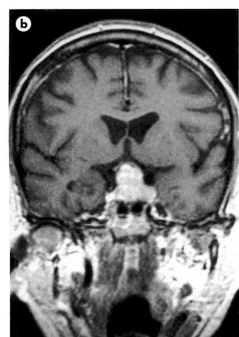

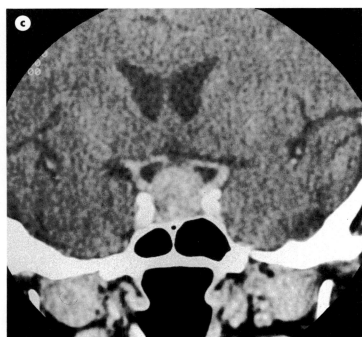

Fig. 24.9 Macroadenoma. Sagittal T1-weighted MR image (a) showing a large sellar/suprasellar macroadenoma. Coronal image (b) following contrast administration shows diffuse homogeneous enhancement with upward displacement of the optic chiasm more clearly identified. Coronal CT (c) of a macroadenoma in a different patient also demonstrating diffuse homogeneous enhancement.

a

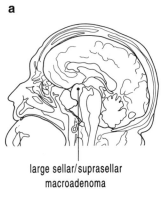

large sellar/suprasellar macroadenoma

b   displaced optic chiasm

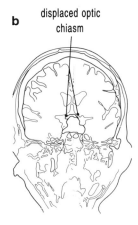

c

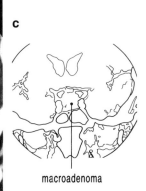

macroadenoma

Macroadenomas, however, may also be heterogeneous in appearance due to necrosis, cystic degeneration or haemorrhage. Necrotic areas show as a lower signal than the surrounding tumour on T1-weighted images. Areas that progress to cystic degeneration show as a signal which is similar to CSF (i.e. low on T1-weighted images and high on T2-weighted images). Acute haemorrhage in these tumours is best seen as high density areas on non-contrast CT studies whilst sub-acute haemorrhage is easier to identify using MR studies, appearing as a high signal on T1-weighted images. Macroadenoma appearance on T2-weighted images varies (Fig. 24.10). A region of high signal intensity would suggest necrosis. Calcification, although rare, may also be seen and is usually curvilinear.

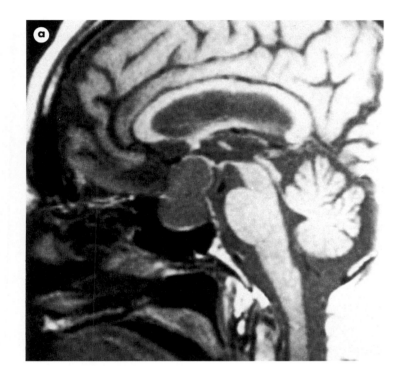

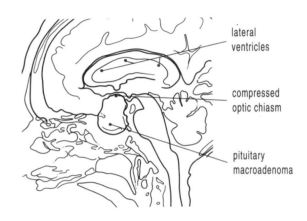

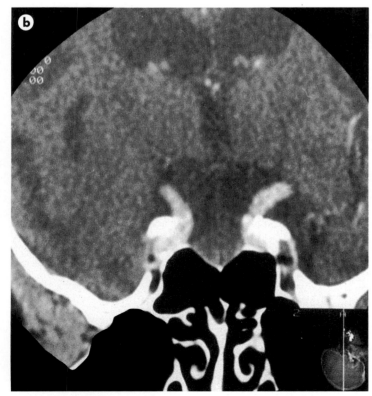

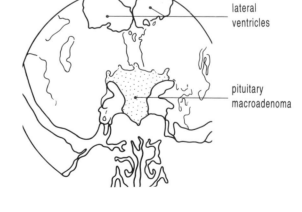

Fig. 24.10 Cystic macroadenoma. Sagittal T1-weighted MR image (a) showing a large pituitary macroadenoma with suprasellar extension, compressing the optic chiasm. The low signal intensity of the mass is similar to the CSF signal in the lateral ventricles suggesting the predominantly cystic nature of the mass. A coronal CT (b) in the same patient showing the mass to be of low density, like the CSF in the lateral ventricles.

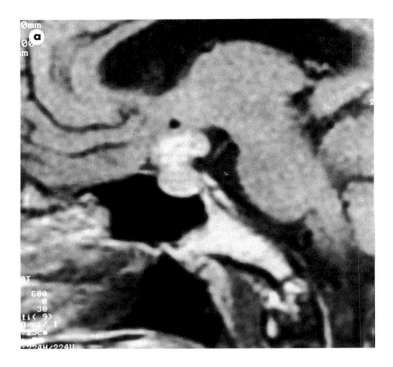

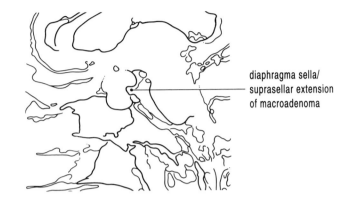

diaphragma sella/
suprasellar extension
of macroadenoma

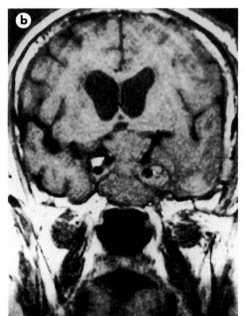

suprasellar extension
of macroadenoma

left cavernous
sinus extension of
macroadenoma

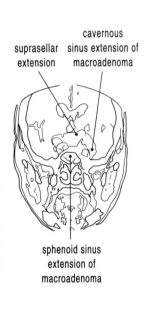

cavernous
sinus extension of
macroadenoma

suprasellar
extension

sphenoid sinus
extension of
macroadenoma

Fig. 24.11 Extrasellar extension of macroadenomas. Sagittal TI-weighted MR image (a) showing suprasellar extension with a 'waist' caused by the diaphragma sellae. Coronal TI-weighted MR image (b) demonstrating suprasellar and left cavernous sinus extension, encasing the left cavernous carotid artery. Coronal CT image (c) showing suprasellar, cavernous sinus, and sphenoid sinus extension.

Extrasellar extension of macroadenoma has important clinical and surgical implications. Suprasellar extension may produce a 'waist' due to compression by the diaphragma sellae (Fig. 24.11). CT best evaluates erosion of the sellar floor and inferior extension into the sphenoid sinus and sphenoid extension is suggested by the appearance of a convex inferior margin of the mass on CT and MR images. However, cavernous sinus extension, particularly when early, is difficult to detect. Unilateral encasement of the carotid artery and distortion of the lateral margins of the cavernous sinus are the most reliable signs (see Fig. 24.11 (b) & (c)).

Post-partum pituitary haemorrhagic infarction may lead to hypopituitarism (Sheehan's syndrome). This appears radiographically as a dense gland on CT examination (Fig. 24.12). Adenomas in other patients may also undergo haemorrhagic infarction. The enlarged haemorrhagic gland may be dysfunctional and compress adjacent structures, producing pituitary apoplexy (Fig. 24.13).

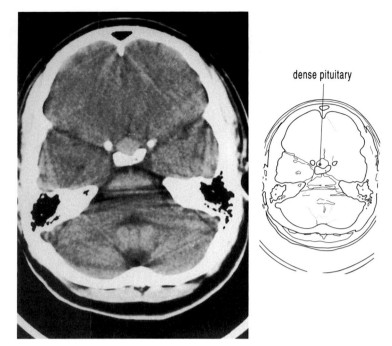

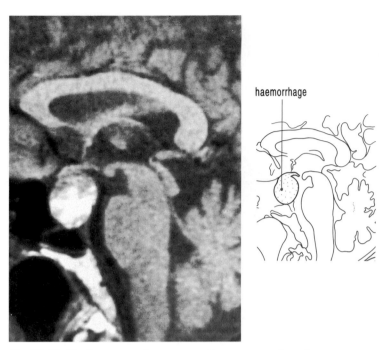

Fig. 24.12 Sheehan's syndrome: computed tomography. Axial CT image showing a dense pituitary due to haemorrhagic infarction following uterine haemorrhage post-partum.

Fig. 24.13 Pituitary apoplexy: magnetic resonance imaging. T1-weighted sagittal MR image showing haemorrhage in a macroadenoma.

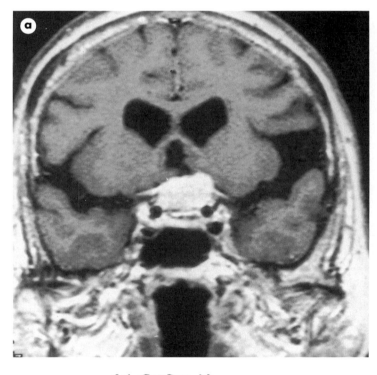

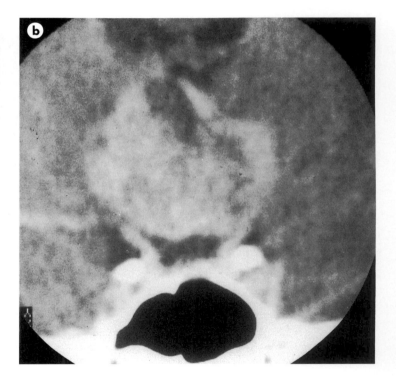

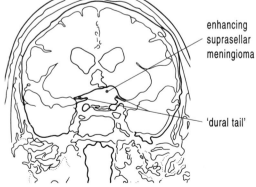

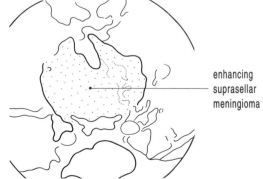

Fig. 24.14 Meningioma. Contrast-enhanced, T1-weighted coronal MR image (a) demonstrating an enhancing suprasellar meningioma with adjacent 'dural tail'. Coronal CT image (b) in a different patient also demonstrating an enhancing suprasellar meningioma.

MENINGIOMAS

Meningiomas are the second most common tumour in the sellar region. These tumours may arise from dural surfaces such as the diaphragma sellae, tuberculum sellae, or cavernous sinuses. They may project into the suprasellar space and rarely arise within the sella. Meningiomas are usually isointense with grey matter on T1- and T2-weighted images and enhance intensely following contrast administration. Differentiation from an adenoma with suprasellar extension may be difficult. A dural 'tail' sign may be produced by adjacent dural enhancement (Fig. 24.14). Coronal images are very helpful in distinguishing the purely suprasellar location of the meningioma from the intrasellar and suprasellar location of the adenoma.

CRANIOPHARYNGIOMAS

Craniopharyngiomas are benign neoplasms which may arise from epithelial remnants of Rathké's pouch. They are the most frequent neoplasm in the sellar region in children and young adults. A second peak also occurs in adults at around the fifth decade. These tumours usually arise in the suprasellar region, however, they may be both suprasellar and intrasellar, or entirely intrasellar. Craniopharyngiomas are radiographically heterogeneous in appearance, often containing cysts and globular calcification (Fig. 24.15). The cystic portions of the mass may appear hypointense on T1-weighted MR images, and hyperintense on T2-weighted images. Craniopharyngiomas may also exhibit both iso- and hyperintense components. The solid portions of

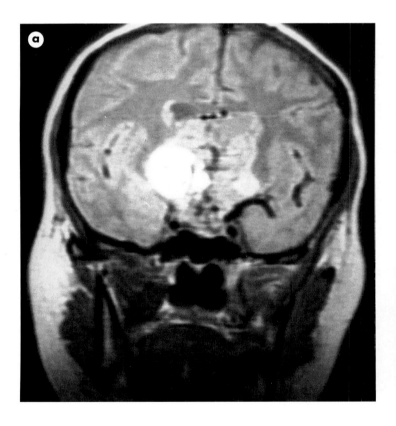

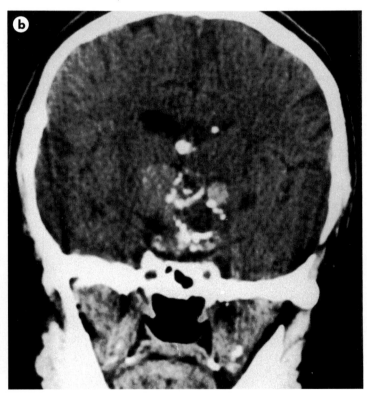

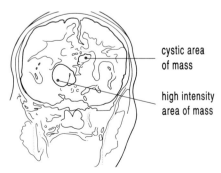

cystic area
of mass

high intensity
area of mass

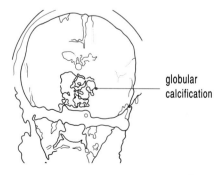

globular
calcification

Fig. 24.15 Craniopharyngioma. Balanced-weighted coronal MR image (a) showing a cystic area and high intensity signal area in a large sellar/suprasellar mass, typical of craniopharyngiomas. Characteristic globular calcification is easier to identify on a coronal CT image (b) of the same patient.

the mass, and the periphery of the cystic components often enhance following contrast administration. MR imaging best shows the mass to be anatomically separate from the pituitary, helping to differentiate the mass from an adenoma. The calcification is much more apparent on CT examination which is often useful in differentiation from other masses. Less commonly, these tumours may appear entirely solid or demonstrate ring calcification surrounding a cystic component (Fig. 24.16).

ANEURYSMS

Aneurysms of the intracavernous or supraclinoid carotid artery appear as dense sellar or juxtasellar masses on CT imaging, with enhancement following contrast administration. However, differentiation from a true neoplasm is often difficult. These lesions are also easily identified on conventional MR examination but unlike stationary tissue, rapidly flowing blood produces little signal. Therefore, MR angiography is another technique that can be used to identify aneurysms (Fig. 24.17).

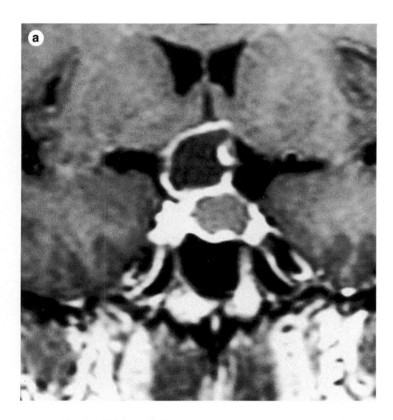

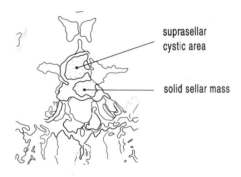

Fig. 24.16 Atypical craniopharyngioma. Coronal T1-weighted MR image (a) following contrast administration showing enhancement of a solid sellar mass with a ring enhancing suprasellar cystic component. A CT image (b) of the same patient shows a ring of calcification around the cystic portion of the mass.

suprasellar cystic area

solid sellar mass

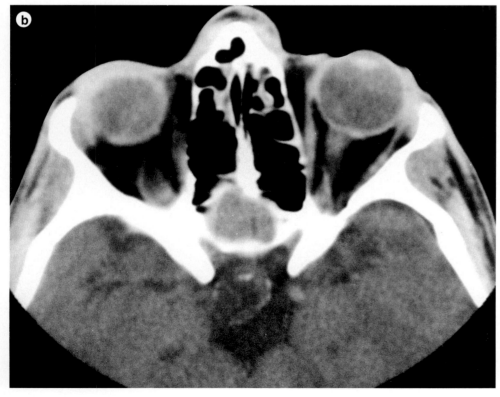

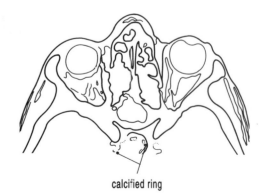

calcified ring

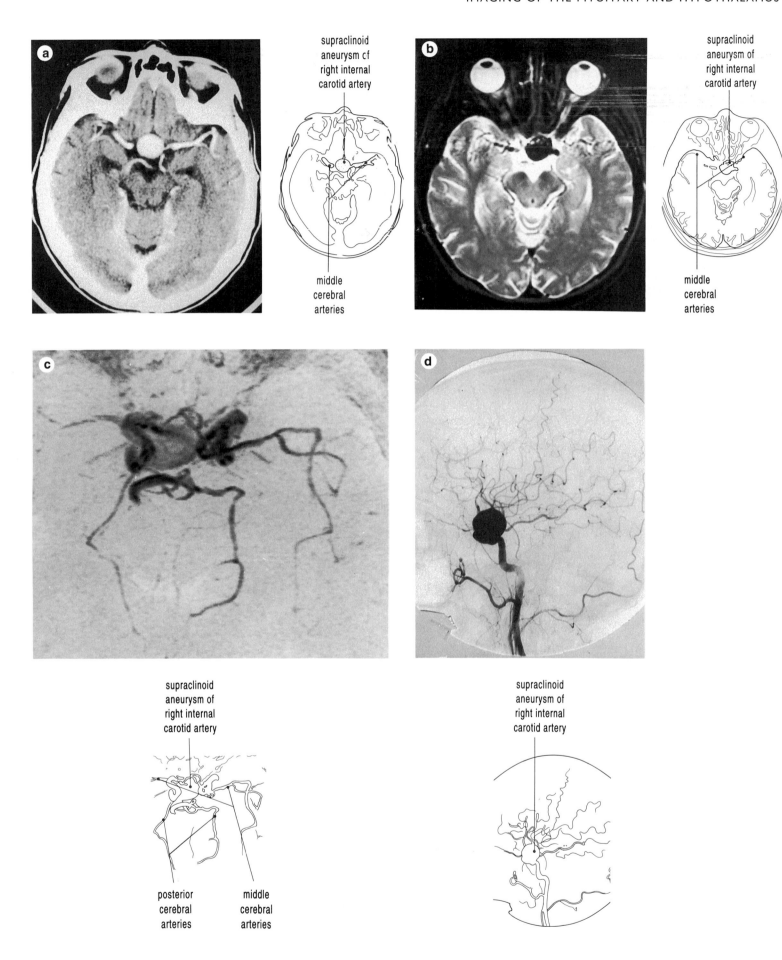

Fig. 24.17 Supraclinoid aneurysm. Multiple studies of the same patient showing a supraclinoid aneurysm of the right internal carotid artery. The middle cerebral arteries are also demonstrated: (a) enhanced CT image; (b) T2-weighted MR image; (c) MR angiogram of similar orientation to (a) and (b), posterior cerebral arteries are also identified; (d) cerebral angiogram.

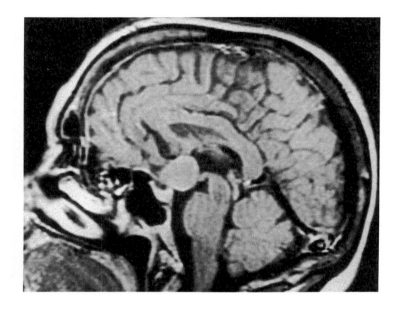

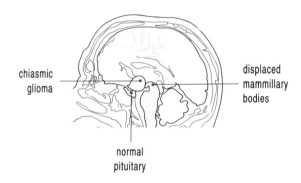

chiasmic glioma

displaced mammillary bodies

normal pituitary

Fig. 24.18 Chiasmic glioma: magnetic resonance imaging.
T1- weighted sagittal MR image showing chiasmic glioma displacing mammillary bodies posteriorly. Note the normal pituitary gland.

GLIOMAS

Gliomas occurring in the sellar region primarily involve the hypothalamus and optic chiasm. Hypothalamic gliomas are tumours of childhood and adolescence, and may extend into the suprasellar cistern. Chiasmic gliomas have a strong association with neurofibromatosis type I when occurring in children. They appear as sharply marginated homogeneous suprasellar masses, clearly separate from the pituitary gland. They are also usually hypointense or isointense with grey matter and may or may not enhance (Fig. 24.18).

CHORDOMAS

Chordomas are neoplasms that develop from intraosseous vestigial remnants of the notochord. The sacrum is the most common site accounting or fifty per cent of occurrences, followed by the clivus at thirty-five per cent. Clival chordomas may project into the sella or suprasellar regions. MR and CT techniques are both important in the differential diagnosis of these tumours. MR imaging best shows tumour infiltration and tumour origin in the clivus. Characteristic tumoural calcification is better identified with CT imaging. These tumours are often slightly hypointense on T1-weighted MR images and intensely enhanced following contrast administrattion (Fig. 24.19). Chondrosarcomas of the clivus may have an identical appearance on CT and MR studies.

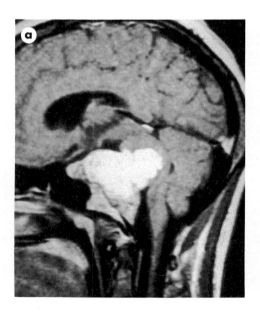

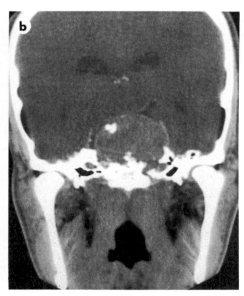

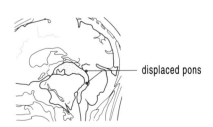

displaced pons

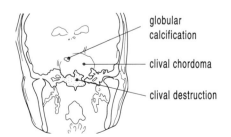

globular calcification

clival chordoma

clival destruction

Fig. 24.19 Clival chordoma. Contrast enhanced T1-weighted sagittal MR image (a) showing an intensely enhancing large clival chordoma. The tumour compresses and displaces the pons posteriorly. Coronal CT image (b) in the same patient demonstrating globular calcification within the mass and clival destruction.

CYSTS

Arachnoid cysts may arise in the suprasellar cistern, or adjacent parasellar regions. Remnants of Rathké's pouch may produce midline epithelial cysts termed Rathké's cleft cysts. These cysts may produce hydrocephalus or compress the optic chiasm, pituitary or infundibulum. These lesions may be difficult to identify because their signal intensities in MR imaging or density in CT is identical to CSF (Fig. 24.20). Rathké's cleft cysts, however, may be hyperintense to CSF on T1-weighted MR images. The diagnosis of arachnoid cysts is made radiologically by noting displacement of the pituitary stalk, chiasm or base of the brain.

INFLAMMATORY DISEASE

Tuberculosis and sarcoidosis may involve the CNS, producing suprasellar masses or thickening of the infundibulum or optic chiasm. These granulomatous lesions are usually isointense with grey matter on T1-weighted MR images. Enhancement of the parenchymal lesions, as well as leptomeningeal enhancement are seen following contrast administration (Fig. 24.21). Other causes of infundibular thickening include lymphoma, metastatic carcinoma, and Langerhans' cell histiocytosis (histiocytosis X) (Fig. 24.22).

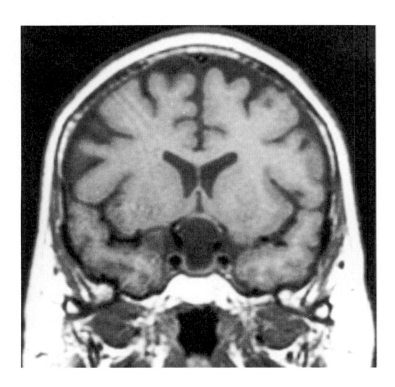

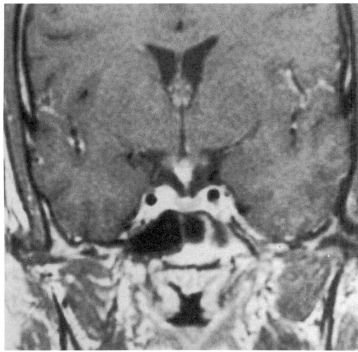

Fig. 24.20 Sellar cyst: magnetic resonance imaging. T1-weighted coronal MR image showing a cystic sellar/suprasellar mass and displacement of the optic chiasm. Absence of an identifiable infundibulum differentiates this mass from an 'empty sella'.

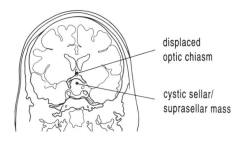

Fig. 24.21 Sarcoidosis: magnetic resonance imaging. Coronal T1-weighted image following contrast administration shows a thickened, enhancing infundibulum typical of CNS granulomatous disease. Enhancement in both sylvian fissures identifies leptomeningeal involvement.

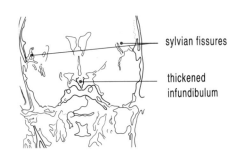

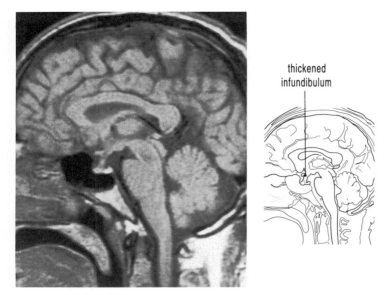

Fig. 24.22 Langerhans' cell histiocytosis: magnetic resonance imaging. Sagittal T1-weighted MR image showing a thickened infundibulum from known histiocytosis.

EXOPHTHALMOS

There are many causes of exophthalmos, however, the majority of cases are due to Graves' disease in adults. MR provides optimal imaging of the orbits, with coronal and axial planes obtained with the patient's head in the neutral position. CT can also be used for orbital imaging by utilizing thin slices (3mm) in the axial and direct coronal planes.

The most common presentation is bilateral and symmetric ocular muscle enlargement with preference for the inferior and medial rectus. Bilateral asymmetric and occasionally unilateral involvement can also occur (Fig. 24.23). Idiopathic inflammation or 'inflammatory pseudotumour' is another frequent cause of exophthalmos which often causes ocular muscle enlargement. Involvement is usually unilateral and tends to involve the muscles' tendinous insertion into the globe or may even present as an orbital mass. Other causes for exophthalmos are usually unilateral and include benign and malignant tumours (Fig. 24.24), vascular malformations, carotid–cavernous fistula, or cavernous sinus thrombosis.

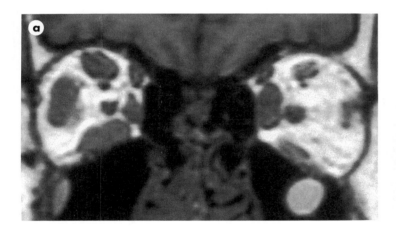

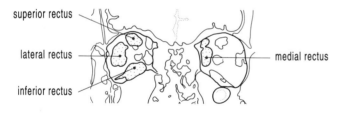

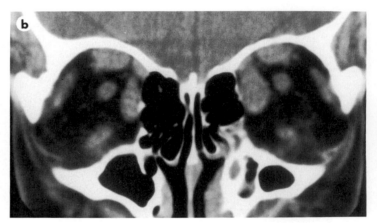

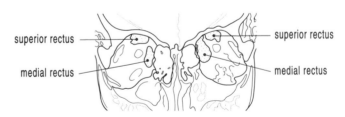

Fig. 24.23 Endocrine ophthalmopathy. Coronal T1-weighted MR image (a) showing extraocular muscle enlargement of the superior rectus, lateral rectus and inferior rectus of the right orbit. Enlargement of the medial rectus in the left orbit is also present. Coronal CT (b) in a different patient with enlargement of the medial rectus and superior rectus of both orbits.

Fig. 24.24 Neurofibroma: magnetic resonance imaging. Large neurofibroma of the left orbit causing exophthalmos of the left globe.

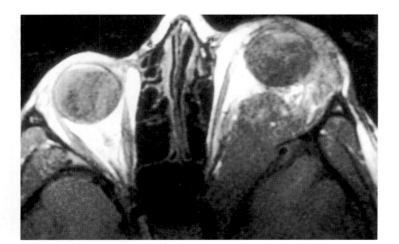

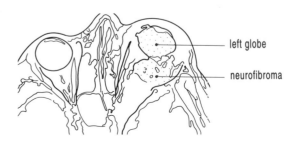

25

Nuclear Medicine Imaging In Endocrinology

Keith E Britton, MD, MSc, FRCP

Jamshed B Bomanji, MD, MSc, PhD

Nuclear medicine is to physiology what radiology is to anatomy. For imaging in endocrinology an agent is chosen whose uptake or metabolism relates to the function of the particular endocrine system. The agent is radiolabelled with a γ-emitting radionuclide so that, after its intravenous or oral administration, it can be detected externally and noninvasively by imaging with a γ-camera. Nuclear medicine techniques may also characterise a tissue by its receptor or antigen expression in ways complementary to radiological and biochemical techniques. It allows in vivo assessment of clinical physiology and pathophysiology and is very sensitive to metabolic disorders Furthermore, stimulation and suppression techniques can be used to enhance its specificity. The absorbed radiation dose equivalent to the patients from diagnostic tests is of the same order as from X-ray studies; usually up to 7.5mSv (0.75rem). One sievert (Sv)

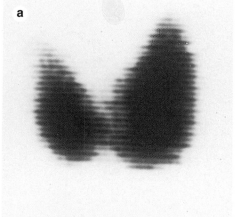

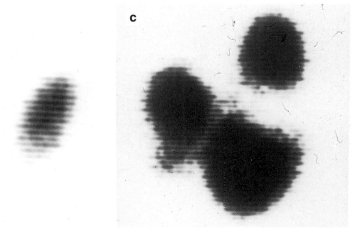

Fig. 25.1 Thyroid images in thyrotoxicosis. These are obtained by γ-camera imaging of the anterior neck 20 minutes after intravenous injection of 80MBq ^{99m}Tc pertechnetate. ^{99m}Tc pertechnetate is trapped but not organified, while radioiodine is trapped and organified by the thyroid gland. (a) Typical image in Graves' disease with homogeneously increased uptake in an enlarged gland; in this case the left lobe is bigger than the right lobe. (b) Typical appearance in an autonomous toxic nodule (Plummer's syndrome) with suppression of uptake in the remaining normal thyroid. (c) Typical appearance of a toxic multinodular goitre with areas of autonomous toxic nodules separated by areas of nodules with no function and areas of normal tissue whose function has been suppressed.

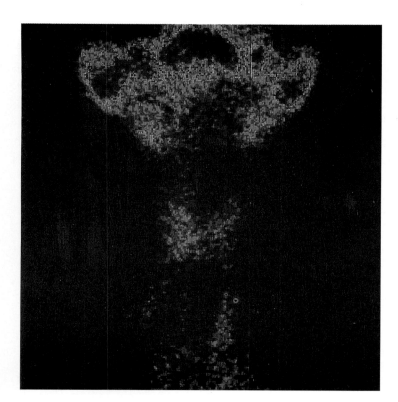

Fig. 25.2 Hyperthyroidism due to subacute thyroiditis.
^{99m}Tc pertechnetate images taken 20 minutes after injection. Using the colour scale 0–100% (blue - green - yellow - red - purple) the thyroid can be seen in green, at the same level as the vascular activity in the aorta and heart inferiorly. Uptake is much reduced below that in the salivary glands and mouth seen superiorly. Normally, thyroid uptake is greater than salivary gland uptake. In this case, with clinical hyperthyroidism, there is severe reduction of uptake due to the inflammation of the thyroid. Autoimmune thyroiditis is a great mimic of the range of thyroid scan abnormalities, from the Hashimoto goitre with inhomogeneous uptake to appearances of 'warm' or 'cold' defects, solitary or multiple, or asymmetric uptake.

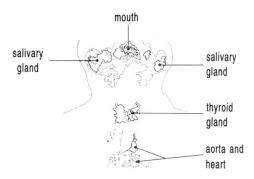

equals one hundred radiation dose equivalents (rem). Natural background radiation from cosmic rays, body potassium, radon, etc. is, in London, about 2mSv (0.2rem) and in Cornwall, 8mSv (0.8rem) annually. Thus, these tests give activities that are considered by the International Committee of Radiation Protection to be of negligible risk to members of the public (up to 5mSv) and to workers using ionising radiation (up to 15mSv).

For therapy, the destructive properties of β-particle (electron) emitting radionuclides are used, so that radiation therapy can be targeted by the chosen carrier agent to the site of the disorder or cancer. This facilitates delivery of therapeutic levels of radiation even more selectively than is possible by external beam therapy.

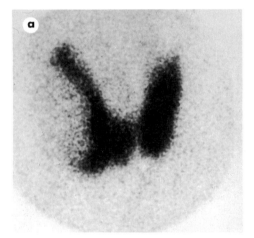 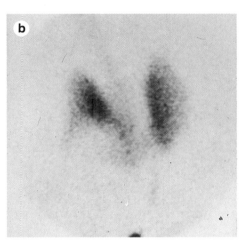 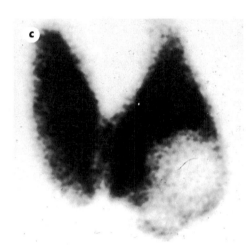

Fig. 25.3 Thyroid images in patients with palpable solitary nodules in their thyroid glands. You will note that the appearances of the scans are similar, each showing an area of deficient or reduced uptake while the rest of the gland shows a homogeneous normal uptake. It is not possible to distinguish between the causes of a solitary nodule: (a) a haemorrhage, (b) a cyst, (c) a follicular thyroid cancer. Ultrasound should be combined with thyroid imaging to demonstrate the simple cyst for aspiration cytology, and to enable fine-needle biopsy for the echogenic (solid) nodule, which is nonfunctional in a thyroid scan. If the mass in the gland is solitary and solid, about 12 per cent of these cases prove to be malignant (see Chapter 16).

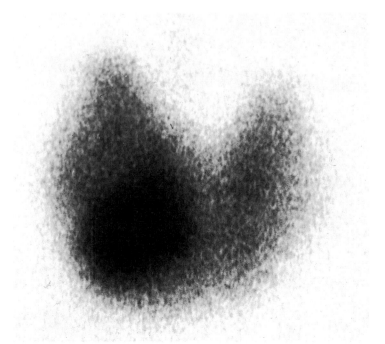

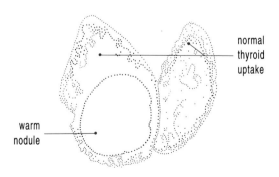

normal
thyroid
uptake

warm
nodule

Fig. 25.4 A 'warm' nodule imaged using ⁹⁹ᵐTc pertechnetate. Uptake in the inferior pole of the enlarged right lobe of the thyroid is greater than that in the surrounding gland and corresponds to the site of a palpable nodule. The study should be repeated using ¹²³I; see scheme in Fig. 25.5.

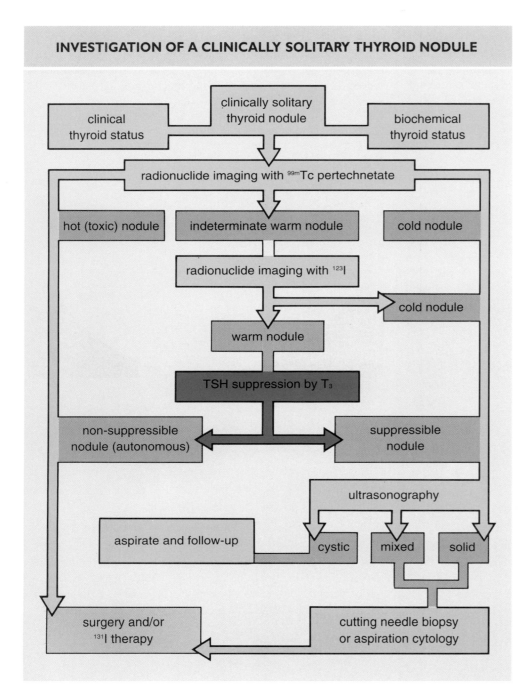

INVESTIGATION OF A CLINICALLY SOLITARY THYROID NODULE

Fig. 25.5 Scheme for investigating a clinically solitary thyroid nodule. It should be noted that the cytopathologist can identify anaplastic, papillary and medullary carcinoma and lymphoma on aspiration biopsy. It is not possible on cytological smears to differentiate follicular adenomas from follicular carcinomas since the latter require identification of vascular invasion for diagnosis (see Chapter 16).

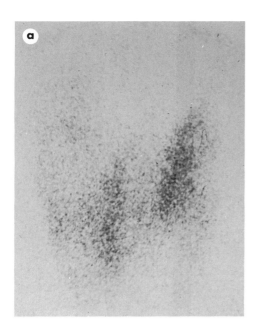

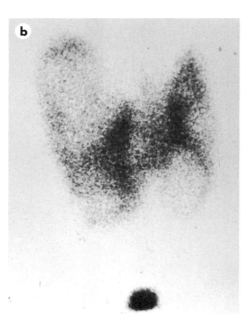

Fig. 25.6 Thyroid imaging in a patient with a multinodular goitre. (a) Using 80MBq 99mTc pertechnetate and (b) using 20MBq 123I sodium iodide. The typical mix of areas of reduced uptake and normal uptake is seen corresponding to the palpable nodules. The incidence of cancer in such a thyroid is low. However, a dominant nonfunctional nodule should be evaluated as a solitary 'cold' nodule.

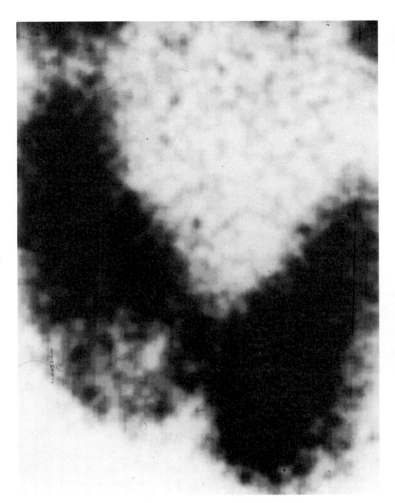

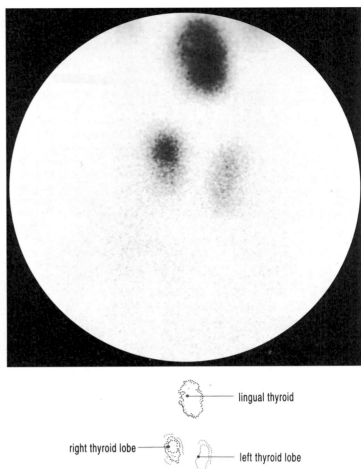

Fig. 25.7 Thyroid image in thyrotoxicosis in a patient with a palpable nodule. This image shows the uniform high uptake seen in Graves' disease with an area of reduced uptake ('cold' area) in the inferior pole of the right thyroid lobe. The incidence of malignancy in a solitary 'cold' nodule in a thyrotoxic gland is greater than that in a euthyroid gland.

Fig. 25.8 Thyroid images in sublingual thyroid. This 77-year-old woman presented with a mass at the back of her tongue. Thyroid ^{99m}Tc pertechnetate imaging shows this to be a source of high uptake. Relatively reduced uptake is seen in the normal thyroid position. Thyroid scanning is an important method for evaluating lumps at the back of the tongue and in the centre of the neck. If there is a doubt about pertechnetate uptake, which vascular lesions can mimic, then ^{123}I should be used. A typical thyroglossal cyst is nonfunctional on a thyroid scan.

Fig. 25.9 Functionally significant thyroid carcinoma imaged three days after ^{131}I therapy (150 mCi, 5.55 GBq). In this case, imaging shows irregular increased uptake in the superior mediastinum, in the paratracheal and supraclavicular nodes, and diffuse high lung uptake. Such uptake may occur rarely when there is a normal chest X-ray, but is usually associated with miliary lung metastases and shows a good response to ^{131}I therapy. High lung uptake may be followed by radiation fibrosis if the dose administered is too great. Indications for ^{131}I therapy are biopsy proven papillary or follicular carcinoma and known or suspected incomplete surgical excision. Differentiated tumours concentrate ^{131}I better than undifferentiated and Hürthle cell cancers. Thyroid carcinoma tissue, which at first appears to take up ^{131}I poorly, may show significant uptake of tracer when all higher avidity normal gland has been ablated (see Chapter 16).

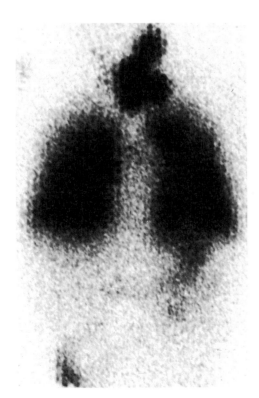

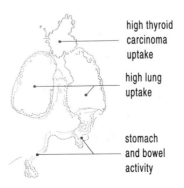

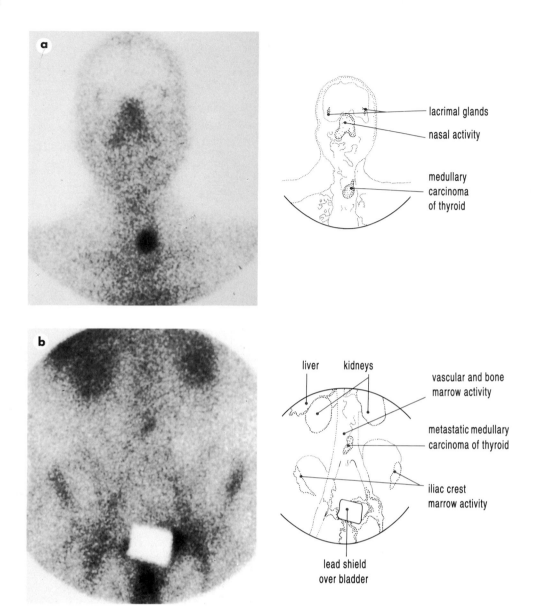

Fig. 25.10 Medullary carcinoma of the thyroid (MCT) imaged with ⁹⁹ᵐTc dimercaptosuccinic acid (DMSA-V). These images were taken four hours after intravenous injection of ⁹⁹ᵐTc DMSA-V. In (a) the head and neck have focally increased uptake in the region of the thyroid to the left of the midline. Note normal thyroid tissue is not shown. Image of the anterior abdomen (b); in the centre of the abdomen a small area of increased uptake is seen which was subsequently shown to be a metastasis of the MCT. ⁹⁹ᵐTc DMSA-V is taken up by several other tumours and by some types of amyloid. Its most consistent uptake is in MCT and it is used to demonstrate primary and recurrent disease. MCT does not take up radioiodine or ⁹⁹ᵐTc pertechnetate and appears as a 'cold' area on a conventional thyroid scan.

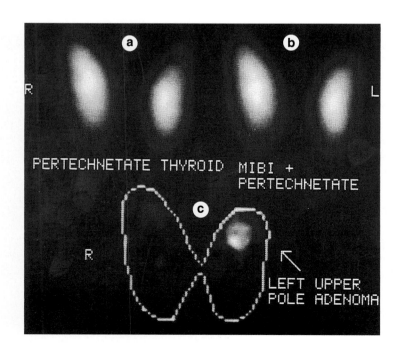

Fig. 25.11 Imaging of a parathyroid adenoma. Image (a) shows a pertechnetate thyroid scan obtained conventionally 10–20 minutes after the intravenous injection of ⁹⁹ᵐTc pertechnetate through an indwelling needle. Without the patient moving, ⁹⁹ᵐTc methoxyisobutylisonitrile (MIBI) is injected and a further series of images taken. In (b) ⁹⁹ᵐTc MIBI is taken up both by the parathyroid adenoma and by normal thyroid so that a combined composite image is seen. Using a change detection algorithm, the change between the two images is determined and the statistical degree of that difference is plotted as a probability. In (c) the high red and orange in the upper pole of the left lobe of the thyroid indicates a change between the two images with a significance of over one in a thousand. This is the site of the upper pole parathyroid adenoma. The outline of the thyroid is also shown. A small area of increased probability of change is also seen in the upper pole of the right lobe of the thyroid. Subsequently a left upper pole thyroid adenoma was removed and a right upper pole hyperplastic gland (100mg) was also removed. Prior to imaging, it is important biochemically to confirm that hypercalcaemia is due to hyperparathyroidism. Imaging of the parathyroid is intended to localise the site of adenomas or hyperplastic glands. Visualisation of a gland depends upon its size. A normal parathyroid gland of less than 20mg will not be visualised by this technique. Earlier attempts to image parathyroid glands using thallium in a similar way has proved less successful than the use of MIBI.

⁷⁵Se SELENOCHOLESTEROL IMAGING IN CONN'S SYNDROME

condition	uptake by adrenals	
	(involved gland)	(contralateral gland)
normal: after dexamethasone suppression:	normal none	normal none
adenoma: after dexamethasone suppression:	high high	none none
bilateral hyperplasia:		
micronodular: after dexamethasone suppression:	high none	high none
macronodular: after dexamethasone suppression:	high high	high high

Fig. 25.12 *⁷⁵Se Selenocholesterol imaging in Conn's syndrome.* Adrenal gland uptake is shown with and without dexamethasone suppression of 2mg per day, starting early on the day of the scan and continuing for two weeks. High uptake is that greater than 0.3 per cent injected activity in an adrenal gland.

⁷⁵Se SELENOCHOLESTEROL IMAGING IN CUSHING'S SYNDROME

condition	uptake by adrenals	
	(involved gland)	(contralateral gland)
normal	normal	normal
adenoma	high	none
bilateral hyperplasia	high uptake by both glands or normal uptake by one and high uptake by the other gland	
carcinoma	no uptake or rarely normal uptake	normal or none
adrenogenital syndrome	high	high

Fig 25.13 *⁷⁵Se Selenocholesterol imaging in Cushing's syndrome.* High uptake is that greater than 0.3 per cent injected activity in an adrenal gland.

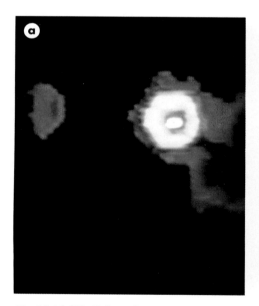 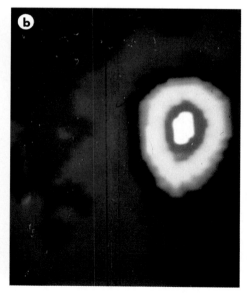

Fig. 25.14 *⁷⁵Se Selenocholesterol adrenocortical imaging in Conn's syndrome and Cushing's syndrome.* Image (a) is a posterior view of the abdomen in a patient with Conn's syndrome (primary aldosteronism). It reveals high uptake of ⁷⁵Se selenocholesterol in the right adrenal cortex, shown in red and yellow, as compared to the normal uptake in the left adrenal cortex, shown in blue. Production of aldosterone by a Conn's adenoma does not suppress the uptake of ⁷⁵Se selenocholesterol by the normal adrenal. The purpose of adrenal cortical imaging is to localise an adenoma or demonstrate bilateral hyperplasia once a positive diagnosis has been made of Conn's or Cushing's syndrome, clinically and biochemically. A second use is to demonstrate whether an adrenal mass, seen incidentally during CT imaging of the abdomen, has a functionally significant abnormality. Image (b) is a posterior view of the abdomen in a patient with Cushing's syndrome due to a solitary cortisol secreting adenoma. A high uptake of ⁷⁵Se selenocholesterol is seen in the cortisol producing adenoma. In this case, the left adrenal is not visualised because of suppression of ACTH by the high cortisol level, thereby reducing the normal uptake of ⁷⁵Se selenocholesterol.

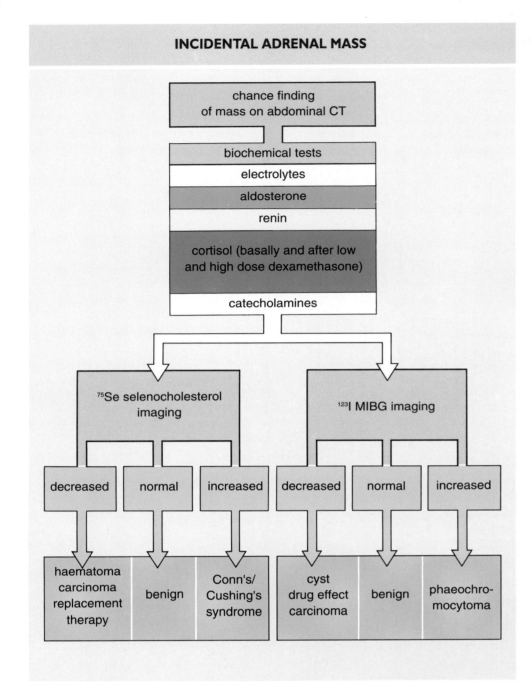

Fig. 25.15 *Incidental adrenal mass (an incidentaloma): a scheme for investigation and diagnosis.*

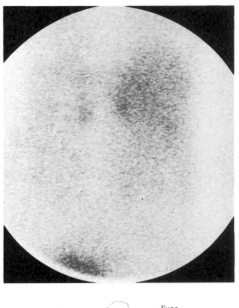

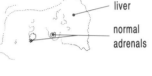
- liver
- normal adrenals

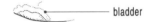
- bladder

Fig. 25.16 *Imaging of the adrenal medulla and neuroendocrine tumours with ^{123}I (MIBG) meta-iodobenzylguanidine at 24 hours, posterior view.* Normal appearance of the liver and two adrenal medullae are seen. Radioiodinated MIBG has been used both for the diagnosis and treatment of phaeochromocytomas, paragangliomas, neuroblastomas, carcinoid tumours and medullary carcinomas of the thyroid. Due to its structural similarity to noradrenaline it is taken up by the adrenal medulla and other tissues with rich sympathetic innervation, mostly via the neuronal uptake-1 system.

Fig. 25.17 *A table of drugs that interfere with radioiodinated MIBG imaging and therapy.* Recommended withdrawal periods prior to study or therapy are given.

DRUGS INTERFERING WITH RADIOIODINATED MIBG UPTAKE AND THERAPY

compound	withdrawal period (days)
inhalers, e.g. salbutamol and related compounds	1
isoprenaline derivatives	1
ephedrine and related compounds	2
noradrenaline and related compounds	2
fenfluramine	2
amitriptyline and related antidepressants	2
chlorpromazine, haloperidol and related compounds	2
guanethidine and related compounds	2
verapamil	2
nasal drops, e.g. containing phenylephedrine	2
reserpine	3
labetalol	3
phenoxybenzamine (high i.v. dose, not standard oral dose)	—

¹²³I MIBG SCINTIGRAPHY OF A NEUROENDOCRINE TUMOUR

Fig. 25.18 Scheme for diagnosis of a suspected neuroendocrine tumour using ¹²³I MIBG scintigraphy.

clinical and biochemical evidence of a neuroendocrine tumour

↓

¹²³I MIBG scan → positive scan

↓

negative scan

↓

re-check for interfering medication → positive scan

↓

negative scan

↓

strong clinical and biochemical evidence

↓

CT scan relevant areas

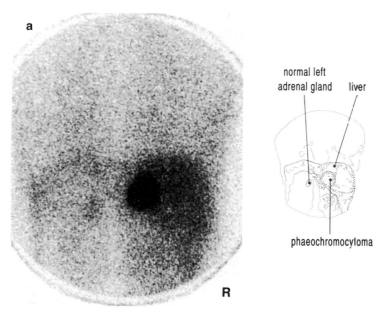

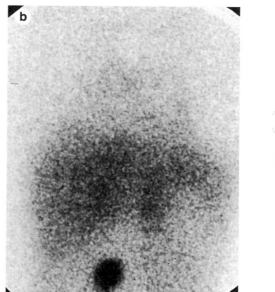

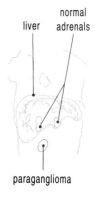

normal left adrenal gland   liver

phaeochromocytoma

R

liver   normal adrenals

paraganglioma

Fig. 25.19 *¹²³I MIBG imaging in a patient with phaeochromocytoma and a patient with paraganglioma.* In (a) focally increased uptake is seen in the right adrenal region (phaeochromocytoma) and normal uptake is seen in the left adrenal gland. Note that the high levels of circulating adrenaline and noradrenaline have not suppressed the uptake and storage of MIBG by the normal adrenal medulla but cardiac uptake is reduced. In (b) high uptake is seen focally in an area in the upper abdomen, inferior to the liver. Uptake in the two normal adrenal medullae is also seen. This technique is 95 per cent accurate in the localisation of paraganglioma and phaeochromocytoma.

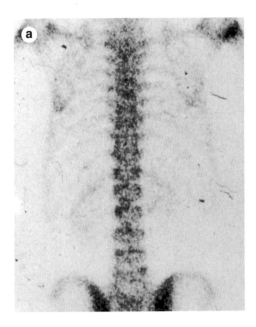

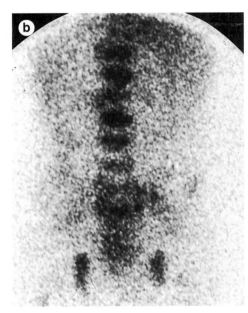

Fig. 25.20 Child with neuroblastoma; a posterior view of the spine. In (a) the bone scan is almost normal and the ¹²³I MIBG image (b) at 24 hours shows multiple sites of increased uptake in the marrow of almost all vertebrae and sacroiliac regions. ¹³¹I MIBG therapy for childhood neuroblastoma is introduced after the initial chemotherapy and surgery for the tumour. Both complete and partial remissions have been obtained, but the therapy is palliative rather than curative.

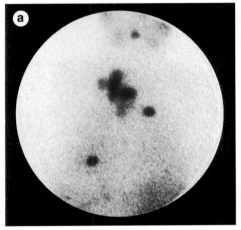

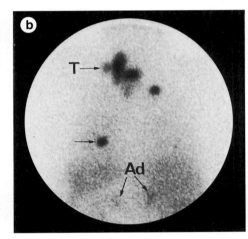

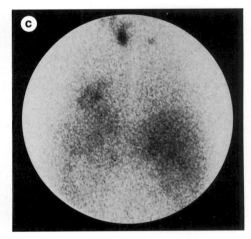

Fig. 25.21 Therapy of malignant paraganglioma with ¹³¹I MIBG. The anterior view (a) of the thorax shows multiple sites of abnormal uptake in the upper mediastinum before therapy. During a course of therapy (b): after a total of two doses of 8.9GBq (240mCi) of ¹³¹I MIBG, six months later (T; mediastinal tumour: arrow; lung metastasis: Ad; adrenal medulla). Image (c) taken after a total of approximately 37GBq (1Ci) of ¹³¹I MIBG, five years later. The reduction in uptake is evident. Before therapy, this patient was incapacitated with symptoms and could not work. After therapy he resumed full-time work, was taken off of all drugs and has fathered three

healthy children. In malignant phaeochromocytoma, paraganglioma and some metastatic carcinoids a good clinical and biochemical response is seen after ¹³¹I MIBG therapy. There is usually reduction of active tumour mass observed on CT. There may be residual sites of uptake seen even though the patient is asymptomatic and catecholamine levels are normal. As the cell turnover in such tumours is slow, so is the interval to response. Thus, benefit may not be clearly established until more than nine months have passed and, therefore, a course of treatment must be planned.

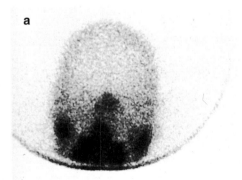

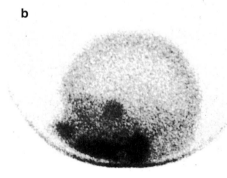

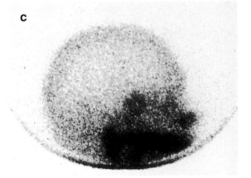

Fig. 25.22 Images in a patient with acromegaly using ¹²³I tyr-3-octreotide (somatostatin analogue). The planar images are taken at 10–20 minutes after injection: (a) anterior view; (b) left lateral view; (c) right lateral image of the head. There is intense focally increased uptake

in the pituitary region due to the presence of somatostatin receptors on the cells of the tumour, which are labelled. Such patients respond to octreotide, therapeutically, with reduction in circulating growth hormone. Indium (¹¹¹In) labelled octreotide analogue may also be used for imaging.

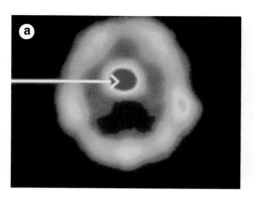
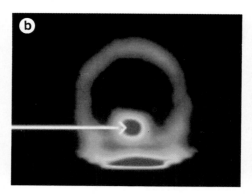
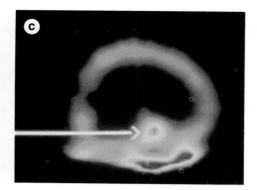

Fig. 25.23 Images of acromegaly taken with single photon emission tomography (SPECT) using ^{123}I octreotide. Image (a) shows a transaxial image through the pituitary adenoma, shown in red; (b) a coronal section; (c) a sagittal section also showing the pituitary adenoma (arrow).

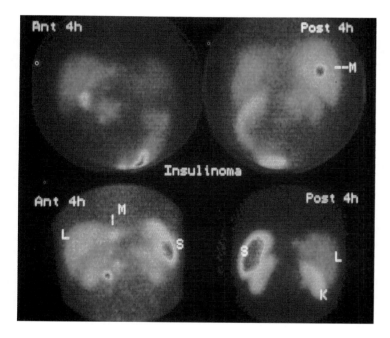

Fig. 25.24 Images of a patient with a metastatic insulinoma before and after chemotherapy. Images above are acquired with ^{123}I octreotide: the upper left image is an anterior view of the abdomen showing the liver outline with some activity in the gall bladder and gut; the upper right image is a posterior view showing the metastatic site (M indicates the tumour) in the posterior part of the liver. Below are images acquired with ^{111}In octreotide after chemotherapy. The lower left image is an anterior view of the abdomen showing the liver (L), spleen (S) and a metastatic site (M) in the left lobe of the liver. Some activity is noted in the kidneys since this is the normal route of excretion for this agent. The lower right image is a posterior view of the abdomen showing the liver (L), spleen (S) and kidney (K). Note that the lesion in the posterior part of the liver, detected with ^{123}I octreotide prior to chemotherapy (upper right), shows complete regression. A majority of gastroendocrine tumours have somatostatin receptors and can be imaged with radiolabelled octreotide. This technique can be used to image insulinomas, carcinoids, vipomas and gastrinomas in principle and to assess these tumours before and after therapy.

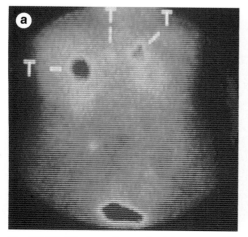
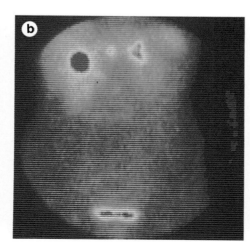
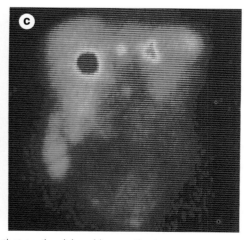

Fig. 25.25 Metastatic carcinoid tumour. ^{111}In octreotide scans taken at (a) 10 minutes, (b) 4 hours and (c) 21 hours show uptake in the metastases (T). Excreted activity is seen in the urinary bladder in the lower part of images (a) and (b). Note that on the delayed images the target to background ratio improves.

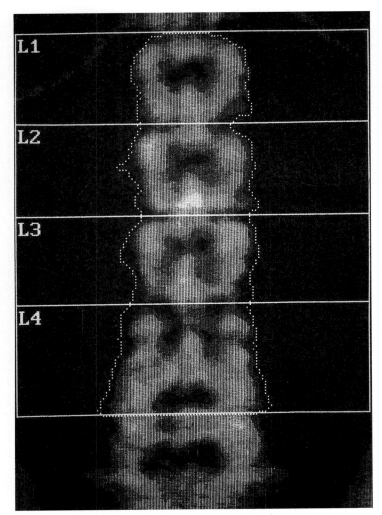

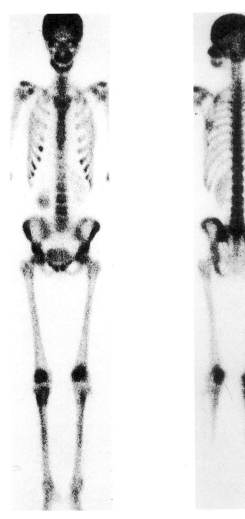

Fig. 25.26 Bone mineral densitometry measurement of the lumbar spine using Dual Energy X-ray Absorptiometry. The method is based on measurement of the radiation transmission of two separate X-ray energies through a medium consisting primarily of two different materials, bone and soft tissue. The total bone mineral content of L2–L4 is measured in grams of hydroxyapatite equivalent (gHA) and expressed as gHA/cm². The normal range depends on age, sex, weight and ethnic origin. Bone mineral measurements from the lumbar spine, femoral neck and radius are used to assess the bone mass and predict the risk of fractures at these sites.

Fig. 25.27 Bone scan in hyperparathyroidism. Images were acquired three hours after injection of ^{99m}Tc MDP (methylene diphosphonate). The bone scan shows increased uptake in the skull, spine and long bones. There is also osteomalacia as shown by the symmetrically increased costochondral uptake. Bone scans with the use of ^{99m}Tc labelled diphosphonates provides a functional display of skeletal metabolic activity. It may be used in conditions such as osteomalacia, renal osteodystrophy, hyperparathyroidism and osteoporosis, to identify focal lesions, e.g. pseudofractures, vertebral collapse, avascular necrosis and generalised increase in bone activity.

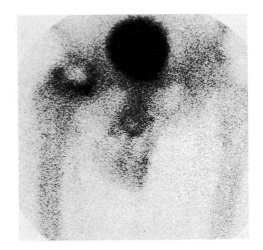

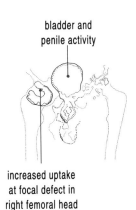

bladder and penile activity

increased uptake at focal defect in right femoral head

Fig. 25.28 Bone scan in avascular necrosis. There is high uptake around a central defect in the head of the right femur. Activity in the bladder and penis is seen centrally. The result is typical of an avascular necrosis of the head of the femur due to prolonged corticosteroid therapy.

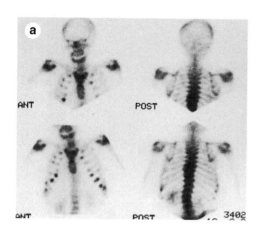

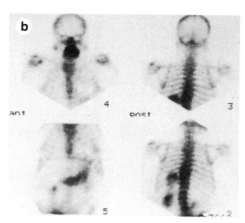

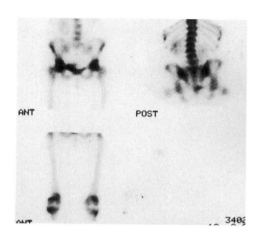

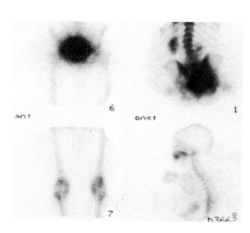

Fig. 25.29 Bone scan in osteomalacia.
Bone scans before and after overtreatment with vitamin D derivatives. The set of images (a) show the following features of osteomalacia: the rickety rosary, symmetrically increased uptake in the costochondral junctions, increased periarticular uptake and increased uptake in the right superior pubic ramus (a pseudofracture). The set of images (b) show that overtreatment has returned all the above features to normal but there is hypercalcaemia, a feature of which is intense uptake of the bone imaging agent in the stomach. Renal uptake is also more intense.

anterior   posterior   anterior   posterior

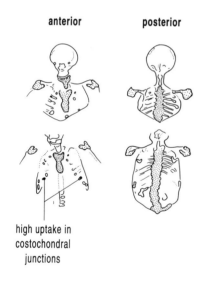

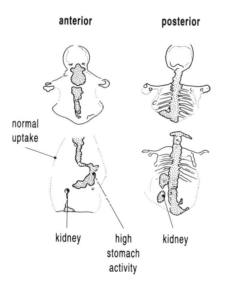

normal uptake

high uptake in costochondral junctions

kidney   high stomach activity   kidney

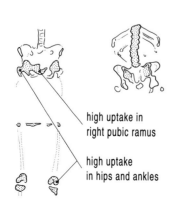

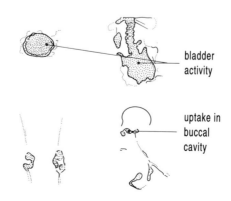

high uptake in right pubic ramus

high uptake in hips and ankles

bladder activity

uptake in buccal cavity

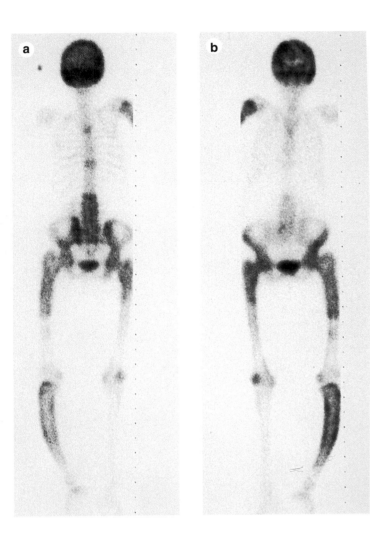

Fig. 25.30 Bone scan in Paget's disease. The ^{99m}Tc MDP bone scan shows high uptake in the skull, sites in the thoracic and lumbar spine, pelvis, proximal femur and left 'sabre' tibia: (a) posterior view; (b) anterior view.

ENDOCRINE NORMAL RANGES

The ranges given here are guidelines only, because laboratories use different reagents and therefore may obtain somewhat different values in the same situations. Each laboratory must derive its own normal ranges. Conversion factor (cf) is shown.

ADRENAL STEROIDS

	Traditional Units	cf	SI Units
Aldosterone			
Normal diet			
upright (4 h)	12–30ng/dl	27.7	330–830pmol/l
supine (30 min)	5–14.5ng/dl		135–400pmol/l
Cortisol			
09.00 h	7–25µg/dl	27.6	200–700nmol/l
18.00 h	3.5–10µg/dl		100–300nmol/l
24.00 h (asleep)	<1.8µg/dl		<50nmol/l
low/dose dexamethasone suppression test (2mg/day for 48 h)	<5µg/dl		<140nmol/l
after insulin-induced hypoglycaemia (blood glucose <2.2mmol/1 or <40ng/dl)	>21µg/dl		>580nmol/l
11-deoxycortisol	0.9–1.6µg/dl	28.8	24–46nmol/l
Dehydroepiandosterone (DHEA)			
09.00	2–9µg/l	3.4	7–31nmol/l
DHEA-sulphate			
women	1100–4400ng/ml	0.0027	3–12µmol/l
men	750–3700ng/ml		2–10µmol/l
pre-pubertal	<185ng/ml		<0.5µmol/l
Androstenedione			
adults	0.9–2.3µg/l	3.49	3–8nmol/l
prepubertal children	<0.3µg/l		<1nmol/l
17-hydroxyprogesterone			
males	0.3–3µg/l	3.3	1–10nmol/l
females			
follicular	0.3–3µg/l		1–10nmol/l
luteal	3–6µg/l		10–20nmol/l
Neonatal (i.e. from 32 weeks gestation to 2 weeks post-partum)	<24µg/l		<80nmol/l
Oestradiol			
prepuberty	<6pg/ml	3.6	<20pmol/l
women:			
postmenopausal	<30pg/ml		<100pmol/l
follicular phase	55–110pg/ml		200–400pmol/l
mid-cycle	110–330pg/ml		400–1200pmol/l
luteal	110–274pg/ml		400–1000pmol/l
men	<50pg/ml		<180pmol/l
Progesterone			
women:			<57pmol/l
follicular phase	<3ng/ml	3.2	<10nmol/l
luteal	>10ng/ml		>30nmol/l/l
men	<2ng/ml		<6nmol/l
Testosterone			
prepubertal children	<0.2ng/ml	3.46	<0.8nmol/l
women	0.14–0.87ng/ml		0.5–3nmol/l (median 18nmol/l)
men	2.5–10ng/ml		9–35nmol/l (median 1.5nmol/l)
Dihydrotestosterone (DHT)			
women	0.087–0.27ng/ml	3.44	0.3–9.3nmol/l
men	0.29–0.76ng/ml		1–2.6nmol/l

PANCREATIC AND GUT HORMONES

	Traditional Units	cf	SI Units
Gastrin	<120pg/ml	0.45	<55pmol/l
Insulin			
overnight fasting	<16µU/ml	7.18	<114µmol/l
after hypoglycaemia (blood glucose < 2.2 mmol/1 or < 40ng/dl)	<3µU/ml		<21µmol/l
Carcinoembryonic antigen (CEA)	<5ng/ml	1	<5µg/l
Vasoactive Intestinal Polypeptide (VIP)	<72pg/ml	0.42	<30pmol/l
Pancreatic Polypeptide (PP)	<1260pg/ml	0.24	<300pmol/l
Glucagon	<175pg/ml	0.28	<50pmolmcl/l

ANTERIOR PITUITARY HORMONES

	Traditional Units	cf	SI Units
Adrenocorticotrophic Hormone (ACTH) (plasma)			
09.00	<80pg/ml	0.22	<18pmol/l
Follicle Stimulating Hormone (FSH)			
women:			
follicular phase	2.5–10mU/ml	1	2.5–10U/l
midcycle	6–25mU/ml		25–70U/l
luteal phase	0.3–2.1mU/ml		>0.32–2.1U/l
postmenopausal	>30mU/ml		>30U/l
men	1–7mU/ml		1–7U/i
prepubertal children	<5mU/ml		<5U/l
Growth Hormone (GH)			
basal, fasting and between pulses	<0.5ng/ml	2	<1mU/l
after hypoglycaemia	>20ng/ml		>40mU/l
Luteinising Hormone (LH)			
women:			
follicular phase	2.5–10mU/ml	1	2.5–10U/l
midcycle	25–70mU/ml		25–70U/l
luteal phase	<1–13mU/ml		<1–13U/l
postmenopausal	>30mU/ml		>30U/l
men	1–10mU/ml		1–10U/l
prepubertal children	<5mU/ml		<5U/l
Prolactin (PRL)	<18ng/ml	20	<360mU/l
Thyroid Stimulating Hormone (TSH)	0.4–5µU/ml	1	0.4–5mU/l

THYROID HORMONES

	Traditional Units	cf	SI Units
Thyroglobulin	<1.2ng/ml		N/A
Thyroxine T$_4$			
free	0.8–1.8ng/ml	12.9	10–22pmol/l
total	5–12µg/ml	12.9	58–174nmol/l
Triiodothyronine T$_3$			
free	3.5–6.5pg/ml	1.54	5–10pmol/l
total	70–220ng/ml	0.015	1.07–3.18nmol/l

CATECHOLAMINES (plasma, lithium heparin)

(lying and with venous catheter in place for 30 min prior to collection of sample)

	Traditional Units	cf	SI Units
Adrenaline (epinephrine)	0.01–0.25ng/ml	5.46	0.03–1.31nmol/l
Noradrenaline (norepinephrine)	0.08–0.75ng/ml	5.99	0.47–4.14nmol/l

Age related insulin-like growth factor-1 (IGF-1)

	Traditional Units	cf	SI Units
0–3yrs	7–100ng/ml	7.5	0.9–13.3nmol/l
4–6yrs	14–175ng/ml		1 9–23.3nmol/l
7–9yrs	42–210ng/ml		5 6–28.0nmol/l
10–12yrs	50–280ng/ml		6 7–37.3nmol/l
13–15yrs	70–420ng/ml		9 3–56.0nmol/l
16–18yrs	70–420ng/ml		9.3–56.0nmol/l
20–40yrs	56–280ng/ml		7.5–37.3nmol/l
40–60yrs	42–175ng/ml		5.6–23.3nmol/l
over 60 yrs	25–175ng/ml		3.3–23.3nmol/l
Parathyroid Hormone (PTH)	9–54ng/l	10	0.9–5.4pmol/l
Alpha-Fetoprotein (AFP)	<10mg/dl	1	<10U/ml
Beta Human Chorionic Gonadotrophin (ß-hCG)	<50mU/ml	1	<50U/l
Calcitonin (plasma lithium heparin)	<80pg/l	1	<80ng/l

URINARY VALUES

	Traditional Units	cf	SI Units
Aldosterone	5–19µg/24h	2.8	14–53nmol/24h
Calcium	<300mg/24h	0.025	<7.5mmol/24h
Cortisol	20–100µg/24h	2.76	55–250nmol/24h
5-Hydroxyindoleacetic Acid (5-HIAA)	<9mg/24h	5.24	<75µmol/24h
Metanephrins	<12mg/24h	5.46	<63µmol/24h
Vanillyl Mandelic Acid (VMA)	1–7mg/24h	5	5–35µmol/24h
Adrenaline (epinephrine)	26µg/24h	5.46	<144nmol/24h
Noradrenaline (norepinephrine)	97µg/24h	5.46	<570nmol/24h
Dopamine	<585µg/24h	5.27	<3100nmol/24h

ACKNOWLEDGEMENTS

1 NEUROENDOCRINE CONTROL OF PITUITARY FUNCTION

Fig 1.1 redrawn from Reichlin S. Introduction. In: Reichlin S, Baldessarini RJ, Martin JB eds., *The Hypothalamus* 1977: 1–14. *Courtesy of Raven Press, New York.*
Fig 1.2 redrawn from Gay VL. The hypothalamus: physiology and clinical use of releasing factors. *Fertil Steril* 1972;23:50–63. *Courtesy of the American Fertility Society, Baltimore.*
Fig 1.3 reproduced from Lechan RM, Nestler JL, Jacobson S. The tuberoinfundibular system of the rat as demonstrated by immunohistochemical localization of retrogradely transported wheat germ agglutinin (WGA) from the median eminence. *Brain Research* 1982;245:1–15. *Courtesy of Elsevier Biomedical Press BV, Amsterdam.*
Fig 1.4b reproduced from Reichlin S. Neuroendocrinology. In: Williams RH ed., *Textbook of Endocrinology*, 6th edition. 1981: 589–645. *Courtesy of WB Saunders Company, Philadelphia.*
Figs 1.5 and 1.6 reproduced from Dyess et al. *Endocrinology* 1988;123:2291–7
Figs 1.13 and 1.19 redrawn from Reichlin S. Neuroendocrinology. In: Wilson JD, Foster DW eds., *Williams - Textbook of Endocrinology.* 7th edition. 1985: 492–567. *Courtesy of WB Saunders Company, Philadelphia.*
Fig 1.16 redrawn from Crowley WF Jr, McArthur JW. Stimulation of the normal menstrual cycle in Kallman's syndrome by pulsatile administration of luteinizing hormone-releasing hormone (LHRH). *J Clin Endocrinoly and Metab* 1980;51:173–175. *Courtesy of Williams and Wilkins Company, Baltimore.*
Fig 1.17 redrawn from Belchetz PE, Plant TM, Nakai Y, et al. Hypophysial responses to continuous and intermittent delivery of hypothalamic gonadotropin-releasing hormone. *Science* 1978;202:631–633. *Courtesy of the American Association for the Advancement of Science, Washington.*
Fig 1.18 redrawn from Thorner MO, Rivier J, Spiess J, et al. Human pancreatic growth-hormone-releasing factor selectively stimulates growth-hormone secretion in man. *Lancet* 1983;1: 24–28. *Courtesy of Lancet Ltd., London.*
Fig 1.22 redrawn from Grossman A, Kruseman ACN, Perry L, et al. New Hypothalamic hormone, corticotropin-releasing factor, specifically stimulates the release of adreno-corticotropic hormone and cotisol in man. *Lancet* 1982;1:921–2. *Courtesy of Lancet Ltd., London.*
Figs 1.23 and 1.24 redrawn from Martin JB, Reichlin S, Brown GM. *Clinical Neuroendocrinology.* 1977: 410pp. *Courtesy of FA Davis Company, Philadelphia.*

For kind provision of slides: Dr RM Lechan, Dr L Alpert and Dr JC King.

2 HYPOPITUITARISM

Fig 2.26 redrawn from Cuneo RC, Salomon F, Sönksen PH. The growth hormone deficiency syndrome in adults. *Clin Endocrinol* 1992;37:387–97. *Courtesy of Blackwell Scientific Publications Ltd, Oxford.*
Fig 2.27. Salomon F, Cuneo RC, Hesp R, Sönsken PH. The effects of treatment with recombinant GH on body compostition and metabolism in adults with GH deficiency. *N Eng J Med* 1989;321:1789–803.
Figs 2.29 and 2.31 redrawn from Cuneo RC, Salomon F, Wilmshurst P, et al. Cardiovascular efect of GH treatment in growth-hormone-deficient adults: Stimulation of the rein-aldosterone system. *Clin Sci* 1991c;81:587–92.
Russell Jones DL, Weissberger AJ, Bowes SB, et al. The effects of growth hormone on protein metabolism in adult growth hormone deficient patients. *Clin Endocrinol* 1993; 38:427–31. *Courtesy Blackwell Scientific Publications Ltd, Oxford.*

For kind provision of slides: Professor I Doniach, Dr B-Å Bengtsson.

3 ACROMEGALY

Fig 3.3 reproduced from Wass JAH. Acromegaly, and Treatment of massive tumours: medical treatment. In: Belchetz PE ed., *Management of Pituitary Disease.* 1984: 123–140 and 415–423. *Courtesy of Chapman and Hall Ltd., London.*
Fig 3.19 redrawn from Laws ER, Piepgras DG, Randall RV, Abboud CF. Neurosurgical management of acromegaly. *J Neurosurgery* 1979;50:454–461. *Courtesy of the American Association of Neurological Surgeons, Hanover.*
Fig 3.16 adapted from Wright AD, Hill DM, Lowy C, Russell-Fraser T. Mortality and acromegaly. *Q J Med* 1970;39:1–16.

4 HYPERPROLACTINAEMIA

Fig 4.20 reproduced from Thorner MO, Martin WH, Rogol AD, et al. Rapid regression of pituitary prolactinomas during bromocriptine treatment. *J Clin Endocrinol Metab* 1980;51:438–445. *Courtesy of Williams and Wilkins, Baltimore.*

For kind provision of slides: Dr G Tindall.

8 CUSHING'S SYNDROME

We thank our many colleagues, clinical, radiological and pathological, for their contributions to this work, and particularly to Professor GM Besser, Professor I Doniach, Dr FE White and Mr GM Rees for permission to use their slides.

9 ADDISON'S DISEASE

Fig 9.7 modified from Takahashi H, Teranishi Y, Nakanishi S, Numa S. Isolation and structural organisation of the human corticotropin-beta-lipotropin gene. *FEBS Letters* 1981;135:97–102, and Whitfield PL, Seeburg PH, Shine J. The human pro-opiomelanocortin gene. organisation, sequence and interspersion with repetitive DNA. *DNA* 1982;1:133-143.

For kind provision of slides: Professor I Doniach.

11 THE TESTIS

Figs 11.2 and 11.3 modified from Griffin JE, Wilson JD. Disorders of the testes and male reproductive tract. In: Wilson JD, Foster DW, eds. *Williams Textbook of Endocrinology.* 7th edn. 1985. *Courtesy of WB Saunders, Philadelphia.*
Fig 11.9 modified from Frantz AG, Wilson JD. Endocrine disorders of the breast. In: Wilson JD, Foster DW, eds. *Williams Textbook of Endocrinology.* 8th edn. 1992. *Courtesy of WB Saunders, Philadelphia.*
Fig 11.11 modified from Griffin JE. Androgen resistance – the clinical and molecular spectrum. *N Engl J Med* 1992;326:611-8. *Courtesy of New England Journal of Medicine.*
Fig 11.15 modified from Griffin JE, Wilson JD. The testis. In: Bondy PK, Rosenberg LE, eds. *Metabolic Control and Disease.* 8th edn. 1980. *Courtesy of WB Saunders, Philadelphia.*
Fig 11.16 modified from Wilson JD, George FW, Griffin JE. The hormonal control of sexual development. *Science* 1981;211:1278. *Courtesy of American Association for the Advancement of Science, Washington DC.*
Fig 11.20 modified from Griffin JE, Wilson JD. The testis. In: Bondy PK, Rosenberg LE, eds. *Metabolic Control and Disease.* 8th edn. 1980. *Courtesy of RM Boyar and WB Saunders, Philadelphia.*
Figs 11.34 and 11.47 modified from Griffin JE, Wilson JD. Disorders of the testes and male reproductive tract. In: Wilson JD, Foster DW, eds. *Williams Textbook of Endocrinology.* 8th edn. 1992. *Courtesy of WB Saunders, Philadelphia.*
Fig 11.45 from Mostofi FK. Pathology of germ cell tumors of testis – a progress report. *Cancer* 1980;45:1745-54. *Courtesy JB Lippincott Compnay, Philadelphia.*

For kind provision of slides: Professor I Doniach and Dr WE Kenyon.

12 THE OVARY

Fig 12.10 modified from Erickson GF. *Semin Reprod Endocrinol* 1986;4:233.
Fig 12.16 reproduced by courtesy of Prof. Dr. med. Hans Fangenheim from Gordon AG, Lewis BV, eds. *Gynaecological Endoscopy* 1988, Gower Medical Publishing, London.
Fig 12.26 redrawn from Judd. *J Clin Endocrinol Metab* 1974;39:1020.© The Endocrine Society. *Courtesy of Williams and Wlkins, Baltimore.*
z
For kind provision of slides: Professor I Doniach, Dr JW Keeling and Dr PR Wheater.

13 NORMAL AND ABNORMAL SEXUAL DEVELOPMENT AND PUBERTY

Figs 13.2 and 13.4 reproduced from Tanner JM. *Growth at Adolescence.* 1962 *Courtesy of Blackwell Scientific Publications, Oxford.*
Fig 13.6 redrawn from Smith DW. Growth and its disorders: basics and standards, approach and classifications, growth deficiency disorders, grwoth excess disorders, obesity. *Major Problems in Clinical Pediatrics* 1977;15:1–155. *Courtesy of WB Saunders Company, Philadelphia.*
Fig 13.13 redrawn from Conte FA, Grumbach MM, Kaplan SL. A diphasic pattern of gonadotropin secretion in patients with the syndrome of gonadal dysgenesis. *J Clin Endocrinol Metab* 1975;40:670–674. *Courtesy of Williams and Wilkins Company, Baltimore.*
Fig 13.14 redrawn from Weitzman ED, Boyar RM, Kapen S, Helman L. The relationship of sleep and sleep stages to neuroendocrine secretion and biological rhythms in man. *Rect Progr Horm Res* 1975;31:399–441. *Courtesy of Academic Press, Orlando.*

15 THYROID PHYSIOLOGY AND HYPOTHYROIDISM

For kind provision of slides: Professor I Doniach.

17 HYPERTHYROIDISM AND GRAVES' DISEASE

Figs 17.9 and 17.10 modified from McGregor AM. Review: Autoimmunity in the thyroid – can the molecular revolution contribute to our understanding? *Q J Med* 1992;82:1–13. *Courtesy of Oxford University Press.*

Professor Mundy would like to acknowledge the advice and provision of some of the slides from my colleagues Professors AM McGregor, AP Weetman, and R Marshall, and Drs JH Lazarus, MD Hourihan, S Renowden, H Adams, P Wise, and B Jasani.

23 RADIOLOGY OF ENDOCRINE DISEASE

Fig 23.20 reproduced from White FE, White MC, Drury PL, et al. Value of computed tomography of the abdomen and chest in the investigation of Cushing's syndrome. *Br Med J* 1982;284:771–774. *Courtesy of the British Medical Journal, London.*

REFERENCES

1 NEUROENDOCRINE CONTROL OF PITUITARY FUNCTION

Brazeau P, Vale W, Burgus R, *et al*. Hypothalmic polypeptide that inhibits the secretion of immunoreactive pituitary growth hormone. *Science* 1973;**179**:77–79.

Campbell HJ, Feuer G, Harris GW. The effect of intrapituitary infusion of median eminence and other brain extracts on anterior pituitary gonadotrophic secretion. *J Physiol* 1964;**170**:474–86.

Du Vigneaud V, Gish DT, Katsoyannis PG, Hess GP. Synthesis of the pressor-antidiuretic hormone, arginine-vasopressin. *J Amer Chem Soc* 1958;**80**:3355.

Du Vigneaud V, Ressler C, Trippett S. The sequence of amino acids in oxytocin, with a proposal for the structure of oxytocin. *J Biol Chem* 1853;**205**:949–57.

Grossman A, Kruseman ACN, Perry L, *et al*. New hypothalamic hormone, corticotropin-releasing factor, specifically stimulates the release of adrenocorticotropic hormone and cortisol in man. *Lancet* 1982;**1**:921–2.

Guillemin R, Brazeau P, Böhlen P, *et al*. Growth hormone-releasing hormone from a human pancreatic tumour that caused acromegaly. *Science* 1982;**218**:585–587.

Guillemin R, Burgus R, Vale W. The hypothalamic hypophysiotropic thyrotropin-releasing factor. *Vit Horm* 1971;**29**:1–39.

Kamberi IA, Mical RS, Proter JC. Hypophysial portal vessel infusion: in vivo demonstration of LRF, FRF and PIF in pituitary stalk plasma. *Endocrinol* 1971;**89**;1042–46.

Krulich L, Dhariwal AP, McCann SM. Stimulatory and inhibitory effects of purified hypothalamic extracts on growth hormone release from rat pituitary in vitro. *Endocrinol* 1968;**83**:783–790.

McCann SM, Taleisnik S, Friedman HM. LH-releasing activity in hypothalamic extracts. *Society for Experimental Biology: Medical Proceedings* 1960;**104**:432–434.

Martin JB, Riechlin S, Brown GM. *Clinical Neuroendocrinology,* 2nd edn. Philadelphia: FA Davis, 1986.

Meites J. Control of mammary growth and lactation. In: Martini L, Ganong WF eds., *Neuroendocrinology*. Volume 1. Academic Press. New York 1966: 669–707.

Reichlin S. Neuroendocrinology. In: Wilson JD, Fosler DW eds., *Williams-Textbook of Endocrinology*. 7th edition. Philadelphia: WB Saunders 1985: 492–567.

Saffran M, Schally Av, Benfrey BG. Stimulation of the release of corticropin from the adenohypophysis by neurohypophysial factor. *Endocrinol* 1955;**57**:439–444.

Schally AV, Kastin AJ, Arimura A. Hypothalamic follicle-stimulating hormone (FSH) and luteinizing hormone (LH)-regulating hormone: structure, physiology and clinical studies. *Fertil Steril* 1971;**22**:703–721.

Scharrer E, Scharrer B. *Neuroendocrinology*. New York: Columbia University Press, 1963.

Thorner MO, Rivier J, Spiess J, *et al*. Human pancreatic growth-hormone-releasing factor selectively stimulates growth-hormone secretion in man. *Lancet* 1983;**1**:24–28.

Vale W, Spiess J, Rivier C, Rivier J. Characterization of a 41-residue ovine hypothalamic peptide that stimulates secretion of corticotropin and beta-endorphin. *Science* 1981;**213**:1394–97.

White WF. On the identity of the LH- and FSH-releasing hormones. In: Gibian H, Plotz EJ eds., *Mammalian Reproduction*. Berlin: Springer Verlag, 1970: 84–87.

2 HYPOPITUITARISM AND GROWTH HORMONE DEFICIENCY

Binnerts A, Swart GR, Wilson JHP, *et al*. The effect of GH administration in GH deficient adults on bone, protein, carbohydrate and lipid homeostasis, as well as on body composition. *Clin Endocrinol* 1992;**37**:79–87.

Cuneo RC, Salomon F, Sönksen PH. The growth hormone deficiency syndrome in adults. *Clin Endocrinol* 1992;**37**:387–97.

Cuneo RC, Salomon F, Wiles CM, *et al*. Growth hormone treatment in GH-deficient adults. I. Effects on muscle mass and strength. *J Appl Physiol* 1991a;**70**:688–94.

Cuneo RC, Salomon F, Wiles CM, *et al*. Growth hormone treatment in GH-deficient adults. II. Effects on exercise performance. *J Appl Physiol* 1991b;**70**:695–700.

Cuneo RC, Salomon F, Wilmshurst P, *et al*. Cardiovascular effects of GH treatment in growth-hormone-deficient adults: Stimulation of the renin–aldosterone system. *Clin Sci* 1991c;**81**:587–92.

Cuneo RC, Wilmshurst P, Lowy C, *et al*. Cardiac failure responding to GH. *Lancet* 1989;**i**:838–9.

Doniach I. Histopathology of the anterior pituitary. *Clin Endocrin Metab* 1977;**6**:21–52.

Frustaci A, Perrone GA, Gentiloni N, Russo MA. Reversible dilated cardiomyopathy due to GH deficiency. *Am J Clin Pathol* 1992;**97**:503–11.

Ho KY, Weissberger AJ. The antinatriuretic action of biosynthetic GH in man involves activation of the renin–angiotensin system. *Metabolism* 1990;**39**:133–7.

Jorgensen JOL, Pedersen SA, Thuesen L, *et al*. Beneficial effects of GH treatment in GH-deficient adults. *Lancet* 1989;**i**:1221–5.

Jorgensen JOL, Pedersen SA, Thuesen L, *et al*. Long-term GH replacement therapy in adult GH deficients for one year. *Horm Res* 1990;**33** (suppl 3):17.

Moller J, Jorgensen JOL, Moller N, *et al*. Expansion of extracellular volume and suppression of natriuretic peptide after GH administration in normal man. *J Clin Endocrinol Metab* 1991;**72**:768–72.

Rosen T, Bengtsson B-A. Premature mortality due to cardiovascular disease in hypopituitarism. *Lancet* 1990;**336**:285–8.

Russell-Jones DL, Weissberger AJ, Bowes SB, *et al*. The effects of GH on protein metabolism in adult GH deficient patients. *Clin Endocrinol* 1993;**38**:427–31.

Salomon F, Cuneo RC, Hesp R, Sönksen PH. The effects of treatment with recombinant GH on body composition and metabolism in adults with GH deficiency. *N Engl J Med* 1989;**321**:1789–803.

Snyder PJ. Gonadotroph cell pituitary adenomas. *Endocrinol Metab Clin North Am* 1987;**16**:755–64.

Sönksen PH, Salomon F, Cuneo RC, *et al*. Cardiac cachexia. *Brit Med J* 1991;**302**:725.

Vallar L, Spada A, Giannattasio G. *Nature* 1987;**330**:566–8.

Wass JAH, Besser GM. Tests of pituitary function. In: De Groot LJ, ed. *Endocrinology*. 2nd edn. Philadelphia: WB Saunders, 1989:492–502.

Whitehead HM, Boreham C, McIlrath EM, *et al*. Growth hormone treatment of adults with growth hormone deficiency: Results of a 13 month placebo controlled crossover study. *Clin Endocrinol* 1992;**36**:45–52.

3 ACROMEGALY

Alexander L, Appleton D, Hall R., *et al*. Epidemiology of acromegaly in the Newcastle region. *Clin Endocrinol* 1980;**12**:71–79.

Battershill PE, Clissold SP. Octreotide, a review of its pharmaco-dynamic properties and therapeutic potential in conditions associated with excessive peptide secretion. *Drugs* 1989;**38**:658–702.

Jones AE. Radiation oncogenesis in relation to the treatment of pituitary tumours. *Clin Endocrinol* 1991;**35**:379–398.

Wass, JAH, Laws ER, Randall, RV, Sheline GE. The treatment of acromegaly. *Clin Endocrin Metab* 1986;**15**:683–707.

Wright AD, Hill DM, Lowy C, Russell-Fraser T. Mortality and acromegaly. *Q J Med* 1970;**39**:1–16.

4 HYPERPROLACTINAEMIA

Chiodini P, Liuzzi A, Cozzi R, *et al*. Size reduction of macroprolactinomas by bromocriptine or lisuride treatment. *J Clin Endocrin Metab* 1981;**53**:737-743.

Hardy J, Le Prolactinome (prolactinoma). *Neurochirurgie* 1981; **27** (suppl. 1):1–110.

Molitch ME, Elton RL, Blackwell RE, *et al*. Bromocriptine as primary therapy for prolactin-secreting macroadenomas: results of a prospective multicenter study. *J Clin Endocrinol Metab* 1985;**60**:698–705.

Thorner MO, Evans WS, MacLeod RM, *et al*. Hyperprolactinaemia: current concepts of management including medical therapy with bromocriptine. In: Goldstein G, Calne DB, Leiberman A, Thorner MO eds., *Ergot Compounds and Brain Functon-Neuroendocrine Aspects*. Raven Press, New York 1980: 165–189.

Thorner MO, Martin WH , Rogol AD, *et al*. Rapid regression of pituitary prolactinomas during bromocriptine treatment. *J Clin Endocrinol Metab* 1980;**51**:438–445.

Thorner MO, Perryman RL, Rogol AD, *et al*. Rapid changes of pro-lactinoma volume after withdrawal and reinstitution of bromocriptine. J *Clin Endocrinol Metab* 1981;**53**:480–483.

Thorner MO, Martin WH, Rogol AD, *et al*. Rapid regression of pituitary prolactinomas during bromocriptine treatment. *J Clin Endocrinol Metab* 1980:**51**:438.45

Thorner MO, Perryman RL, Rogol AD, *et al*. Rapid changes of pro-lactinoma volume after withdrawal and reinstitution of bromocriptine. *J Clin Endocrinol Metab* 1981;**53**:480–3.

Thorner MO, Vance ML, Horvath E, Kovacs K. In: Wilson JD, Foster DW, eds. *Williams' Textbook of endocrinology*. Philadelphia: WB Saunders. 1991: 221–310.

5 THE POSTERIOR PITUITARY

Bartter FC, Schwartz WB. The syndrome of inappropriate secretion of antidiuretic hormone. *Am J Med* 1967;**42**:790–806.

Baylis PH, Thompson CJ. Osmoregulation of vasopressin secretion and thirst in health and disease. *Clin Endocrinol* 1988;**29**:549–76.

Chard T. Oxytocin: Physiology and pathophysiology. In: Baylis PH, Padfield PL, eds. *The posterior pituitary: Hormone secretion in health and disease*. New York: Marcel Dekker, 1985:361–90.

Robertson GL. Posterior pituitary. In: Felig P, Baxter JD, Broadus AE, Frohman LA, eds. *Endocrinology and metabolism*. New York: McGraw-Hill, 1987:338–85.

Stearns RH, Riggs J, Schochet SS. Osmotic demyelination syndrome following correction of hyponatraemia. *New Engl J Med* 1986; **314**: 1535–42.

Verbalis JG. Inappropriate antidiuresis and other hypoosmolar states. In: Becker KL, ed. *Principles and practice of endocrinology and metabolism*. Philadelphia: JB Lippincott, 1990:237–47.

6 LIPIDS AND LIPOPROTEINS

Breslow JL. Familial disorders of high density lipoprotein metabolism. In: Scriver CR, Beaudet AL, Sly WS, Valle D, eds. *Metabolic basis of inherited diseases*. 6th edn. New York: McGraw-Hill, 1989:1251–66.

Brunzell JD. The hyperlipoproteinemias. In: Wyngaarden JD, Smith LH, Bennett JC, eds. *Cecil textbook of medicine*. 19th edn. Philadelphia: WB Saunders, 1992:1082–90.

Chait A. Hyperlipidemia. In: Rakel RE, ed. *Conn's current therapy*. Philadelphia, WB Saunders.1992:504–9.

Chait A, Brunzell JD. Chylomicronemia syndrome. *Adv Int Med* 1991;**37**:249–73.

Goldstein JL, Brown MS. Familial hypercholesterolemia. In: Scriver CR, Beaudet AL, Sly WS, Valle D, eds. *Metabolic basis of inherited diseases*. 6th edn. New York: McGraw-Hill, 1989:1215–60.

LaRosa JC. Disorders of lipid metabolism. *Endocrinol Metab Clin N Am* 1991;19:211–467.

Study Group, European Atherosclerosis Society. The recognition and management of hyperlipidaemia in adults: A policy statement of the European Atherosclerosis Society. *Eur Heart J* 1988;**9**:571–600.

The Expert Panel. Report of the National Cholesterol Education Program Expert Panel on detection, evaluation, and treatment of high blood cholesterol in adults. *Arch Int Med* 1988;**18**:36–69.

Thompson GR. *A handbook of hyperlipidaemia*. London: Current Science, 1989.

7 ADRENAL CORTEX PHYSIOLOGY

Beato M. Gene regulation by steroid hormones. *Cell* 1989; **56**:335–44.

Brown MS, Kovanen PT, Goldstein JL. Receptor-mediated uptake of lipoprotein-cholesterol and its utilization for steroid synthesis in the adrenal cortex. *Recent Prog Horm Res* 1979;**35**:215–57.

Dallman MF, Akana SF, Cascio CS, *et al*. Regulation of ACTH secretion. *Recent Prog Horm Res* 1987;**43**:113–74.

James VHT. *Comprehensive endocrinology: The adrenal gland*. New York: Raven Press, 1992.

Lieberman S, Prasad VVK. Heterox notions on pathways of steroidogenesis. *Endocr Rev* 1990;**11**:469–93.

Makin HJL. *Biochemistry of steroid hormones*. 2nd edn. Oxford: Blackwell Scientific Publications, 1984.

Miller WM. Molecular biology of steroid hormone synthesis. *Endocr Rev* 1988;**9**:295–318.

Moore CCD, Miller WL. The role of transcriptional regulation in steroid hormone biosynthesis. *J Steroid Biochem Mol Biol* 1991;**40**:517–25.

Muller J. *Regulation of aldosterone biosynthesis*. Berlin: Springer, 1988.

Parker LN. *Adrenal androgens in clinical medicine*. San Diego: Academic Press, 1989.

8 CUSHING'S SYNDROME

Beardwell C, Robertson GL eds., *The Pituitary*. Butterworth's International Medical Reviews, London 1981: 337pp.

Crapo L. Cushing's syndrome: a review of diagnostic tests. *Metabolism* 1979;**28**:955-977.Faiman C. The etiology and management of Cushing's syndrome. In: Anderson DC, Winter JSD eds., *Adrenal Cortex*. Butterworth's International Medical Reviews, London 1985:154–168.

Howlett TA, Rees LH, Besser GM. Cushing's syndrome. *Clinics in Endocrinology and Metabolism* 1985;**14**:911–945.

Krieger DT. Physiopathology of Cushing's disease. *Endocrine Reviews* 1983;**4**:22–43.

Nelson DH. Cushing's Syndrome. In: De Groot LJ, ed. *Endocrinology*. Philadelphia: WB Saunders, 1989.

Ross EJ, Linch DC. Cushing's syndrome - killing disease: discriminatory values of signs and symptoms aiding early diagnosis. *Lancet* 1982;**2**:646-649.

Trainer PJ, Besser GM. The diagnosis and differential diagnosis of Cushing's syndrome. *Clin Endocrinol* 1991;**34**:317–30.

Trainer PJ, Lawrie HS, Verhelst J *et al*. Transsphenoidal resection in Cushing's disease: undetectable serum cortisol as the definition of successful treatment. *Clin Endocrinol* 1993;**38**:73–78.

Verhelst JA, Trainer PJ, Howlett TA *et al*. Short and long-term responses to metyrapone in the medical management of 91 patients with Cushing's syndrome. *Clin Endocrinol* 1991;**35**:169–78.

9 ADDISON'S DISEASE

Bondy PK. Disorders of the adrenal cortex. In: Wilson JD, Foster DW eds., *Williams - Textbook of Endocrinology. 7th edition*. WB Saunders Company, Philadelphia 1985: 816–890.

Gilkes JJH, Rees LH, Besser GM. Plasma immunoreactive corticotrophin and lipotrophin in Cushing's syndrome and Addison's disease. *Br Med J* 1977;**1**:966–998.

Hornsby PH. The regulation of adrenocortical function by control of growth and structure. In: Anderson DC, Winter JSD eds., *Adrenal Cortex*. Butterworth's International Medical Reviews, London 1985: 1–31.

Irvine WJ, TOft Ad, Feek CM. Addison's disease. In: James VHT ed., *Comprehensive Endocrinology. The Adrenal Gland*. Raven Press, New York 1979: 131–164.

Takahashi H, Teranishi Y, Nakanishi S, Numa S. Isolation and structural organisation of the human corticotropin-beta-lipotropin gene. *FEBS Letters* 1981;**135**:97–102.

Whitfeld PL, Seeburg PH, Shine J. The human pro-opiomelancortin gene: organisation, sequence and interspersion with repetitive DNA. *DNA* 1982;**1**:133–143.

10 ENDOCRINE HYPERTENSION

Biglieri EG, Herron MA, Brust N. 17-hydroxylation deficiency in man. *Journal of Clinical Investigation* 1966;**45**;1946–1954.

Breslin DJ, Swinton NW, Libertino JA, Zinman L, eds., *Renovascular Hypertension*. Williams and Wilkins Company, Baltimore 1982: 210pp.

Edwards CRW, Carey RM eds., *Essential Hypertension as an Endocrine Disease*. Butterworth's International Medical Reviews, London 1985: 380pp.

Edwards CRW, Stewart PM, Burt D, *et al*. Tissue localisation of 11β-hydroxysteroid dehydrogenase - Tissue-specific protector of the mineralocorticoid receptor. *Lancet* 1988;**ii**:986–9.

Mantero F. Biglieri EG, Edwards CRW eds., Endocrinology of Hypertension. *Proceedings of the Serono Symposium*, Volume 50. Academic Press, London 1982: 434pp.

Stewart PM, Corrie JET, Shackleton CHL, Edwards CRW. The syndrome of "apparent mineralocorticoid excess": a defect in the cortisol cortisone shuttle. *J Clin Invest* 1988;**82**:340–9.

Stewart PM, Wallace AM, Valention R, *et al*. Mineralocorticoid activity of liquorice: 11b-hydroxysteroid dehydrogenase deficiency comes of age. *Lancet* 1987;**ii**:821–4.

Vallotton MB, Favre L,. The adrenal cortex and hypertension. In: Anderson DC, Winter JSD eds., *Adrenal Cortex*. Butterworth's International Medical Reviews, London 1985: 169–187.

11 THE TESTIS

Frantz AG, Wilson JD. Endocrine disorders of the breast. In: Wilson JD, Foster DW, eds. *Williams textbook of endocrinology.* 8th edn. Philadelphia: WB Saunders, 1991:953–75.

Griffin JE. Androgen resistance–the clinical and molecular spectrum. *N Engl J Med* 1992;**326**:611–618.

Griffin JE, Wilson JD. The androgen resistance syndromes: 5α-reductase deficiency, testicular feminization, and related disorders. In: Scriver CR, Beaudet AL, Sly WS, Valle D, eds. *The metabolic basis of inherited disease.* 6th edn. New York: McGraw-Hill, 1989:1919–44.

Griffin JE, Wilson JD. Disorders of the testes and the male reproductive tract. In: Wilson JD, Foster DW, eds. *Williams textbook of endocrinology.* 8th edn. Philadelphia: WB Saunders, 1991:799–852.

Griffin JE, Wilson JD. Disorders of sexual differentiation. In: Walsh PC, Retik AB, Stamey TA, Vaughan ED, eds. *Campbell's textbook of urology.* 6th edn. Philadelphia: WB Saunders Company, 1992.

Grumbach MM, Conte FA. Disorders of sex differentiation. In: Wilson JD, Foster DW, eds. *Williams textbook of endocrinology.* 8th edn. Philadelphia: WB Saunders, 1991:853–951.

McPhaul MJ, Marcelli M, Tilley WD, *et al.* Androgen resistance caused by mutations in the androgen receptor gene. FASEB J 1991;**5**:2910–15.

Wilson JD. Androgen abuse by athletes. *Endocr Rev* 1988;**9**:181–99.

12 THE OVARY

Adashi EYY, Rosenwaks Z. Hirsutism and virilization. In: Rosenwaks Z, Benjamin F, Stone ML, eds. *Gynecology Principles and Practice.* New York: MacMillan, 1988:611–646.

Adashi EY. The climacteric ovary: a viable endocrine organ. *Sem Reproduct Endocrinol* 1991; **9(3)**: 200–206.

Adashi EY. The ovarian cycle. In: Yen SSC, Jaffe RB eds. *Reproduct Endocrinol.* Volume 3. New York: Saunders, 1991: 181–237.

Gougeon A, Dynamics of follicular growth in the human: a model from preliminary results. *Human Reproduct* 1986; **1**: 81–87.

Judd, *et al. J Clin Endocrin Metab* 1974; **39**: 1020.

13 NORMAL AND ABNORMAL SEXUAL DEVELOPMENT AND PUBERTY

Beitins IZ, Padmanabhan V. Bioactivity of gonadotropins. Styne DM, ed. *Endocrinology and Metabolism Clinics of North America.* Philadelphia: WB Saunders, 1991.

Boepple PA, Mansfield MJ, Wierman ME, *et al.* Use of a potent long-acting agonist of gonadotropin-releasing hormone in the treatment of precocious puberty. *Endocrinology Review* 1986;7:24-33.

Conte FA, Grumbach MM, Kaplan SL. A disphasic pattern of gonadotropin secretion in patients with the syndrome of gonadal dysgenesis. *J Clin Endocrinol Metab* 1975;**40**:670-4.

Crowley WF, Filicori M, Spratt DI, Santoro NF. The physiology of gonadotropin-releasing hormone (GnRH) secretion in men and women. *Recent Prog Horm Res* 1985;**41**:473–526

Feuillan PP, Foster CM, Pescovitz OH, *et al.* Treatment of precocious puberty in the McCune–Albright syndrome with the aromatase inhibitor testolactone. *N Engl J Med* 1986;**313**:1115–19.

Finkelstein JW, Kapan S, Weitzman ED, *et al.* Twenty-four-hour plasma prolactin patterns in prepubertal and adolescent boys. *J Clin Endocrinol Metab* 1978;**47**:1123–28.

Greulich WS, Pyle SI. *Radiographic atlas of skeletal development of the hand and wrist.* Stanford: Stanford University Press, 1959.

Grumbach MM, Styne DM. Puberty: ontogeny, neuroendocrinology, physiology, and disorders. *Textbook of Endocrinology.* 8th edn. Philadelphia: WB Saunders, 1992: 1139–1221.

Harris DA, van Vliet G, Egli CA, *et al.* Somatomedin-C in normal puberty and in true precocious puberty before and after treatment with a potent luteinizing hormone-releasing hormone agonist. *J Clin Endocrinol Metab* 1985;**61**;152–9.

Kaplan SLK, Grumbach MM. Clinical review 14: Pathophysiology and treatment of sexual precocity. *J Clin Endocrinol Metab* 1990;**71**;785–9.

Kelch RP, Foster CM, Kletter GB, Marshall JC. Neuroendocrine regulation of puberty in boys. Sizonenko PC, Aubert ML, eds. *Developmental Endocrinology.* New York: Raven Press, 1990: 103–15.

Marshall WA, Tanner JM. Variations in pattern of pubertal changes in girls. *Arch Dis Child* 1969;**44**:291–303.

Marshall WA, Tanner JM. Variations in the pattern of pubertal changes in boys. *Arch Dis Child* 1970;**45**:13–23.

McKusick VA. Heritable disorders of connective tissue. St Louis: CV Mosby, 1972: 73–4.

Relter EO, Fuldauer VG, Root AW. Secretion of the adrenalandrogen, dehydroepiandrosterone sulfate, during normal infancy, childhood, and adolescence, in sick infants, and in children with endocrinologic abnormalities. *J Pediatr* 1977;**90**:766.

Rosenfield RL. Diagnosis and management of delayed puberty. *J Clin Endocrinol Metab* 1990;**70**:559–62.

Rosenthal SM, Grumbach MM, Kaplan SL. Gonadotropin-independent familial sexual precocity with premature Leydig and germinal cell maturation (familial testoxicosis): effects of a potent luteinizing hormone-releasing factor agonist and medroxyprogesterone acetate therapy in four cases. *J Clin Endocrinol Metab* 1983;**57**:571–9.

Styne DM, Grumbach MM. Disorders of puberty in the male and female. *Reproductive Endocrinology.* 3rd edn. 1991: 511–54.

Van Dop C, Burstein S, Conte FA, Grumbach MM. Isolated gonadotropin deficiency in boys: clinical charasteristics and growth. *J Pediatr* 1987;**111**:684–92.

14 GROWTH DISORDERS

Brook CGD, ed. Clinical paediatric endocrinology. 2nd edn. Oxford: Blackwell Scientific Publications, 1989.

Brook CGD. A guide to the practice of paediatric endocrinology. Cambridge: Cambridge University Press, 1993.

Hindmarsh PC, Brook CGD. Disorders of stature. In: Grossman A, ed. Clinical endocrinology. Oxford: Blackwell Scientific Publications 1992: 810–36.

15 THYROID PHYSIOLOGY AND HYPOTHYROIDISM

Amino N. Autoimmune thyroid disease/thyroiditis. In: DeGroot LJ, Besser GM, Burger HG, *et al.* eds. *Endocrinology* 3rd edn. Philadelphia: WB Saunders, 1994.

DeGroot LJ, Larsen PR, Refetoff S, Stanbury JB. *The thyroid and its diseases.* New York: John Wiley, 1984.

Retetoff S, Sarne D. Thyroid tests. In: DeGroot LJ, Besser GM, Burger HG, *et al.* eds. *Endocrinology* 3rd edn. Philadelphia: WB Saunders, 1994.

Salvatore G. T4 formation/T4 secretion. In: DeGroot LJ, Besser GM, Burger HG, *et al.* eds. *Endocrinology* 3rd edn. Philadelphia: WB Saunders, 1994.

Utiger R. Hypothyroidism. In: DeGroot LJ, Besser GM, Burger HG, *et al.* eds. *Endocrinology* 3rd edn. Philadelphia: WB Saunders, 1994.

Vassart G, Dumont J. Thyroid regulation. In: DeGroot LJ, Besser GM, Burger HG, *et al.* eds. *Endocrinology* 3rd edn. Philadelphia: WB Saunders, 1994.

Werner and Ingbar's *The Thyroid.* 6th edn. Philadelphia: JB Lippincott, 1991.

16 CARCINOMA OF THE THYROID

Hedinger C, Williams ED, Sobin LH. *Histological typing of thyroid tumours. World Health Organization, International histological classification of tumours.* 2nd ed. Berlin: Springer Verlag, 1988.

Kaplan M. Thyroid carcinoma. *Endocrinol Metab Clin N Am* 1990;**19(3)**.

17 HYPERTHYROIDISM AND GRAVES' DISEASE

Gordon A, Gross J, Hennemann G, eds. Progress in thyroid research. Proceedings of the 10th international thyroid conferGordon ence, The Hague, 4–18 Feb 1991. Rotterdam: AA Balkema, 1991.

Hall R. Fluctuating thyroid function [Commentary]. Clin Endocrinol 1992;**36**:214–160.

McGregor AM. Autoantibodies to the TSH receptor in patients with autoimmunity thyroid disease [Commentary]. Clin Endocrinol 1990;**33**:683–5.

McGregor AM. Immuno-endocrine interactions and autoimmunity. *N Engl J Med* 1990;**322**:1739-41.

Weetman AP. Autoimmune endocrine disease. Cambridge: University Press Cambridge, 1991.

Braverman LE, Utiger RV, eds. Werner and Ingbar's. The Thyroid, a fundamental and clinical text. 6th edn. Philadelphia: JB Lippincott, 1991.

18 CALCIUM AND COMMON ENDOCRINE DISORDERS

Favus MJ. *Primer on the metabolic bone disease and disorder of mineral metabolism.* 1990.

Mundy GR. *Calcium homeostasis: Hypercalcemia and hypocalcemia.* 2nd edn. London: Martin Dunitz, 1990.

Mundy GR. The hypercalcaemia of malignancy. In: Avioli LV, Krane SM, eds. *Metabolic bone disease and clinical related disorders.* 2nd edn 1990:793–803.

Mundy GR, Martin TJ. *Physiology and pharmacology of bone. Handbook of experimental pharmacology.* Berlin: Springer Verlag.

19 ENDOCRINOLOGY OF THE GASTROINTESTINAL TRACT

Bloom SR, Long RG. *Radioimmunoassay of gut regulatory peptides.* London: WB Saunders, 1982.

Jensen RT. Gastrointestinal endocrinology. *Gastroenterol Clin N Am* 1989;**18**:671–931.

Mazzaferri EL, O'Dorisio TMO. Endocrine tumours. *Semin Oncol* 1987;**14**:235–91.

Oberg K. Neuroendocrine gut and pancreatic tumours. *Acta Oncol* 1989;**28**:301–449.

Krejs G. Gastrointestinal endocrine tumours. *Am J Med* 1987;**82**(suppl 5B).

Rossi P, Allison DJ, Bezzi M, Kennedy A, Maccioni F, Wynick D, Maradci A, Bloom SR. Endocrine tumors of the pancreas. *Radiol Clin N Am* 1989;**27**:129–61.

20 HYPOGLYCAEMIA AND INSULINOMAS

Field JB, ed. Hypoglycemia. *Endocrinol Metab Clin North Am* 1989;**18**.

Marks V, Rose FC. *Hypoglycaemia.* 2nd edn. Oxford: Blackwell,1981.

Service FJ, ed. *Hypoglycemic disorders: Pathogenesis, diagnosis, and treatment.* Boston: GK Hall, 1983.

21 ECTOPIC HUMORAL SYNDROMES

Bondy PK. Hormonal and metabolic manifestations of tumors. In: Moossa AR, Robson MC, Schimpff SC, eds. *Comprehensive textbook of oncology.* Baltimore: Williams & Wilkins, 1986:386–96.

Bunn PA Jr, Ridgway EC. Paraneoplastic syndromes. In: Devita VT, Hellman S, Rosenberg SA, eds. *Cancer — principles and practice of oncology.* 3rd edn. Philadelphia: JB Lippincott, 1989:1896–940.

Odell WD, Appleton WS. Humoral manifestations of cancer. In: Wilson JD, Foster DW, eds. *Textbook of endocrinology.* 8th edn. Philadelphia: WB Saunders, 1992:1599–1617.

Orth DN. Ectopic hormone production. In: Felig P, Baxter JD, Broadus AE, Frohman LA, eds. *Endocrinology and metabolism.* 2nd edn. New York: McGraw-Hill, 1987:1692–1735.

22 HORMONE ASSAY TECHNIQUES

Berson SA, Yalow RS. Immunoassay of protein hormones. In: Pincus G, Thimann KV, Astwood EB, eds. *The hormones.* Volume 4. New York: Academic Press, 1964:557–630.

Ekins RP. General principles of hormone assay. In: Loraine JA, Bell ET, eds. *Hormone assays and their clinical application.* 4th edn. Edinburgh: Churchill Livingstone, 1976:1–72.

Hemmilä I. Fluoroimmunoassays and immunofluorometric assays. *Clin Chem* 1985;**31**:359–70.

Miyai K, Ishibashi K, Ogihara T, Tanizawa O, Nishi K, Kwashima M, Kumahara Y. Evaluation of EIA of hormones for clinical applications. In: Pal SB, ed. *Enzyme-linked immunoassay of hormones and drugs.* Berlin: Walter de Gruyter, 1978:287–99.

Torresani TE, Scherz R. Thyroid screening of neonates without use of radioactivity: Evaluation of time-resolved fluoroimmunoassay of thyrotropin. *Clin Chem* 1986;**32**:1013–16.

Weeks I, Woodhead JS. Chemiluminescence immunoassay. *J Clin Immunoassay* 1984;7:82–9.

Yalow RS, Berson SA. Assay of plasma insulin in human subjects by immunological methods. *Nature* 1959;**184**:1648.

23 RADIOLOGY OF ENDOCRINE DISORDERS

Grainger RG, Allison DJ, eds. *Diagnostic radiology: an Anglo-American textbook of imaging* . Volumes 1, 2 and 3. 2nd edn. Edinburgh: Churchill Livingstone, 1992.

Ross EJ, Prichard BNC, Kaufman L, Robertson AIG, Harries BJ. Preoperative and operative management of patients with phaeochromocytoma. *Br Med J* 1967;**1**:191–8.

Siegelman SS, Gatewood OMB, Goldman SM. *Computed tomography of the kidneys and adrenals.* New York: Churchill Livingstone, 1984.

24 IMAGING OF THE PITUITARY AND HYPOTHALAMUS

Ahmadi H, Larsson EM, Jinkins JR. Normal pituitary gland: coronal MR imaring of infundibular tilt. *Radiology* 1990;**177**:389–92.

Chakeres VW, Curtin A, Ford G. Magnetic resonance imaging of pituitary and parasellar abnormalities. *Radiol Clin N Am* 1989;**27**(2):265–81.

Elster AB, Chen MYM, Williams DW, Key LL. Pituitary gland: MR imaging of the physiologic hypertrophy in adolescents. *Radiology* 1990;**174**:681–5.

Goldsher D, Litt AW, Pinto RS, *et al.* Dural 'tail' associated with meningiomas on GD-DTPA-enhanced MR images: characteristics, differential diagnostic value, and possible implications for treatment. *Radiology* 1990;**176**:447–50.

Ostrov SG, Quencer RM, Hoffman JC *et al.* Hemorrhage within pituitary adenomas: how often associated with pituitary apoplexy syndrome? *Am J Neuroradiol* 1989;**10**:503–10.

Pusey E, Kortman KE, Flannigan BB, *et al.* MR of cranial pharyngiomas: tumor delineation and characterization. *Am J Neuroradiol* 1987;**8**:439–44.

Sherman JL, Stern BJ. Sarcoidosis of the CNS: comparison of unenhanced and enhanced MR images. *Am J Neuroradiol* 1990;**11**:915–23.

Zimmerman RA. Imaging of intrasellar, suprasellar, and parasellar tumors. *Sem Roentgenol* 1990;**25**(2):174–97.

25 NUCLEAR MEDICINE IMAGING IN ENDOCRINOLOGY

Bomanji J, Levison DA, Flatman WD, *et al.* Uptake of ^{123}I MIBG by phaeochromocytomas, paragangliomas and neuroblastomas, a histopathological comparison. *J Nuclear Med* 1987;**28**:973–8.

Chan TYK, Serpall JW, Chan O. *et al.* Misinterpretation of the upper parathyroid adenoma on Thallium 201/Technetium-99m subtraction scintigraphy. *Br J Radiol* 1990;**64**:1–4.

Fogelman I. The bone scan in metabolic bone disease. In: Fogelman I, ed. *Bone scanning in clinical practice.* Berlin: Springer Verlag, 1987:73–88.

Fogelman I, Maisey MN. The thyroid scan in the management of thyroid disease. In: *Nuclear Medicine Annual 1989.* New York: Raven Press, 1989: 1–48.

Goris ML, Basso LV, Keling G. Parathyroid imaging. *J Nuclear Med* 1991;**32**:887–9.

Hofnagel CA. Radionuclide therapy revisited. *Eur J Nuclear Med* 1991;**18**:408–31.

Khafagi FA, Shapiro B, Cross MD. The Adrenal Gland. In: Maisey MN, Britton KE, Gilday DL, eds. *Clinical Nuclear Medicine.* 2nd edn. London: Chapman and Hall, 1991:271–91.

Lamberts SWJ, Bakkar WH, Reubi JC, Krenning EP. Somatostatin receptor imaging in the localisation of endocrine tumours. *New Engl J Med* 1990;**323**:1246–9.

Ramtoola S, Maisey MN, Clarke SEM, Fogelman I. The thyroid scan in Hashimoto's thyroiditis; the great mimic. *Nucl Med Comm* 1988;**9**:639–45.

ReschiniE, Catania A. Clinical experience with the adrenal scanning agents Iodine 131-19-iodocholesterol and Selenium 75 selenomethylcholesterol. *Eur J Nucl Med* 1991;**18**:817-23.

Shapiro B, Britton KE, Hawkins LA, Edwards CRW. Clinical experience with ^{75}Se selenomethylcholesterol adrenal imaging. *Clin Endocrinol* 1981;**15**:19-27.

INDEX